MOSBY'S

GUIDE TO

NURSING
DIAGNOSIS

MOSBY'S

GUIDE TO

NURSING
DIAGNOSIS

Fourth Edition

Gail B. Ladwig, MSN, RN
Betty J. Ackley, MSN, EdS, RN

ELSEVIER

ELSEVIER
SAUNDERS

3251 Riverport Lane
Maryland Heights, Missouri 63043

Mosby's Guide to Nursing Diagnosis, Fourth Edition   ISBN: 978-0-323-08920-3

Notice

Knowledge and best practice in this field are constantly changing. As new research and experience broaden our knowledge, changes in practice, treatment and drug therapy may become necessary or appropriate. Readers are advised to check the most current information provided (i) on procedures featured or (ii) by the manufacturer of each product to be administered, to verify the recommended dose or formula, the method and duration of administration, and contraindications. It is the responsibility of the practitioner, relying on their own experience and knowledge of the patient, to make diagnoses, to determine dosages and the best treatment for each individual patient, and to take all appropriate safety precautions. To the fullest extent of the law, neither the Publisher nor the Editors assumes any liability for any injury and/or damage to persons or property arising out of or related to any use of the material contained in this book.

The Publisher

Library of Congress Cataloging-in-Publication Data
ISBN: 978-0-323-08920-3

Senior Content Strategist: Sandra Clark
Associate Content Development Specialist: Jennifer Wade
Publishing Services Manager: Jeffrey Patterson
Senior Project Manager: Jeanne Genz
Design Direction: Paula Catalano

Printed in China
Last digit is the print number: 9 8 7 6 5 4 3 2

Working together to grow
libraries in developing countries
www.elsevier.com | www.bookaid.org | www.sabre.org

ELSEVIER   BOOK AID International   Sabre Foundation

To

Dale Ackley, the greatest guy in the world, without whose support
this book would have never happened; and my daughter Dawn, and
her husband Cameron Goulding.
And the absolute joys of my life, granddaughter Althea Goulding
and grandson Emmett Goulding.

B. Ackley

Jerry Ladwig, my wonderful husband, who after 48 years is still
supportive and helpful—he has been "my right-hand man"
in every revision of this book. Also to my very special children,
their spouses, and all of my grandchildren: Jerry, Timothy, Alexandra,
Elizabeth, and Benjamin Ladwig; Christina, John, Sean, Ciara,
and Bridget McMahon; Jennifer, Jim, Abby, Katelyn, Blake, and
Connor Martin; Amy, Scott, Ford, and Vaughn Bertram
—the greatest family anyone could ever hope for.

Gift

to teach
is
to learn
to learn
is
to teach
the greatest moment
is when
the teacher
becomes the student
and
the student becomes the teacher

G. Ladwig

The authors would like to thank the following individuals for their contributions to *Nursing Diagnosis Handbook: An Evidence-Based Guide to Planning Care*, Tenth Edition, by Betty J. Ackley and Gail B. Ladwig, from which this book has been developed:

Betty J. Ackley, MSN, EdS, RN
Risk for Aspiration; Risk for Sudden Infant Death Syndrome; Impaired Dentition; Risk for complicated Grieving; Noncompliance; Imbalanced Nutrition: less than body requirements; Imbalanced Nutrition: more than body requirements; Risk for imbalanced Nutrition: more than body requirements; Readiness for enhanced Nutrition; Impaired Oral mucous membrane; Risk for Poisoning; Hearing loss; Vision loss; Risk for Suffocation; Overflow urinary Incontinence; Reflex urinary Incontinence; Impaired Urinary elimination; Readiness for enhanced Urinary elimination; Urinary retention

Keith A. Anderson, PhD
Readiness for enhanced family Coping

Sharon Baranoski, MSN, RN, CWCN, APN-CCNS, FAAN
Impaired Skin integrity; Risk for impaired Skin integrity; Impaired Tissue integrity

Nancy Albright Beyer, RN, CEN, MSN
Diarrhea; Risk for impaired Liver function; Dysfunctional gastrointestinal Motility

Kathaleen C. Bloom, PhD, CNM
Ineffective Health maintenance; Impaired Home maintenance; Deficient Knowledge; Readiness for enhanced Knowledge

Lisa Burkhart, PhD, RN
Moral Distress; Impaired Religiosity; Readiness for enhanced Religiosity; Spiritual distress; Readiness for enhanced Spiritual well-being

Emilia Campos de Carvalho, RN, PhD
Risk for vascular Trauma

Stacey M. Carroll, PhD, ANP-BC
Readiness for enhanced Communication; Impaired verbal Communication

Stephanie C. Christensen, PhD, CCC-SLP
Impaired Swallowing

June M. Como, RN, MSA, MS, EdD(c), CNS
Stress overload, Risk for Shock, Risk for Bleeding

Elizabeth Crago, RN, MSN, PhD
Autonomic dysreflexia

Maryanne Crowther, DNP, APN, CCRN
Decreased Cardiac output; Risk for decreased Cardiac perfusion

Ruth M. Curchoe, RN, MSN, CIC
Risk for Infection; Ineffective Protection

Helen de Graaf-Waar, CNS, RN
Grieving

Mary DeWys, RN, BS, CIMI
Risk for impaired Attachment; Disorganized Infant behavior

Susan Dirkes, BSN, MSA, CCRN
Excess fluid volume; Deficient fluid volume; Readiness for enhanced fluid balance; Risk for electrolyte imbalance

Roberta B. Dobrzanski, MSN, RN
Risk for disproportionate Growth

Julianne E. Doubet, BSN, RN, CEN, NREMT-P
Ineffective Denial; Risk for Loneliness; Rape-Trauma syndrome; Social isolation; Risk for Trauma

Lorraine Duggan, MSN, RN, ACNP, AHNP
Activity Intolerance; Ineffective peripheral tissue Perfusion

Shelly Eisbach, PhD, RN
Risk for compromised Resilience; Impaired individual Resilience; Readiness for enhanced Resilience

Dawn Fairlie, ANP, FNP, GNP, DNS(c)
Decisional Conflict; Ineffective community Coping; Readiness for enhanced community Coping; Readiness for enhanced Decision-Making; Ineffective family Therapeutic regimen management

Arlene T. Farren, RN, PhD, AOCN, CTN-A
Ineffective Coping; Readiness for enhanced Coping

Patricia Ferreira, RN, MSN
Defensive Coping; Disturbed person identity

Debora Y. Fields, RN, BSN, MA, CARN, LICDC, CM
Dysfunctional Family processes

Natalie Fischetti, PhD, RN
Readiness for enhanced Comfort

Judith A. Floyd, PhD, RN, FAAN
Insomnia; Sleep deprivation; Readiness for enhanced Sleep; Disturbed Sleep pattern

Terri A. Foster, BSN, RN, CNOR
Risk for imbalanced Fluid volume; Risk for perioperative positioning Injury

Shari Froelich, DNP(c), MSN, MSBA, RN
Risk for compromised human Dignity

Susanne W. Gibbons, PhD, C-ANP, C-GNP/Self Neglect
Self-Neglect

Marie Giordano, RN, DNS(c)
Ineffective Self-Health Management; Readiness for enhanced Self-Health Management; Powerlessness; Readiness for enhanced Power

Barbara A. Given, PhD, RN, FAAN
Caregiver role strain; Fatigue

Mila W. Grady, MSN, RN
Adult failure to thrive; Acute Confusion; Chronic Confusion; Deficient diversional activity;
Functional incontinence; Stress urinary incontinence; Urge urinary incontinence

Pauline M. Green, PhD, RN, CNE
Contamination; Risk for Contamination

Sherry A. Greenberg, MSN, GNP-BC
Risk for Falls

Jennifer Hafner, RN, BSN, CCRN, TNCC
Risk for ineffective renal Perfusion; Risk for decreased gastrointestinal perfusion

Elizabeth A. Henneman, RN, PhD, CCNS, FAAN
Risk for Poisoning

Sheri Holmes, RN, MSN, ACNS-C
Risk for disturbed Maternal/Fetal dyad

Paula D. Hopper, MSN, RN
Risk for unstable blood Glucose level

Teresa Howell, DNP, RN, CNE
Effective Breastfeeding; Ineffective Breastfeeding; Interrupted Breastfeeding

Jean D. Humphries, PhD(c), MS, RN
Insomnia; Sleep deprivation; Readiness for enhanced Sleep; Disturbed Sleep pattern

Teresa James, MSN, RN, CNE
Ineffective infant Feeding pattern

Dena L. Jarog, DNP
Delayed Growth and development

Elizabeth S. Jenuwine, PhD, MLIS
Insomnia; Sleep deprivation; Readiness for enhanced Sleep; Disturbed Sleep pattern

Kimberly J. Johnson-Crisanti, MSN, CNM
Ineffective childbearing; Risk for ineffective childbearing

Rebecca Johnson, PhD, RN, FAAN
Relocation stress syndrome

Michelangelo Juvenale, Biologist/Immunologist, MSc, PhD
Defensive Coping; Disturbed personal Identity

Kathleen Karsten, DNS(c), RN-BC
Readiness for enhanced Immunization status

Helen Kelley, MSN, RN
Section I: Revision L–Z

Joan Klehr, RNC, BS, MPH
Risk for ineffective Gastrointestinal Perfusion; Risk for decreased renal Perfusion

Kathy Kolcaba, RN, PhD
Impaired Comfort

Beverly Kopala, PhD, RN
Moral Distress

Gail B. Ladwig, MSN, RN
Ineffective Activity Planning; Risk for Ineffective Activity Planning; Risk for Allergy Response; Readiness for enhanced organized Infant Behavior; Risk for Disorganized Infant Behavior; Insufficient Breast Milk; Readiness for enhanced Childbearing Process; Deficient Community Health; Readiness for enhanced Hope; Hopelessness; Risk for impaired Parenting; Risk for Disturbed Personal Identity; Risk for Powerlessness; Risk for Ineffective Relationship; Readiness for Enhanced Relationship; Ineffective Relationship; Risk for impaired Religiosity; Ineffective Role Performance; Readiness for Enhanced Self-Concept; Chronic Low Self-Esteem; Situational Low Self-Esteem; Risk for Chronic Low Self-Esteem; Risk for Situational Low Self-Esteem; Risk for Spiritual Distress

Mary Beth Flynn Makic, RN, PhD, CNS, CCNS
Hyperthermia; Hypothermia; Ineffective Thermoregulation; Bowel Incontinence

Marina Martinez-Kratz, RN, MS
Ineffective Impulse Control

Ruth McCaffrey, DNP, ARNP, FNP-BC, GNP-BC
Anxiety; Death Anxiety; Fear

Dr. Graham J. McDougall, Jr., PhD, RN, FAAN, FGSA
Impaired Memory

Marsha McKenzie, BSN, RN
Disturbed Body Image; Risk for delayed development; Disabled Family Coping

Laura Mcilvoy, PhD, RN, CCRN, CNRN
Decreased Intracranial adaptive capacity; Risk for ineffective cerebral tissue perfusion

Noreen C. Miller, RN, MSN, FNP-C
Risk for Peripheral neurovascular dysfunction; Impaired bed Mobility; Impaired wheelchair Mobility; Impaired Transfer ability; Impaired Walking; Risk for Disuse Syndrome

DeLancey Nicoll, BSN
Latex Allergy response; Risk for latex Allergy response; Delayed Surgical recovery

Leslie H. Nicoll, PhD, MBA, RN
Latex Allergy response; Risk for latex Allergy response; Delayed Surgical recovery

Katherina A. Nikzad-Terhune, PhD, LCSW
Compromised family Coping

Barbara J. Olinzock, EdD, RN
Ineffective Health maintenance; Impaired Home maintenance; Deficient Knowledge; Readiness for enhanced Knowledge

Peg Padnos, AB, BSN, RN
Risk for impaired Attachment; Disorganized Infant behavior

Chris Pasero, MS, RN-BC, FAAN
Acute Pain; Chronic Pain

Kathleen L. Patusky, MA, PhD, RN, CNS
Self-Mutilation; Risk for Self-Mutilation; Risk for Suicide; Risk for other-directed Violence; Risk for self-directed Violence

Laura V. Polk, PhD, RN
Contamination; Risk for Contamination

Sherry H. Pomeroy, PhD, RN
Sedentary Lifestyle; Impaired physical Mobility

Lori M. Rhudy, PhD, RN, CNRN, ACNS-BC
Unilateral Neglect

Chad D. Rogers, MSN, RN
Risk for Injury; Risk for Trauma

Mary Jane Roth, BSN, MA, RN
Post-Trauma Syndrome; Risk for Post-Trauma Syndrome

Vanessa Sammons, MSN, RN, PHCNS-BC, CNE
Interrupted Family Processes

Marilee Schmelzer, PhD, RN
Constipation; Perceived Constipation

Paula Sherwood, RN, PhD, CNRN, FAAN
Autonomic dysreflexia; Caregiver role strain; Fatigue

Debra Siela, PhD, RN, CCNS, ACNS-BC, CCRN, CNE, RRT
Ineffective airway clearance; Impaired gas exchange; Ineffective breathing pattern; Dysfunctional ventilator weaning response; Impaired spontaneous ventilation

Kim Silvey, MSN, RN
Parental role Conflict; Interrupted Family processes; Readiness for enhanced Family processes; Impaired parenting; Readiness for enhanced Parenting

Elaine E. Steinke, PhD, RN, CNS-BC, FAHA
Sexual dysfunction; Ineffective Sexuality pattern

Laura Struble, PhD, GNP-BC
Wandering

Dennis Tanner, PhD
Impaired Swallowing

Janelle M. Tipton, MSN, RN, AOCN
Nausea

Dr. Terry Ward, BSN, MSN, RN
Risk for compromised Resilience; Impaired individual Resilience; Readiness for enhanced Resilience

Diane Wind Wardell, PhD, RN, WHNP-BC, AHN-BC
Disturbed Energy field

Patricia White, PhD, ANP-BC
Grieving; Complicated grieving; Chronic Sorrow

Suzanne White, MSN, RN, PHCNS-BC
Multicultural and Pediatrics for Impaired Verbal Communication; Readiness for enhanced Communication

Linda S. Williams, MSN, RN
*Bathing Self-Care deficit; Dressing Self-Care deficit; Feeding Self-Care deficit;
Toileting Self-Care deficit*

David Wilson, MS, RNC (NIC)
Neonatal Jaundice; Risk for Neonatal Jaundice

ASSESS

Assess the client using the format provided by the clinical setting. Collect data including client's symptoms, clinical state, and known medical or psychiatric diagnoses.

DIAGNOSIS

Use Section I, Guide to Nursing Diagnoses, and locate the client's symptoms, clinical state, medical or psychiatric diagnoses, and anticipated or prescribed diagnostic studies or surgical interventions (listed in alphabetical order). Note suggestions for appropriate nursing diagnoses.

Then use Section II, Guide to Planning Care, to evaluate each suggested nursing diagnosis and "related to" etiology statement. Section II is a listing of care plans according to NANDA-I, arranged alphabetically by diagnostic concept, for each nursing diagnosis referred to in Section I. Determine the appropriateness of each nursing diagnosis by comparing the Defining Characteristics and/or Risk Factors to the client data collected.

DETERMINE OUTCOMES

Use Section II, Guide to Planning Care, to find appropriate outcomes for the client.

PLAN INTERVENTIONS

Use Section II, Guide to Planning Care, to find appropriate interventions for the client.

GIVE NURSING CARE

Administer nursing care following the plan of care based on the interventions.

EVALUATE NURSING CARE

Evaluate nursing care administered using the Client Outcomes. If the outcomes were not met, and the nursing interventions were not effective, reassess the client and determine if the appropriate nursing diagnoses were made.

DOCUMENT

Document all of the previous steps using the format provided in the clinical setting.

CONTENTS

SECTION

I

Guide to Nursing Diagnoses

Section I is an alphabetical listing of client symptoms, client problems, medical diagnoses, psychosocial diagnoses, and clinical states. Each of these will have a list of possible nursing diagnoses. You may use this section to find suggestions for nursing diagnoses for your client.

- Assess the client using the format provided by the clinical setting.
- Locate the client's symptoms, problems, clinical state, diagnoses, surgeries, and diagnostic testing in the alphabetical listing contained in this section.
- Note suggestions given for appropriate nursing diagnoses.
- Evaluate the suggested nursing diagnoses to determine if they are appropriate for the client and have information that was found in the assessment.
- Use Section II (which contains an alphabetized list of all NANDA-I approved nursing diagnoses) to validate this information and check the definition, related factors, and defining characteristics. Determine if the nursing diagnosis you have selected is appropriate for the client.

A

ABDOMINAL DISTENTION

Constipation r/t decreased activity, decreased fluid intake, decreased fiber intake, pathological process

Dysfunctional **Gastrointestinal Motility** r/t decreased perfusion of intestines, medication effect

Nausea r/t irritation of gastrointestinal tract

Imbalanced **Nutrition:** less than body requirements r/t nausea, vomiting

Acute **Pain** r/t retention of air, gastrointestinal secretions

Delayed **Surgical Recovery** r/t retention of gas, secretions

ABDOMINAL HYSTERECTOMY

See Hysterectomy

ABDOMINAL PAIN

Dysfunctional **Gastrointestinal Motility** r/t decreased perfusion, medication effect

Acute **Pain** r/t injury, pathological process

See cause of Abdominal Pain

ABDOMINAL SURGERY

Constipation r/t decreased activity, decreased fluid intake, anesthesia, opioids

Dysfunctional **Gastrointestinal Motility** r/t medication or anesthesia effect, trauma from surgery

Imbalanced **Nutrition:** less than body requirements r/t high metabolic needs, decreased ability to ingest or digest food

Acute **Pain** r/t surgical procedure

Ineffective peripheral **Tissue Perfusion** r/t immobility, abdominal surgery

Risk for **Infection:** Risk factor: invasive procedure

Readiness for enhanced **Knowledge:** expresses an interest in learning

See Surgery, Perioperative Care; Surgery, Postoperative Care; Surgery, Preoperative Care

ABDOMINAL TRAUMA

Disturbed **Body Image** r/t scarring, change in body function, need for temporary colostomy

Ineffective **Breathing Pattern** r/t abdominal distention, pain

Deficient **Fluid Volume** r/t hemorrhage

Dysfunctional **Gastrointestinal Motility** r/t decreased perfusion

Acute **Pain** r/t abdominal trauma

Risk for **Bleeding:** Risk factor: trauma and possible rupture of abdominal organs

Risk for **Infection:** Risk factor: possible perforation of abdominal structures

ABLATION, RADIOFREQUENCY CATHETER

Fear r/t invasive procedure

Risk for decreased **Cardiac** tissue perfusion: Risk factor: catheterization of heart

ABORTION, INDUCED

Compromised family **Coping** r/t unresolved feelings about decision

Acute **Pain** r/t surgical intervention

Chronic low **Self-Esteem** r/t feelings of guilt

Chronic **Sorrow** r/t loss of potential child

Risk for **Bleeding:** Risk factor: trauma from abortion

Risk for delayed **Development:** Risk factors: unplanned or unwanted pregnancy

Risk for **Infection:** Risk factors: open uterine blood vessels, dilated cervix

Risk for **Post-Trauma Syndrome:** Risk factor: psychological trauma of abortion

Risk for **Spiritual Distress:** Risk factor: perceived moral implications of decision

Readiness for enhanced **Knowledge:** expresses an interest in learning

ABORTION, SPONTANEOUS

Disturbed **Body Image** r/t perceived inability to carry pregnancy, produce child

Disabled family **Coping** r/t unresolved feelings about loss

Ineffective **Coping** r/t personal vulnerability

Interrupted **Family Processes** r/t unmet expectations for pregnancy and childbirth

Fear r/t implications for future pregnancies

Grieving r/t loss of fetus

Acute **Pain** r/t uterine contractions, surgical intervention

Situational low **Self-Esteem** r/t feelings about loss of fetus

Chronic **Sorrow** r/t loss of potential child

Risk for **Bleeding:** Risk factor: trauma from abortion

Risk for **Infection:** Risk factors: septic or incomplete abortion of products of conception, open uterine blood vessels, dilated cervix

Risk for **Post-Trauma Syndrome:** Risk factor: psychological trauma of abortion

Risk for **Spiritual Distress:** Risk factor: loss of fetus

Readiness for enhanced **Knowledge:** expresses an interest in learning

ABRUPTIO PLACENTAE <36 WEEKS

Anxiety r/t unknown outcome, change in birth plans

Death **Anxiety** r/t unknown outcome, hemorrhage, or pain

Interrupted **Family Processes** r/t unmet expectations for pregnancy and childbirth

Fear r/t threat to well-being of self and fetus

Impaired **Gas Exchange:** placental r/t decreased uteroplacental area

Acute **Pain** r/t irritable uterus, hypertonic uterus

Impaired **Tissue Integrity:** maternal r/t possible uterine rupture

Risk for **Bleeding:** Risk factor: separation of placenta from uterus causing bleeding

Risk for disproportionate **Growth:** Risk factor: uteroplacental insufficiency

Risk for **Infection:** Risk factor: partial separation of placenta

Risk for disturbed **Maternal/Fetal Dyad:** Risk factors: trauma of process, lack of energy of mother

Risk for **Shock:** Risk factors: separation of placenta from uterus

Readiness for enhanced **Knowledge:** expresses an interest in learning

ABSCESS FORMATION

Ineffective **Protection** r/t inadequate nutrition, abnormal blood profile, drug therapy, depressed immune function

Impaired **Tissue Integrity** r/t altered circulation, nutritional deficit or excess

Readiness for enhanced **Knowledge:** expresses an interest in learning

ABUSE, CHILD

See Child Abuse

ABUSE, SPOUSE, PARENT, OR SIGNIFICANT OTHER

Anxiety r/t threat to self-concept, situational crisis of abuse

Caregiver Role Strain r/t chronic illness, self-care deficits, lack of respite care, extent of caregiving required

Impaired verbal **Communication** r/t psychological barriers of fear

Compromised family **Coping** r/t abusive patterns

Defensive **Coping** r/t low self-esteem

A

Dysfunctional **Family Processes** r/t inadequate coping skills

Insomnia r/t psychological stress

Post-Trauma Syndrome r/t history of abuse

Powerlessness r/t lifestyle of helplessness

Chronic low **Self-Esteem** r/t negative family interactions

Risk for self-directed **Violence:** Risk factor: history of abuse

ACCESSORY MUSCLE USE (TO BREATHE)

Ineffective **Breathing Pattern** (See **Breathing Pattern,** ineffective, Section II)

See Asthma; Bronchitis; COPD (Chronic Obstructive Pulmonary Disease); Respiratory Infections, Acute Childhood

ACCIDENT PRONE

Adult **Failure to Thrive** r/t fatigue

Acute **Confusion** r/t altered level of consciousness

Ineffective **Coping** r/t personal vulnerability, situational crises

Ineffective **Impulse Control** (See **Impulse Control,** ineffective, Section II)

Risk for **Injury:** Risk factor: history of accidents

ACHALASIA

Ineffective **Coping** r/t chronic disease

Acute **Pain** r/t stasis of food in esophagus

Impaired **Swallowing** r/t neuromuscular impairment

Risk for **Aspiration:** Risk factor: nocturnal regurgitation

ACID-BASE IMBALANCES

Risk for **Electrolyte Imbalance:** Risk factors: renal dysfunction, diarrhea, treatment-related side effects (e.g., medications, drains)

ACIDOSIS, METABOLIC

Acute **Confusion** r/t acid-base imbalance, associated electrolyte imbalance

Impaired **Memory** r/t effect of metabolic acidosis on brain function

Imbalanced **Nutrition:** less than body requirements r/t inability to ingest, absorb nutrients

Risk for **Electrolyte Imbalance:** Risk factor: effect of metabolic acidosis on renal function

Risk for **Injury:** Risk factors: disorientation, weakness, stupor

Risk for decreased **Cardiac** tissue perfusion: Risk factor: dysrhythmias from hyperkalemia

Risk for **Shock:** Risk factors: abnormal metabolic state, presence of acid state impairing function

ACIDOSIS, RESPIRATORY

Activity Intolerance r/t imbalance between oxygen supply and demand

Impaired **Gas Exchange** r/t ventilation-perfusion imbalance

Impaired **Memory** r/t hypoxia

Risk for decreased **Cardiac** tissue perfusion: Risk factor: dysrhythmias associated with respiratory acidosis

ACNE

Disturbed **Body Image** r/t biophysical changes associated with skin disorder

Ineffective **Self-Health Management** r/t deficient knowledge (medications, personal care, cause)

Impaired **Skin Integrity** r/t hormonal changes (adolescence, menstrual cycle)

ACS (ACUTE CORONARY SYNDROME)

See (MI) Myocardial Infarction

ACQUIRED IMMUNODEFICIENCY SYNDROME

See AIDS (Acquired Immunodeficiency Syndrome)

ACROMEGALY

Activity Intolerance (See **Activity Intolerance**, Section II)

Ineffective **Airway Clearance** r/t airway obstruction by enlarged tongue

Disturbed **Body Image** r/t changes in body function and appearance

Impaired physical **Mobility** r/t joint pain

Risk for decreased **Cardiac** tissue perfusion: Risk factor: r/t increased atherosclerosis from abnormal health status

Risk for unstable blood **Glucose** level: Risk factor: abnormal physical health status

Sexual Dysfunction r/t changes in hormonal secretions

ACTIVITY INTOLERANCE, POTENTIAL TO DEVELOP

Risk for **Activity Intolerance** (See **Activity Intolerance**, risk for, Section II)

ACUTE ABDOMINAL PAIN

Deficient **Fluid Volume** r/t air and fluids trapped in bowel, inability to drink

Acute **Pain** r/t pathological process

Risk for dysfunctional **Gastrointestinal Motility**: Risk factor: ineffective gastrointestinal tissue perfusion

See cause of Abdominal Pain

ACUTE ALCOHOL INTOXICATION

Ineffective **Breathing Pattern** r/t depression of the respiratory center from excessive alcohol intake

Acute **Confusion** r/t central nervous system depression

Dysfunctional **Family Processes** r/t abuse of alcohol

Risk for **Aspiration**: Risk factor: depressed reflexes with acute vomiting

Risk for **Infection**: Risk factor: impaired immune system from malnutrition associated with chronic excessive alcohol intake

ACUTE BACK PAIN

Anxiety r/t situational crisis, back injury

Constipation r/t decreased activity, effect of pain medication

Ineffective **Coping** r/t situational crisis, back injury

Impaired physical **Mobility** r/t pain

Acute **Pain** r/t back injury

Readiness for enhanced **Knowledge**: expresses an interest in learning

ACUTE CONFUSION

See Confusion, Acute

ACUTE CORONARY SYNDROME

Risk for decreased **Cardiac** tissue perfusion: Risk factor: (See **Cardiac** tissue perfusion, risk for decreased)

ACUTE LYMPHOCYTIC LEUKEMIA (ALL)

See Cancer; Chemotherapy; Child with Chronic Condition; Leukemia

ACUTE RENAL FAILURE

See Renal Failure

ACUTE RESPIRATORY DISTRESS SYNDROME

See ARDS (Acute Respiratory Distress Syndrome)

ADAMS-STOKES SYNDROME

See Dysrhythmia

ADDICTION

See Alcoholism; Drug Abuse

A

ADDISON'S DISEASE

Activity Intolerance r/t weakness, fatigue

Disturbed **Body Image** r/t increased skin pigmentation

Deficient **Fluid Volume** r/t failure of regulatory mechanisms

Imbalanced **Nutrition:** less than body requirements r/t chronic illness

Risk for **Injury:** Risk factor: weakness

Readiness for enhanced **Knowledge:** expresses an interest in learning

ADENOIDECTOMY

Acute **Pain** r/t surgical incision

Ineffective **Airway Clearance** r/t hesitation or reluctance to cough as a result of pain, fear

Nausea r/t anesthesia effects, drainage from surgery

Acute **Pain** r/t surgical incision

Risk for **Aspiration:** Risk factors: postoperative drainage, impaired swallowing

Risk for **Bleeding:** Risk factors: surgical incision

Risk for deficient **Fluid Volume:** Risk factors: decreased intake as a result of painful swallowing, effects of anesthesia

Risk for imbalanced **Nutrition:** less than body requirements: Risk factors: reluctance to swallow

Readiness for enhanced **Knowledge:** expresses an interest in learning

ADHESIONS, LYSIS OF

See Abdominal Surgery

ADJUSTMENT DISORDER

Anxiety r/t inability to cope with psychosocial stressor

Risk-prone **Health Behavior** r/t assault to self-esteem

Disturbed personal **Identity** r/t psychosocial stressor (specific to individual)

Situational low **Self-Esteem** r/t change in role function

Impaired **Social Interaction** r/t absence of significant others or peers

ADJUSTMENT IMPAIRMENT

Risk-prone **Health Behavior** (See **Health Behavior,** risk-prone, Section III)

ADOLESCENT, PREGNANT

Anxiety r/t situational and maturational crisis, pregnancy

Disturbed **Body Image** r/t pregnancy superimposed on developing body

Decisional Conflict: keeping child versus giving up child versus abortion r/t lack of experience with decision-making, interference with decision-making, multiple or divergent sources of information, lack of support system

Disabled family **Coping** r/t highly ambivalent family relationships, chronically unresolved feelings of guilt, anger, despair

Ineffective **Coping** r/t situational and maturational crisis, personal vulnerability

Ineffective **Denial** r/t fear of consequences of pregnancy becoming known

Interrupted **Family Processes** r/t unmet expectations for adolescent, situational crisis

Fear r/t labor and delivery

Delayed **Growth and Development** r/t pregnancy

Deficient **Knowledge** r/t pregnancy, infant growth and development, parenting

Imbalanced **Nutrition:** less than body requirements r/t lack of knowledge of nutritional needs during pregnancy and as growing adolescent

Ineffective **Role Performance** r/t pregnancy

Situational low **Self-Esteem** r/t feelings of shame and guilt about becoming or being pregnant

Impaired **Social Interaction** r/t self-concept disturbance

Social Isolation r/t absence of supportive significant others

Risk for impaired **Attachment**: Risk factor: anxiety associated with the parent role

Risk for delayed **Development**: Risk factor: unplanned or unwanted pregnancy

Risk for urge urinary **Incontinence**: Risk factor: pressure on bladder by growing uterus

Risk for disturbed **Maternal/Fetal Dyad**: Risk factors: immaturity, substance use

Risk for impaired **Parenting**: Risk factors: adolescent parent, unplanned or unwanted pregnancy, single parent

Readiness for enhanced **Childbearing Process**: reports appropriate prenatal lifestyle

Readiness for enhanced **Knowledge**: expresses an interest in learning

ADOPTION, GIVING CHILD UP FOR

Decisional Conflict r/t unclear personal values or beliefs, perceived threat to value system, support system deficit

Ineffective **Coping** r/t stress of loss of child

Interrupted **Family Processes** r/t conflict within family regarding relinquishment of child

Grieving r/t loss of child, loss of role of parent

Insomnia r/t depression or trauma of relinquishment of child

Social Isolation r/t making choice that goes against values of significant others

Chronic **Sorrow** r/t loss of relationship with child

Risk for **Spiritual Distress**: Risk factor: perceived moral implications of decision

Readiness for enhanced **Spiritual Well-Being**: harmony with self regarding final decision

ADRENOCORTICAL INSUFFICIENCY

Deficient **Fluid Volume** r/t insufficient ability to reabsorb water

Ineffective **Protection** r/t inability to tolerate stress

Delayed **Surgical Recovery** r/t inability to respond to stress

Risk for **Shock**: Risk factor: deficient **Fluid Volume,** decreased cortisol to initiate stress response to insult to body

See Addison's Disease; Shock, Hypovolemic

ADVANCE DIRECTIVES

Death **Anxiety** r/t planning for end-of-life health decisions

Decisional Conflict r/t unclear personal values or beliefs, perceived threat to value system, support system deficit

Grieving r/t possible loss of self, significant other

Readiness for enhanced **Spiritual Well-Being**: harmonious interconnectedness with self, others, higher power, God

AFFECTIVE DISORDERS

See specific disorder: Depression (Major Depressive Disorder); Dysthymic Disorder; Manic Disorder, Bipolar I, Seasonal Affective Disorder

AGE-RELATED MACULAR DEGENERATION

See Macular Degeneration

AGGRESSIVE BEHAVIOR

Fear r/t real or imagined threat to own well-being

Risk for other-directed **Violence** (See **Violence**, other-directed, risk for, Section II)

AGING

Death **Anxiety** r/t fear of unknown, loss of self, impact on significant others

A

Impaired **Dentition** r/t ineffective oral hygiene

Adult **Failure to Thrive** r/t depression, apathy, fatigue

Grieving r/t multiple losses, impending death

Ineffective **Self-Health Management** r/t deficient knowledge: medication, nutrition, exercise, coping strategies

Hearing Loss r/t exposure to loud noises, aging

Functional urinary **Incontinence** r/t impaired vision, impaired cognition, neuromuscular limitations, altered environmental factors

Impaired individual **Resilience** r/t aging, multiple losses

Sleep deprivation r/t aging-related sleep-stage shifts

Ineffective **Thermoregulation** r/t aging

Vision Loss r/t aging (see care plan on Evolve)

Risk for **Caregiver Role Strain**: Risk factor: inability to handle increasing needs of significant other

Risk for **Injury**: Risk factor: vision loss, hearing loss, decreased balance, decreased sensation in feet

Risk for **Loneliness**: Risk factors: inadequate support system, role transition, health alterations, depression, fatigue

Readiness for enhanced community **Coping**: providing social support and other resources identified as needed for elderly client

Readiness for enhanced family **Coping**: ability to gratify needs, address adaptive tasks

Readiness for enhanced **Knowledge**: specify need to improve health

Readiness for enhanced **Nutrition**: need to improve health

Readiness for enhanced **Relationship**: demonstrates understanding of partner's insufficient function

Readiness for enhanced **Self-Health Management**: knowledge about medication, nutrition, exercise, coping strategies

Readiness for enhanced **Sleep**: need to improve sleep

Readiness for enhanced **Spiritual Well-Being**: one's experience of life's meaning, harmony with self, others, higher power, God, environment

Readiness for enhanced **Urinary Elimination**: need to improve health

AGITATION

Acute **Confusion** r/t side effects of medication, hypoxia, decreased cerebral perfusion, alcohol abuse or withdrawal, substance abuse or withdrawal, sensory deprivation or overload

Sleep deprivation r/t sundown syndrome

See cause of Agitation

AGORAPHOBIA

Anxiety r/t real or perceived threat to physical integrity

Ineffective **Coping** r/t inadequate support systems

Fear r/t leaving home, going out in public places

Impaired **Social Interaction** r/t disturbance in self-concept

Social Isolation r/t altered thought process

AGRANULOCYTOSIS

Delayed **Surgical Recovery** r/t abnormal blood profile

Risk for **Infection**: Risk factor: abnormal blood profile

Readiness for enhanced **Knowledge**: expresses an interest in learning

AIDS (ACQUIRED IMMUNODEFICIENCY SYNDROME)

Death **Anxiety** r/t fear of premature death

Disturbed **Body Image** r/t chronic contagious illness, cachexia

Caregiver Role Strain r/t unpredictable illness course, presence of situation stressors

Diarrhea r/t inflammatory bowel changes

Disturbed **Energy Field** r/t chronic illness

Interrupted **Family Processes** r/t distress about diagnosis of human immunodeficiency virus (HIV) infection

Fatigue r/t disease process, stress, decreased nutritional intake

Fear r/t powerlessness, threat to well-being

Grieving: family/parental r/t potential or impending death of loved one

Grieving: individual r/t loss of physical and psychosocial well-being

Hopelessness r/t deteriorating physical condition

Imbalanced **Nutrition:** less than body requirements r/t decreased ability to eat and absorb nutrients as a result of anorexia, nausea, diarrhea; oral candidiasis

Chronic **Pain** r/t tissue inflammation and destruction

Impaired individual **Resilience** r/t chronic illness

Situational low **Self-Esteem** r/t crisis of chronic contagious illness

Ineffective **Sexuality Pattern** r/t possible transmission of disease

Social Isolation r/t self-concept disturbance, therapeutic isolation

Spiritual Distress r/t challenged beliefs or moral system

Risk for deficient **Fluid Volume:** Risk factors: diarrhea, vomiting, fever, bleeding

Risk for **Infection:** Risk factor: inadequate immune system

Risk for **Loneliness:** Risk factor: social isolation

Risk for impaired **Oral Mucous Membrane:** Risk factor: immunological deficit

Risk for impaired **Skin Integrity:** Risk factors: immunological deficit, diarrhea

Risk for **Spiritual Distress:** Risk factor: physical illness

Readiness for enhanced **Knowledge:** expresses an interest in learning

See AIDS, Child; Cancer; Pneumonia

AIDS DEMENTIA

Chronic **Confusion** r/t viral invasion of nervous system

See Dementia

AIDS, CHILD

Impaired **Parenting** r/t congenital acquisition of infection secondary to intravenous (IV) drug use, multiple sexual partners, history of contaminated blood transfusion

See AIDS (Acquired Immunodeficiency Syndrome); Child with Chronic Condition; Hospitalized Child; Terminally Ill Child, Adolescent; Terminally Ill Child, Infant/Toddler; Terminally Ill Child, Preschool Child; Terminally Ill Child, School-Age Child/ Preadolescent; Terminally Ill Child/ Death of Child, Parent

AIRWAY OBSTRUCTION/ SECRETIONS

Ineffective **Airway Clearance** (See **Airway Clearance**, ineffective, Section II)

ALCOHOL WITHDRAWAL

Anxiety r/t situational crisis, withdrawal

Acute **Confusion** r/t effects of alcohol withdrawal

Ineffective **Coping** r/t personal vulnerability

Dysfunctional **Family Processes** r/t abuse of alcohol

A

Insomnia r/t effect of alcohol withdrawal, anxiety

Imbalanced **Nutrition:** less than body requirements r/t poor dietary habits

Chronic low **Self-Esteem** r/t repeated unmet expectations

Risk for deficient **Fluid Volume:** Risk factors: excessive diaphoresis, agitation, decreased fluid intake

Risk for other-directed **Violence:** Risk factor: substance withdrawal

Risk for self-directed **Violence:** Risk factor: substance withdrawal

Readiness for enhanced **Knowledge:** expresses an interest in learning

ALCOHOLISM

Anxiety r/t loss of control

Risk-prone **Health Behavior** r/t lack of motivation to change behaviors, addiction

Acute **Confusion** r/t alcohol abuse

Chronic **Confusion** r/t neurological effects of chronic alcohol intake

Defensive **Coping** r/t denial of reality of addiction

Disabled family **Coping** r/t codependency issues due to alcoholism

Ineffective **Coping** r/t use of alcohol to cope with life events

Ineffective **Denial** r/t refusal to acknowledge addiction

Dysfunctional **Family Process** r/t alcohol abuse

Impaired **Home Maintenance** r/t memory deficits, fatigue

Insomnia r/t irritability, nightmares, tremors

Impaired **Memory** r/t alcohol abuse

Self-Neglect r/t effects of alcohol abuse

Imbalanced **Nutrition:** less than body requirements r/t anorexia, inappropriate diet with increased carbohydrates

Powerlessness r/t alcohol addiction

Ineffective **Protection** r/t malnutrition, sleep deprivation

Chronic low **Self-Esteem** r/t failure at life events

Social Isolation r/t unacceptable social behavior, values

Risk for **Injury:** Risk factor: alteration in sensory or perceptual function

Risk for **Loneliness:** Risk factor: unacceptable social behavior

Risk for other-directed **Violence:** Risk factors: reactions to substances used, impulsive behavior, disorientation, impaired judgment

Risk for self-directed **Violence:** Risk factors: reactions to substances used, impulsive behavior, disorientation, impaired judgment

ALCOHOLISM, DYSFUNCTIONAL FAMILY PROCESSES

Dysfunctional **Family Processes** (See **Family Processes,** dysfunctional, Section II)

ALKALOSIS

See Metabolic Alkalosis

ALL (ACUTE LYMPHOCYTIC LEUKEMIA)

See Cancer; Chemotherapy; Child with a Chronic Condition; Leukemia

ALLERGIES

Latex Allergy Response r/t hypersensitivity to natural rubber latex

Risk for **Allergy Response:** Risk factor: chemical factors, dander, environmental substances, foods, insect stings, medications

Risk for **Latex Allergy Response:** Risk factor: repeated exposure to products containing latex

Readiness for enhanced **Knowledge:** expresses an interest in learning

ALOPECIA

Disturbed **Body Image** r/t loss of hair, change in appearance

Readiness for enhanced **Knowledge:** expresses an interest in learning

ALTERED MENTAL STATUS

See Confusion, Acute; Confusion, Chronic; Memory Deficit

ALS (AMYOTROPHIC LATERAL SCLEROSIS)

See Amyotrophic Lateral Sclerosis (ALS)

ALZHEIMER'S DISEASE

Caregiver Role Strain r/t duration and extent of caregiving required

Chronic **Confusion** r/t loss of cognitive function

Compromised family **Coping** r/t interrupted family processes

Adult **Failure to Thrive** r/t difficulty in reasoning, judgment, memory, concentration

Fear r/t loss of self

Impaired **Home Maintenance** r/t impaired cognitive function, inadequate support systems

Hopelessness r/t deteriorating condition

Insomnia r/t neurological impairment, daytime naps

Impaired **Memory** r/t neurological disturbance

Impaired physical **Mobility** r/t severe neurological dysfunction

Self-Neglect r/t loss of cognitive function

Powerlessness r/t deteriorating condition

Self-Care deficit: specify r/t loss of cognitive function, psychological impairment

Social Isolation r/t fear of disclosure of memory loss

Wandering r/t cognitive impairment, frustration, physiological state

Risk for **Injury:** Risk factor: confusion

Risk for **Loneliness:** Risk factor: potential social isolation

Risk for **Relocation Stress Syndrome:** Risk factors: impaired psychosocial health, decreased health status

Risk for other-directed **Violence:** Risk factors: frustration, fear, anger, loss of cognitive function

Readiness for enhanced **Knowledge:** Caregiver: expresses an interest in learning

See Dementia

AMD (AGE-RELATED MACULAR DEGENERATION)

See Macular Degeneration

AMENORRHEA

Imbalanced **Nutrition:** less than body requirements r/t inadequate food intake

See Sexuality, Adolescent

AMI (ACUTE MYOCARDIAL INFARCTION)

See MI (Myocardial Infarction)

AMNESIA

Acute **Confusion** r/t alcohol abuse, delirium, dementia, drug abuse

Dysfunctional **Family Processes** r/t alcohol abuse, inadequate coping skills

Impaired **Memory** r/t excessive environmental disturbance, neurological disturbance

Post-Trauma Syndrome r/t history of abuse, catastrophic illness, disaster, accident

AMNIOCENTESIS

Anxiety r/t threat to self and fetus, unknown future

Decisional Conflict r/t choice of treatment pending results of test

Risk for **Infection:** Risk factor: invasive procedure

A

AMNIONITIS

See Chorioamnionitis

AMNIOTIC MEMBRANE RUPTURE

See Premature Rupture of Membranes

AMPUTATION

Disturbed **Body Image** r/t negative effects of amputation, response from others

Grieving r/t loss of body part, future lifestyle changes

Impaired physical **Mobility** r/t musculoskeletal impairment, limited movement

Acute **Pain** r/t surgery, phantom limb sensation

Chronic **Pain** r/t surgery, phantom limb sensation

Ineffective peripheral **Tissue Perfusion** r/t impaired arterial circulation

Impaired **Skin** integrity r/t poor healing, prosthesis rubbing

Risk for **Bleeding**: Risk factor: vulnerable surgical site

Readiness for enhanced **Knowledge**: expresses an interest in learning

AMYOTROPHIC LATERAL SCLEROSIS (ALS)

Death **Anxiety** r/t impending progressive loss of function leading to death

Ineffective **Breathing Pattern** r/t compromised muscles of respiration

Impaired verbal **Communication** r/t weakness of muscles of speech, deficient knowledge of ways to compensate and alternative communication devices

Decisional Conflict: ventilator therapy r/t unclear personal values or beliefs, lack of relevant information

Impaired individual **Resilience** r/t chronic debilitating illness

Chronic **Sorrow** r/t chronic illness

Impaired **Swallowing** r/t weakness of muscles involved in swallowing

Impaired **Spontaneous Ventilation** r/t weakness of muscles of respiration

Risk for **Aspiration**: Risk factor: impaired swallowing

Risk for **Spiritual Distress**: Risk factor: chronic debilitating condition

See Neurologic Disorders

ANAL FISTULA

See Hemorrhoidectomy

ANAPHYLACTIC SHOCK

Ineffective **Airway Clearance** r/t laryngeal edema, bronchospasm

Latex Allergy Response r/t abnormal immune mechanism response

Impaired **Spontaneous Ventilation** r/t acute airway obstruction from anaphylaxis process

ANAPHYLAXIS PREVENTION

Risk for **Allergy Response** (See **Allergy Response**, risk for, Section III)

ANASARCA

Excess **Fluid Volume** r/t excessive fluid intake, cardiac/renal dysfunction, loss of plasma proteins

Risk for impaired **Skin Integrity**: Risk factor: impaired circulation to skin from edema

See cause of Anasarca

ANEMIA

Anxiety r/t cause of disease

Impaired **Comfort** r/t feelings of always being cold from decreased hemoglobin and decreased metabolism

Fatigue r/t decreased oxygen supply to the body, increased cardiac workload

Impaired **Memory** r/t change in cognition from decreased oxygen supply to the body

Delayed **Surgical Recovery** r/t decreased oxygen supply to body, increased cardiac workload

Risk for **Bleeding** (See **Bleeding**, risk for, Section II)

Risk for **Injury:** Risk factor: alteration in peripheral sensory perception

Readiness for enhanced **Knowledge:** expresses an interest in learning

ANEMIA, IN PREGNANCY

Anxiety r/t concerns about health of self and fetus

Fatigue r/t decreased oxygen supply to the body, increased cardiac workload

Risk for delayed **Development:** Risk factor: reduction in the oxygen-carrying capacity of blood

Risk for **Infection:** Risk factor: reduction in oxygen-carrying capacity of blood

Risk for disturbed **Maternal/Fetal Dyad:** Risk factor: compromised oxygen transport

Readiness for enhanced **Knowledge:** expresses an interest in learning

ANEMIA, SICKLE CELL

See Anemia, Sickle Cell Anemia/Crisis

ANENCEPHALY

See Neural Tube Defects

ANEURYSM, ABDOMINAL SURGERY

Risk for deficient **Fluid Volume:** Risk factor: hemorrhage r/t potential abnormal blood loss

Risk for **Infection:** Risk factor: invasive procedure

Risk for ineffective **Gastrointestinal Perfusion** (See **Gastrointestinal Perfusion**, ineffective, risk for, Section II)

Risk for ineffective **Renal Perfusion:** Risk factor: prolonged ischemia of kidneys

See Abdominal Surgery

ANEURYSM, CEREBRAL

See Craniectomy/Craniotomy; Subarachnoid Hemorrhage (if aneurysm has ruptured)

ANGER

Anxiety r/t situational crisis

Risk-prone **Health Behavior** r/t assault to self-esteem, disability requiring change in lifestyle, inadequate support system

Defensive **Coping** r/t inability to acknowledge responsibility for actions and results of actions

Fear r/t environmental stressor, hospitalization

Grieving r/t significant loss

Powerlessness r/t health care environment

Risk for compromised **Human Dignity:** Risk factors: inadequate participation in decision-making, perceived dehumanizing treatment, perceived humiliation, exposure of the body, cultural incongruity

Risk for **Post-Trauma Syndrome:** Risk factor: inadequate social support

Risk for other-directed **Violence:** Risk factors: history of violence, rage reaction

Risk for self-directed **Violence:** Risk factors: history of violence, history of abuse, rage reaction

ANGINA

Activity Intolerance r/t acute pain, dysrhythmias

Anxiety r/t situational crisis

Decreased **Cardiac Output** r/t myocardial ischemia, medication effect, dysrhythmia

Ineffective **Coping** r/t personal vulnerability to situational crisis of new diagnosis, deteriorating health

Ineffective **Denial** r/t deficient knowledge of need to seek help with symptoms

Grieving r/t pain, loss of health

Acute **Pain** r/t myocardial ischemia

A

Ineffective **Sexuality Pattern** r/t disease process, medications, loss of libido

Readiness for enhanced **Knowledge:** expresses an interest in learning

ANGIOCARDIOGRAPHY (CARDIAC CATHETERIZATION)

See Cardiac Catheterization

ANGIOPLASTY, CORONARY

Fear r/t possible outcome of interventional procedure

Ineffective peripheral **Tissue Perfusion** r/t vasospasm, hematoma formation

Risk for **Bleeding:** Risk factors: possible damage to coronary artery, hematoma formation

Risk for decreased **Cardiac** tissue perfusion: Risk factors: ventricular ischemia, dysrhythmias

Readiness for enhanced **Knowledge:** expresses an interest in learning

ANOMALY, FETAL/NEWBORN (PARENT DEALING WITH)

Anxiety r/t threat to role functioning, situational crisis

Decisional Conflict: interventions for fetus or newborn r/t lack of relevant information, spiritual distress, threat to value system

Parental **Role Conflict** r/t separation from newborn, intimidation with invasive or restrictive modalities, specialized care center policies

Disabled family **Coping** r/t chronically unresolved feelings about loss of perfect baby

Ineffective **Coping** r/t personal vulnerability in situational crisis

Interrupted **Family Processes** r/t unmet expectations for perfect baby, lack of adequate support systems

Fear r/t real or imagined threat to baby, implications for future pregnancies, powerlessness

Grieving r/t loss of ideal child

Hopelessness r/t long-term stress, deteriorating physical condition of child, lost spiritual belief

Deficient **Knowledge** r/t limited exposure to situation

Impaired **Parenting** r/t interruption of bonding process

Powerlessness r/t complication threatening fetus or newborn

Situational low **Self-Esteem** r/t perceived inability to produce a perfect child

Social Isolation r/t alterations in child's physical appearance, altered state of wellness

Chronic **Sorrow** r/t loss of ideal child, inadequate bereavement support

Spiritual Distress r/t test of spiritual beliefs

Risk for impaired **Attachment:** Risk factor: ill infant unable to effectively initiate parental contact as result of altered behavioral organization

Risk for disorganized **Infant** behavior: Risk factor: congenital disorder

Risk for impaired **Parenting:** Risk factors: interruption of bonding process; unrealistic expectations for self, infant, or partner; perceived threat to own emotional survival; severe stress; lack of knowledge

Risk for **Spiritual Distress:** Risk factor: lack of normal child to raise and carry on family name

ANORECTAL ABSCESS

Disturbed **Body Image** r/t odor and drainage from rectal area

Acute **Pain** r/t inflammation of perirectal area

Risk for **Constipation:** Risk factor: fear of painful elimination

Readiness for Enhanced **Knowledge:** expresses an interest in learning

ANOREXIA

Deficient **Fluid Volume** r/t inability to drink

Imbalanced **Nutrition:** less than body requirements r/t loss of appetite, nausea, vomiting, laxative abuse.

Delayed **Surgical Recovery** r/t inadequate nutritional intake

ANOREXIA NERVOSA

Activity Intolerance r/t fatigue, weakness

Disturbed **Body Image** r/t misconception of actual body appearance

Constipation r/t lack of adequate food, fiber, and fluid intake

Defensive **Coping** r/t psychological impairment, eating disorder

Disabled family **Coping** r/t highly ambivalent family relationships

Ineffective **Denial** r/t fear of consequences of therapy, possible weight gain

Diarrhea r/t laxative abuse

Interrupted **Family Processes** r/t situational crisis

Imbalanced **Nutrition:** less than body requirements r/t inadequate food intake, excessive exercise

Chronic low **Self-Esteem** r/t repeated unmet expectations

Ineffective **Sexuality Pattern** r/t loss of libido from malnutrition

Ineffective family **Therapeutic Regimen Management** r/t family conflict, excessive demands on family associated with complexity of condition and treatment

Risk for **Infection:** Risk factor: malnutrition resulting in depressed immune system

Risk for **Spiritual Distress:** Risk factor: low self-esteem

See Maturational Issues, Adolescent

ANOSMIA (SMELL, LOSS OF ABILITY TO)

Imbalanced **Nutrition:** less than body requirements r/t loss of appetite associated with loss of smell

ANTEPARTUM PERIOD

See Pregnancy, Normal; Prenatal Care, Normal

ANTERIOR REPAIR, ANTERIOR COLPORRHAPHY

Urinary Retention r/t edema of urinary structures

Risk for urge urinary **Incontinence:** Risk factor: trauma to bladder

Readiness for enhanced **Knowledge:** expresses an interest in learning

See Vaginal Hysterectomy

ANTICOAGULANT THERAPY

Risk for **Bleeding:** Risk factors: altered clotting function from anticoagulant

Risk for deficient **Fluid Volume:** hemorrhage: Risk factor: altered clotting mechanism

Readiness for enhanced **Knowledge:** expresses an interest in learning

ANTISOCIAL PERSONALITY DISORDER

Defensive **Coping** r/t excessive use of projection

Ineffective **Coping** r/t frequently violating the norms and rules of society

Hopelessness r/t abandonment

Impaired **Social Interaction** r/t sociocultural conflict, chemical dependence, inability to form relationships

Spiritual Distress r/t separation from religious or cultural ties

Ineffective family **Therapeutic Regimen Management** r/t excessive demands on family

A

Risk for **Loneliness:** Risk factor: inability to interact appropriately with others

Risk for impaired **Parenting:** Risk factors: inability to function as parent or guardian, emotional instability

Risk for **Self-Mutilation:** Risk factors: self-hatred, depersonalization

Risk for other-directed **Violence:** Risk factor: history of violence, altered thought patterns

ANURIA

See Renal Failure

ANXIETY

*See **Anxiety**, Section II*

ANXIETY DISORDER

Ineffective **Activity Planning** r/t unrealistic perception of events

Anxiety r/t unmet security and safety needs

Death **Anxiety** r/t fears of unknown, powerlessness

Decisional Conflict r/t low self-esteem, fear of making a mistake

Defensive **Coping** r/t overwhelming feelings of dread

Disabled family **Coping** r/t ritualistic behavior, actions

Ineffective **Coping** r/t inability to express feelings appropriately

Ineffective **Denial** r/t overwhelming feelings of hopelessness, fear, threat to self

Disturbed **Energy Field** r/t hopelessness, helplessness

Insomnia r/t psychological impairment, emotional instability

Powerlessness r/t lifestyle of helplessness

Self-Care deficit r/t ritualistic behavior, activities

Sleep deprivation r/t prolonged psychological discomfort

Risk for **Spiritual Distress:** Risk factor: psychological distress

Readiness for enhanced **Knowledge:** expresses an interest in learning

AORTIC ANEURYSM REPAIR (ABDOMINAL SURGERY)

See Abdominal Surgery; Aneurysm, Abdominal Surgery

AORTIC VALVULAR STENOSIS

See Congenital Heart Disease/Cardiac Anomalies

APHASIA

Anxiety r/t situational crisis of aphasia

Impaired verbal **Communication** r/t decrease in circulation to brain

Ineffective **Coping** r/t loss of speech

Ineffective **Health Maintenance** r/t deficient knowledge regarding information on aphasia and alternative communication techniques

APLASTIC ANEMIA

Activity Intolerance r/t imbalance between oxygen supply and demand

Fear r/t ability to live with serious disease

Risk for **Bleeding:** Risk factor: inadequate clotting factors

Risk for **Infection:** Risk factor: inadequate immune function

Readiness for enhanced **Knowledge:** expresses an interest in learning

APNEA IN INFANCY

See Premature Infant (Child); Premature Infant (Parent); SIDS (Sudden Infant Death Syndrome)

APNEUSTIC RESPIRATIONS

Ineffective **Breathing Pattern** r/t perception or cognitive impairment, neurological impairment

See cause of Apneustic Respirations

APPENDECTOMY

Deficient **Fluid Volume** r/t fluid restriction, hypermetabolic state, nausea, vomiting

Acute **Pain** r/t surgical incision

Delayed **Surgical Recovery** r/t rupture of appendix

Risk for **Infection:** Risk factors: perforation or rupture of appendix, surgical incision, peritonitis

Readiness for enhanced **Knowledge:** expresses an interest in learning

See Hospitalized Child; Surgery, Postoperative

APPENDICITIS

Deficient **Fluid Volume** r/t anorexia, nausea, vomiting

Acute **Pain** r/t inflammation

Risk for **Infection:** Risk factor: possible perforation of appendix

Readiness for enhanced **Knowledge:** expresses an interest in learning

APPREHENSION

Anxiety r/t threat to self-concept, threat to health status, situational crisis

Death **Anxiety** r/t apprehension over loss of self, consequences to significant others

ARDS (ACUTE RESPIRATORY DISTRESS SYNDROME)

Ineffective **Airway Clearance** r/t excessive tracheobronchial secretions

Death **Anxiety** r/t seriousness of physical disease

Impaired **Gas Exchange** r/t damage to alveolar capillary membrane, change in lung compliance

Impaired **Spontaneous Ventilation** r/t damage to alveolar capillary membrane

See Ventilator Client

ARRHYTHMIA

See Dysrhythmia

ARTERIAL INSUFFICIENCY

Ineffective peripheral **Tissue Perfusion** r/t interruption of arterial flow

Delayed **Surgical Recovery** r/t ineffective tissue perfusion

ARTHRITIS

Activity Intolerance r/t chronic pain, fatigue, weakness

Disturbed **Body Image** r/t ineffective coping with joint abnormalities

Impaired physical **Mobility** r/t joint impairment

Chronic **Pain** r/t progression of joint deterioration

Self-Care deficit: specify r/t pain with movement, damage to joints

Readiness for enhanced **Knowledge:** expresses an interest in learning

See JRA (Juvenile Rheumatoid Arthritis)

ARTHROCENTESIS

Acute **Pain** r/t invasive procedure

ARTHROPLASTY (TOTAL HIP REPLACEMENT)

See Total Joint Replacement (Total Knee, Total Hip, Shoulder); Surgery, Perioperative; Surgery, Postoperative; Surgery, Preoperative

ARTHROSCOPY

Impaired physical **Mobility** r/t surgical trauma of knee

Readiness for enhanced **Knowledge:** expresses an interest in learning

ASCITES

Ineffective **Breathing Pattern** r/t increased abdominal girth

Imbalanced **Nutrition:** less than body requirements r/t loss of appetite

Chronic **Pain** r/t altered body function

Readiness for enhanced **Knowledge:** expresses an interest in learning

A *See cause of Ascites; Cancer; Cirrhosis*

ASPERGER'S SYNDROME

Ineffective **Relationship** r/t poor communication skills, lack of empathy

See Autism

ASPHYXIA, BIRTH

Ineffective **Breathing Pattern** r/t depression of breathing reflex secondary to anoxia

Ineffective **Coping** r/t uncertainty of child outcome

Fear (parental) r/t concern over safety of infant

Impaired **Gas Exchange** r/t poor placental perfusion, lack of initiation of breathing by newborn

Grieving r/t loss of "perfect" child, concern of loss of future abilities

Impaired **Spontaneous Ventilation** r/t brain injury

Risk for impaired **Attachment**: Risk factors: ill infant who is unable to initiate parental contact, hospitalization in critical care environment

Risk for delayed **Development**: Risk factor: lack of oxygen to brain

Risk for disproportionate **Growth**: Risk factor: lack of oxygen to brain

Risk for disorganized **Infant** behavior: Risk factor: lack of oxygen to brain

Risk for **Injury**: Risk factor: lack of oxygen to brain

Risk for ineffective **Cerebral** tissue perfusion: Risk factor: poor placental perfusion or cord compression resulting in lack of oxygen to brain

ASPIRATION, DANGER OF

Risk for **Aspiration** (See **Aspiration**, risk for, Section II)

ASSAULT VICTIM

Post-Trauma Syndrome r/t assault

Rape-Trauma Syndrome r/t rape

Impaired individual **Resilience** r/t frightening experience, post-trauma stress response

Risk for **Post-Trauma Syndrome:** Risk factors: perception of event, inadequate social support, unsupportive environment, diminished ego strength, duration of event

Risk for **Spiritual Distress:** Risk factors: physical, psychological stress

ASSAULTIVE CLIENT

Risk for **Injury:** Risk factors: confused thought process, impaired judgment

Risk for other-directed **Violence:** Risk factors: paranoid ideation, anger

ASTHMA

Activity Intolerance r/t fatigue, energy shift to meet muscle needs for breathing to overcome airway obstruction

Ineffective **Airway Clearance** r/t tracheobronchial narrowing, excessive secretions

Anxiety r/t inability to breathe effectively, fear of suffocation

Disturbed **Body Image** r/t decreased participation in physical activities

Ineffective **Breathing Pattern** r/t anxiety

Ineffective **Coping** r/t personal vulnerability to situational crisis

Ineffective **Self-Health Management** (See **Self-Health Management,** ineffective, in Section II)

Impaired **Home Maintenance** r/t deficient knowledge regarding control of environmental triggers

Sleep deprivation r/t ineffective breathing pattern, cough

Readiness for enhanced **Self-Health Management** (See **Self-Health Management,** readiness for enhanced, Section II)

Readiness for enhanced **Knowledge:** expresses an interest in learning

See Child with Chronic Condition; Hospitalized Child

ATAXIA

Anxiety r/t change in health status

Disturbed **Body Image** r/t staggering gait

Impaired physical **Mobility** r/t neuromuscular impairment

Risk for **Falls:** Risk factors: gait alteration, instability

ATELECTASIS

Ineffective **Breathing Pattern** r/t loss of functional lung tissue, depression of respiratory function or hypoventilation because of pain

Impaired **Gas Exchange** r/t decreased alveolar-capillary surface

See condition causing Atelectasis

ATHEROSCLEROSIS

See MI (Myocardial Infarction); CVA (Cerebrovascular Accident); Peripheral Vascular Disease (PVD)

ATHLETE'S FOOT

Impaired **Skin Integrity** r/t effects of fungal agent

Readiness for enhanced **Knowledge:** expresses an interest in learning

See Itching; Pruritus

ATN (ACUTE TUBULAR NECROSIS)

See Renal Failure

ATRIAL FIBRILLATION

See Dysrhythmia

ATRIAL SEPTAL DEFECT

See Congenital Heart Disease/Cardiac Anomalies

ATTENTION DEFICIT DISORDER

Risk-prone **Health Behavior** r/t intense emotional state

Disabled family **Coping** r/t significant person with chronically unexpressed feelings of guilt, anxiety, hostility, and despair

Ineffective **Impulse Control** r/t (See **Impulse Control,** ineffective, Section II)

Chronic low **Self-Esteem** r/t difficulty in participating in expected activities, poor school performance

Social Isolation r/t unacceptable social behavior

Risk for delayed **Development:** Risk factor: behavior disorders

Risk for **Falls:** Risk factor: rapid non-thinking behavior

Risk for **Loneliness:** Risk factor: social isolation

Risk for impaired **Parenting:** Risk factor: lack of knowledge of factors contributing to child's behavior

Risk for **Spiritual Distress:** Risk factor: poor relationships

AUDITORY PROBLEMS

See Hearing Impairment

AUTISM

Impaired verbal **Communication** r/t speech and language delays

Compromised family **Coping** r/t parental guilt over etiology of disease, inability to accept or adapt to child's condition, inability to help child and other family members seek treatment

Delayed **Growth and Development** r/t difficulty developing relationships with other human beings, inability to identify own body as separate from those of other people, inability to integrate concept of self

Disturbed personal **Identity** r/t inability to distinguish between self and environment, inability to identify own body as separate from those of other people, inability to integrate concept of self

B

Self-Neglect r/t impaired socialization

Impaired **Social Interaction** r/t communication barriers, inability to relate to others, failure to develop peer relationships

Risk for delayed **Development**: Risk factor: autism

Risk for **Loneliness**: Risk factors: difficulty developing relationships with other people

Risk for **Self-Mutilation**: Risk factor: autistic state

Risk for other-directed **Violence**: Risk factors: frequent destructive rages toward others secondary to extreme response to changes in routine, fear of harmless things

Risk for self-directed **Violence**: Risk factors: frequent destructive rages toward self, secondary to extreme response to changes in routine, fear of harmless things

See Child with Chronic Condition; Mental Retardation

AUTONOMIC DYSREFLEXIA

Autonomic Dysreflexia r/t bladder distention, bowel distention, noxious stimuli

Risk for **Autonomic Dysreflexia**: Risk factors: bladder distention, bowel distention, noxious stimuli

AUTONOMIC HYPERREFLEXIA

See Autonomic Dysreflexia

B

BABY CARE

Readiness for enhanced **Childbearing Process**: demonstrates appropriate feeding and baby care techniques, along with attachment to infant and providing a safe environment

BACK PAIN

Anxiety r/t situational crisis, back injury

Ineffective **Coping** r/t situational crisis, back injury

Disturbed **Energy Field** r/t chronic pain

Impaired physical **Mobility** r/t pain

Acute **Pain** r/t back injury

Chronic **Pain** r/t back injury

Risk for **Constipation**: Risk factors: decreased activity, side effect of pain medication

Risk for **Disuse Syndrome**: Risk factor: severe pain

Readiness for enhanced **Knowledge**: expresses an interest in learning

BACTEREMIA

Risk for **Infection**: Risk factor: compromised immune system

Risk for **Shock**: Risk factor: development of systemic inflammatory response from presence of bacteria in blood stream

See Infection; Infection, Potential for

BARREL CHEST

See Aging (if appropriate); COPD (Chronic Obstructive Pulmonary Disease)

BATHING/HYGIENE PROBLEMS

Impaired **Mobility** r/t chronic physically limiting condition

Self-Neglect (See **Neglect**, self, Section II)

Bathing **Self-Care** deficit (See **Self-Care** deficit, bathing, Section II)

BATTERED CHILD SYNDROME

Dysfunctional **Family Processes** r/t inadequate coping skills

Sleep deprivation r/t prolonged psychological discomfort

Chronic **Sorrow** r/t situational crises

Risk for **Post-Trauma Syndrome:** Risk factors: physical abuse, incest, rape, molestation

Risk for **Self-Mutilation:** Risk factors: feelings of rejection, dysfunctional family

Risk for **Suicide:** Risk factor: childhood abuse.

See Child Abuse

BATTERED PERSON

See Abuse, Spouse, Parent, or Significant Other

BEDBUGS, INFESTATION

Impaired **Home Maintenance** r/t deficient knowledge regarding prevention of bedbug infestation

Impaired **Skin Integrity** r/t bites of bedbugs

See Itching; Pruritus

BED MOBILITY, IMPAIRED

Impaired bed **Mobility** (See **Mobility**, bed, impaired, Section II)

BED REST, PROLONGED

Deficient **Diversional Activity** r/t prolonged bed rest

Impaired bed **Mobility** r/t neuromuscular impairment

Social Isolation r/t prolonged bed rest

Risk for **Disuse Syndrome:** Risk factor: prolonged immobility

Risk for **Loneliness:** Risk factor: prolonged bed rest

BEDSORES

See Pressure Ulcer

BEDWETTING

Ineffective **Health Maintenance** r/t unachieved developmental level, neuromuscular immaturity, diseases of the urinary system.

BELL'S PALSY

Disturbed **Body Image** r/t loss of motor control on one side of face

Imbalanced **Nutrition:** less than body requirements r/t difficulty with chewing

Acute **Pain** r/t inflammation of facial nerve

Risk for **Injury** (eye): Risk factor: decreased tears, decreased blinking of eye

Readiness for enhanced **Knowledge:** expresses an interest in learning

BENIGN PROSTATIC HYPERTROPHY

See BPH (Benign Prostatic Hypertrophy); Prostatic Hypertrophy

BEREAVEMENT

Grieving r/t loss of significant person

Insomnia r/t grief

Risk for complicated **Grieving:** Risk factor: emotional instability, lack of social support

Risk for **Spiritual Distress:** Risk factor: death of a loved one

BILIARY ATRESIA

Anxiety r/t surgical intervention, possible liver transplantation

Impaired **Comfort** r/t inflammation of skin, itching

Imbalanced **Nutrition:** less than body requirements r/t decreased absorption of fat and fat-soluble vitamins, poor feeding

Risk for **Bleeding:** Risk factors: vitamin K deficiency, altered clotting mechanisms

Risk for ineffective **Breathing Pattern:** Risk factors: enlarged liver, development of ascites

Risk for impaired **Skin Integrity:** Risk factor: pruritus

See Child with Chronic Condition; Cirrhosis (as complication); Hospitalized Child; Terminally Ill Child,

B

Adolescent; Infant/Toddler; Preschool Child; School-Age Child/Preadolescent; Death of Child, Parent

BILIARY CALCULUS

See Cholelithiasis

BILIARY OBSTRUCTION

See Jaundice

BILIRUBIN ELEVATION IN NEONATE

Neonatal **Jaundice** (See **Jaundice**, Neonatal, Section II)

BIOPSY

Fear r/t outcome of biopsy

Readiness for enhanced **Knowledge:** expresses an interest in learning

BIOTERRORISM

Contamination r/t exposure to bioterrorism

Risk for **Infection:** Risk factor: exposure to harmful biological agent

Risk for **Post-Trauma Syndrome:** Risk factor: perception of event of bioterrorism

BIPOLAR DISORDER I (MOST RECENT EPISODE, DEPRESSED OR MANIC)

Ineffective **Activity Planning** r/t unrealistic perception of events

Risk-prone **Health Behavior** r/t low state of optimism

Disturbed **Energy Field** r/t disharmony of mind, body, spirit

Fatigue r/t psychological demands

Ineffective **Health Maintenance** r/t lack of ability to make good judgments regarding ways to obtain help

Self-Care deficit: specify r/t depression, cognitive impairment

Chronic low **Self-Esteem** r/t repeated unmet expectations

Social Isolation r/t ineffective coping

Risk for complicated **Grieving:** Risk factor: lack of previous resolution of former grieving response

Risk for **Loneliness:** Risk factors: stress, conflict

Risk for **Spiritual Distress:** Risk factor: mental illness

Risk for **Suicide:** Risk factor: psychiatric disorder, poor support system

See Depression (Major Depressive Disorder); Manic Disorder, Bipolar I

BIRTH ASPHYXIA

See Asphyxia, Birth

BIRTH CONTROL

See Contraceptive Method

BLADDER CANCER

Urinary Retention r/t clots obstructing urethra

See Cancer; TURP (Transurethral Resection of the Prostate)

BLADDER DISTENTION

Urinary Retention r/t high urethral pressure caused by weak detrusor, inhibition of reflex arc, blockage, strong sphincter

BLADDER TRAINING

Disturbed **Body Image** r/t difficulty maintaining control of urinary elimination

Functional urinary **Incontinence** r/t altered environment; sensory, cognitive, mobility deficit

Stress urinary **Incontinence** r/t degenerative change in pelvic muscles and structural supports

Urge urinary **Incontinence** r/t decreased bladder capacity, increased urine concentration, overdistention of bladder

Readiness for enhanced **Knowledge:** expresses an interest in learning

BLADDER TRAINING, CHILD

See Toilet Training

BLEEDING TENDENCY

Risk for **Bleeding** (See **Bleeding**, risk for, Section III)

Risk for delayed **Surgical Recovery**: Risk factor: bleeding tendency

BLEPHAROPLASTY

Disturbed **Body Image** r/t effects of surgery

Readiness for enhanced **Knowledge**: expresses an interest in learning

BLINDNESS

Interrupted **Family Processes** r/t shift in health status of family member (change in visual acuity)

Impaired **Home Maintenance** r/t decreased vision

Ineffective **Role Performance** r/t alteration in health status (change in visual acuity)

Self-Care deficit: specify r/t inability to see to be able to perform activities of daily living

Vision Loss r/t impaired sensory reception, transmission, or integration

Risk for delayed **Development**: Risk factor: vision impairment

Risk for **Injury**: Risk factor: sensory dysfunction

Readiness for enhanced **Knowledge**: expresses an interest in learning

See Vision Impairment

BLOOD DISORDER

Ineffective **Protection** r/t abnormal blood profile

Risk for **Bleeding**: Risk factor: abnormal blood profile

See cause of Blood Disorder

BLOOD PRESSURE ALTERATION

See Hypotension; HTN (Hypertension)

BLOOD SUGAR CONTROL

Risk for unstable blood **Glucose** level (See **Glucose** level, blood, unstable, risk for, Section II)

BLOOD TRANSFUSION

Anxiety r/t possibility of harm from transfusion

See Anemia

BODY DYSMORPHIC DISORDER

Anxiety r/t perceived defect of body

Disturbed **Body Image** r/t overinvolvement in physical appearance

Chronic low **Self-Esteem** r/t lack of self-valuing because of perceived body defects

Social Isolation r/t distancing self from others because of perceived self body defects

Risk for **Suicide**: Risk factor: perceived defects of body affecting self-valuing and hopes

BODY IMAGE CHANGE

Disturbed **Body Image** (See **Body Image**, disturbed, Section II)

BODY TEMPERATURE, ALTERED

Ineffective **Thermoregulation** (See **Thermoregulation**, ineffective, Section II)

BONE MARROW BIOPSY

Fear r/t unknown outcome of results of biopsy

Acute **Pain** r/t bone marrow aspiration

Readiness for Enhanced **Knowledge**: expresses an interest in learning

See disease necessitating bone marrow biopsy (e.g., Leukemia)

BORDERLINE PERSONALITY DISORDER

Ineffective **Activity Planning** r/t unrealistic perception of events

B

Anxiety r/t perceived threat to self-concept

Defensive **Coping** r/t difficulty with relationships, inability to accept blame for own behavior

Ineffective **Coping** r/t use of maladjusted defense mechanisms (e.g., projection, denial)

Powerlessness r/t lifestyle of helplessness

Social Isolation r/t immature interests

Ineffective family **Therapeutic Regimen Management** r/t manipulative behavior of client

Risk for **Caregiver Role Strain**: Risk factors: inability of care receiver to accept criticism, care receiver taking advantage of others to meet own needs or having unreasonable expectations

Risk for **Self-Mutilation**: Risk factors: ineffective coping, feelings of self-hatred

Risk for **Spiritual Distress**: Risk factor: poor relationships associated with abnormal behaviors

Risk for self-directed **Violence**: Risk factors: feelings of need to punish self, manipulative behavior

BOREDOM

Deficient **Diversional Activity** r/t environmental lack of diversional activity

Social Isolation r/t altered state of wellness

BOTULISM

Deficient **Fluid Volume** r/t profuse diarrhea

Readiness for enhanced **Knowledge**: expresses an interest in learning

BOWEL INCONTINENCE

Bowel **Incontinence** r/t decreased awareness of need to defecate, loss of sphincter control, fecal impaction

Readiness for enhanced **Knowledge**: expresses an interest in learning

BOWEL OBSTRUCTION

Constipation r/t decreased motility, intestinal obstruction

Deficient **Fluid Volume** r/t inadequate fluid volume intake, fluid loss in bowel

Imbalanced **Nutrition**: less than body requirements r/t nausea, vomiting

Acute **Pain** r/t pressure from distended abdomen

BOWEL RESECTION

See Abdominal Surgery

BOWEL SOUNDS, ABSENT OR DIMINISHED

Constipation r/t decreased or absent peristalsis

Deficient **Fluid Volume** r/t inability to ingest fluids, loss of fluids in bowel

Delayed **Surgical Recovery** r/t inability to obtain adequate nutritional status

Risk for dysfunctional **Gastrointestinal Motility** (See **Gastrointestinal Motility**, dysfunctional, risk for, Section II)

BOWEL SOUNDS, HYPERACTIVE

Diarrhea r/t increased gastrointestinal motility

BOWEL TRAINING

Bowel **Incontinence** r/t loss of control of rectal sphincter

Readiness for enhanced **Knowledge**: expresses an interest in learning

BOWEL TRAINING, CHILD

See Toilet Training

BPH (BENIGN PROSTATIC HYPERTROPHY)

Ineffective **Health Maintenance** r/t deficient knowledge regarding self-care with prostatic hypertrophy

Insomnia r/t nocturia

Urinary Retention r/t obstruction of urethra

Risk for urge urinary Incontinence: Risk factors: detrusor muscle instability with impaired contractility, involuntary sphincter relaxation

Risk for Infection: Risk factors: urinary residual after voiding, bacterial invasion of bladder

Readiness for enhanced Knowledge: expresses an interest in learning

See Prostatic Hypertrophy

BRADYCARDIA

Decreased Cardiac Output r/t slow heart rate supplying inadequate amount of blood for body function

Risk for ineffective Cerebral tissue perfusion: Risk factors: decreased cardiac output secondary to bradycardia, vagal response

Readiness for enhanced Knowledge: expresses an interest in learning

BRADYPNEA

Ineffective Breathing Pattern r/t neuromuscular impairment, pain, musculoskeletal impairment, perception or cognitive impairment, anxiety, fatigue or decreased energy, effects of drugs

See cause of Bradypnea

BRAIN INJURY

See Intracranial Pressure, Increased

BRAIN SURGERY

See Craniectomy/Craniotomy

BRAIN TUMOR

Acute Confusion r/t pressure from tumor

Fear r/t threat to well-being

Grieving r/t potential loss of physiosocial-psychosocial well-being

Decreased Intracranial Adaptive Capacity r/t presence of brain tumor

Acute Pain r/t pressure from tumor

Vision Loss r/t tumor growth compressing optic nerve and/or brain tissue

Risk for Injury: Risk factors: sensory-perceptual alterations, weakness

See Cancer; Chemotherapy; Child with Chronic Condition; Craniectomy/ Craniotomy; Hospitalized Child; Radiation Therapy; Terminally Ill Child, Adolescent; Terminally Ill Child, Infant/ Toddler; Terminally Ill Child, Preschool Child; Terminally Ill Child, School-Age Child/Preadolescent; Terminally Ill Child/Death of Child, Parent

BRAXTON HICKS CONTRACTIONS

Activity Intolerance r/t increased contractions with increased gestation

Anxiety r/t uncertainty about beginning labor

Fatigue r/t lack of sleep

Stress urinary Incontinence r/t increased pressure on bladder with contractions

Insomnia r/t contractions when lying down

Ineffective Sexuality Pattern r/t fear of contractions associated with loss of infant

BREAST BIOPSY

Fear r/t potential for diagnosis of cancer

Risk for Spiritual Distress: Risk factor: fear of diagnosis of cancer

Readiness for enhanced Knowledge: expresses an interest in learning

BREAST CANCER

Death Anxiety r/t diagnosis of cancer

Ineffective Coping r/t treatment, prognosis

Fear r/t diagnosis of cancer

Sexual Dysfunction r/t loss of body part, partner's reaction to loss

Chronic Sorrow r/t diagnosis of cancer, loss of body integrity

B

B

Risk for **Spiritual Distress**: Risk factor: fear of diagnosis of cancer

Readiness for enhanced **Knowledge**: expresses an interest in learning

See Cancer; Chemotherapy; Mastectomy; Radiation Therapy

BREAST EXAMINATION, SELF

See SBE (Self-Breast Examination)

BREAST LUMPS

Fear r/t potential for diagnosis of cancer

Readiness for enhanced **Knowledge**: expresses an interest in learning

BREAST MILK, INSUFFICIENT

Insufficient **Breast Milk** (See **Breast Milk,** insufficient, Section II)

BREAST PUMPING

Risk for **Infection**: Risk factors: possible contaminated breast pump, incomplete emptying of breast

Risk for impaired **Skin Integrity**: Risk factor: high suction

Readiness for enhanced **Knowledge**: expresses an interest in learning

BREASTFEEDING, EFFECTIVE

Readiness for enhanced **Breastfeeding** (See **Breastfeeding,** readiness for enhanced, Section II)

BREASTFEEDING, INEFFECTIVE

Ineffective **Breastfeeding** (See **Breastfeeding,** ineffective, Section II)

See Infant Feeding Pattern, Ineffective; Painful Breasts, Engorgement; Painful Breasts, Sore Nipples

BREASTFEEDING, INTERRUPTED

Interrupted **Breastfeeding** (See **Breastfeeding,** interrupted, Section II)

BREATH SOUNDS, DECREASED OR ABSENT

See Atelectasis; Pneumothorax

BREATHING PATTERN ALTERATION

Ineffective **Breathing Pattern** r/t neuromuscular impairment, pain, musculoskeletal impairment, perception or cognitive impairment, anxiety, decreased energy or fatigue

BREECH BIRTH

Fear: maternal r/t danger to infant, self

Impaired **Gas Exchange**: fetal r/t compressed umbilical cord

Risk for **Aspiration**: fetal: Risk factor: birth of body before head

Risk for delayed **Development**: Risk factor: compressed umbilical cord

Risk for impaired **Tissue Integrity**: fetal: Risk factor: difficult birth

Risk for impaired **Tissue Integrity**: maternal: Risk factor: difficult birth

BRONCHITIS

Ineffective **Airway Clearance** r/t excessive thickened mucus secretion

Readiness for enhanced **Self-Health Management**: wishes to stop smoking

Readiness for enhanced **Knowledge**: expresses an interest in learning

BRONCHOPULMONARY DYSPLASIA

Activity Intolerance r/t imbalance between oxygen supply and demand

Excess **Fluid Volume** r/t sodium and water retention

Imbalanced **Nutrition**: less than body requirements r/t poor feeding, increased caloric needs as a result of increased work of breathing

See Child with Chronic Condition; Hospitalized Child; Respiratory Conditions of the Neonate

BRONCHOSCOPY

Risk for **Aspiration**: Risk factor: temporary loss of gag reflex

Risk for **Injury**: Risk factors: complication of pneumothorax, laryngeal edema, hemorrhage (if biopsy done)

BRUITS, CAROTID

Risk for ineffective **Cerebral** tissue perfusion: Risk factors: interruption of carotid blood flow to brain

BRYANT'S TRACTION

See Traction and Casts

BUCK'S TRACTION

See Traction and Casts

BUERGER'S DISEASE

See Peripheral Vascular Disease (PVD)

BULIMIA

Disturbed **Body Image** r/t misperception about actual appearance, body weight

Compromised family **Coping** r/t chronically unresolved feelings of guilt, anger, hostility

Defensive **Coping** r/t eating disorder

Diarrhea r/t laxative abuse

Fear r/t food ingestion, weight gain

Imbalanced **Nutrition**: less than body requirements r/t induced vomiting, excessive exercise, laxative abuse.

Powerlessness r/t urge to purge self after eating

Chronic low **Self-Esteem** r/t lack of positive feedback

See Maturational Issues, Adolescent

BUNION

Readiness for enhanced **Knowledge**: expresses an interest in learning

BUNIONECTOMY

Impaired physical **Mobility** r/t sore foot

Impaired **Walking** r/t pain associated with surgery

Risk for **Infection**: Risk factors: surgical incision, advanced age

Readiness for enhanced **Knowledge**: expresses an interest in learning

BURN RISK

Risk for **Thermal Injury**: Risk factors (See **Thermal Injury**, risk for, Section II)

BURNS

Disturbed **Body Image** r/t altered physical appearance

Deficient **Diversional Activity** r/t long-term hospitalization

Fear r/t pain from treatments, possible permanent disfigurement

Deficient **Fluid Volume** r/t loss of protective skin

Grieving r/t loss of bodily function, loss of future hopes and plans

Hypothermia r/t impaired skin integrity

Impaired physical **Mobility** r/t pain, musculoskeletal impairment, contracture formation

Imbalanced **Nutrition**: less than body requirements r/t increased metabolic needs, anorexia, protein and fluid loss

Acute **Pain** r/t burn injury, treatments

Ineffective peripheral **Tissue Perfusion** r/t circumferential burns, impaired arterial/venous circulation

Post-Trauma Syndrome r/t life-threatening event

Impaired **Skin Integrity** r/t injury of skin

Delayed **Surgical Recovery** r/t ineffective tissue perfusion

Risk for ineffective **Airway Clearance**: Risk factors: potential tracheobronchial obstruction, edema

Risk for deficient **Fluid Volume**: Risk factors: loss from skin surface, fluid shift

Risk for **Infection**: Risk factors: loss of intact skin, trauma, invasive sites

Risk for **Peripheral Neurovascular Dysfunction:** Risk factor: eschar formation with circumferential burn

Risk for **Post-Trauma Syndrome:** Risk factors: perception, duration of event that caused burns

Readiness for enhanced **Knowledge:** expresses an interest in learning

See Hospitalized Child; Safety, Childhood

BURSITIS

Impaired physical **Mobility** r/t inflammation in joint

Acute **Pain** r/t inflammation in joint

BYPASS GRAFT

See Coronary Artery Bypass Grafting (CABG)

C

CABG (CORONARY ARTERY BYPASS GRAFTING)

See Coronary Artery Bypass Grafting (CABG)

CACHEXIA

Adult **Failure to Thrive** r/t (See Thrive, failure to, Section II)

Imbalanced **Nutrition:** less than body requirements r/t inability to ingest food because of physiological factors

Risk for **Infection:** Risk factor: inadequate nutrition

CALCIUM ALTERATION

See Hypercalcemia; Hypocalcemia

CANCER

Activity Intolerance r/t side effects of treatment, weakness from cancer

Death **Anxiety** r/t unresolved issues regarding dying

Disturbed **Body Image** r/t side effects of treatment, cachexia

Decisional Conflict r/t selection of treatment choices, continuation or discontinuation of treatment, "do not resuscitate" decision

Constipation r/t side effects of medication, altered nutrition, decreased activity

Compromised family **Coping** r/t prolonged disease or disability progression that exhausts supportive ability of significant others

Ineffective **Coping** r/t personal vulnerability in situational crisis, terminal illness

Ineffective **Denial** r/t complicated grieving process

Fear r/t serious threat to well-being

Grieving r/t potential loss of significant others, high risk for infertility

Ineffective **Health Maintenance** r/t deficient knowledge regarding prescribed treatment

Hopelessness r/t loss of control, terminal illness

Insomnia r/t anxiety, pain

Impaired physical **Mobility** r/t weakness, neuromusculoskeletal impairment, pain

Imbalanced **Nutrition:** less than body requirements r/t loss of appetite, difficulty swallowing, side effects of chemotherapy, obstruction by tumor

Impaired **Oral Mucous Membrane** r/t chemotherapy, effects of radiation, oral pH changes, decreased oral secretions

Chronic **Pain** r/t metastatic cancer

Powerlessness r/t treatment, progression of disease

Ineffective **Protection** r/t cancer suppressing immune system

Ineffective **Role Performance** r/t change in physical capacity, inability to resume prior role

Self-Care deficit: specify r/t pain, intolerance to activity, decreased strength

Impaired **Skin Integrity** r/t immunological deficit, immobility

Social Isolation r/t hospitalization, lifestyle changes

Chronic **Sorrow** r/t chronic illness of cancer

Spiritual Distress r/t test of spiritual beliefs

Risk for **Bleeding:** Risk factor: bone marrow depression from chemotherapy

Risk for **Disuse Syndrome:** Risk factors: immobility, fatigue

Risk for impaired **Home Maintenance:** Risk factor: lack of familiarity with community resources

Risk for **Infection:** Risk factor: inadequate immune system

Risk for compromised **Resilience:** Risk factors: multiple stressors, pain, chronic illness

Risk for **Spiritual Distress:** Risk factor: physical illness of cancer

Readiness for enhanced **Knowledge:** expresses an interest in learning

Readiness for enhanced **Spiritual Well-Being:** desire for harmony with self, others, higher power, God, when faced with serious illness

See Chemotherapy; Child with Chronic Condition; Hospitalized Child; Leukemia; Radiation Therapy; Terminally Ill Child, Adolescent; Terminally Ill Child, Infant/Toddler; Terminally Ill Child, Preschool Child; Terminally Ill Child, School-Age Child/Preadolescent; Terminally Ill Child/Death of Child, Parent

CANDIDIASIS, ORAL

Readiness for enhanced **Knowledge:** expresses an interest in learning

Impaired **Oral Mucous Membrane** r/t overgrowth of infectious agent, depressed immune function

CAPILLARY REFILL TIME, PROLONGED

Impaired **Gas Exchange** r/t ventilation-perfusion imbalance

Ineffective peripheral **Tissue Perfusion** r/t interruption of arterial flow

See Shock, Hypovolemic

CARBON MONOXIDE POISONING

See Smoke Inhalation

CARDIAC ARREST

Post-Trauma Syndrome r/t experiencing serious life event

See cause of Cardiac Arrest

CARDIAC CATHETERIZATION

Fear r/t invasive procedure, uncertainty of outcome of procedure

Risk for **Injury:** hematoma: Risk factor: invasive procedure

Risk for decreased **Cardiac** tissue perfusion: Risk factors: ventricular ischemia, dysrhythmia

Risk for **Peripheral Neurovascular Dysfunction:** Risk factor: vascular obstruction

Readiness for enhanced **Knowledge:** expresses an interest in learning postprocedure care, treatment, and prevention of coronary artery disease

CARDIAC DISORDERS

Decreased **Cardiac Output** r/t cardiac disorder

Risk for decreased **Cardiac** tissue perfusion: Risk factor: cardiac disorder

See specific cardiac disorder

CARDIAC DISORDERS IN PREGNANCY

Activity Intolerance r/t cardiac pathophysiology, increased demand for cardiac output because of pregnancy, weakness, fatigue

Death **Anxiety** r/t potential danger of condition

Compromised family **Coping** r/t prolonged hospitalization or maternal incapacitation that exhausts supportive capacity of significant others

Ineffective **Coping** r/t personal vulnerability

Interrupted **Family Processes** r/t hospitalization, maternal incapacitation, changes in roles

Fatigue r/t physiological, psychological, and emotional demands

Fear r/t potential maternal effects, potential poor fetal or maternal outcome

Powerlessness r/t illness-related regimen

Ineffective **Role Performance** r/t changes in lifestyle, expectations from disease process with superimposed pregnancy

Situational low **Self-Esteem** r/t situational crisis, pregnancy

Social Isolation r/t limitations of activity, bed rest or hospitalization, separation from family and friends

Risk for delayed **Development**: Risk factor: poor maternal oxygenation

Risk for deficient **Fluid Volume**: Risk factor: sudden changes in circulation after delivery of placenta

Risk for excess **Fluid Volume**: Risk factors: compromised regulatory mechanism with increased afterload, preload, circulating blood volume

Risk for impaired **Gas Exchange**: Risk factor: pulmonary edema

Risk for disproportionate **Growth**: Risk factor: poor maternal oxygenation

Risk for disturbed **Maternal/Fetal Dyad**: Risk factor: compromised oxygen transport

Risk for decreased **Cardiac** tissue perfusion: Risk factor: strain on compromised heart from work of pregnancy, delivery

Risk for compromised **Resilience**: Risk factors: multiple stressors, fear

Risk for **Spiritual Distress**: Risk factor: fear of diagnosis for self and infant

Readiness for enhanced **Knowledge**: expresses an interest in learning

CARDIAC DYSRHYTHMIA

See Dysrhythmia

CARDIAC OUTPUT, DECREASED

Decreased **Cardiac Output** r/t cardiac dysfunction

CARDIAC TAMPONADE

Decreased **Cardiac Output** r/t fluid in pericardial sac

See Pericarditis

CARDIOGENIC SHOCK

See Shock, Cardiogenic

CAREGIVER ROLE STRAIN

Caregiver Role Strain (See **Caregiver Role Strain**, Section II)

Risk for compromised **Resilience**: Risk factor: stress of prolonged caregiving

CARIOUS TEETH

See Cavities in Teeth

CAROTID ENDARTERECTOMY

Fear r/t surgery in vital area

Risk for ineffective **Airway Clearance**: Risk factor: hematoma compressing trachea

Risk for **Bleeding**: Risk factor: possible hematoma formation, trauma to region

Risk for ineffective **Cerebral** tissue perfusion: Risk factors: hemorrhage, clot formation

Readiness for enhanced **Knowledge**: expresses an interest in learning

CARPAL TUNNEL SYNDROME

Impaired physical **Mobility** r/t neuromuscular impairment

Chronic **Pain** r/t unrelieved pressure on median nerve

Self-Care deficit: bathing, dressing, feeding r/t pain

CARPOPEDAL SPASM

See Hypocalcemia

CASTS

Deficient **Diversional Activity** r/t physical limitations from cast

Impaired physical **Mobility** r/t limb immobilization

Self-Care deficit: bathing, dressing, feeding r/t presence of cast(s) on upper extremities

Self-Care deficit: toileting r/t presence of cast(s) on lower extremities

Impaired **Walking** r/t cast(s) on lower extremities, fracture of bones

Risk for **Peripheral Neurovascular Dysfunction:** Risk factor: mechanical compression from cast, trauma from fracture

Risk for impaired **Skin Integrity:** Risk factor: unrelieved pressure on skin from cast

Readiness for enhanced **Knowledge:** expresses an interest in learning

See Traction and Casts

CATARACT EXTRACTION

Anxiety r/t threat of permanent vision loss, surgical procedure

Vision Loss r/t edema from surgery

Risk for **Injury:** Risk factors: increased intraocular pressure, accommodation to new visual field

Readiness for enhanced **Knowledge:** expresses an interest in learning

See Vision Impairment

CATARACTS

Vision Loss r/t impaired sensory input

See Vision Impairment

CATATONIC SCHIZOPHRENIA

Impaired verbal **Communication** r/t cognitive impairment

Impaired **Memory** r/t cognitive impairment

Impaired physical **Mobility** r/t cognitive impairment, maintenance of rigid posture, inappropriate or bizarre postures

Imbalanced **Nutrition:** less than body requirements r/t decrease in outside stimulation, loss of perception of hunger, resistance to instructions to eat

Social Isolation r/t inability to communicate, immobility

See Schizophrenia

CATHETERIZATION, URINARY

Risk for **Infection:** Risk factor: invasive procedure

Readiness for enhanced **Knowledge:** expresses an interest in learning

CAVITIES IN TEETH

Impaired **Dentition** r/t ineffective oral hygiene, barriers to self-care, economic barriers to professional care, nutritional deficits, dietary habits

CELIAC DISEASE

Imbalanced **Nutrition:** less than body requirements r/t malabsorption due to immune effects of gluten

Diarrhea r/t malabsorption of food, immune effects of gluten on gastrointestinal system

Readiness for enhanced **Knowledge:** expresses an interest in learning

CELLULITIS

Acute **Pain** r/t inflammatory changes in tissues from infection

Ineffective peripheral **Tissue Perfusion** r/t edema of extremities

Impaired **Tissue Integrity** r/t inflammatory process damaging skin and underlying tissue

Risk for **Vascular Trauma:** Risk factor: infusion of antibiotics

Readiness for enhanced **Knowledge:** expresses an interest in learning

CELLULITIS, PERIORBITAL

Acute **Pain** r/t edema and inflammation of skin/tissues

Vision Loss r/t decreased visual field secondary to edema of eyelids

Impaired **Skin Integrity** r/t inflammation or infection of skin, tissues

Readiness for enhanced **Knowledge:** expresses an interest in learning

See Hospitalized Child

CENTRAL LINE INSERTION

Risk for **Infection:** Risk factor: invasive procedure

Risk for **Vascular Trauma** (See **Vascular Trauma,** risk for, Section II)

Readiness for enhanced **Knowledge:** expresses an interest in learning

CEREBRAL ANEURYSM

See Craniectomy/Craniotomy; Intracranial Pressure, Increased; Subarachnoid Hemorrhage

CEREBRAL PALSY

Impaired verbal **Communication** r/t impaired ability to articulate or speak words because of facial muscle involvement

Deficient **Diversional Activity** r/t physical impairments, limitations on ability to participate in recreational activities

Impaired physical **Mobility** r/t spasticity, neuromuscular impairment or weakness

Imbalanced **Nutrition:** less than body requirements r/t spasticity, feeding or swallowing difficulties

Self-Care deficit: specify r/t neuromuscular impairments, sensory deficits

Impaired **Social Interaction** r/t impaired communication skills, limited physical activity, perceived differences from peers

Chronic **Sorrow** r/t presence of chronic disability

Risk for **Falls:** Risk factor: impaired physical mobility

Risk for **Injury:** Risk factors: muscle weakness, inability to control spasticity

Risk for impaired **Parenting:** Risk factor: caring for child with overwhelming needs resulting from chronic change in health status

Risk for **Spiritual Distress:** Risk factors: psychological stress associated with chronic illness

See Child with Chronic Condition

CEREBRAL PERFUSION

Risk for ineffective **Cerebral** tissue perfusion (See **Cerebral** tissue perfusion, ineffective, risk for, Section II)

CEREBROVASCULAR ACCIDENT (CVA)

See CVA (Cerebrovascular Accident)

CERVICITIS

Ineffective **Health Maintenance** r/t deficient knowledge regarding care and prevention of condition

Ineffective **Sexuality Pattern** r/t abstinence during acute stage

Risk for **Infection:** Risk factors: spread of infection, recurrence of infection

CESAREAN DELIVERY

Disturbed **Body Image** r/t surgery, unmet expectations for childbirth

Interrupted **Family Processes** r/t unmet expectations for childbirth

Fear r/t perceived threat to own well-being, outcome of birth

Impaired physical **Mobility** r/t pain

Acute **Pain** r/t surgical incision

Ineffective **Role Performance** r/t unmet expectations for childbirth

Situational low **Self-Esteem** r/t inability to deliver child vaginally

Risk for **Bleeding**: Risk factor: surgery

Risk for imbalanced **Fluid Volume**: Risk factors: loss of blood, fluid shifts

Risk for **Infection**: Risk factor: surgical incision

Risk for **Urinary Retention**: Risk factor: regional anesthesia

Readiness for enhanced **Childbearing Process**: a pattern of preparing for, maintaining, and strengthening care of newborn

Readiness for Enhanced **Knowledge**: expresses an interest in learning

CHEMICAL DEPENDENCE

See Alcoholism; Drug Abuse; Cocaine Abuse; Substance Abuse

CHEMOTHERAPY

Death **Anxiety** r/t chemotherapy not accomplishing desired results

Disturbed **Body Image** r/t loss of weight, loss of hair

Fatigue r/t disease process, anemia, drug effects

Nausea r/t effects of chemotherapy

Imbalanced **Nutrition**: less than body requirements r/t side effects of chemotherapy

Impaired **Oral Mucous Membrane** r/t effects of chemotherapy

Ineffective **Protection** r/t suppressed immune system, decreased platelets

Risk for **Bleeding**: Risk factors: tumor eroding blood vessel, stress effects on GI system

Risk for **Infection**: Risk factor: immunosuppression

Risk for **Vascular Trauma**: Risk factor: infusion of irritating medications

Readiness for enhanced **Knowledge**: expresses an interest in learning

See Cancer

CHEST PAIN

Fear r/t potential threat of death

Acute **Pain** r/t myocardial injury, ischemia

Risk for decreased **Cardiac** tissue perfusion: Risk factor: ventricular ischemia

See Angina; MI (Myocardial Infarction)

CHEST TUBES

Ineffective **Breathing Pattern** r/t asymmetrical lung expansion secondary to pain

Impaired **Gas Exchange** r/t decreased functional lung tissue

Acute **Pain** r/t presence of chest tubes, injury

Risk for **Injury**: Risk factor: presence of invasive chest tube

CHEYNE-STOKES RESPIRATION

Ineffective **Breathing Pattern** r/t critical illness

See cause of Cheyne-Stokes Respiration

CHF (CONGESTIVE HEART FAILURE)

Activity Intolerance r/t weakness, fatigue

Decreased **Cardiac Output** r/t impaired cardiac function, increased preload, decreased contractility, increased afterload

Constipation r/t activity intolerance

Fatigue r/t disease process with decreased cardiac output

Fear r/t threat to one's own well-being

Excess **Fluid Volume** r/t impaired excretion of sodium and water

C

Impaired **Gas Exchange** r/t excessive fluid in interstitial space of lungs

Powerlessness r/t illness-related regimen

Risk for **Shock** (Cardiogenic): Risk factors: decreased contractility of heart, increased afterload

Readiness for enhanced **Self-Health Management** (See **Self-Health Management**, readiness for enhanced, Section II)

See Child with Chronic Condition; Congenital Heart Disease/Cardiac Anomalies; Hospitalized Child

CHICKENPOX

See Communicable Diseases, Childhood

CHILD ABUSE

Interrupted **Family Processes** r/t inadequate coping skills

Fear r/t threat of punishment for perceived wrongdoing

Delayed **Growth and Development** r/t inadequate caretaking, stimulation deficiencies

Insomnia r/t hypervigilance, fear

Imbalanced **Nutrition:** less than body requirements r/t inadequate caretaking

Acute **Pain** r/t physical injuries

Impaired **Parenting** r/t psychological impairment, physical or emotional abuse of parent, substance abuse, unrealistic expectations of child

Post-Trauma Syndrome r/t physical abuse, incest, rape, molestation

Chronic low **Self-Esteem** r/t lack of positive feedback, excessive negative feedback

Impaired **Skin Integrity** r/t altered nutritional state, physical abuse

Social Isolation: family imposed r/t fear of disclosure of family dysfunction and abuse

Risk for delayed **Development:** Risk factors: shaken baby syndrome, abuse

Risk for disproportionate **Growth:** Risk factor: abuse

Risk for **Poisoning:** Risk factors: inadequate safeguards, lack of proper safety precautions, accessibility of illicit substances because of impaired home maintenance

Risk for **Suffocation:** Risk factors: unattended child, unsafe environment

Risk for **Trauma:** Risk factors: inadequate precautions, cognitive or emotional difficulties

CHILDBEARING PROBLEMS

Ineffective **Childbearing Process** (See **Childbearing Process**, ineffective, Section II)

Risk for ineffective **Childbearing Process:** Risk factors: (See **Childbearing Process**, risk for ineffective, Section II)

CHILD NEGLECT

See Child Abuse; Failure to Thrive, Nonorganic

CHILD WITH CHRONIC CONDITION

Activity Intolerance r/t fatigue associated with chronic illness

Decisional Conflict r/t treatment options, conflicting values

Parental **Role Conflict** r/t separation from child as a result of chronic illness, home care of child with special needs, interruptions of family life resulting from home care regimen

Compromised family **Coping** r/t prolonged overconcern for child; distortion of reality regarding child's health problem, including extreme denial about its existence or severity

Disabled family **Coping** r/t prolonged disease or disability progression that exhausts supportive capacity of significant others

Ineffective **Coping:** child r/t situational or maturational crises

Deficient **Diversional Activity** r/t immobility, monotonous environment, frequent or lengthy treatments, reluctance to participate, self-imposed social isolation

Interrupted **Family Processes** r/t intermittent situational crisis of illness, disease, hospitalization

Delayed **Growth and Development** r/t effects of physical disability, prescribed dependence, separation from significant others

Ineffective **Health Maintenance** r/t exhausting family resources (finances, physical energy, support systems)

Impaired **Home Maintenance** r/t overtaxed family members (e.g., exhausted, anxious)

Hopelessness: child r/t prolonged activity restriction, long-term stress, lack of involvement in or passively allowing care as a result of parental overprotection

Insomnia: child or parent r/t time-intensive treatments, exacerbation of condition, 24-hour care needs

Deficient **Knowledge** r/t knowledge or skill acquisition regarding health practices, acceptance of limitations, promotion of maximal potential of child, self-actualization of rest of family

Imbalanced **Nutrition:** less than body requirements r/t anorexia, fatigue from physical exertion

Imbalanced **Nutrition:** more than body requirements r/t effects of steroid medications on appetite

Chronic **Pain** r/t physical, biological, chemical, or psychological factors

Powerlessness: child r/t health care environment, illness-related regimen, lifestyle of learned helplessness

Chronic low **Self-Esteem** r/t actual or perceived differences; peer acceptance; decreased ability to participate in physical, school, and social activities

Ineffective **Sexuality Pattern:** parental r/t disrupted relationship with sexual partner

Impaired **Social Interaction** r/t developmental lag or delay, perceived differences

Social Isolation: family r/t actual or perceived social stigmatization, complex care requirements

Chronic **Sorrow** r/t developmental stages and missed opportunities or milestones that bring comparisons with social or personal norms, unending caregiving as reminder of loss

Risk for delayed **Development:** Risk factor: chronic illness

Risk for disproportionate **Growth:** Risk factor: chronic illness

Risk for **Infection:** Risk factor: debilitating physical condition

Risk for impaired **Parenting:** Risk factors: impaired or disrupted bonding, caring for child with perceived overwhelming care needs

Readiness for enhanced family **Coping:** impact of crisis on family values, priorities, goals, or relationships; changes in family choices to optimize wellness

CHILDBIRTH

Readiness for enhanced **Childbearing Process** (See **Childbearing Process,** readiness for enhanced, Section II)

See Labor, Normal; Postpartum, Normal Care

CHILLS

Hyperthermia r/t infectious process

CHLAMYDIA INFECTION

See STD (Sexually Transmitted Disease)

CHLOASMA

Disturbed **Body Image** r/t change in skin color

C

CHOKING OR COUGHING WITH EATING

Impaired **Swallowing** r/t neuromuscular impairment

Risk for **Aspiration**: Risk factors: depressed cough and gag reflexes

CHOLECYSTECTOMY

Imbalanced **Nutrition**: less than body requirements r/t high metabolic needs, decreased ability to digest fatty foods

Acute **Pain** r/t trauma from surgery

Risk for deficient **Fluid Volume**: Risk factors: restricted intake, nausea, vomiting

Readiness for enhanced **Knowledge**: expresses an interest in learning

See Abdominal Surgery

CHOLELITHIASIS

Imbalanced **Nutrition**: less than body requirements r/t anorexia, nausea, vomiting

Acute **Pain** r/t obstruction of bile flow, inflammation in gallbladder

Readiness for enhanced **Knowledge**: expresses an interest in learning

CHORIOAMNIONITIS

Anxiety r/t threat to self and infant

Grieving r/t guilt about potential loss of ideal pregnancy and birth

Hyperthermia r/t infectious process

Situational low **Self-Esteem** r/t guilt about threat to infant's health

Risk for delayed **Growth and Development**: Risk factor: risk of preterm birth

Risk for **Infection**: Risk factor: infection transmission from mother to fetus; infection in fetal environment

CHRONIC CONFUSION

See Confusion, Chronic

CHRONIC LYMPHOCYTIC LEUKEMIA

See Cancer; Chemotherapy; Leukemia

CHRONIC OBSTRUCTIVE PULMONARY DISEASE (COPD)

See COPD (Chronic Obstructive Pulmonary Disease)

CHRONIC PAIN

See Pain, Chronic

CHRONIC RENAL FAILURE

See Renal Failure

CHVOSTEK'S SIGN

See Hypocalcemia

CIRCUMCISION

Acute **Pain** r/t surgical intervention

Risk for **Bleeding**: Risk factor: surgical trauma

Risk for **Infection**: Risk factor: surgical wound

Readiness for enhanced **Knowledge**: parent: expresses an interest in learning

CIRRHOSIS

Chronic **Confusion** r/t chronic organic disorder with increased ammonia levels, substance abuse

Defensive **Coping** r/t inability to accept responsibility to stop drinking

Fatigue r/t malnutrition

Ineffective **Health Maintenance** r/t deficient knowledge regarding correlation between lifestyle habits and disease process

Nausea r/t irritation to gastrointestinal system

Imbalanced **Nutrition**: less than body requirements r/t loss of appetite, nausea, vomiting

Chronic **Pain** r/t liver enlargement

Chronic low **Self-Esteem** r/t chronic illness

Chronic **Sorrow** r/t presence of chronic illness

Risk for **Bleeding:** Risk factors: impaired blood coagulation, bleeding from portal hypertension

Risk for **Injury:** Risk factors: substance intoxication, potential delirium tremens

Risk for impaired **Oral Mucous Membrane:** Risk factors: altered nutrition, inadequate oral care

Risk for impaired **Skin Integrity:** Risk factors: altered nutritional state, altered metabolic state

CLEFT LIP/CLEFT PALATE

Ineffective **Airway Clearance** r/t common feeding and breathing passage, postoperative laryngeal, incisional edema

Ineffective **Breastfeeding** r/t infant anomaly

Impaired verbal **Communication** r/t inadequate palate function, possible hearing loss from infected eustachian tubes

Fear: parental r/t special care needs, surgery

Grieving r/t loss of perfect child

Ineffective infant **Feeding Pattern** r/t cleft lip, cleft palate

Impaired physical **Mobility** r/t imposed restricted activity, use of elbow restraints

Impaired **Oral Mucous Membrane** r/t surgical correction

Acute **Pain** r/t surgical correction, elbow restraints

Impaired **Skin Integrity** r/t incomplete joining of lip, palate ridges

Chronic **Sorrow** r/t birth of child with congenital defect

Risk for **Aspiration:** Risk factor: common feeding and breathing passage

Risk for disturbed **Body Image:** Risk factors: disfigurement, speech impediment

Risk for delayed **Development:** Risk factor: inadequate nutrition resulting from difficulty feeding

Risk for deficient **Fluid Volume:** Risk factor: inability to take liquids in usual manner

Risk for disproportionate **Growth:** Risk factor: inability to feed with normal techniques

Risk for **Infection:** Risk factors: invasive procedure, disruption of eustachian tube development, aspiration

Readiness for enhanced **Knowledge:** Parent: expresses an interest in learning

CLOTTING DISORDER

Fear r/t threat to well-being

Risk for **Bleeding:** Risk factor: impaired clotting

Readiness for enhanced **Knowledge:** expresses an interest in learning

See Anticoagulant Therapy; DIC (Disseminated Intravascular Coagulation); Hemophilia

COCAINE ABUSE

Ineffective **Breathing Pattern** r/t drug effect on respiratory center

Chronic **Confusion** r/t excessive stimulation of nervous system by cocaine

Ineffective **Coping** r/t inability to deal with life stresses

Risk for decreased **Cardiac** tissue perfusion r/t increase in sympathetic response in the body damaging the heart

See Drug Abuse; Substance Abuse

COCAINE BABY

See Crack Baby; Infant of Substance-Abusing Mother

CODEPENDENCY

Caregiver Role Strain r/t codependency

Impaired verbal **Communication** r/t psychological barriers

Decisional Conflict r/t support system deficit

Ineffective **Coping** r/t inadequate support systems

Ineffective **Denial** r/t unmet self-needs

Powerlessness r/t lifestyle of helplessness

COLD, VIRAL

Readiness for enhanced **Comfort** (See **Comfort,** readiness for enhanced, Section II)

Readiness for enhanced **Knowledge:** expresses an interest in learning

COLECTOMY

Constipation r/t decreased activity, decreased fluid intake

Imbalanced **Nutrition:** less than body requirements r/t high metabolic needs, decreased ability to ingest or digest food

Acute **Pain** r/t recent surgery

Risk for **Infection:** Risk factor: invasive procedure

Readiness for enhanced **Knowledge:** expresses an interest in learning

See Abdominal Surgery

COLITIS

Diarrhea r/t inflammation in colon

Deficient **Fluid Volume** r/t frequent stools

Acute **Pain** r/t inflammation in colon

Readiness for enhanced **Knowledge:** expresses an interest in learning

See Crohn's Disease; Inflammatory Bowel Disease (Child and Adult)

COLLAGEN DISEASE

See specific disease (e.g., Lupus Erythematosus; JRA [Juvenile Rheumatoid Arthritis]); Congenital Heart Disease/Cardiac Anomalies

COLOSTOMY

Disturbed **Body Image** r/t presence of stoma, daily care of fecal material

Ineffective **Sexuality Pattern** r/t altered body image, self-concept

Social Isolation r/t anxiety about appearance of stoma and possible leakage of stool

Risk for **Constipation:** Risk factor: inappropriate diet

Risk for **Diarrhea:** Risk factor: inappropriate diet

Risk for impaired **Skin Integrity:** Risk factor: irritation from bowel contents

Readiness for enhanced **Knowledge:** expresses an interest in learning

COLPORRHAPHY, ANTERIOR

See Vaginal Hysterectomy

COMA

Death **Anxiety:** significant others r/t unknown outcome of coma state

Interrupted **Family Processes** r/t illness or disability of family member

Functional urinary **Incontinence** r/t presence of comatose state

Self-Care deficit: specify r/t neuromuscular impairment

Ineffective family **Therapeutic Regimen Management** r/t complexity of therapeutic regimen

Risk for **Aspiration:** Risk factors: impaired swallowing, loss of cough or gag reflex

Risk for **Disuse Syndrome:** Risk factor: altered level of consciousness impairing mobility

Risk for **Injury:** Risk factor: potential seizure activity

Risk for impaired **Oral Mucous Membrane:** Risk factor: dry mouth, inability to do own mouth care

Risk for impaired **Skin Integrity:** Risk factor: immobility

Risk for **Spiritual Distress:** significant others: Risk factors: loss of ability to relate to loved one, unknown outcome of coma

See cause of Coma

COMFORT, LOSS OF

Impaired **Comfort** (See **Comfort,** impaired, Section II)

Readiness for enhanced **Comfort** (See **Comfort,** readiness for enhanced, Section II)

COMMUNICABLE DISEASES, CHILDHOOD (E.G., MEASLES, MUMPS, RUBELLA, CHICKENPOX, SCABIES, LICE, IMPETIGO)

Impaired **Comfort** r/t pruritus, inflammation or infection of skin, subdermal organisms

Deficient **Diversional Activity** r/t imposed isolation from peers, disruption in usual play activities, fatigue, activity intolerance

Ineffective **Health Maintenance** r/t nonadherence to appropriate immunization schedules, lack of prevention of transmission of infection

Acute **Pain** r/t impaired skin integrity, edema

Risk for **Infection:** transmission to others: Risk factor: contagious organisms

Readiness for enhanced **Immunization Status** (See **Immunization Status,** readiness for enhanced, Section II)

See Meningitis/Encephalitis; Respiratory Infections, Acute Childhood; Reye's Syndrome

COMMUNICATION

Readiness for enhanced **Communication** (See **Communication,** readiness for enhanced, Section II)

COMMUNICATION PROBLEMS

Impaired verbal **Communication** (See **Communication,** verbal, impaired, Section II)

COMMUNITY COPING

Ineffective community **Coping** (See **Coping,** community, ineffective, Section II)

Readiness for enhanced community **Coping:** community sense of power to manage stressors, social supports available, resources available for problem solving

COMMUNITY HEALTH PROBLEMS

Deficient community **Health** r/t (See **Health,** deficient, community, Section II)

COMPARTMENT SYNDROME

Fear r/t possible loss of limb, damage to limb

Acute **Pain** r/t pressure in compromised body part

Ineffective peripheral **Tissue Perfusion** r/t increased pressure within compartment

COMPULSION

See OCD (Obsessive-Compulsive Disorder)

CONDUCTION DISORDERS (CARDIAC)

See Dysrhythmia

CONFUSION, ACUTE

Acute **Confusion** r/t older than 70 years of age with hospitalization, alcohol abuse, delirium, dementia, drug abuse

Adult **Failure to Thrive** r/t confusion

CONFUSION, CHRONIC

Chronic **Confusion** r/t dementia, Korsakoff's psychosis, multi-infarct dementia, cerebrovascular accident, head injury

Adult **Failure to Thrive** r/t confusion

Impaired **Memory** r/t fluid and electrolyte imbalance, neurological disturbances, excessive environmental disturbances, anemia, acute or chronic hypoxia, decreased cardiac output

See Alzheimer's Disease; Dementia

CONFUSION, POSSIBLE

Risk for acute **Confusion**: Risk factor (See **Confusion**, acute, risk for, Section II)

CONGENITAL HEART DISEASE/CARDIAC ANOMALIES

Activity Intolerance r/t fatigue, generalized weakness, lack of adequate oxygenation

Ineffective **Breathing Pattern** r/t pulmonary vascular disease

Decreased **Cardiac Output** r/t cardiac dysfunction

Excess **Fluid Volume** r/t cardiac dysfunction, side effects of medication

Impaired **Gas Exchange** r/t cardiac dysfunction, pulmonary congestion

Delayed **Growth** and **Development** r/t inadequate oxygen and nutrients to tissues

Imbalanced **Nutrition**: less than body requirements r/t fatigue, generalized weakness, inability of infant to suck and feed, increased caloric requirements

Risk for delayed **Development**: Risk factor: inadequate oxygen and nutrients to tissues

Risk for deficient **Fluid Volume**: Risk factor: side effects of diuretics

Risk for disproportionate **Growth**: Risk factor: inadequate oxygen and nutrients to tissues

Risk for disorganized **Infant** behavior: Risk factor: invasive procedures

Risk for **Poisoning**: Risk factor: potential toxicity of cardiac medications

Risk for ineffective **Thermoregulation**: Risk factor: neonatal age

See Child with Chronic Condition; Hospitalized Child

CONGESTIVE HEART FAILURE (CHF)

See CHF (Congestive Heart Failure)

CONJUNCTIVITIS

Acute **Pain** r/t inflammatory process

Vision Loss r/t change in visual acuity resulting from inflammation

CONSCIOUSNESS, ALTERED LEVEL OF

Acute **Confusion** r/t alcohol abuse, delirium, dementia, drug abuse, head injury

Chronic **Confusion** r/t multi-infarct dementia, Korsakoff's psychosis, head injury, cerebrovascular accident, neurological deficit

Adult **Failure to Thrive** r/t altered level of consciousness

Functional urinary **Incontinence** r/t neurological dysfunction

Decreased **Intracranial Adaptive Capacity** r/t brain injury

Impaired **Memory** r/t neurological disturbances

Self-Care deficit: specify r/t neuromuscular impairment

Risk for **Aspiration**: Risk factors: impaired swallowing, loss of cough or gag reflex

Risk for **Disuse Syndrome**: Risk factors: impaired mobility resulting from altered level of consciousness

Risk for impaired **Oral Mucous Membrane**: Risk factor: dry mouth, interrupted oral care

Risk for ineffective **Cerebral** tissue perfusion: Risk factor: increased intracranial pressure, altered cerebral perfusion

Risk for impaired **Skin Integrity**: Risk factor: immobility

See cause of Altered Level of Consciousness

CONSTIPATION

Constipation (See **Constipation**, Section II)

CONSTIPATION, PERCEIVED

Perceived **Constipation** r/t (See **Constipation**, perceived, Section II)

CONSTIPATION, RISK FOR

Risk for **Constipation**: Risk factors (See **Constipation**, risk for, Section II)

CONTAMINATION

Contamination (See **Contamination**, Section II)

Risk for **Contamination**: Risk factors (See **Contamination**, risk for, Section II)

CONTINENT ILEOSTOMY (KOCK POUCH)

Ineffective **Coping** r/t stress of disease, exacerbations caused by stress

Imbalanced **Nutrition**: less than body requirements r/t malabsorption from disease process

Risk for **Injury**: Risk factors: failure of valve, stomal cyanosis, intestinal obstruction

Readiness for enhanced **Knowledge**: expresses an interest in learning

See Abdominal Surgery, Crohn's Disease

CONTRACEPTIVE METHOD

Decisional Conflict: method of contraception r/t unclear personal values or beliefs, lack of experience or interference with decision-making, lack of relevant information, support system deficit

Ineffective **Sexuality Pattern** r/t fear of pregnancy

Readiness for enhanced **Self-Health Management**: requesting information about available and appropriate birth control methods

CONVULSIONS

Anxiety r/t concern over controlling convulsions

Impaired **Memory** r/t neurological disturbance

Risk for **Aspiration**: Risk factor: impaired swallowing

Risk for delayed **Development**: Risk factor: seizures

Risk for **Injury**: Risk factor: seizure activity

Readiness for enhanced **Knowledge**: expresses an interest in learning

See Seizure Disorders, Adult; Seizure Disorders, Childhood

COPD (CHRONIC OBSTRUCTIVE PULMONARY DISEASE)

Activity Intolerance r/t imbalance between oxygen supply and demand

Ineffective **Airway Clearance** r/t bronchoconstriction, increased mucus, ineffective cough, infection

Anxiety r/t breathlessness, change in health status

Death **Anxiety** r/t seriousness of medical condition, difficulty being able to "catch breath," feeling of suffocation

Interrupted **Family Processes** r/t role changes

Impaired **Gas Exchange** r/t ventilation-perfusion inequality

Ineffective **Self-Health Management** (See **Self-Health Management**, ineffective, Section II)

Imbalanced **Nutrition**: less than body requirements r/t decreased intake because of dyspnea, unpleasant taste in mouth left by medications, increased need for calories from work of breathing

Powerlessness r/t progressive nature of disease

C

Self Care deficit: specify: r/t fatigue from the increased work of breathing

Chronic low **Self-Esteem** r/t chronic illness

Sleep deprivation r/t breathing difficulties when lying down

Impaired **Social Interaction** r/t social isolation because of oxygen use, activity intolerance

Chronic **Sorrow** r/t presence of chronic illness

Risk for **Infection**: Risk factor: stasis of respiratory secretions

Readiness for enhanced **Self-Health Management** (See **Self-Health Management**, readiness for enhanced, Section II)

Readiness for enhanced **Coping** (See **Coping**, readiness for enhanced, Section II)

Defensive **Coping** (See **Coping**, defensive, Section II)

Ineffective **Coping** (See **Coping**, ineffective, Section II) *See Community Coping; Family Problems*

Risk for **Injury**: Risk factors: accidental corneal abrasion, drying of cornea

Risk for **Infection**: Risk factors: invasive procedure, surgery

Readiness for enhanced **Self-Health Management**: describes need to rest and avoid strenuous activities during healing phase

Decreased **Cardiac Output** r/t dysrhythmia, depressed cardiac function,

change in preload, contractility or afterload

Fear r/t outcome of surgical procedure

Deficient **Fluid Volume** r/t intraoperative blood loss, use of diuretics in surgery

Acute **Pain** r/t traumatic surgery

Risk for **Perioperative Positioning Injury**: Risk factors: hypothermia, extended supine position

Readiness for enhanced **Knowledge**: expresses an interest in learning

See Kidney Stone; Pyelonephritis

Ineffective **Airway Clearance** r/t decreased energy, fatigue, normal aging changes

See Bronchitis; COPD (Chronic Obstructive Pulmonary Disease); Pulmonary Edema

See Cocaine Abuse; Drug Abuse; Substance Abuse

Disorganized **Infant** behavior r/t prematurity, drug withdrawal, lack of attachment

Risk for impaired **Attachment**: Risk factors: parent's inability to meet infant's needs, substance abuse

Risk for disturbed **Maternal/Fetal Dyad**: Risk factor: substance abuse

See Infant of Substance-Abusing Mother

Ineffective **Airway Clearance** r/t excessive secretions in airways, ineffective cough

See cause of Coarse Crackles in Lungs

CRACKLES IN LUNGS, FINE

Ineffective **Breathing Pattern** r/t fatigue, surgery, decreased energy

See Bronchitis or Pneumonia (if from pulmonary infection); CHF (Congestive Heart Failure) (if cardiac in origin); Infection

CRANIECTOMY/ CRANIOTOMY

Adult **Failure to Thrive** r/t altered cerebral tissue perfusion, decreased cognition

Fear r/t threat to well-being

Decreased **Intracranial Adaptive Capacity** r/t brain injury, intracranial hypertension

Impaired **Memory** r/t neurological surgery

Acute **Pain** r/t recent brain surgery, increased intracranial pressure

Risk for **Injury**: Risk factor: potential confusion

Risk for ineffective **Cerebral** tissue perfusion: Risk factors: cerebral edema, increased intracranial pressure

See Coma (if relevant)

CREPITATION, SUBCUTANEOUS

See Pneumothorax

CRISIS

Anxiety r/t threat to or change in environment, health status, interaction patterns, situation, self-concept, or role functioning; threat of death of self or significant other

Death **Anxiety** r/t feelings of hopelessness associated with crisis

Compromised family **Coping** r/t situational or developmental crisis

Ineffective **Coping** r/t situational or maturational crisis

Disturbed **Energy Field** r/t disharmony caused by crisis

Fear r/t crisis situation

Grieving r/t potential significant loss

Impaired individual **Resilience** r/t onset of crisis

Situational low **Self-Esteem** r/t perception of inability to handle crisis

Stress overload (See **Stress** overload, Section II)

Risk for **Spiritual Distress**: Risk factors: physical or psychological stress, natural disasters, situational losses, maturational losses

CROHN'S DISEASE

Anxiety r/t change in health status

Ineffective **Coping** r/t repeated episodes of diarrhea

Diarrhea r/t inflammatory process

Ineffective **Health Maintenance** r/t deficient knowledge regarding management of disease

Imbalanced **Nutrition**: less than body requirements r/t diarrhea, altered ability to digest and absorb food

Acute **Pain** r/t increased peristalsis

Powerlessness r/t chronic disease

Risk for deficient **Fluid Volume**: Risk factor: abnormal fluid loss with diarrhea

CROUP

See Respiratory Infections, Acute Childhood

CRYOSURGERY FOR RETINAL DETACHMENT

See Retinal Detachment

CUSHING'S SYNDROME

Activity Intolerance r/t fatigue, weakness

Disturbed **Body Image** r/t change in appearance from disease process

Excess **Fluid Volume** r/t failure of regulatory mechanisms

Sexual Dysfunction r/t loss of libido

Impaired **Skin Integrity** r/t thin vulnerable skin from effects of increased cortisol

Risk for **Infection**: Risk factor: suppression of immune system caused by increased cortisol levels

Risk for **Injury**: Risk factors: decreased muscle strength, brittle bones

Readiness for enhanced **Knowledge**: expresses an interest in learning

CUTS (WOUNDS)

See Lacerations

CVA (CEREBROVASCULAR ACCIDENT)

Anxiety r/t situational crisis, change in physical or emotional condition

Disturbed **Body Image** r/t chronic illness, paralysis

Caregiver Role Strain r/t cognitive problems of care receiver, need for significant home care

Impaired verbal **Communication** r/t pressure damage, decreased circulation to brain in speech center informational sources

Chronic **Confusion** r/t neurological changes

Constipation r/t decreased activity

Ineffective **Coping** r/t disability

Adult **Failure to Thrive** r/t neurophysiological changes

Interrupted **Family Processes** r/t illness, disability of family member

Grieving r/t loss of health

Impaired **Home Maintenance** r/t neurological disease affecting ability to perform activities of daily living

Functional urinary **Incontinence** r/t neurological dysfunction

Reflex urinary **Incontinence** r/t loss of feeling to void

Impaired **Memory** r/t neurological disturbances

Impaired physical **Mobility** r/t loss of balance and coordination

Unilateral Neglect r/t disturbed perception from neurological damage

Self-Care deficit: specify r/t decreased strength and endurance, paralysis

Impaired **Social Interaction** r/t limited physical mobility, limited ability to communicate

Impaired **Swallowing** r/t neuromuscular dysfunction

Impaired **Transfer Ability** r/t limited physical mobility

Vision Loss r/t pressure damage to visual centers in the brain

Impaired **Walking** r/t loss of balance and coordination

Risk for **Aspiration**: Risk factors: impaired swallowing, loss of gag reflex

Risk for **Disuse Syndrome**: Risk factor: paralysis

Risk for **Falls**: Risk factor: paralysis, decreased balance

Risk for **Injury**: Risk factor: vision loss, decreased tissue perfusion with loss of sensation

Risk for ineffective **Cerebral** tissue perfusion: Risk factor: clot, emboli, or hemorrhage from cerebral vessel

Risk for impaired **Skin Integrity**: Risk factor: immobility

Readiness for enhanced **Knowledge**: expresses an interest in learning

CYANOSIS, CENTRAL WITH CYANOSIS OF ORAL MUCOUS MEMBRANES

Impaired **Gas Exchange** r/t alveolar-capillary membrane changes

CYANOSIS, PERIPHERAL WITH CYANOSIS OF NAIL BEDS

Ineffective peripheral **Tissue Perfusion** r/t interruption of arterial flow, severe vasoconstriction, cold temperatures

CYSTIC FIBROSIS

Activity Intolerance r/t imbalance between oxygen supply and demand

Ineffective **Airway** clearance r/t increased production of thick mucus

Anxiety r/t dyspnea, oxygen deprivation

Disturbed **Body Image** r/t changes in physical appearance, treatment of chronic lung disease (clubbing, barrel chest, home oxygen therapy)

Impaired **Gas Exchange** r/t ventilation-perfusion imbalance

Impaired **Home Maintenance** r/t extensive daily treatment, medications necessary for health

Imbalanced **Nutrition:** less than body requirements r/t anorexia; decreased absorption of nutrients, fat; increased work of breathing

Chronic **Sorrow** r/t presence of chronic disease

Risk for **Caregiver Role Strain:** Risk factors: illness severity of care receiver, unpredictable course of illness

Risk for deficient **Fluid Volume:** Risk factors: decreased fluid intake, increased work of breathing

Risk for **Infection:** Risk factors: thick, tenacious mucus; harboring of bacterial organisms; immunocompromised state

Risk for **Spiritual Distress:** Risk factor: presence of chronic disease

See Child with Chronic Condition; Hospitalized Child; Terminally Ill Child, Adolescent; Terminally Ill Child, Infant/ Toddler; Terminally Ill Child, Preschool Child; Terminally Ill Child, School-Age Child/Preadolescent; Terminally Ill Child/Death of Child, Parent

CYSTITIS

Acute **Pain:** dysuria r/t inflammatory process in bladder and urethra

Impaired **Urinary Elimination:** frequency r/t urinary tract infection

Urge urinary **Incontinence:** Risk factor: infection in bladder

Readiness for enhanced **Knowledge:** expresses an interest in learning

CYSTOCELE

Stress urinary **Incontinence** r/t prolapsed bladder

Readiness for enhanced **Knowledge:** expresses an interest in learning

CYSTOSCOPY

Urinary Retention r/t edema in urethra obstructing flow of urine

Risk for **Infection:** Risk factor: invasive procedure

Readiness for enhanced **Knowledge:** expresses an interest in learning

D

DEAFNESS

Hearing Loss r/t alteration in sensory reception, transmission, integration

Impaired verbal **Communication** r/t impaired hearing

Risk for delayed **Development:** Risk factor: impaired hearing

Risk for **Injury** r/t alteration in sensory perception

DEATH

Risk for **Sudden Infant Death Syndrome** (SIDS) (See **Death Syndrome,** infant, sudden, Risk for, Section II)

DEATH, ONCOMING

Death **Anxiety** r/t unresolved issues surrounding dying

Compromised family **Coping** r/t client's inability to provide support to family

Ineffective **Coping** r/t personal vulnerability

Fear r/t threat of death

Grieving r/t loss of significant other

D

Powerlessness r/t effects of illness, oncoming death

Social Isolation r/t altered state of wellness

Spiritual Distress r/t intense suffering

Readiness for enhanced **Spiritual Well-Being:** desire of client and family to be in harmony with each other and higher power, God

See Terminally Ill Child, Adolescent; Terminally Ill Child, Infant/Toddler; Terminally Ill Child, Preschool Child; Terminally Ill Child, School-Age Child/Preadolescent; Terminally Ill Child/Death of Child, Parent

DECISIONS, DIFFICULTY MAKING

Decisional Conflict r/t support system deficit, perceived threat to value system, multiple or divergent sources of information, lack of relevant information, unclear personal values or beliefs

Readiness for enhanced **Decision-Making** (See **Decision-Making,** readiness for enhanced, Section II)

DECUBITUS ULCER

See Pressure Ulcer

DEEP VEIN THROMBOSIS (DVT)

See DVT (Deep Vein Thrombosis)

DEFENSIVE BEHAVIOR

Defensive **Coping** r/t nonacceptance of blame, denial of problems or weakness

Ineffective **Denial** r/t inability to face situation realistically

DEHISCENCE, ABDOMINAL

Fear r/t threat of death, severe dysfunction

Acute **Pain** r/t stretching of abdominal wall

Impaired **Skin Integrity** r/t altered circulation, malnutrition, opening in incision

Delayed **Surgical Recovery** r/t altered circulation, malnutrition, opening in incision

Impaired **Tissue Integrity** r/t exposure of abdominal contents to external environment

Risk for deficient **Fluid Volume:** Risk factor: altered circulation associated with opening of wound and exposure of abdominal contents

Risk for **Infection:** Risk factor: loss of skin integrity, open surgical wound

DEHYDRATION

Deficient **Fluid Volume** r/t active fluid volume loss

Impaired **Oral Mucous Membrane** r/t decreased salivation, fluid deficit

Readiness for enhanced **Knowledge:** expresses an interest in learning

See cause of Dehydration

DELIRIUM

Acute **Confusion** r/t effects of medication, response to hospitalization, alcohol abuse, substance abuse, sensory deprivation or overload, infection, polypharmacy

Adult **Failure to Thrive** r/t delirium

Impaired **Memory** r/t delirium

Sleep deprivation r/t nightmares

Risk for **Injury:** Risk factor: altered level of consciousness

DELIRIUM TREMENS (DT)

See Alcohol Withdrawal

DELIVERY

See Labor, Normal

DELUSIONS

Impaired verbal **Communication** r/t psychological impairment, delusional thinking

Acute **Confusion** r/t alcohol abuse, delirium, dementia, drug abuse

Ineffective **Coping** r/t distortion and insecurity of life events

Adult **Failure to Thrive** r/t delusional state

Fear r/t content of intrusive thoughts

Risk for other-directed **Violence**: Risk factor: delusional thinking

Risk for self-directed **Violence**: Risk factor: delusional thinking

DEMENTIA

Chronic **Confusion** r/t neurological dysfunction

Impaired **Environmental Interpretation Syndrome** r/t dementia

Adult **Failure to Thrive** r/t depression, apathy

Interrupted **Family Processes** r/t disability of family member

Impaired **Home Maintenance** r/t inadequate support system, neurological dysfunction

Functional urinary **Incontinence** r/t neurological dysfunction

Insomnia r/t neurological impairment, naps during the day

Impaired physical **Mobility** r/t neuromuscular impairment

Self-Neglect r/t cognitive impairment

Imbalanced **Nutrition**: less than body requirements r/t neurological impairment

Self-Care deficit: specify r/t psychological or neuromuscular impairment

Impaired **Swallowing** r/t neuromuscular changes associated with long-standing dementia

Chronic **Sorrow**: Significant other r/t chronic long-standing disability, loss of mental function

Risk for **Caregiver Role Strain**: Risk factors: number of caregiving tasks, duration of caregiving required

Risk for **Falls**: Risk factor: diminished mental status

Risk for **Injury**: Risk factors: confusion, decreased muscle coordination

Risk for impaired **Skin Integrity**: Risk factors: altered nutritional status, immobility

DENIAL OF HEALTH STATUS

Ineffective **Denial** r/t lack of perception about the health status effects of illness

Ineffective **Self-Health Management** r/t denial of seriousness of health situation

DENTAL CARIES

Impaired **Dentition** r/t ineffective oral hygiene, barriers to self-care, economic barriers to professional care, nutritional deficits, dietary habits

Ineffective **Self-Health Maintenance** r/t lack of knowledge regarding prevention of dental disease

DEPRESSION (MAJOR DEPRESSIVE DISORDER)

Death **Anxiety** r/t feelings of lack of self-worth

Constipation r/t inactivity, decreased fluid intake

Disturbed **Energy Field** r/t disharmony

Impaired **Environmental Interpretation Syndrome** r/t severe mental functional impairment

Adult **Failure to Thrive** r/t depression

Fatigue r/t psychological demands

Ineffective **Health Maintenance** r/t lack of ability to make good judgments regarding ways to obtain help

Hopelessness r/t feeling of abandonment, long-term stress

Insomnia r/t inactivity

Self-Neglect r/t depression, cognitive impairment

Powerlessness r/t pattern of helplessness

Chronic low **Self-Esteem** r/t repeated unmet expectations

D

Sexual Dysfunction r/t loss of sexual desire

Social Isolation r/t ineffective coping

Chronic **Sorrow** r/t unresolved grief

Risk for complicated **Grieving:** Risk factor: lack of previous resolution of former grieving response

Risk for **Suicide:** Risk factor: grieving, hopelessness

DERMATITIS

Anxiety r/t situational crisis imposed by illness

Impaired **Comfort** r/t itching

Impaired **Skin Integrity** r/t side effect of medication, allergic reaction

Readiness for enhanced **Knowledge:** expresses an interest in learning

See Itching

DESPONDENCY

Hopelessness r/t long-term stress

See Depression (Major Depressive Disorder)

DESTRUCTIVE BEHAVIOR TOWARD OTHERS

Risk-prone **Health Behavior** r/t intense emotional state

Ineffective **Coping** r/t situational crises, maturational crises, disturbance in pattern of appraisal of threat

Risk for other-directed **Violence** (See **Violence,** other-directed, risk for, Section II)

DEVELOPMENTAL CONCERNS

Delayed **Growth and Development** (See **Growth and Development,** delayed, Section II)

Risk for delayed **Development** (See **Development,** delayed, risk for, Section II)

See Growth and Development Lag

DIABETES IN PREGNANCY

See Gestational Diabetes (Diabetes in Pregnancy)

DIABETES INSIPIDUS

Deficient **Fluid Volume** r/t inability to conserve fluid

Ineffective **Health Maintenance** r/t deficient knowledge regarding care of disease, importance of medications

DIABETES MELLITUS

Adult **Failure to Thrive** r/t undetected disease process

Ineffective **Health Maintenance** r/t complexity of therapeutic regimen

Ineffective **Self-Health Management** (See **Self-Health Management,** ineffective, Section II)

Imbalanced **Nutrition:** less than body requirements r/t inability to use glucose (type 1 [insulin-dependent] diabetes)

Imbalanced **Nutrition:** more than body requirements r/t excessive intake of nutrients (type 2 diabetes)

Ineffective peripheral **Tissue Perfusion** r/t impaired arterial circulation

Powerlessness r/t perceived lack of personal control

Sexual Dysfunction r/t neuropathy associated with disease

Vision Loss r/t ineffective tissue perfusion of retina

Risk for unstable blood **Glucose** level (See **Glucose** level, blood, unstable, risk for, Section II)

Risk for **Infection:** Risk factors: hyperglycemia, impaired healing, circulatory changes

Risk for **Injury:** Risk factors: hypoglycemia or hyperglycemia from failure to consume adequate calories, failure to take insulin

Risk for dysfunctional **Gastrointestinal Motility:** Risk factor: complication of diabetes

Risk for impaired **Skin Integrity:** Risk factor: loss of pain perception in extremities

Readiness for enhanced **Self-Health Management** (See **Self-Health Management,** readiness for enhanced, Section II)

Readiness for enhanced **Knowledge:** expresses an interest in learning

See Hyperglycemia; Hypoglycemia

DIABETES MELLITUS, JUVENILE (IDDM TYPE 1)

Risk-prone **Health Behavior** r/t inadequate comprehension, inadequate social support, low self-efficacy, impaired adjustment attributable to adolescent maturational crises

Disturbed **Body Image** r/t imposed deviations from biophysical and psychosocial norm, perceived differences from peers

Impaired **Comfort** r/t insulin injections, peripheral blood glucose testing

Ineffective **Health Maintenance** r/t (See **Health Maintenance,** ineffective, Section II)

Imbalanced **Nutrition:** less than body requirements r/t inability of body to adequately metabolize and use glucose and nutrients, increased caloric needs of child to promote growth and physical activity participation with peers

Readiness for enhanced **Knowledge:** expresses an interest in learning

See Diabetes Mellitus; Child with Chronic Condition; Hospitalized Child

DIABETIC COMA

Acute **Confusion** r/t hyperglycemia, presence of excessive metabolic acids

Deficient **Fluid Volume** r/t hyperglycemia resulting in polyuria

Ineffective **Self-Health Management** r/t lack of understanding of preventive measures, adequate blood sugar control

Risk for unstable blood **Glucose** level (See **Glucose** level, blood, unstable, risk for, Section II)

Risk for **Infection:** Risk factors: hyperglycemia, changes in vascular system

See Diabetes Mellitus

DIABETIC KETOACIDOSIS

See Ketoacidosis, Diabetic

DIABETIC RETINOPATHY

Grieving r/t loss of vision

Ineffective **Health Maintenance** r/t deficient knowledge regarding preserving vision with treatment if possible, use of low-vision aids

Vision Loss r/t change in sensory reception

See Vision Impairment; Blindness

DIALYSIS

See Hemodialysis; Peritoneal Dialysis

DIAPHRAGMATIC HERNIA

See Hiatal Hernia

DIARRHEA

Diarrhea r/t infection, change in diet, gastrointestinal disorders, stress, medication effect, impaction

Deficient **Fluid Volume** r/t excessive loss of fluids in liquid stools.

Risk for **Electrolyte Imbalance:** Risk factor: effect of loss of electrolytes from frequent stools

DIC (DISSEMINATED INTRAVASCULAR COAGULATION)

Fear r/t threat to well-being

Deficient **Fluid Volume:** hemorrhage r/t depletion of clotting factors

D

Risk for **Bleeding**: Risk factors: microclotting within vascular system, depleted clotting factors

Risk for ineffective **Gastrointestinal Perfusion** (See **Gastrointestinal Perfusion,** ineffective, risk for, Section II)

DIGITALIS TOXICITY

Decreased **Cardiac Output** r/t drug toxicity affecting cardiac rhythm, rate

Ineffective **Self-Health Management** r/t deficient knowledge regarding action, appropriate method of administration of digitalis

DIGNITY, LOSS OF

Risk for compromised **Human Dignity** (See **Human Dignity,** compromised, risk for, Section II)

DILATION AND CURETTAGE (D&C)

Acute **Pain** r/t uterine contractions

Risk for **Bleeding**: Risk factor: surgical procedure

Risk for **Infection**: Risk factor: surgical procedure

Risk for ineffective **Sexuality Pattern**: Risk factors: painful coitus, fear associated with surgery on genital area

Readiness for enhanced **Knowledge**: expresses an interest in learning

DIRTY BODY (FOR PROLONGED PERIOD)

Self-Neglect r/t mental illness, substance abuse, cognitive impairment

DISCHARGE PLANNING

Impaired **Home Maintenance** r/t family member's disease or injury interfering with home maintenance

Deficient **Knowledge** r/t lack of exposure to information for home care

Readiness for enhanced **Knowledge**: expresses an interest in learning

DISCOMFORTS OF PREGNANCY

Disturbed **Body Image** r/t pregnancy-induced body changes

Impaired **Comfort** r/t enlarged abdomen, swollen feet

Fatigue r/t hormonal, metabolic, body changes

Stress urinary **Incontinence** r/t enlarged uterus, fetal movement

Insomnia r/t psychological stress, fetal movement, muscular cramping, urinary frequency, shortness of breath

Nausea r/t hormone effect

Acute **Pain**: headache r/t hormonal changes of pregnancy

Acute **Pain**: leg cramps r/t nerve compression, calcium/phosphorus/potassium imbalance

Risk for **Constipation**: Risk factors: decreased intestinal motility, inadequate fiber in diet

Risk for **Injury**: Risk factors: faintness and/or syncope caused by vasomotor lability or postural hypotension, venous stasis in lower extremities

DISLOCATION OF JOINT

Acute Pain r/t dislocation of a joint

Self-Care deficit: specify r/t inability to use a joint

Risk for **Injury**: Risk factor: unstable joint

DISSECTING ANEURYSM

Fear r/t threat to well-being

See Abdominal Surgery; Aneurysm, Abdominal Surgery

DISSEMINATED INTRAVASCULAR COAGULATION (DIC)

See DIC (Disseminated Intravascular Coagulation)

DISSOCIATIVE IDENTITY DISORDER (NOT OTHERWISE SPECIFIED)

Anxiety r/t psychosocial stress

Ineffective **Coping** r/t personal vulnerability in crisis of accurate self-perception

Disturbed personal **Identity** r/t inability to distinguish self caused by multiple personality disorder, depersonalization, disturbance in memory

Impaired **Memory** r/t altered state of consciousness

See Multiple Personality Disorder (Dissociative Identity Disorder)

DISTRESS

Anxiety r/t situational crises, maturational crises

Death **Anxiety** r/t denial of one's own mortality or impending death

Disturbed **Energy Field** r/t disruption in flow of energy as result of pain, depression, fatigue, anxiety, stress

DISUSE SYNDROME, POTENTIAL TO DEVELOP

Risk for **Disuse Syndrome**: Risk factors: paralysis, mechanical immobilization, prescribed immobilization, severe pain, altered level of consciousness

DIVERSIONAL ACTIVITY, LACK OF

Deficient **Diversional Activity** r/t environmental lack of diversional activity as in frequent hospitalizations, lengthy treatments

DIVERTICULITIS

Constipation r/t dietary deficiency of fiber and roughage

Diarrhea r/t increased intestinal motility caused by inflammation

Deficient **Knowledge** r/t diet needed to control disease, medication regimen

Imbalanced **Nutrition**: less than body requirements r/t loss of appetite

Acute **Pain** r/t inflammation of bowel

Risk for deficient **Fluid Volume**: Risk factor: diarrhea

DIZZINESS

Decreased **Cardiac Output** r/t dysfunctional electrical conduction

Deficient **Knowledge** r/t actions to take to prevent or modify dizziness and prevent falls

Impaired physical **Mobility** r/t dizziness

Risk for **Falls**: Risk factor: difficulty maintaining balance

Risk for ineffective **Cerebral** tissue perfusion: Risk factor: interruption of cerebral arterial blood flow

DOMESTIC VIOLENCE

Impaired verbal **Communication** r/t psychological barriers of fear

Compromised family **Coping** r/t abusive patterns

Defensive **Coping** r/t low self-esteem

Dysfunctional **Family Processes** r/t inadequate coping skills

Fear r/t threat to self-concept, situational crisis of abuse

Insomnia r/t psychological stress

Post-Trauma Syndrome r/t history of abuse

Powerlessness r/t lifestyle of helplessness

Situational low **Self-Esteem** r/t negative family interactions

Risk for compromised **Resilience**: Risk factor: effects of abuse

Risk for other-directed **Violence**: Risk factor: history of abuse

DOWN SYNDROME

See Child with Chronic Condition; Mental Retardation

D

DRESS SELF (INABILITY TO)

Dressing **Self-Care** deficit r/t intolerance to activity, decreased strength and endurance, pain, discomfort, perceptual or cognitive impairment, neuromuscular impairment, musculoskeletal impairment, depression, severe anxiety

DRIBBLING OF URINE

Overflow urinary **Incontinence** r/t degenerative changes in pelvic muscles and urinary structures

Stress urinary **Incontinence** r/t degenerative changes in pelvic muscles and urinary structures

DROOLING

Impaired **Swallowing** r/t neuromuscular impairment, mechanical obstruction

Risk for **Aspiration**: Risk factor: impaired swallowing

DROPOUT FROM SCHOOL

Impaired individual **Resilience** (See **Resilience**, individual, impaired, Section II)

DRUG ABUSE

Anxiety r/t threat to self-concept, lack of control of drug use

Risk-prone **Health Behavior** r/t addiction

Ineffective **Coping** r/t situational crisis

Ineffective **Denial** r/t use of drugs affecting quality of own life and that of significant others

Insomnia r/t effects of drugs

Imbalanced **Nutrition**: less than body requirements r/t poor eating habits

Powerlessness r/t feeling unable to change patterns of drug abuse

Impaired individual **Resilience** (See **Resilience**, individual, impaired, Section III)

Sexual Dysfunction r/t actions and side effects of drug abuse

Sleep deprivation r/t prolonged psychological discomfort

Impaired **Social Interaction** r/t disturbed thought processes from drug abuse

Spiritual Distress r/t separation from religious, cultural ties

Risk for **Injury**: Risk factors: hallucinations, drug effects

Risk for other-directed **Violence**: Risk factor: poor impulse control

See Cocaine Abuse; Substance Abuse

DRUG WITHDRAWAL

Anxiety r/t physiological withdrawal

Acute **Confusion** r/t effects of substance withdrawal

Ineffective **Coping** r/t situational crisis, withdrawal

Insomnia r/t effects of medication withdrawal

Imbalanced **Nutrition**: less than body requirements r/t poor eating habits

Risk for other-directed **Violence**: Risk factors: poor impulse control, hallucinations

Risk for self-directed **Violence**: Risk factors: poor impulse control, hallucinations

See Drug Abuse

DRY EYE

Risk for dry **Eye**: Risk factors: (See dry **Eye**, risk for, Section II)

Readiness for enhanced **Knowledge**: expresses an interest in learning

See Conjunctivitis; Keratoconjunctivitis Sicca

DT (DELIRIUM TREMENS)

See Alcohol Withdrawal

DVT (DEEP VEIN THROMBOSIS)

Constipation r/t inactivity, bed rest

Impaired physical **Mobility** r/t pain in extremity

Acute **Pain** r/t vascular inflammation, edema

Ineffective peripheral **Tissue Perfusion** r/t deficient knowledge of aggravating factors

Delayed **Surgical Recovery** r/t impaired physical mobility

Readiness for enhanced **Knowledge:** expresses an interest in learning

See Anticoagulant Therapy

DYING CLIENT

See Terminally Ill Adult; Terminally Ill Adolescent; Terminally Ill Child, Infant/Toddler; Terminally Ill Child, Preschool Child; Terminally Ill Child, School-Age Child/Preadolescent; Terminally Ill Child/Death of Child, Parent

DYSFUNCTIONAL EATING PATTERN

Imbalanced **Nutrition:** less than body requirements r/t psychological factors

Imbalanced **Nutrition:** more than body requirements r/t psychological factors

See Anorexia Nervosa; Bulimia; Maturational Issues, Adolescent; Obesity

DYSFUNCTIONAL FAMILY UNIT

See Family Problems

DYSFUNCTIONAL VENTILATORY WEANING

Dysfunctional **Ventilatory Weaning Response** r/t physical, psychological, situational factors

DYSMENORRHEA

Nausea r/t prostaglandin effect

Acute **Pain** r/t cramping from hormonal effects

Readiness for enhanced **Knowledge:** expresses an interest in learning

DYSPAREUNIA

Sexual Dysfunction r/t lack of lubrication during intercourse, alteration in reproductive organ function

D

DYSPEPSIA

Anxiety r/t pressures of personal role

Acute **Pain** r/t gastrointestinal disease, consumption of irritating foods

Readiness for enhanced **Knowledge:** expresses an interest in learning

DYSPHAGIA

Impaired **Swallowing** r/t neuromuscular impairment

Risk for **Aspiration:** Risk factor: loss of gag or cough reflex

DYSPHASIA

Impaired verbal **Communication** r/t decrease in circulation to brain

Impaired **Social Interaction** r/t difficulty in communicating

DYSPNEA

Activity Intolerance r/t imbalance between oxygen supply and demand

Ineffective **Breathing Pattern** r/t compromised cardiac or pulmonary function, decreased lung expansion, neurological impairment affecting respiratory center, extreme anxiety

Fear r/t threat to state of well-being, potential death

Impaired **Gas Exchange** r/t alveolar-capillary damage

Insomnia r/t difficulty breathing, positioning required for effective breathing

Sleep deprivation r/t ineffective breathing pattern

DYSRHYTHMIA

Activity Intolerance r/t decreased cardiac output

Decreased **Cardiac Output** r/t altered electrical conduction

Fear r/t threat of death, change in health status

Risk for ineffective **Cerebral** tissue perfusion: Risk factor: decreased blood supply to the brain from dysrhythmia

Readiness for enhanced **Knowledge:** expresses an interest in learning

DYSTHYMIC DISORDER

Ineffective **Coping** r/t impaired social interaction

Ineffective **Health Maintenance** r/t inability to make good judgments regarding ways to obtain help

Insomnia r/t anxious thoughts

Chronic low **Self-Esteem** r/t repeated unmet expectations

Ineffective **Sexuality Pattern** r/t loss of sexual desire

Social Isolation r/t ineffective coping

See Depression (Major Depressive Disorder)

DYSTOCIA

Anxiety r/t difficult labor, deficient knowledge regarding normal labor pattern

Ineffective **Coping** r/t situational crisis

Fatigue r/t prolonged labor

Grieving r/t loss of ideal labor experience

Acute **Pain** r/t difficult labor, medical interventions

Powerlessness r/t perceived inability to control outcome of labor

Risk for **Bleeding:** Risk factor: hemorrhage secondary to uterine atony

Risk for delayed **Development** (Infant): Risk factor: difficult labor and birth

Risk for disproportionate **Growth:** Risk factor: difficult labor and birth

Risk for **Infection:** Risk factor: prolonged rupture of membranes

Risk for ineffective **Cerebral** tissue perfusion (fetal): Risk factor: difficult labor and birth

Risk for impaired **Tissue Integrity** (maternal and fetal): Risk factor: difficult labor

DYSURIA

Impaired **Urinary Elimination** r/t infection/inflammation of the urinary tract

Risk for urge urinary **Incontinence:** Risk factor: detrusor hyperreflexia from infection in the urinary tract

E

EARACHE

Acute **Pain** r/t trauma, edema, infection

Hearing Loss r/t altered sensory reception, transmission

ECMO (EXTRACORPOREAL MEMBRANE OXYGENATOR)

Death **Anxiety** r/t emergency condition, hemorrhage

Decreased **Cardiac Output** r/t ineffective function of the heart

Impaired **Gas Exchange** (See **Gas Exchange,** impaired, Section II)

See condition necessitating use of ECMO

E. COLI INFECTION

Fear r/t serious illness, unknown outcome

Deficient **Knowledge** r/t how to prevent disease; care of self with serious illness

See Gastroenteritis; Gastroenteritis, Child; Hospitalized Child

EAR SURGERY

Acute **Pain** r/t edema in ears from surgery

Hearing Loss r/t invasive surgery of ears, dressings

Risk for delayed **Development**: Risk factor: hearing impairment

Risk for **Falls**: Risk factor: dizziness from excessive stimuli to vestibular apparatus

Readiness for enhanced **Knowledge**: Expresses an interest in learning

See Hospitalized Child

ECLAMPSIA

Interrupted **Family Processes** r/t unmet expectations for pregnancy and childbirth

Fear r/t threat of well-being to self and fetus

Risk for **Aspiration**: Risk factor: seizure activity

Risk for delayed **Development**: Risk factor: uteroplacental insufficiency

Risk for excess **Fluid Volume**: Risk factor: decreased urine output as a result of renal dysfunction

Risk for disproportionate **Growth**: Risk factor: uteroplacental insufficiency

Risk for ineffective **Cerebral** tissue perfusion: fetal: Risk factor: uteroplacental insufficiency

ECT (ELECTROCONVULSIVE THERAPY)

Decisional Conflict r/t lack of relevant information

Fear r/t real or imagined threat to well-being

Impaired **Memory** r/t effects of treatment

See Depression (Major Depressive Disorder)

ECTOPIC PREGNANCY

Death **Anxiety** r/t emergency condition, hemorrhage

Disturbed **Body Image** r/t negative feelings about body and reproductive functioning

Fear r/t threat to self, surgery, implications for future pregnancy

Acute **Pain** r/t stretching or rupture of implantation site

Ineffective **Role Performance** r/t loss of pregnancy

Situational low **Self-Esteem** r/t loss of pregnancy, inability to carry pregnancy to term

Chronic **Sorrow** r/t loss of pregnancy, potential loss of fertility

Risk for **Bleeding**: Risk factor: possible rupture of implantation site, surgical trauma

Risk for ineffective **Coping**: Risk factor: loss of pregnancy

Risk for interrupted **Family Processes**: Risk factor: situational crisis

Risk for **Infection**: Risk factors: traumatized tissue, surgical procedure

Risk for **Spiritual Distress**: Risk factor: grief process

ECZEMA

Disturbed **Body Image** r/t change in appearance from inflamed skin

Impaired **Comfort**: pruritus r/t inflammation of skin

Impaired **Skin Integrity** r/t side effect of medication, allergic reaction

Readiness for enhanced **Knowledge**: expresses an interest in learning

ED (ERECTILE DYSFUNCTION)

See Erectile Dysfunction (ED); Impotence

EDEMA

Excess **Fluid Volume** r/t excessive fluid intake, cardiac dysfunction, renal dysfunction, loss of plasma proteins

Ineffective **Health Maintenance** r/t deficient knowledge regarding treatment of edema

Risk for impaired **Skin Integrity**: Risk factors: impaired circulation, fragility of skin

See cause of Edema

E

ELDER ABUSE

See Abuse, Spouse, Parent, or Significant Other

ELDERLY

See Aging

ELECTROCONVULSIVE THERAPY

See ECT (Electroconvulsive Therapy)

ELECTROLYTE IMBALANCE

Risk for **Electrolyte Imbalance** (See **Electrolyte Imbalance,** risk for, Section II)

EMACIATED PERSON

Adult **Failure to Thrive** r/t (See **Failure to Thrive,** adult, Section II)

Imbalanced **Nutrition:** less than body requirements r/t inability to ingest food, digest food, absorb nutrients because of biological, psychological, economic factors

EMBOLECTOMY

Fear r/t threat of great bodily harm from embolus

Ineffective peripheral **Tissue Perfusion** r/t presence of embolus

Risk for **Bleeding:** Risk factors: postoperative complication, surgical area

See Surgery, Postoperative Care

EMBOLI

See Pulmonary Embolism

EMBOLISM IN LEG OR ARM

Ineffective peripheral **Tissue Perfusion** r/t arterial obstruction from clot

EMESIS

Nausea (See **Nausea,** Section II)

See Vomiting

EMOTIONAL PROBLEMS

See Coping Problems

EMPATHY

Readiness for enhanced community **Coping:** social supports, being available for problem solving

Readiness for enhanced family **Coping:** basic needs met, desire to move to higher level of health

Readiness for enhanced **Spiritual Well-Being:** desire to establish interconnectedness through spirituality

EMPHYSEMA

See COPD (Chronic Obstructive Pulmonary Disease)

EMPTINESS

Social Isolation r/t inability to engage in satisfying personal relationships

Chronic **Sorrow** r/t unresolved grief

Spiritual Distress r/t separation from religious or cultural ties

ENCEPHALITIS

See Meningitis/Encephalitis

ENDOCARDIAL CUSHION DEFECT

See Congenital Heart Disease/Cardiac Anomalies

ENDOCARDITIS

Activity Intolerance r/t reduced cardiac reserve, prescribed bed rest

Decreased **Cardiac Output** r/t inflammation of lining of heart and change in structure of valve leaflets, increased myocardial workload

Risk for imbalanced **Nutrition:** less than body requirements: Risk factors: fever, hypermetabolic state associated with fever

Risk for ineffective **Cerebral** tissue perfusion: Risk factor: possible presence of emboli in cerebral circulation

Risk for ineffective peripheral **Tissue Perfusion:** Risk factor: possible presence of emboli in peripheral circulation

Readiness for enhanced **Knowledge:** expresses an interest in learning

ENDOMETRIOSIS

Grieving r/t possible infertility

Nausea r/t prostaglandin effect

Acute **Pain** r/t onset of menses with distention of endometrial tissue

Sexual Dysfunction r/t painful intercourse

Readiness for enhanced **Knowledge:** expresses an interest in learning

ENDOMETRITIS

Anxiety r/t, fear of unknown

Ineffective **Thermoregulation** r/t infectious process

Acute **Pain** r/t infectious process in reproductive tract

Readiness for enhanced **Knowledge:** expresses an interest in learning

ENURESIS

Ineffective **Health Maintenance** r/t unachieved developmental task, neuromuscular immaturity, diseases of urinary system

See Toilet Training

ENVIRONMENTAL INTERPRETATION PROBLEMS

(See chronic **Confusion**)

EPIDIDYMITIS

Anxiety r/t situational crisis, pain, threat to future fertility

Acute **Pain** r/t inflammation in scrotal sac

Ineffective **Sexuality Pattern** r/t edema of epididymis and testes

Readiness for enhanced **Knowledge:** expresses an interest in learning

EPIGLOTTITIS

See Respiratory Infections, Acute Childhood (Croup, Epiglottis, Pertussis, Pneumonia, Respiratory Syncytial Virus)

EPILEPSY

Anxiety r/t threat to role functioning

Ineffective **Self-Health Management** r/t deficient knowledge regarding seizure control

Impaired **Memory** r/t seizure activity

Risk for **Aspiration:** Risk factors: impaired swallowing, excessive secretions

Risk for delayed **Development:** Risk factor: seizure disorder

Risk for **Injury:** Risk factor: environmental factors during seizure

Readiness for enhanced **Knowledge:** expresses an interest in learning

See Seizure Disorders, Adult; Seizure Disorders, Childhood

EPISIOTOMY

Anxiety r/t fear of pain

Disturbed **Body Image** r/t fear of resuming sexual relations

Impaired physical **Mobility** r/t pain, swelling, tissue trauma

Acute **Pain** r/t tissue trauma

Sexual Dysfunction r/t altered body structure, tissue trauma

Impaired **Skin Integrity** r/t perineal incision

Risk for **Infection:** Risk factor: tissue trauma

EPISTAXIS

Fear r/t large amount of blood loss

Risk for deficient **Fluid Volume:** Risk factor: excessive blood loss

EPSTEIN-BARR VIRUS

See Mononucleosis

ERECTILE DYSFUNCTION (ED)

Situational low **Self-Esteem** r/t physiological crisis, inability to practice usual sexual activity

E

Sexual Dysfunction r/t altered body function

Readiness for enhanced **Knowledge:** information regarding treatment for erectile dysfunction

See Impotence

ESOPHAGEAL VARICES

Fear r/t threat of death from hematemesis

Risk for **Bleeding:** Risk factor: portal hypertension, distended variceal vessels that can easily rupture

See Cirrhosis

ESOPHAGITIS

Acute **Pain** r/t inflammation of esophagus

Readiness for enhanced **Knowledge:** Expresses an interest in learning

ETOH WITHDRAWAL

See Alcohol Withdrawal

EVISCERATION

See Debiscence, Abdominal

EXHAUSTION

Impaired individual **Resilience** (See **Resilience,** individual, impaired, Section II)

Disturbed **Sleep Pattern** (See **Sleep Pattern,** disturbed, Section II)

EXPOSURE TO HOT OR COLD ENVIRONMENT

Hyperthermia r/t exposure to hot environment, abnormal reaction to anesthetics

Hypothermia r/t exposure to cold environment

EXTERNAL FIXATION

Disturbed **Body Image** r/t trauma, change to affected part

Risk for **Infection:** Risk factor: presence of pins inserted into bone

See Fracture

EXTRACORPOREAL MEMBRANE OXYGENATOR (ECMO)

See ECMO (Extracorporeal Membrane Oxygenator)

EYE DISCOMFORT

Risk for dry **Eye:** Risk factors (See **Eye,** risk for dry, Section II)

EYE SURGERY

Anxiety r/t possible loss of vision

Self-Care deficit: Specify r/t impaired vision

Vision Loss r/t surgical procedure, eye pathology

Risk for **Injury:** Risk factor: impaired vision

Readiness for enhanced **Knowledge:** Expresses an interest in learning

See Hospitalized Child; Vision Impairment

F

FAILURE TO THRIVE, ADULT

Adult **Failure to Thrive** r/t depression, apathy, fatigue

FAILURE TO THRIVE, CHILD

Delayed **Growth and Development** r/t parental deficient knowledge, lack of stimulation, nutritional deficit, long-term hospitalization

Disorganized **Infant** behavior (See **Infant** behavior, disorganized, Section II)

Insomnia r/t inconsistency of caretaker; lack of quiet, consistent environment

Imbalanced **Nutrition:** less than body requirements r/t inadequate type or amounts of food for infant or child, inappropriate feeding techniques

Impaired **Parenting** r/t lack of parenting skills, inadequate role modeling

Chronic low **Self-Esteem:** parental r/t feelings of inadequacy, support system deficiencies, inadequate role model

Social Isolation r/t limited support systems, self-imposed situation

Risk for impaired **Attachment:** Risk factor: inability of parents to meet infant's needs

Risk for delayed **Development** (See **Development,** delayed, risk for, Section II)

Risk for disproportionate **Growth** (See **Growth,** disproportionate, risk for, Section II)

FALLS, RISK FOR

Risk for **Falls** (See **Falls,** risk for, Section II)

FAMILY PROBLEMS

Compromised family **Coping** (See **Coping,** family, compromised, Section II)

Disabled family **Coping** (See **Coping,** family, disabled, Section II)

Interrupted **Family Processes** r/t situation transition and/or crises, developmental transition and/or crises

Ineffective family **Therapeutic Regimen Management** r/t (See **Therapeutic Regimen Management,** ineffective family, Section II)

Readiness for enhanced family **Coping:** needs sufficiently gratified, adaptive tasks effectively addressed to enable goals of self-actualization to surface

FAMILY PROCESS

Dysfunctional **Family Processes** r/t (See **Family Processes,** dysfunctional, Section II)

Interrupted **Family Processes** r/t (see **Family Processes,** interrupted, Section II)

Readiness for enhanced **Family Processes** (See **Family Processes,** readiness for enhanced, Section II)

Readiness for enhanced **Relationship** (See **Relationship,** readiness for enhanced, Section II)

FATIGUE

Disturbed **Energy Field** r/t disharmony

Fatigue (See **Fatigue,** Section II)

FEAR

Death **Anxiety** r/t fear of death

Fear r/t identifiable physical or psychological threat to person

FEBRILE SEIZURES

See Seizure Disorders, Childhood

FECAL IMPACTION

See Impaction of Stool

FECAL INCONTINENCE

Bowel **Incontinence** r/t neurological impairment, gastrointestinal disorders, anorectal trauma, weakened perineal muscles

FEEDING PROBLEMS, NEWBORN

Ineffective **Breastfeeding** (See **Breastfeeding,** ineffective, Section II)

Insufficient **Breastfeeding** (See **Breastfeeding,** insufficient, Section II)

Disorganized **Infant** behavior r/t prematurity, immature neurological system

Ineffective infant **Feeding Pattern** r/t prematurity, neurological impairment or delay, oral hypersensitivity, prolonged nothing-by-mouth status

Impaired **Swallowing** r/t prematurity

Risk for delayed **Development:** Risk factor: inadequate nutrition

Risk for deficient **Fluid Volume:** Risk factor: inability to take in adequate amount of fluids

Risk for disproportionate **Growth:** Risk factor: feeding problems

F

F

FEMORAL POPLITEAL BYPASS

Anxiety r/t threat to or change in health status

Acute **Pain** r/t surgical trauma, edema in surgical area

Ineffective peripheral **Tissue Perfusion** r/t impaired arterial circulation

Risk for **Bleeding:** Risk factor: surgery on arteries

Risk for **Infection:** Risk factor: invasive procedure

FETAL ALCOHOL SYNDROME

See Infant of Substance-Abusing Mother

FETAL DISTRESS/ NONREASSURING FETAL HEART RATE PATTERN

Fear r/t threat to fetus

Ineffective peripheral **Tissue Perfusion:** fetal r/t interruption of umbilical cord blood flow

FEVER

Ineffective **Thermoregulation** r/t infectious process

FIBROCYSTIC BREAST DISEASE

See Breast Lumps

FILTHY HOME ENVIRONMENT

Impaired **Home Maintenance** (See **Home Maintenance,** impaired, Section II)

Self-Neglect r/t mental illness, substance abuse, cognitive impairment

FINANCIAL CRISIS IN THE HOME ENVIRONMENT

Impaired **Home Maintenance** r/t insufficient finances

FISTULECTOMY

See Hemorrhoidectomy

FLAIL CHEST

Ineffective **Breathing Pattern** r/t chest trauma

Fear r/t difficulty breathing

Impaired **Gas Exchange** r/t loss of effective lung function

Impaired **Spontaneous Ventilation** r/t paradoxical respirations

FLASHBACKS

Post-Trauma Syndrome r/t catastrophic event

FLAT AFFECT

Adult **Failure to Thrive** r/t apathy

Hopelessness r/t prolonged activity restriction creating isolation, failing or deteriorating physiological condition, long-term stress, abandonment, lost belief in transcendent values or higher power or God

Risk for **Loneliness:** Risk factors: social isolation, lack of interest in surroundings

See Depression (Major Depressive Disorder); Dysthymic Disorder

FLESH-EATING BACTERIA (NECROTIZING FASCIITIS)

See Necrotizing Fasciitis (Flesh-Eating Bacteria)

FLUID BALANCE

Readiness for enhanced **Fluid Balance** (See **Fluid Balance,** readiness for enhanced, Section II)

FLUID VOLUME DEFICIT

Deficient **Fluid Volume** r/t active fluid loss, vomiting, diarrhea, failure of regulatory mechanisms

Risk for **Shock:** Risk factor: hypovolemia

FLUID VOLUME EXCESS

Excess **Fluid Volume** r/t compromised regulatory mechanism, excess sodium intake

FLUID VOLUME IMBALANCE, RISK FOR

Risk for imbalanced **Fluid Volume**: Risk factor: major invasive surgeries

FOOD ALLERGIES

Diarrhea r/t immune effects of offending food on gastrointestinal system

Risk for **Allergy Response**: Risk factor: specific foods

Readiness for enhanced **Knowledge**: expresses an interest in learning

See Anaphylactic Shock if relevant

FOODBORNE ILLNESS

Diarrhea r/t infectious material in gastrointestinal tract

Deficient **Fluid Volume** r/t active fluid loss from vomiting and diarrhea

Deficient **Knowledge** r/t care of self with serious illness, prevention of further incidences of foodborne illness

Nausea r/t contamination irritating stomach

Risk for dysfunctional **Gastrointestinal Motility**: Risk factor: contaminated food

See Gastroenteritis; Gastroenteritis, Child; Hospitalized Child; E. coli Infection

FOOD INTOLERANCE

Risk for dysfunctional **Gastrointestinal Motility**: Risk factor: food intolerance

FOREIGN BODY ASPIRATION

Ineffective **Airway Clearance** r/t obstruction of airway

Ineffective **Health Maintenance** r/t parental deficient knowledge regarding high-risk items

Risk for **Suffocation**: Risk factor: inhalation of small objects

See Safety, Childhood

FORMULA FEEDING OF INFANT

Grieving: maternal r/t loss of desired breastfeeding experience

Risk for **Constipation**: infant: Risk factor: iron-fortified formula

Risk for **Infection**: infant: Risk factors: lack of passive maternal immunity, supine feeding position, contamination of formula

Readiness for enhanced **Knowledge**: expresses an interest in learning

FRACTURE

Deficient **Diversional Activity** r/t immobility

Impaired physical **Mobility** r/t limb immobilization

Acute **Pain** r/t muscle spasm, edema, trauma

Impaired **Walking** r/t limb immobility

Risk for ineffective peripheral **Tissue Perfusion**: Risk factors: immobility, presence of cast

Risk for **Peripheral Neurovascular Dysfunction**: Risk factors: mechanical compression, treatment of fracture

Risk for impaired **Skin Integrity**: Risk factors: immobility, presence of cast

Readiness for enhanced **Knowledge**: expresses an interest in learning

FRACTURED HIP

See Hip Fracture

FREQUENCY OF URINATION

Stress urinary **Incontinence** r/t degenerative change in pelvic muscles and structural support

Urge urinary **Incontinence** r/t decreased bladder capacity, irritation of bladder stretch receptors causing spasm, alcohol, caffeine, increased fluids, increased urine concentration, overdistended bladder

Urinary Retention r/t high urethral pressure caused by weak detrusor, inhibition of reflex arc, strong sphincter, blockage

Impaired **Urinary Elimination** r/t urinary tract infection

F

FRIENDSHIP

Readiness for enhanced **Relationship:** express desire to enhance communication between partners

FROSTBITE

Acute **Pain** r/t decreased circulation from prolonged exposure to cold

Ineffective peripheral **Tissue Perfusion** r/t damage to extremities from prolonged exposure to cold

Impaired **Tissue Integrity** r/t freezing of skin and tissues

See Hypothermia

FROTHY SPUTUM

See CHF (Congestive Heart Failure); Pulmonary Edema; Seizure Disorders, Adult; Seizure Disorders, Childhood

FUSION, LUMBAR

Anxiety r/t fear of surgical procedure, possible recurring problems

Impaired physical **Mobility** r/t limitations from surgical procedure, presence of brace

Acute **Pain** r/t discomfort at bone donor site, surgical operation

Risk for **Injury:** Risk factor: improper body mechanics

Risk for **Perioperative Positioning Injury:** Risk factor: immobilization during surgery

Readiness for enhanced **Knowledge:** expresses an interest in learning

G

GAG REFLEX, DEPRESSED OR ABSENT

Impaired **Swallowing** r/t neuromuscular impairment

Risk for **Aspiration:** Risk factors: depressed cough or gag reflex

GALLOP RHYTHM

Decreased **Cardiac Output** r/t decreased contractility of heart

GALLSTONES

See Cholelithiasis

GANG MEMBER

Impaired individual **Resilience** (See **Resilience,** individual, impaired, Section II)

GANGRENE

Fear r/t possible loss of extremity

Ineffective peripheral **Tissue Perfusion** r/t obstruction of arterial flow

See condition causing gangrene, Diabetes, Peripheral Vascular Disease

GAS EXCHANGE, IMPAIRED

Impaired **Gas Exchange** r/t ventilation-perfusion imbalance

GASTRIC ULCER

See GI Bleed (Gastrointestinal Bleeding); Ulcer, Peptic (Duodenal or Gastric)

GASTRITIS

Imbalanced **Nutrition:** less than body requirements r/t vomiting, inadequate intestinal absorption of nutrients, restricted dietary regimen

Acute **Pain** r/t inflammation of gastric mucosa

Risk for deficient **Fluid Volume:** Risk factors: excessive loss from gastrointestinal tract from vomiting, decreased intake

GASTROENTERITIS

Diarrhea r/t infectious process involving intestinal tract

Deficient **Fluid Volume** r/t excessive loss from gastrointestinal tract from diarrhea, vomiting

Nausea r/t irritation to gastrointestinal system

Imbalanced **Nutrition:** less than body requirements r/t vomiting, inadequate intestinal absorption of nutrients, restricted dietary intake

Acute **Pain** r/t increased peristalsis causing cramping

Risk for **Electrolyte Imbalance:** Risk factor: loss of gastrointestinal fluids high in electrolytes

Readiness for enhanced **Knowledge:** expresses an interest in learning

See Gastroenteritis, Child

GASTROENTERITIS, CHILD

Impaired **Skin Integrity:** diaper rash r/t acidic excretions on perineal tissues

Readiness for enhanced **Knowledge:** expresses an interest in learning

See Gastroenteritis; Hospitalized Child

GASTROESOPHAGEAL REFLUX

Ineffective **Airway Clearance** r/t reflux of gastric contents into esophagus and tracheal or bronchial tree

Ineffective **Health Maintenance** r/t deficient knowledge regarding anti-reflux regimen (e.g., positioning, change in diet)

Acute **Pain** r/t irritation of esophagus from gastric acids

Risk for **Aspiration:** Risk factor: entry of gastric contents in tracheal or bronchial tree

GASTROESOPHAGEAL REFLUX, CHILD

Ineffective **Airway Clearance** r/t reflux of gastric contents into esophagus and tracheal or bronchial tree

Anxiety: parental r/t possible need for surgical intervention

Deficient **Fluid Volume** r/t persistent vomiting

Imbalanced **Nutrition:** less than body requirements r/t poor feeding, vomiting

Risk for **Aspiration:** Risk factor: entry of gastric contents in tracheal or bronchial tree

Risk for impaired **Parenting:** Risk factors: disruption in bonding as a result of irritable or inconsolable infant; lack of sleep for parents

Readiness for enhanced **Knowledge:** expresses an interest in learning

See Child with Chronic Condition; Hospitalized Child

GASTROINTESTINAL BLEEDING (GI BLEED)

See GI Bleed (Gastrointestinal Bleeding)

GASTROINTESTINAL HEMORRHAGE

See GI Bleed (Gastrointestinal Bleeding)

GASTROINTESTINAL SURGERY

Risk for **Injury:** Risk factor: inadvertent insertion of nasogastric tube through gastric incision line

Risk for Ineffective **Gastrointestinal Perfusion** (See **Gastrointestinal Perfusion,** ineffective, risk for, Section II)

See Abdominal Surgery

GASTROSCHISIS/ OMPHALOCELE

Ineffective **Airway Clearance** r/t complications of anesthetic effects

Impaired **Gas Exchange** r/t effects of anesthesia, subsequent atelectasis

Grieving r/t threatened loss of infant, loss of perfect birth or infant because of serious medical condition

Risk for deficient **Fluid Volume:** Risk factors: inability to feed because of condition, subsequent electrolyte imbalance

G

Risk for **Infection**: Risk factor: disrupted skin integrity with exposure of abdominal contents

Risk for **Injury**: Risk factors: disrupted skin integrity, ineffective protection

GASTROSTOMY

Risk for impaired **Skin Integrity**: Risk factor: presence of gastric contents on skin

See Tube Feeding

GENITAL HERPES

See Herpes Simplex II

GENITAL WARTS

See STD (Sexually Transmitted Disease)

GERD

See Gastroesophageal Reflux

GESTATIONAL DIABETES (DIABETES IN PREGNANCY)

Anxiety r/t threat to self and/or fetus

Impaired **Nutrition**: less than body requirements r/t decreased insulin production and glucose uptake in cells

Impaired **Nutrition**: more than body requirements: fetal r/t excessive glucose uptake

Risk for delayed **Development**: fetal: Risk factor: endocrine disorder of mother

Risk for disproportionate **Growth**: fetal: Risk factor: endocrine disorder of mother

Risk for disturbed **Maternal/Fetal Dyad**: Risk factor: impaired glucose metabolism

Risk for impaired **Tissue Integrity**: fetal: Risk factors: large infant, congenital defects, birth injury

Risk for impaired **Tissue Integrity**: maternal: Risk factor: delivery of large infant

Risk for unstable blood **Glucose**: Risk factor: excessive intake of carbohydrates

Readiness for enhanced **Knowledge**: expresses an interest in learning

See Diabetes Mellitus

GI BLEED (GASTROINTESTINAL BLEEDING)

Fatigue r/t loss of circulating blood volume, decreased ability to transport oxygen

Fear r/t threat to well-being, potential death

Deficient **Fluid Volume** r/t gastrointestinal bleeding

Imbalanced **Nutrition**: less than body requirements r/t nausea, vomiting

Acute **Pain** r/t irritated mucosa from acid secretion

Risk for ineffective **Coping**: Risk factors: personal vulnerability in crisis, bleeding, hospitalization

Readiness for enhanced **Knowledge**: Expresses an interest in learning

GINGIVITIS

Impaired **Oral Mucous Membrane** r/t ineffective oral hygiene

GLAUCOMA

Deficient **Knowledge** r/t treatment and self-care for disease

Vision Loss r/t untreated increased intraocular pressure

See Vision Impairment

GLOMERULONEPHRITIS

Excess **Fluid Volume** r/t renal impairment

Imbalanced **Nutrition**: less than body requirements r/t anorexia, restrictive diet

Acute **Pain** r/t edema of kidney

Readiness for enhanced **Knowledge**: expresses an interest in learning

GLUTEN ALLERGY

See Celiac Disease

GONORRHEA

Acute **Pain** r/t inflammation of reproductive organs

Risk for **Infection:** Risk factor: spread of organism throughout reproductive organs

Readiness for enhanced **Knowledge:** expresses an interest in learning

See STD (Sexually Transmitted Disease)

GOUT

Impaired physical **Mobility** r/t musculoskeletal impairment

Chronic **Pain** r/t inflammation of affected joint

Readiness for enhanced **Knowledge:** expresses an interest in learning

GRANDIOSITY

Defensive **Coping** r/t inaccurate perception of self and abilities

GRAND MAL SEIZURE

See Seizure Disorders, Adult; Seizure Disorders, Childhood

GRANDPARENTS RAISING GRANDCHILDREN

Anxiety r/t change in role status

Decisional Conflict r/t support system deficit

Parental **Role Conflict** r/t change in parental role

Compromised family **Coping** r/t family role changes

Interrupted **Family Processes** r/t family roles shift

Ineffective **Role Performance** r/t role transition, aging

Ineffective family **Therapeutic Regimen Management** r/t excessive demands on individual or family

Risk for impaired **Parenting:** Risk factor: role strain

Risk for **Powerlessness:** Risk factors: role strain, situational crisis, aging

Risk for **Spiritual Distress:** Risk factor: life change

Readiness for enhanced **Parenting:** physical and emotional needs of children are met

GRAVES' DISEASE

See Hyperthyroidism

GRIEVING

Grieving r/t anticipated or actual significant loss, change in life status, style, or function

GRIEVING, COMPLICATED

Complicated **Grieving** r/t expected or sudden death of a significant other with whom had a volatile relationship, emotional instability, lack of social support

Risk for complicated **Grieving:** Risk factors: death of a significant other with whom had volatile relationship, emotional instability, lack of social support

GROOM SELF (INABILITY TO)

Bathing **Self-Care** deficit (See **Self-Care** deficit, bathing, Section II)

Dressing **Self-Care** deficit (See **Self-Care** deficit, dressing, Section II)

GROWTH AND DEVELOPMENT LAG

Delayed **Growth and Development** (See **Growth and Development,** delayed, Section II)

Risk for disproportionate **Growth** (See **Growth,** disproportionate, risk for, Section II)

GUILLAIN-BARRÉ SYNDROME

Impaired **Spontaneous Ventilation** r/t weak respiratory muscles

See Neurologic Disorders

GUILT

Grieving r/t potential loss of significant person, animal, prized material possession, change in life role

G

Impaired individual **Resilience**
(See **Resilience,** individual, impaired,
Section II)

Situational low **Self-Esteem** r/t unmet
expectations of self

Risk for complicated **Grieving:** Risk
factors: actual loss of significant person,
animal, prized material possession,
change in life role

Risk for **Post-Trauma Syndrome:** Risk
factor: exaggerated sense of responsibility
for traumatic event

Readiness for enhanced **Spiritual Well-
Being:** desire to be in harmony with self,
others, higher power or God

H

H1N1

See Influenza

HAIR LOSS

Disturbed **Body Image** r/t psychological
reaction to loss of hair

Imbalanced **Nutrition:** less than body
requirements r/t inability to ingest food
because of biological, psychological,
economic factors

HALITOSIS

Impaired **Dentition** r/t ineffective oral
hygiene

Impaired **Oral Mucous Membrane** r/t
ineffective oral hygiene

HALLUCINATIONS

Anxiety r/t threat to self-concept

Acute **Confusion** r/t alcohol abuse,
delirium, dementia, mental illness, drug
abuse

Ineffective **Coping** r/t distortion and
insecurity of life events

Adult **Failure to Thrive** r/t altered mental
status

Risk for **Self-Mutilation:** Risk factor:
command hallucinations

Risk for other-directed **Violence:** Risk
factors: catatonic excitement, manic
excitement, rage or panic reactions,
response to violent internal stimuli

Risk for self-directed **Violence:** Risk
factors: catatonic excitement, manic
excitement, rage or panic reactions,
response to violent internal stimuli

HEAD INJURY

Ineffective **Breathing Pattern** r/t pressure
damage to breathing center in brainstem

Acute **Confusion** r/t increased
intracranial pressure

Decreased **Intracranial Adaptive Capacity**
r/t increased intracranial pressure

Risk for ineffective **Cerebral** tissue
perfusion: Risk factors: effects of
increased intracranial pressure, trauma
to brain

Vision Loss r/t pressure damage to
sensory centers in brain

See Neurologic Disorders

HEADACHE

Disturbed **Energy Field** r/t disharmony

Acute **Pain** r/t lack of knowledge of pain
control techniques or methods to prevent
headaches

Ineffective **Self-Health Management**
r/t lack of knowledge, identification,
elimination of aggravating factors

HEALTH BEHAVIOR, RISK-PRONE

Risk-prone **Health Behavior:** Risk
factors: (See **Health Behavior,** risk-
prone, Section II)

HEALTH MAINTENANCE PROBLEMS

Ineffective **Health Maintenance**
(See **Health Maintenance,** ineffective,
Section II)

Ineffective **Self-Health Management**
(See **Self-Health Management,**
ineffective, Section II)

HEALTH-SEEKING PERSON

Readiness for enhanced **Self-Health Management** (See **Self-Health Management,** readiness for enhanced, Section II)

HEARING IMPAIRMENT

Hearing Loss r/t (See **Hearing Loss,** Section II)

Impaired verbal **Communication** r/t inability to hear own voice

Social Isolation r/t difficulty with communication

HEART ATTACK

See MI (Myocardial Infarction)

HEARTBURN

Nausea r/t gastrointestinal irritation

Acute **Pain:** heartburn r/t inflammation of stomach and esophagus

Risk for imbalanced **Nutrition:** less than body requirements: Risk factor: pain after eating

Readiness for enhanced **Knowledge:** expresses an interest in learning

HEART FAILURE

See CHF (Congestive Heart Failure)

HEART SURGERY

See Coronary Artery Bypass Grafting (CABG)

HEAT STROKE

Deficient **Fluid Volume** r/t profuse diaphoresis from high environmental temperature

Hyperthermia r/t vigorous activity, hot environment

HEMATEMESIS

See GI Bleed (Gastrointestinal Bleeding)

HEMATURIA

See Kidney Stone; UTI (Urinary Tract Infection)

HEMIANOPIA

Anxiety r/t change in vision

Unilateral Neglect r/t effects of disturbed perceptual abilities

Visual Loss r/t impaired sensory reception, transmission, integration

Risk for **Injury:** Risk factor: disturbed sensory perception

HEMIPLEGIA

H

Anxiety r/t change in health status

Disturbed **Body Image** r/t functional loss of one side of body

Impaired physical **Mobility** r/t loss of neurological control of involved extremities

Unilateral Neglect r/t effects of disturbed perceptual abilities

Self-Care deficit: specify: r/t neuromuscular impairment

Impaired **Transfer Ability** r/t partial paralysis

Impaired **Walking** r/t loss of neurological control of involved extremities

Risk for **Falls:** Risk factor: impaired mobility

Risk for impaired **Skin Integrity:** Risk factors: alteration in sensation, immobility

See CVA (Cerebrovascular Accident)

HEMODIALYSIS

Ineffective **Coping** r/t situational crisis

Interrupted **Family Processes** r/t changes in role responsibilities as a result of therapy regimen

Excess **Fluid Volume** r/t renal disease with minimal urine output

Powerlessness r/t treatment regimen

Risk for **Caregiver Role Strain:** Risk factor: complexity of care receiver treatment

Risk for **Electrolyte Imbalance:** Risk factor: effect of metabolic state on kidney function

Risk for deficient **Fluid Volume:** Risk factor: excessive removal of fluid during dialysis

Risk for **Infection:** Risk factors: exposure to blood products, risk for developing hepatitis B or C, impaired immune system

Risk for **Injury:** Risk factor: clotting of blood access: Risk factor: abnormal surface for blood flow

Readiness for enhanced **Knowledge:** expresses an interest in learning

See Renal Failure; Renal Failure, Child with Chronic Condition

HEMODYNAMIC MONITORING

Risk for **Infection:** Risk factor: invasive procedure

Risk for **Injury:** Risk factors: inadvertent wedging of catheter, dislodgement of catheter, disconnection of catheter

See Cardiogenic Shock

HEMOLYTIC UREMIC SYNDROME

Deficient **Fluid Volume** r/t vomiting, diarrhea

Fear r/t serious condition with unknown outcome

Fatigue r/t decreased red blood cells

Nausea r/t effects of uremia

Risk for **Injury:** Risk factors: decreased platelet count, seizure activity

Risk for impaired **Skin Integrity:** Risk factor: diarrhea

See Hospitalized Child; Renal Failure, Acute/Chronic, Child

HEMOPHILIA

Fear r/t high risk for AIDS infection from contaminated blood products

Impaired physical **Mobility** r/t pain from acute bleeds, imposed activity restrictions, joint pain

Acute **Pain** r/t bleeding into body tissues

Risk for **Bleeding:** Risk factors: deficient clotting factors, child's developmental level, age-appropriate play, inappropriate use of toys or sports equipment

Readiness for enhanced **Knowledge:** expresses an interest in learning

See Child with Chronic Condition; Hospitalized Child; Maturational Issues, Adolescent

HEMOPTYSIS

Fear r/t serious threat to well-being

Risk for ineffective **Airway Clearance:** Risk factor: obstruction of airway with blood and mucus

Risk for deficient **Fluid Volume:** Risk factor: excessive loss of blood

HEMORRHAGE

Fear r/t threat to well-being

Deficient **Fluid Volume** r/t massive blood loss

See cause of Hemorrhage; Hypovolemic Shock

HEMORRHOIDECTOMY

Anxiety r/t embarrassment, need for privacy

Constipation r/t fear of pain with defecation

Acute **Pain** r/t surgical procedure

Urinary Retention r/t pain, anesthetic effect

Risk for **Bleeding:** Risk factors: inadequate clotting, trauma from surgery

Readiness for enhanced **Knowledge:** expresses an interest in learning

HEMORRHOIDS

Impaired **Comfort** r/t itching in rectal area

Constipation r/t painful defecation, poor bowel habits

Readiness for enhanced **Knowledge:** expresses an interest in learning

HEMOTHORAX

Deficient **Fluid Volume** r/t blood in pleural space

See Pneumothorax

HEPATITIS

Activity Intolerance r/t weakness or fatigue caused by infection

Deficient **Diversional Activity** r/t isolation

Fatigue r/t infectious process, altered body chemistry

Imbalanced **Nutrition:** less than body requirements r/t anorexia, impaired use of proteins and carbohydrates

Acute **Pain** r/t edema of liver, bile irritating skin

Social Isolation r/t treatment-imposed isolation

Risk for deficient **Fluid Volume:** Risk factor: excessive loss of fluids from vomiting and diarrhea

Readiness for enhanced **Knowledge:** expresses an interest in learning

HERNIA

See Hiatal Hernia; Inguinal Hernia Repair

HERNIATED DISK

See Low Back Pain

HERNIORRHAPHY

See Inguinal Hernia Repair

HERPES IN PREGNANCY

Fear r/t threat to fetus, impending surgery

Situational low **Self-Esteem** r/t threat to fetus as a result of disease process

Risk for **Infection** (Infant): Risk factors: transplacental transfer during primary herpes, exposure to active herpes during birth process

See Herpes Simplex II

HERPES SIMPLEX I

Impaired **Oral Mucous Membrane** r/t inflammatory changes in mouth

HERPES SIMPLEX II

Ineffective **Health Maintenance** r/t deficient knowledge regarding treatment, prevention, spread of disease

Acute **Pain** r/t active herpes lesion

Situational low **Self-Esteem** r/t expressions of shame or guilt

Sexual Dysfunction r/t disease process

Impaired **Tissue Integrity** r/t active herpes lesion

Impaired **Urinary Elimination** r/t pain with urination

HERPES ZOSTER

See Shingles

HHNC (HYPEROSMOLAR HYPERGLYCEMIC NONKETOTIC COMA)

See Hyperosmolar Hyperglycemic Nonketotic Coma (HHNC)

HIATAL HERNIA

Ineffective **Health Maintenance** r/t deficient knowledge regarding care of disease

Nausea r/t effects of gastric contents in esophagus

Imbalanced **Nutrition:** less than body requirements r/t pain after eating

Acute **Pain** r/t gastroesophageal reflux

HIP FRACTURE

Acute Confusion r/t sensory overload, sensory deprivation, medication side effects, advanced age, pain

Constipation r/t immobility, opioids, anesthesia

Fear r/t outcome of treatment, future mobility, present helplessness

Impaired physical **Mobility** r/t surgical incision, temporary absence of weight bearing, pain when walking

H

Acute **Pain** r/t injury, surgical procedure, movement

Powerlessness r/t health care environment

Self-Care deficit: specify r/t musculoskeletal impairment

Impaired **Transfer Ability** r/t immobilization of hip

Impaired **Walking** r/t temporary absence of weight bearing

Risk for **Bleeding:** Risk factors: postoperative complication, surgical blood loss

Risk for **Infection:** Risk factor: invasive procedure

Risk for **Injury:** Risk factors: activities such as greater than 90-degree flexion of hips that can result in dislodged prosthesis, unsteadiness when ambulating

Risk for **Perioperative Positioning Injury:** Risk factors: immobilization, muscle weakness, emaciation

Risk for **Peripheral Neurovascular Dysfunction:** Risk factor: trauma, vascular obstruction, fracture

Risk for impaired **Skin Integrity:** Risk factor: immobility

HIP REPLACEMENT

See Total Joint Replacement (Total Hip/ Total Knee/Shoulder)

HIRSCHSPRUNG'S DISEASE

Constipation: bowel obstruction r/t inhibited peristalsis as a result of congenital absence of parasympathetic ganglion cells in distal colon

Grieving r/t loss of perfect child, birth of child with congenital defect even though child expected to be normal within 2 years

Imbalanced **Nutrition:** less than body requirements r/t anorexia, pain from distended colon

Acute **Pain** r/t distended colon, incisional postoperative pain

Impaired **Skin Integrity** r/t stoma, potential skin care problems associated with stoma

Readiness for enhanced **Knowledge:** expresses an interest in learning

See Hospitalized Child

HIRSUTISM

Disturbed **Body Image** r/t excessive hair

HITTING BEHAVIOR

Acute **Confusion** r/t dementia, alcohol abuse, drug abuse, delirium

Risk for other-directed **Violence** (See **Violence,** other-directed, risk for, Section II)

HIV (HUMAN IMMUNODEFICIENCY VIRUS)

Fear r/t possible death

Ineffective **Protection** r/t depressed immune system

See AIDS (Acquired Immunodeficiency Syndrome)

HODGKIN'S DISEASE

See Anemia; Cancer; Chemotherapy

HOMELESSNESS

Impaired **Home Maintenance** r/t impaired cognitive or emotional functioning, inadequate support system, insufficient finances

Self-Neglect r/t mental illness, substance abuse, cognitive impairment

Powerlessness r/t interpersonal interactions

Risk for **Trauma:** Risk factor: being in high-crime neighborhood

HOME MAINTENANCE PROBLEMS

Impaired **Home Maintenance** (See **Home Maintenance,** impaired, Section II)

HOPE

Readiness for enhanced **Hope** (See **Hope,** readiness for enhanced, Section II)

HOPELESSNESS

Hopelessness (See **Hopelessness,** Section II)

HOSPITALIZED CHILD

Activity Intolerance r/t fatigue associated with acute illness

Anxiety: separation (child) r/t familiar surroundings and separation from family and friends

Compromised family **Coping** r/t possible prolonged hospitalization that exhausts supportive capacity of significant people

Ineffective **Coping:** parent r/t possible guilt regarding hospitalization of child, parental inadequacies

Deficient **Diversional Activity** r/t immobility, monotonous environment, frequent or lengthy treatments, reluctance to participate, therapeutic isolation, separation from peers

Interrupted **Family Processes** r/t situational crisis of illness, disease, hospitalization

Fear r/t deficient knowledge or maturational level with fear of unknown, mutilation, painful procedures, surgery

Delayed **Growth and Development** r/t regression or lack of progression toward developmental milestones as a result of frequent or prolonged hospitalization, inadequate or inappropriate stimulation, cerebral insult, chronic illness, effects of physical disability, prescribed dependence

Hopelessness: child r/t prolonged activity restriction, uncertain prognosis

Insomnia: child or parent r/t 24-hour care needs of hospitalization

Acute **Pain** r/t treatments, diagnostic or therapeutic procedures, disease process

Powerlessness: child r/t health care environment, illness-related regimen

Risk for impaired **Attachment:** Risk factor: separation

Risk for delayed **Growth and Development:** regression: Risk factors: disruption of normal routine, unfamiliar environment or caregivers, developmental vulnerability of young children

Risk for **Injury:** Risk factors: unfamiliar environment, developmental age, lack of parental knowledge regarding safety (e.g., side rails, IV site/pole)

Risk for imbalanced **Nutrition:** less than body requirements: Risk factors: anorexia, absence of familiar foods, cultural preferences

Readiness for enhanced family **Coping:** impact of crisis on family values, priorities, goals, relationships in family

See Child with Chronic Condition

HOSTILE BEHAVIOR

Risk for other-directed **Violence:** Risk factor: antisocial personality disorder

HTN (HYPERTENSION)

Ineffective **Self-Health Management** (See **Self-Health Management,** ineffective, Section II)

Imbalanced **Nutrition:** more than body requirements r/t lack of knowledge of relationship between diet and disease process

Readiness for enhanced **Self-Health Management** (See **Self-Health Management,** readiness for enhanced, Section II)

HUMAN IMMUNODEFICIENCY VIRUS (HIV)

See AIDS (Acquired Immunodeficiency Syndrome); HIV (Human Immunodeficiency Virus)

H

HUMILIATING EXPERIENCE

Risk for compromised **Human Dignity** (See **Human Dignity**, compromised, risk for, Section II)

HUNTINGTON'S DISEASE

Decisional Conflict r/t whether to have children

See Neurologic Disorders

HYDROCELE

Acute Pain r/t severely enlarged hydrocele

Ineffective **Sexuality Pattern** r/t recent surgery on area of scrotum

HYDROCEPHALUS

Decisional Conflict r/t unclear or conflicting values regarding selection of treatment modality

Interrupted **Family Processes** r/t situational crisis

Delayed **Growth and Development** r/t sequelae of increased intracranial pressure

Imbalanced **Nutrition:** less than body requirements r/t inadequate intake as a result of anorexia, nausea, vomiting, feeding difficulties

Risk for delayed **Development:** Risk factor: sequelae of increased intracranial pressure

Risk for disproportionate **Growth:** Risk factor: sequelae of increased intracranial pressure

Risk for **Infection:** Risk factor: sequelae of invasive procedure (shunt placement)

Risk for ineffective **Cerebral t**issue perfusion: Risk factors: interrupted flow, hypervolemia of cerebral ventricles

See Normal Pressure Hydrocephalus (NPH); Child with Chronic Condition; Hospitalized Child; Mental Retardation (if appropriate); Premature Infant (Child); Premature Infant (Parent)

HYGIENE, INABILITY TO PROVIDE OWN

Adult **Failure to Thrive** r/t depression, apathy as evidenced by inability to perform self-care

Self-Neglect (See **Self-Neglect**, Section II)

Bathing **Self-Care** deficit (See **Self-Care** deficit, bathing, Section II)

HYPERACTIVE SYNDROME

Decisional Conflict r/t multiple or divergent sources of information regarding education, nutrition, medication regimens; willingness to change own food habits; limited resources

Parental **Role Conflict:** when siblings present r/t increased attention toward hyperactive child

Compromised family **Coping** r/t unsuccessful strategies to control excessive activity, behaviors, frustration, anger

Ineffective **Impulse Control** r/t disorder of development, environment that might cause frustration or irritation

Ineffective **Role Performance:** parent r/t stressors associated with dealing with hyperactive child, perceived or projected blame for causes of child's behavior, unmet needs for support or care, lack of energy to provide for those needs

Chronic low **Self-Esteem** r/t inability to achieve socially acceptable behaviors; frustration; frequent reprimands, punishment, or scolding for uncontrolled activity and behaviors; mood fluctuations and restlessness; inability to succeed academically; lack of peer support

Impaired **Social Interaction** r/t impulsive and overactive behaviors, concomitant emotional difficulties, distractibility and excitability

Risk for delayed **Development:** Risk factor: behavior disorders

Risk for impaired **Parenting**: Risk factor: disruptive or uncontrollable behaviors of child

Risk for other-directed **Violence**: parent or child: Risk factors: frustration with disruptive behavior, anger, unsuccessful relationships

HYPERBILIRUBINEMIA

Anxiety: parent r/t threat to infant, unknown future

Parental **Role Conflict** r/t interruption of family life because of care regimen

Neonatal **Jaundice** r/t abnormal breakdown of red blood cells following birth

Imbalanced **Nutrition**: less than body requirements (infant) r/t disinterest in feeding because of jaundice-related lethargy

Risk for disproportionate **Growth**: infant: Risk factor: disinterest in feeding because of jaundice-related lethargy

Risk for imbalanced body **Temperature**: infant: Risk factor: phototherapy

Risk for **Injury**: infant: Risk factors: kernicterus, phototherapy lights

HYPERCALCEMIA

Decreased **Cardiac Output** r/t bradydysrhythmia

Impaired physical **Mobility** r/t decreased muscle tone

Imbalanced **Nutrition**: less than body requirements r/t gastrointestinal manifestations of hypercalcemia (nausea, anorexia, ileus)

Risk for **Disuse Syndrome**: Risk factor: comatose state impairing mobility

HYPERCAPNIA

Fear r/t difficulty breathing

Impaired **Gas Exchange** r/t ventilation-perfusion imbalance, retention of carbon dioxide

See cause of Hypercapnia

HYPEREMESIS GRAVIDARUM

Anxiety r/t threat to self and infant, hospitalization

Deficient **Fluid Volume** r/t excessive vomiting

Impaired **Home Maintenance** r/t chronic nausea, inability to function

Nausea r/t hormonal changes of pregnancy

Imbalanced **Nutrition**: less than body requirements r/t excessive vomiting

Powerlessness r/t health care regimen

Social Isolation r/t hospitalization

HYPERGLYCEMIA

Ineffective **Self-Health Management** r/t complexity of therapeutic regimen, decisional conflicts, economic difficulties, unsupportive family, insufficient cues to action, deficient knowledge, mistrust, lack of acknowledgment of seriousness of condition

Risk for unstable blood **Glucose** level (See **Glucose** level, blood, unstable, risk for, Section II)

See Diabetes Mellitus

HYPERKALEMIA

Risk for **Activity Intolerance**: Risk factor: muscle weakness

Risk for excess **Fluid Volume**: Risk factor: untreated renal failure

Risk for decreased **Cardiac tissue** perfusion: Risk factor: abnormal electrolyte level affecting heart electrical conduction

HYPERNATREMIA

Risk for deficient **Fluid Volume**: Risk factors: abnormal water loss, inadequate water intake

HYPEROSMOLAR HYPERGLYCEMIC NONKETOTIC COMA (HHNC)

Acute **Confusion** r/t dehydration, electrolyte imbalance

H

Deficient **Fluid Volume** r/t polyuria, inadequate fluid intake

Risk for **Electrolyte Imbalance**: Risk factors: effect of metabolic state on kidney function

Risk for **Injury**: seizures: Risk factors: hyperosmolar state, electrolyte imbalance

See Diabetes Mellitus; Diabetes Mellitus, Juvenile

HYPERPHOSPHATEMIA

Deficient **Knowledge** r/t dietary changes needed to control phosphate levels

See Renal Failure

HYPERSENSITIVITY TO SLIGHT CRITICISM

Defensive **Coping** r/t situational crisis, psychological impairment, substance abuse

HYPERTENSION (HTN)

See HTN (Hypertension)

HYPERTHERMIA

Hyperthermia (See **Hyperthermia**, Section II)

HYPERTHYROIDISM

Anxiety r/t increased stimulation, loss of control

Diarrhea r/t increased gastric motility

Insomnia r/t anxiety, excessive sympathetic discharge

Imbalanced **Nutrition**: less than body requirements r/t increased metabolic rate, increased gastrointestinal activity

Risk for **Injury**: eye damage: Risk factor: protruding eyes without sufficient lubrication

Readiness for enhanced **Knowledge**: expresses an interest in learning

HYPERVENTILATION

Ineffective **Breathing Pattern** r/t anxiety, acid-base imbalance

See cause of Hyperventilation

HYPOCALCEMIA

Activity Intolerance r/t neuromuscular irritability

Ineffective **Breathing Pattern** r/t laryngospasm

Imbalanced **Nutrition**: less than body requirements r/t effects of vitamin D deficiency, renal failure, malabsorption, laxative use

HYPOGLYCEMIA

Acute **Confusion** r/t insufficient blood glucose to brain

Ineffective **Self-Health Management** r/t deficient knowledge regarding disease process, self-care

Imbalanced **Nutrition**: less than body requirements r/t imbalance of glucose and insulin level

Risk for unstable blood **Glucose** level (See **Glucose** level, blood, unstable, risk for, Section II)

See Diabetes Mellitus; Diabetes Mellitus, Juvenile

HYPOKALEMIA

Activity Intolerance r/t muscle weakness

Risk for decreased **Cardiac** tissue perfusion: Risk factor: possible dysrhythmia from electrolyte imbalance

HYPOMAGNESEMIA

Imbalanced **Nutrition**: less than body requirements r/t deficient knowledge of nutrition, alcoholism

See Alcoholism

HYPOMANIA

Insomnia r/t psychological stimulus

See Manic Disorder, Bipolar I

HYPONATREMIA

Acute **Confusion** r/t electrolyte imbalance

Excess **Fluid Volume** r/t excessive intake of hypotonic fluids

Risk for **Injury:** Risk factors: seizures, new onset of confusion

See Congenital Heart Disease/Cardiac Anomalies

Decreased **Cardiac Output** r/t decreased preload, decreased contractility

Risk for deficient **Fluid Volume:** Risk factor: excessive fluid loss

Risk for ineffective **Cerebral** tissue perfusion: Risk factors: hypovolemia, decreased contractility, decreased afterload

Risk for ineffective **Gastrointestinal Perfusion** (See **Gastrointestinal Perfusion,** ineffective, risk for, Section II)

Risk for ineffective **Renal Perfusion:** Risk factor: prolonged ischemia of kidneys

Risk for **Shock** (See **Shock,** risk for, Section II)

See cause of Hypotension

Hypothermia (See **Hypothermia,** Section II)

Activity Intolerance r/t muscular stiffness, shortness of breath on exertion

Constipation r/t decreased gastric motility

Impaired **Gas Exchange** r/t respiratory depression

Imbalanced **Nutrition:** more than body requirements r/t decreased metabolic process

Impaired **Skin Integrity** r/t edema, dry or scaly skin

See Shock, Hypovolemic

Acute **Confusion** r/t decreased oxygen supply to brain

Fear r/t breathlessness

Impaired **Gas Exchange** r/t altered oxygen supply, inability to transport oxygen

Risk for **Shock** (See **Shock,** risk for, Section II)

Constipation r/t opioids, anesthesia, bowel manipulation during surgery

Ineffective **Coping** r/t situational crisis of surgery

Grieving r/t change in body image, loss of reproductive status

Acute **Pain** r/t surgical injury

Sexual Dysfunction r/t disturbance in self-concept

Urinary Retention r/t edema in area, anesthesia, opioids, pain

Risk for **Bleeding:** Risk factor: surgical procedure

Risk for **Constipation:** Risk factors: opioids, anesthesia, bowel manipulation during surgery

Risk for ineffective peripheral **Tissue Perfusion:** Risk factor: deficient knowledge of aggravating factors

Readiness for enhanced **Knowledge:** expresses an interest in learning

See Surgery, Perioperative; Surgery, Preoperative; Surgery, Postoperative

Constipation r/t low-residue diet, stress

Diarrhea r/t increased motility of intestines associated with disease process, stress

Ineffective **Self-Health Management** r/t deficient knowledge, powerlessness

Chronic **Pain** r/t spasms, increased motility of bowel

Readiness for enhanced **Self-Health Management**: expressed desire to manage illness and prevent onset of symptoms

ICD (IMPLANTABLE CARDIOVERTER/ DEFIBRILLATOR)

Decreased **Cardiac Output** r/t possible dysrhythmia

Readiness for enhanced **Knowledge**: expresses an interest in learning

IDDM (INSULIN-DEPENDENT DIABETES)

See Diabetes Mellitus

IDENTITY DISTURBANCE/ PROBLEMS

Disturbed personal **Identity** r/t situational crisis, psychological impairment, chronic illness, pain

Risk for disturbed personal **Identity** (See **Identity,** personal, risk for disturbed, in Section II)

IDIOPATHIC THROMBOCYTOPENIC PURPURA (ITP)

See ITP (Idiopathic Thrombocytopenic Purpura)

ILEAL CONDUIT

Disturbed **Body Image** r/t presence of stoma

Ineffective **Self-Health Management** r/t new skills required to care for appliance and self

Ineffective **Sexuality Pattern** r/t altered body function and structure

Social Isolation r/t alteration in physical appearance, fear of accidental spill of urine

Risk for **Latex Allergy Response:** Risk factor: repeated exposures to latex associated with treatment and management of disease

Risk for impaired **Skin Integrity:** Risk factor: difficulty obtaining tight seal of appliance

Readiness for enhanced **Knowledge:** expresses an interest in learning

ILEOSTOMY

Disturbed **Body Image** r/t presence of stoma

Diarrhea r/t dietary changes, alteration in intestinal motility

Deficient **Knowledge** r/t limited practice of stoma care, dietary modifications

Ineffective **Sexuality Pattern** r/t altered body function and structure

Social Isolation r/t alteration in physical appearance, fear of accidental spill of ostomy contents

Risk for impaired **Skin Integrity:** Risk factors: difficulty obtaining tight seal of appliance, caustic drainage

Readiness for enhanced **Knowledge:** expresses an interest in learning

ILEUS

Deficient **Fluid Volume** r/t loss of fluids from vomiting, fluids trapped in bowel

Dysfunctional **Gastrointestinal Motility** r/t effects of surgery, decreased perfusion of intestines, medication effect, immobility

Nausea r/t gastrointestinal irritation

Acute **Pain** r/t pressure, abdominal distention

Readiness for enhanced **Knowledge:** expresses an interest in learning

IMMOBILITY

Ineffective **Breathing Pattern** r/t inability to deep breathe in supine position

Acute **Confusion:** elderly r/t sensory deprivation from immobility

Constipation r/t immobility

Adult **Failure to Thrive** r/t limited physical mobility

Impaired physical **Mobility** r/t medically imposed bed rest

Ineffective peripheral **Tissue Perfusion** r/t interruption of venous flow

Powerlessness r/t forced immobility from health care environment

Impaired **Walking** r/t limited physical mobility, deconditioning of body

Risk for **Disuse Syndrome:** Risk factor: immobilization

Risk for impaired **Skin Integrity:** Risk factors: pressure on immobile parts, shearing forces when moved

Readiness for enhanced **Knowledge:** expresses an interest in learning

IMMUNIZATION

Readiness for enhanced **Immunization Status** (See **Immunization Status**, readiness for enhanced, Section II)

IMMUNOSUPPRESSION

Risk for **Infection:** Risk factor: immunosuppression

IMPACTION OF STOOL

Constipation r/t decreased fluid intake, less than adequate amounts of fiber and bulk-forming foods in diet, medication effect, or immobility

IMPERFORATE ANUS

Anxiety r/t ability to care for newborn

Deficient **Knowledge** r/t home care for newborn

Impaired **Skin Integrity** r/t pruritus

IMPETIGO

Impaired **Skin Integrity** r/t infectious disease

Readiness for enhanced **Knowledge:** expresses an interest in learning

See Communicable Diseases, Childhood

IMPLANTABLE CARDIOVERTER/ DEFIBRILLATOR (ICD)

See ICD (Implantable Cardioverter/ Defibrillator)

IMPOTENCE

Situational low **Self-Esteem** r/t physiological crisis, inability to practice usual sexual activity

Sexual Dysfunction r/t altered body function

Readiness for enhanced **Knowledge:** treatment information for erectile dysfunction

See Erectile Dysfunction (ED)

IMPULSIVENESS

Ineffective **Impulse Control** r/t (See **Impulse Control**, ineffective, Section II)

INACTIVITY

Activity Intolerance r/t imbalance between oxygen supply and demand, sedentary lifestyle, weakness, immobility

Hopelessness r/t deteriorating physiological condition, long-term stress, social isolation

Impaired physical **Mobility** r/t intolerance to activity, decreased strength and endurance, depression, severe anxiety, musculoskeletal impairment, perceptual or cognitive impairment, neuromuscular impairment, pain, discomfort

Risk for **Constipation:** Risk factor: insufficient physical activity

INCOMPETENT CERVIX

See Premature Dilation of the Cervix (Incompetent Cervix)

INCONTINENCE OF STOOL

Disturbed **Body Image** r/t inability to control elimination of stool

Bowel **Incontinence** r/t decreased awareness of need to defecate, loss of sphincter control

Toileting **Self-Care** deficit r/t cognitive impairment, neuromuscular impairment, perceptual impairment, weakness.

Situational low **Self-Esteem** r/t inability to control elimination of stool

Risk for impaired **Skin Integrity:** Risk factor: presence of stool

INCONTINENCE OF URINE

Functional urinary **Incontinence** r/t altered environment; sensory, cognitive, or mobility deficits

Overflow urinary **Incontinence** r/t relaxation of pelvic muscles and changes in urinary structures

Reflex urinary **Incontinence** r/t neurological impairment

Stress urinary **Incontinence** (See **Incontinence,** urinary, stress, Section II)

Urge urinary **Incontinence** (See **Incontinence,** urinary, urge, Section II)

Toileting **Self-Care** deficit r/t cognitive impairment

Situational low **Self-Esteem** r/t inability to control passage of urine

Risk for impaired **Skin Integrity:** Risk factor: presence of urine on perineal skin

INDIGESTION

Nausea r/t gastrointestinal irritation

Imbalanced **Nutrition:** less than body requirements r/t discomfort when eating

INDUCTION OF LABOR

Anxiety r/t medical interventions, powerlessness

Decisional Conflict r/t perceived threat to idealized birth

Ineffective **Coping** r/t situational crisis of medical intervention in birthing process

Acute **Pain** r/t contractions

Situational low **Self-Esteem** r/t inability to carry out normal labor

Risk for **Injury:** maternal and fetal: Risk factors: hypertonic uterus, potential prematurity of newborn

Readiness for enhanced **Family Processes:** family support during induction of labor

INFANT APNEA

See Premature Infant (Child); Respiratory Conditions of the Neonate; SIDS (Sudden Infant Death Syndrome)

INFANT BEHAVIOR

Disorganized **Infant** behavior r/t pain, oral/motor problems, feeding intolerance, environmental overstimulation, lack of containment or boundaries, prematurity, invasive or painful procedures

Risk for disorganized **Infant** behavior: Risk factors: pain, oral/motor problems, environmental overstimulation, lack of containment or boundaries

Readiness for enhanced organized **Infant** behavior: stable physiological measures, use of some self-regulatory measures

INFANT CARE

Readiness for enhanced **Childbearing Process:** a pattern of preparing for, maintaining, and strengthening care of newborn infant

INFANT FEEDING PATTERN, INEFFECTIVE

Ineffective infant **Feeding Pattern** r/t prematurity, neurological impairment or delay, oral hypersensitivity, prolonged nothing-by-mouth order

INFANT OF DIABETIC MOTHER

Decreased **Cardiac Output** r/t cardiomegaly

Deficient **Fluid Volume** r/t increased urinary excretion and osmotic diuresis

Delayed **Growth and Development** r/t prolonged and severe postnatal hypoglycemia

Imbalanced **Nutrition**: less than body requirements r/t hypotonia, lethargy, poor sucking, postnatal metabolic changes from hyperglycemia to hypoglycemia and hyperinsulinism

Risk for delayed **Development**: Risk factors: prolonged and severe postnatal hypoglycemia

Risk for impaired **Gas Exchange**: Risk factors: increased incidence of cardiomegaly, prematurity

Risk for unstable blood **Glucose** level: Risk factor: metabolic change from hyperglycemia to hypoglycemia and hyperinsulinism

Risk for disproportionate **Growth**: Risk factors: prolonged and severe postnatal hypoglycemia

Risk for disturbed **Maternal/Fetal Dyad**: Risk factor: impaired glucose metabolism

See Premature Infant (Child); Respiratory Conditions of the Neonate

INFANT OF SUBSTANCE-ABUSING MOTHER (FETAL ALCOHOL SYNDROME, CRACK BABY, OTHER DRUG WITHDRAWAL INFANTS)

Ineffective **Airway Clearance** r/t pooling of secretions from the lack of adequate cough reflex, effects of viral or bacterial lower airway infection as a result of altered protective state

Interrupted **Breastfeeding** r/t use of drugs or alcohol by mother

Diarrhea r/t effects of withdrawal, increased peristalsis from hyperirritability

Ineffective infant **Feeding Pattern** r/t uncoordinated or ineffective sucking reflex

Delayed **Growth and Development** r/t effects of maternal use of drugs, effects of neurological impairment, decreased attentiveness to environmental stimuli or inadequate stimuli

Disorganized **Infant** behavior r/t exposure and or withdrawal from toxic substances (alcohol and drugs)

Ineffective **Childbearing Process** r/t inconsistent prenatal health visits, suboptimal maternal nutrition, substance abuse

Insomnia r/t hyperirritability or hypersensitivity to environmental stimuli

Imbalanced **Nutrition**: less than body requirements r/t feeding problems; uncoordinated or ineffective suck and swallow; effects of diarrhea, vomiting, or colic associated with maternal substance abuse

Impaired **Parenting** r/t impaired or absent attachment behaviors, inadequate support systems

Risk for delayed **Development**: Risk factor: substance abuse

Risk for disproportionate **Growth**: Risk factor: substance abuse

Risk for **Infection**: skin, meningeal, respiratory: Risk factor: stress effects of withdrawal

See Cerebral Palsy; Child with Chronic Condition; Crack Baby; Failure to Thrive, Nonorganic; Hospitalized Child; Hyperactive Syndrome; Premature Infant (Child); SIDS (Sudden Infant Death Syndrome)

INFANTILE POLYARTERITIS

See Kawasaki Disease

INFECTION

Hyperthermia r/t increased metabolic rate

Ineffective **Protection** r/t inadequate nutrition, abnormal blood profiles, drug therapies, treatments

Risk for **Vascular Trauma**: Risk factor: infusion of antibiotics

I

INFECTION, POTENTIAL FOR

Risk for **Infection** (See **Infection**, risk for, Section II)

INFERTILITY

Ineffective **Self-Health Management** r/t deficient knowledge about infertility

Powerlessness r/t infertility

Chronic **Sorrow** r/t inability to conceive a child

Spiritual Distress r/t inability to conceive a child

INFLAMMATORY BOWEL DISEASE (CHILD AND ADULT)

Ineffective **Coping** r/t repeated episodes of diarrhea

Diarrhea r/t effects of inflammatory changes of the bowel

Deficient **Fluid Volume** r/t frequent and loose stools

Imbalanced **Nutrition**: less than body requirements r/t anorexia, decreased absorption of nutrients from gastrointestinal tract

Acute **Pain** r/t abdominal cramping and anal irritation

Impaired **Skin Integrity** r/t frequent stools, development of anal fissures

Social Isolation r/t diarrhea

See Child with Chronic Condition; Crohn's Disease; Hospitalized Child; Maturational Issues, Adolescent

INFLUENZA

Deficient **Fluid Volume** r/t inadequate fluid intake

Ineffective **Self-Health Management** r/t lack of knowledge regarding preventive immunizations

Ineffective **Thermoregulation** r/t infectious process

Acute **Pain** r/t inflammatory changes in joints

Readiness for enhanced **Knowledge**: about information to prevent or treat influenza

INGUINAL HERNIA REPAIR

Impaired physical **Mobility** r/t pain at surgical site and fear of causing hernia to rupture

Acute **Pain** r/t surgical procedure

Urinary Retention r/t possible edema at surgical site

Risk for **Infection**: Risk factor: surgical procedure

INJURY

Risk for **Falls**: Risk factors: orthostatic hypotension, impaired physical mobility, diminished mental status

Risk for **Injury**: Risk factor: environmental conditions interacting with client's adaptive and defensive resources

Risk for **Thermal Injury**: Risk factor: cognitive impairment, inadequate supervision, developmental level

INSANITY

See Mental Illness, Psychosis

INSOMNIA

*See **Insomnia** (Section II)*

INSULIN SHOCK

See Hypoglycemia

INTERMITTENT CLAUDICATION

Deficient **Knowledge** r/t lack of knowledge of cause and treatment of peripheral vascular diseases

Acute **Pain** r/t decreased circulation to extremities with activity

Ineffective peripheral **Tissue Perfusion** r/t interruption of arterial flow

Risk for **Injury**: Risk factor: tissue hypoxia

Readiness for enhanced **Knowledge:** prevention of pain and impaired circulation

See Peripheral Vascular Disease (PVD)

INTERNAL CARDIOVERTER/ DEFIBRILLATOR (ICD)

See ICD (Implantable Cardioverter/ Defibrillator)

INTERNAL FIXATION

Impaired **Walking** r/t repair of fracture

Risk for **Infection:** Risk factors: traumatized tissue, broken skin

See Fracture

INTERSTITIAL CYSTITIS

Acute **Pain** r/t inflammatory process

Impaired **Urinary Elimination** r/t inflammation of bladder

Risk for **Infection:** Risk factor: suppressed inflammatory response

Readiness for enhanced **Knowledge:** expresses an interest in learning

INTERVERTEBRAL DISK EXCISION

See Laminectomy

INTESTINAL OBSTRUCTION

See Ileus, Bowel Obstruction

INTESTINAL PERFORATION

See Peritonitis

INTOXICATION

Anxiety r/t loss of control of actions

Acute **Confusion** r/t alcohol abuse

Ineffective **Coping** r/t use of mind-altering substances as a means of coping

Impaired **Memory** r/t effects of alcohol on mind

Risk for **Aspiration:** Risk factors: diminished mental status, vomiting

Risk for **Falls:** Risk factor: diminished mental status

Risk for other-directed **Violence:** Risk factor: inability to control thoughts and actions

INTRAAORTIC BALLOON COUNTERPULSATION

Anxiety r/t device providing cardiovascular assistance

Decreased **Cardiac Output** r/t failing heart needing counterpulsation

Compromised family **Coping** r/t seriousness of significant other's medical condition

Impaired physical **Mobility** r/t restriction of movement because of mechanical device

Risk for **Peripheral Neurovascular Dysfunction:** Risk factors: vascular obstruction of balloon catheter, thrombus formation, emboli, edema

INTRACRANIAL PRESSURE, INCREASED

Ineffective **Breathing Pattern** r/t pressure damage to breathing center in brainstem

Acute **Confusion** r/t increased intracranial pressure

Adult **Failure to Thrive** r/t undetected changes from increased intracranial pressure

Decreased **Intracranial Adaptive Capacity** r/t sustained increase in intracranial pressure

Impaired **Memory** r/t neurological disturbance

Vision Loss r/t pressure damage to sensory centers in brain

Risk for ineffective **Cerebral tissue** perfusion: Risk factors: body position, cerebral vessel circulation deficits

See cause of Increased Intracranial Pressure

INTRAUTERINE GROWTH RETARDATION

Anxiety: maternal r/t threat to fetus

Ineffective **Coping:** maternal r/t situational crisis, threat to fetus

Impaired **Gas** exchange r/t insufficient placental perfusion

Delayed **Growth and Development** r/t insufficient supply of oxygen and nutrients

Imbalanced **Nutrition:** less than body requirements r/t insufficient placenta

Situational low **Self-Esteem:** maternal r/t guilt about threat to fetus

Spiritual Distress r/t unknown outcome of fetus

Risk for **Powerlessness:** Risk factor: unknown outcome of fetus

INTRAVENOUS THERAPY

Risk for **Vascular Trauma:** Risk factor: infusion of irritating chemicals

INTUBATION, ENDOTRACHEAL OR NASOGASTRIC

Disturbed **Body Image** r/t altered appearance with mechanical devices

Impaired verbal **Communication** r/t endotracheal tube

Imbalanced **Nutrition:** less than body requirements r/t inability to ingest food because of the presence of tubes

Impaired **Oral Mucous Membrane** r/t presence of tubes

Acute **Pain** r/t presence of tube

IODINE REACTION WITH DIAGNOSTIC TESTING

Risk for adverse reaction to iodinated **Contrast** media: Risk factor (See reaction to iodinated **Contrast** media, risk for adverse, Section II)

IRREGULAR PULSE

See Dysrhythmia

IRRITABLE BOWEL SYNDROME (IBS)

See IBS (Irritable Bowel Syndrome)

ISOLATION

Impaired individual **Resilience** (See **Resilience,** individual, impaired, Section II)

Social Isolation (See **Social Isolation,** Section II)

ITCHING

Impaired **Comfort** r/t inflammation of skin causing itching

Risk for impaired **Skin Integrity:** Risk factor: scratching, dry skin

ITP (IDIOPATHIC THROMBOCYTOPENIC PURPURA)

Deficient **Diversional Activity** r/t activity restrictions, safety precautions

Ineffective **Protection** r/t decreased platelet count

Risk for **Bleeding:** Risk factors: decreased platelet count, developmental level, age-appropriate play

See Hospitalized Child

J

JAUNDICE

Imbalanced **Nutrition,** less than body requirements r/t decreased appetite with liver disorder

Risk for **Bleeding:** Risk factor: impaired liver function

Risk for impaired **Liver Function:** Risk factors: possible viral infection, medication effect

Risk for impaired **Skin Integrity:** Risk factors: pruritus, itching

See Cirrhosis; Hepatitis

JAUNDICE, NEONATAL

Neonatal **Jaundice** (See **Jaundice,** neonatal, Section II)

Risk for ineffective **Gastrointestinal Perfusion:** Risk factor: liver dysfunction

Readiness for enhanced **Self-Health Management** (parents): expresses desire to manage treatment: assessment of jaundice when infant is discharged from the hospital, when to call the physician, and possible preventive measures such as frequent breastfeeding

See Hyperbilirubinemia

JAW PAIN AND HEART ATTACKS

See Angina; Chest Pain; MI (Myocardial Infarction)

JAW SURGERY

Deficient **Knowledge** r/t emergency care for wired jaws (e.g., cutting bands and wires), oral care

Imbalanced **Nutrition:** less than body requirements r/t jaws wired closed, difficulty eating

Acute **Pain** r/t surgical procedure

Impaired **Swallowing** r/t edema from surgery

Risk for **Aspiration:** Risk factor: wired jaws

JITTERY

Anxiety r/t unconscious conflict about essential values and goals, threat to or change in health status

Death **Anxiety** r/t unresolved issues relating to end of life

Risk for **Post-Trauma Syndrome:** Risk factors: occupation, survivor's role in event, inadequate social support

JOCK ITCH

Ineffective **Self-Health Management** r/t prevention and treatment of disorder

Impaired **Skin Integrity** r/t moisture and irritating or tight-fitting clothing

See Itching

JOINT DISLOCATION

See Dislocation of Joint

JOINT PAIN

See Arthritis; Bursitis; JRA (Juvenile Rheumatoid Arthritis); Osteoarthritis; Rheumatoid Arthritis

JOINT REPLACEMENT

Risk for **Peripheral Neurovascular Dysfunction:** Risk factor: orthopedic surgery

See Total Joint Replacement (Total Hip/ Total Knee/Shoulder)

JRA (JUVENILE RHEUMATOID ARTHRITIS)

Impaired **Comfort** r/t altered health status

Fatigue r/t chronic inflammatory disease

Delayed **Growth and Development** r/t effects of physical disability, chronic illness

Impaired physical **Mobility** r/t pain, restricted joint movement

Acute **Pain** r/t swollen or inflamed joints, restricted movement, physical therapy

Self-Care deficit. feeding, bathing, dressing, toileting r/t restricted joint movement, pain

Risk for compromised **Human Dignity:** Risk factors. perceived intrusion by clinicians, invasion of privacy

Risk for **Injury:** Risk factors: impaired physical mobility, splints, adaptive devices, increased bleeding potential from antiinflammatory medications

Risk for compromised **Resilience:** Risk factor: chronic condition

Risk for situational low **Self-Esteem:** Risk factor: disturbed body image

Risk for impaired **Skin Integrity:** Risk factors: splints, adaptive devices

See Child with Chronic Condition; Hospitalized Child

JUVENILE ONSET DIABETES

See Diabetes Mellitus, Juvenile

K

KAPOSI'S SARCOMA

Risk for complicated **Grieving:** Risk factor: loss of social support

Risk for impaired **Religiosity:** Risk factors: illness/hospitalization, ineffective coping

Risk for compromised **Resilience:** Risk factor: serious illness

See AIDS (Acquired Immunodeficiency Syndrome)

KAWASAKI DISEASE

Anxiety: parental r/t progression of disease, complications of arthritis, and cardiac involvement

Impaired **Comfort** r/t altered health status

Hyperthermia r/t inflammatory disease process

Imbalanced **Nutrition:** less than body requirements r/t impaired oral mucous membranes

Impaired **Oral Mucous Membrane** r/t inflamed mouth and pharynx; swollen lips that become dry, cracked, fissured

Acute **Pain** r/t enlarged lymph nodes; erythematous skin rash that progresses to desquamation, peeling, denuding of skin

Impaired **Skin Integrity** r/t inflammatory skin changes

Risk for imbalanced **Fluid Volume:** Risk factor: hypovolemia

Risk for decreased **Cardiac** tissue perfusion: Risk factor: cardiac involvement

See Hospitalized Child

KEGEL EXERCISE

Stress urinary **Incontinence** r/t degenerative change in pelvic muscles

Urge urinary **Incontinence** r/t inflammation of bladder

Risk for urge urinary **Incontinence:** Risk factors: overactive bladder dysfunction; urinary tract infection; dietary risk factors: consumption of caffeine

Readiness for enhanced **Self-Health Management:** desires information to relieve incontinence

KELOIDS

Disturbed **Body Image** r/t presence of scar tissue at site of a healed skin injury

Readiness for enhanced **Self-Health Management:** desire to have information to manage condition

KERATOCONJUNCTIVITIS SICCA (DRY EYE SYNDROME)

Risk for **Infection:** Risk factor: dry eyes that are more vulnerable to infection

Vision Loss r/t dry eye resulting in film or obstruction of vision

See Conjunctivitis

KERATOPLASTY

See Corneal Transplant

KETOACIDOSIS, ALCOHOLIC

See Alcohol Withdrawal; Alcoholism

KETOACIDOSIS, DIABETIC

Deficient **Fluid Volume** r/t excess excretion of urine, nausea, vomiting, increased respiration

Impaired **Memory** r/t fluid and electrolyte imbalance

Imbalanced **Nutrition:** less than body requirements r/t body's inability to use nutrients

Risk for unstable blood **Glucose** level: Risk factor: deficient knowledge of diabetes management (e.g., action plan)

Risk for **Powerlessness:** Risk factor: illness-related regimen

Risk for compromised **Resilience:** Risk factor: complications of disease

See Diabetes Mellitus

KEYHOLE HEART SURGERY

See MIDCAB (Minimally Invasive Direct Coronary Artery Bypass)

KIDNEY DISEASE SCREENING

Readiness for enhanced **Self-Health Management:** seeks information for screening

KIDNEY FAILURE

See Renal Failure

KIDNEY STONE

Overflow urinary **Incontinence** r/t bladder outlet obstruction

Acute **Pain** r/t obstruction from renal calculi

Impaired **Urinary Elimination:** urgency and frequency r/t anatomical obstruction, irritation caused by stone

Risk for **Infection:** Risk factor: obstruction of urinary tract with stasis of urine

Readiness for enhanced **Knowledge:** Expresses an interest in learning

KIDNEY TRANSPLANT

Ineffective **Protection** r/t immunosuppressive therapy

Risk for ineffective **Renal Perfusion.** Risk factor: complications from transplant procedure

Readiness for enhanced **Decision-Making:** expresses desire to enhance understanding of choices

Readiness for enhanced **Family Processes:** adapting to life without dialysis

Readiness for enhanced **Self-Health Management:** desire to manage the treatment and prevention of complications post transplant

Readiness for enhanced **Spiritual Well-Being:** heightened coping, living without dialysis

See Nephrectomy; Renal Failure; Renal Transplantation, Donor; Renal Transplantation, Recipient; Surgery, Perioperative Care; Surgery, Postoperative Care; Surgery, Preoperative Care

KIDNEY TUMOR

See Wilms' Tumor

KISSING DISEASE

See Mononucleosis

KNEE REPLACEMENT

See Total Joint Replacement (Total Hip/ Total Knee/Shoulder)

KNOWLEDGE

Readiness for enhanced **Knowledge** (See **Knowledge,** readiness for enhanced, Section II)

KNOWLEDGE, DEFICIENT

Ineffective **Health Maintenance** r/t lack of or significant alteration in communication skills (written, verbal, and/or gestural)

Deficient **Knowledge** (See **Knowledge,** deficient, Section II)

Readiness for enhanced **Knowledge** (See **Knowledge,** readiness for enhanced, Section II)

KOCK POUCH

See Continent Ileostomy (Kock Pouch)

KORSAKOFF'S SYNDROME

Acute **Confusion** r/t alcohol abuse

Dysfunctional **Family Processes** r/t alcoholism as possible cause of syndrome

Impaired **Memory** r/t neurological changes associated with excessive alcohol intake

Self-Neglect r/t cognitive impairment from chronic alcohol abuse

Risk for **Falls:** Risk factor: cognitive impairment from chronic alcohol abuse

Risk for **Injury:** Risk factors: sensory dysfunction, lack of coordination when ambulating from chronic alcohol abuse

Risk for impaired **Liver Function:** Risk factor: substance abuse (alcohol)

Risk for imbalanced **Nutrition:** less than body requirements: Risk factor: lack of adequate balanced intake from chronic alcohol abuse

L

LABOR, INDUCTION OF

See Induction of Labor

LABOR, NORMAL

Anxiety r/t fear of the unknown, situational crisis

Impaired **Comfort** r/t labor

Fatigue r/t childbirth

Deficient **Knowledge** r/t lack of preparation for labor

Acute **Pain** r/t uterine contractions, stretching of cervix and birth canal

Impaired **Tissue Integrity** r/t passage of infant through birth canal, episiotomy

Risk for deficient **Fluid Volume:** Risk factor: excessive loss of blood

Risk for **Infection:** Risk factors: multiple vaginal examinations, tissue trauma, prolonged rupture of membranes

Risk for **Injury:** fetal: Risk factor: hypoxia

Risk for **Post-Trauma Syndrome:** Risk factors: trauma or violence associated with labor pains, medical or surgical interventions, history of sexual abuse

Risk for **Powerlessness:** Risk factor: labor process

Readiness for enhanced **Childbearing Process:** responds appropriately, is proactive, bonds with infant and uses support systems

Readiness for enhanced family **Coping:** significant other providing support during labor

Readiness for enhanced **Power:** expresses readiness to enhance participation in choices regarding treatment during labor

Readiness for enhanced **Self-Health Management:** prenatal care and childbirth education birth process

LABYRINTHITIS

Ineffective **Self-Health Management** r/t delay in seeking treatment for respiratory and ear infections

Risk for **Injury** r/t dizziness

Readiness for enhanced **Self-Health Management:** management of episodes

See Ménière's Disease

LACERATIONS

Risk for **Infection:** Risk factor: broken skin

Risk for **Trauma:** Risk factor: children playing with dangerous objects

Readiness for enhanced **Self-Health Management:** proper care of injury

LACTATION

See Breastfeeding, Ineffective; Breastfeeding, Interrupted; Breastfeeding, Readiness for Enhanced

LACTIC ACIDOSIS

Decreased **Cardiac Output** r/t altered heart rate/rhythm, preload, and contractility

Risk for **Electrolyte Imbalance:** Risk factor: impaired regulatory mechanism

Risk for decreased **Cardiac** tissue perfusion: Risk factor: hypoxia

See Ketoacidosis, Diabetic

LACTOSE INTOLERANCE

Readiness for enhanced **Knowledge:** interest in identifying lactose intolerance, treatment, and substitutes for milk products

See Abdominal Distention; Diarrhea

LAMINECTOMY

Anxiety r/t change in health status, surgical procedure

Impaired **Comfort** r/t surgical procedure

Deficient **Knowledge** r/t appropriate postoperative and postdischarge activities

Impaired physical **Mobility** r/t neuromuscular impairment

Acute **Pain** r/t localized inflammation and edema

Urinary Retention r/t competing sensory impulses, effects of opioids or anesthesia

Risk for **Bleeding:** Risk factor: surgery

Risk for **Infection:** Risk factor: invasive procedure

Risk for **Perioperative Positioning Injury:** Risk factor: prone position

Risk for ineffective, cerebral, peripheral tissue and or decreased cardiac **Tissue Perfusion:** Risk factors: edema, hemorrhage, embolism

See Scoliosis; Surgery, Perioperative; Surgery, Postoperative; Surgery, Preoperative

LANGUAGE IMPAIRMENT

See Speech Disorders

LAPAROSCOPIC LASER CHOLECYSTECTOMY

See Cholecystectomy; Laser Surgery

LAPAROSCOPY

Urge urinary **Incontinence** r/t pressure on the bladder from gas

Acute **Pain:** shoulder r/t gas irritating the diaphragm

Risk for ineffective **Gastrointestinal Perfusion:** Risk factor: complications from procedure

LAPAROTOMY

See Abdominal Surgery

LARGE BOWEL RESECTION

See Abdominal Surgery

LARYNGECTOMY

Ineffective **Airway Clearance** r/t surgical removal of glottis, decreased humidification of air

Disturbed **Body Image** r/t change in body structure and function

Impaired **Comfort** r/t surgery

Death **Anxiety** r/t unknown results of surgery

Interrupted **Family Processes** r/t surgery, serious condition of family member, difficulty communicating

Grieving r/t loss of voice, fear of death

Imbalanced **Nutrition:** less than body requirements r/t absence of oral feeding, difficulty swallowing, increased need for fluids

Impaired **Oral Mucous Membrane** r/t absence of oral feeding

Chronic **Sorrow** r/t change in body image

Ineffective **Self-Health Management** r/t deficient knowledge regarding self-care with laryngectomy

Impaired **Swallowing** r/t edema, laryngectomy tube

Impaired verbal **Communication** r/t removal of larynx

Risk for **Electrolyte Imbalance:** Risk factor: fluid imbalance

Risk for complicated **Grieving:** Risk factors: loss, major life event

Risk for compromised **Human Dignity:** Risk factor: loss of control of body function

Risk for **Infection:** Risk factors: invasive procedure, surgery

Risk for **Powerlessness:** Risk factors: chronic illness, change in communication

L

Risk for compromised **Resilience:** Risk factor: change in health status

Risk for situational low **Self-Esteem:** Risk factor: disturbed body image

LASER SURGERY

Impaired **Comfort** r/t surgery

Constipation r/t laser intervention in vulval and perianal areas

Deficient **Knowledge** r/t preoperative and postoperative care associated with laser procedure

Acute **Pain** r/t heat from laser

Risk for **Bleeding:** Risk factor: surgery

Risk for **Infection:** Risk factor: delayed heating reaction of tissue exposed to laser

Risk for **Injury:** Risk factor: accidental exposure to laser beam

LASIK EYE SURGERY (LASER-ASSISTED IN SITU KERATOMILEUSIS)

Impaired **Comfort** r/t surgery

Decisional Conflict r/t decision to have the surgery

Risk for **Infection** r/t surgery

Readiness for enhanced **Self-Health Management:** surgical procedure pre- and postoperative teaching and expectations

LATEX ALLERGY

Latex Allergy Response (See **Latex Allergy Response,** Section II)

Risk for **Latex Allergy Response** (See **Latex Allergy Response,** risk for, Section II)

Readiness for enhanced **Knowledge:** prevention and treatment of exposure to latex products

LAXATIVE ABUSE

Perceived **Constipation** r/t health belief, faulty appraisal, impaired thought processes

LEAD POISONING

Contamination r/t flaking, peeling paint in presence of young children

Impaired **Home Maintenance** r/t presence of lead paint

Risk for delayed **Development:** Risk factor: lead poisoning

LEFT HEART CATHETERIZATION

See Cardiac Catheterization

LEGIONNAIRES' DISEASE

Contamination r/t contaminated water in air-conditioning systems

See Pneumonia

LENS IMPLANT

See Cataract Extraction; Vision Impairment

LETHARGY/LISTLESSNESS

Adult **Failure to Thrive** r/t apathy

Fatigue r/t decreased metabolic energy production

Insomnia r/t internal or external stressors

Risk for ineffective **Cerebral** tissue perfusion: Risk factor: lack of oxygen supply to brain

See cause of Lethargy/Listlessness

LEUKEMIA

Ineffective **Protection** r/t abnormal blood profile

Risk for imbalanced **Fluid Volume:** Risk factors: nausea, vomiting, bleeding, side effects of treatment

Risk for **Infection:** Risk factor: ineffective immune system

Risk for compromised **Resilience:** Risk factor: serious illness

See Cancer; Chemotherapy

LEUKOPENIA

Ineffective **Protection** r/t leukopenia

Risk for **Infection:** Risk factor: low white blood cell count

LEVEL OF CONSCIOUSNESS, DECREASED

See Confusion, Acute; Confusion, Chronic

LICE

Impaired **Comfort** r/t inflammation, pruritus

Impaired **Home Maintenance** r/t close unsanitary, overcrowded conditions

Self-Neglect r/t lifestyle

Readiness for enhanced **Self-Health Management:** preventing and treating infestation

See Communicable Diseases, Childhood

LIFESTYLE, SEDENTARY

Sedentary lifestyle (See **Sedentary** lifestyle, Section II)

Risk for ineffective peripheral **Tissue Perfusion** r/t lack of movement

LIGHTHEADEDNESS

See Dizziness; Vertigo

LIMB REATTACHMENT PROCEDURES

Anxiety r/t unknown outcome of reattachment procedure, use and appearance of limb

Disturbed **Body Image** r/t unpredictability of function and appearance of reattached body part

Grieving r/t unknown outcome of reattachment procedure

Spiritual Distress r/t anxiety about condition

Stress overload r/t multiple coexisting stressors, physical demands

Risk for **Bleeding:** Risk factor: severed vessels

Risk for **Perioperative Positioning Injury:** Risk factor: immobilization

Risk for **Peripheral Neurovascular Dysfunction:** Risk factors: trauma, orthopedic and neurovascular surgery, compression of nerves and blood vessels

Risk for **Powerlessness:** Risk factor: unknown outcome of procedure

Risk for impaired **Religiosity:** Risk factors: suffering, hospitalization

See Surgery, Postoperative Care

LIPOSUCTION

Disturbed **Body Image** r/t dissatisfaction with unwanted fat deposits in body

Risk for compromised **Resilience:** Risk factor: body image disturbance

Readiness for enhanced **Decision-Making:** expresses desire to make decision regarding liposuction

Readiness for enhanced **Self-Concept:** satisfaction with new body image

See Surgery, Perioperative Care; Surgery, Postoperative Care; Surgery, Preoperative Care

LITHOTRIPSY

Readiness for enhanced **Self-Health Management:** expresses desire for information related to procedure and aftercare and prevention of stones

See Kidney Stone

LIVER BIOPSY

Anxiety r/t procedure and results

Risk for deficient **Fluid Volume:** Risk factor: hemorrhage from biopsy site

Risk for **Powerlessness:** Risk factor: inability to control outcome of procedure

LIVER CANCER

Risk for ineffective **Gastrointestinal Perfusion:** Risk factor: liver dysfunction

Risk for impaired **Liver Function:** Risk factor: disease process

Risk for compromised **Resilience:** Risk factor: serious illness

See Cancer; Chemotherapy; Radiation Therapy

LIVER DISEASE

See Cirrhosis; Hepatitis

LIVER FUNCTION

Risk for impaired **Liver Function** (See **Liver Function**, impaired, risk for, Section II)

LIVER TRANSPLANT

Impaired **Comfort** r/t surgical pain

Decisional Conflict r/t acceptance of donor liver

Ineffective **Protection** r/t immunosuppressive therapy

Risk for impaired **Liver Function:** Risk factors: possible rejection, infection

Readiness for enhanced **Family Processes:** change in physical needs of family member

Readiness for enhanced **Self-Health Management:** desire to manage the treatment and prevention of complications posttransplant

Readiness for enhanced **Spiritual Well-Being:** heightened coping

See Surgery, Perioperative Care; Surgery, Postoperative Care; Surgery, Preoperative Care

LIVING WILL

Moral Distress r/t end-of-life decisions

Readiness for enhanced **Decision-Making:** expresses desire to enhance understanding of choices for decision-making

Readiness for enhanced **Relationship:** shares information with others

Readiness for enhanced **Religiosity:** request to meet with religious leaders or facilitators

Readiness for enhanced **Resilience:** uses effective communication

Readiness for enhanced **Spiritual Well-Being:** acceptance of and preparation for end of life

See Advance Directives

LOBECTOMY

See Thoracotomy

LONELINESS

Spiritual Distress r/t loneliness, social alienation

Risk for **Loneliness** (See **Loneliness**, risk for, Section II)

Risk for impaired **Religiosity:** Risk factor: lack of social interaction

Risk for situational low **Self-Esteem:** Risk factors: failure, rejection

Readiness for enhanced **Hope:** expresses desire to enhance interconnectedness with others

Readiness for enhanced **Relationship:** expresses satisfaction with complementary relationship between partners

LOOSE STOOLS (BOWEL MOVEMENTS)

Diarrhea r/t increased gastric motility

Risk for dysfunctional **Gastrointestinal Motility:** Risk factor: diarrhea

See cause of Loose Stools; Diarrhea

LOSS OF BLADDER CONTROL

See Incontinence of Urine

LOSS OF BOWEL CONTROL

See Incontinence of Stool

LOU GEHRIG'S DISEASE

See Amyotrophic Lateral Sclerosis (ALS)

LOW BACK PAIN

Impaired **Comfort** r/t back pain

Ineffective **Health Maintenance** r/t deficient knowledge regarding self-care with back pain

L

Impaired physical **Mobility** r/t back pain

Chronic **Pain** r/t degenerative processes, musculotendinous strain, injury, inflammation, congenital deformities

Urinary Retention r/t possible spinal cord compression

Risk for **Powerlessness:** Risk factor: living with chronic pain

Readiness for enhanced **Self-Health Management:** expressed desire for information to manage pain

LOW BLOOD PRESSURE

See Hypotension

LOW BLOOD SUGAR

See Hypoglycemia

LOWER GI BLEEDING

See GI Bleed (Gastrointestinal Bleeding)

LUMBAR PUNCTURE

Anxiety r/t invasive procedure and unknown results

Deficient **Knowledge** r/t information about procedure

Acute **Pain** r/t possible loss of cerebrospinal fluid

Risk for **Infection:** Risk factor: invasive procedure

Risk for ineffective **Cerebral** tissue perfusion: Risk factor: treatment-related side effects

LUMPECTOMY

Decisional Conflict r/t treatment choices

Readiness for enhanced **Knowledge:** preoperative and postoperative care

Readiness for enhanced **Spiritual Well-Being:** hope of benign diagnosis

See Cancer

LUNG CANCER

See Cancer; Chemotherapy; Radiation Therapy; Thoracotomy

LUNG SURGERY

See Thoracotomy

LUPUS ERYTHEMATOSUS

Disturbed **Body Image** r/t change in skin, rash, lesions, ulcers, mottled erythema

Fatigue r/t increased metabolic requirements

Ineffective **Health Maintenance** r/t deficient knowledge regarding medication, diet, activity

Acute **Pain** r/t inflammatory process

Powerlessness r/t unpredictability of course of disease

Impaired **Religiosity** r/t ineffective coping with disease

Chronic **Sorrow** r/t presence of chronic illness

Spiritual Distress r/t chronicity of disease, unknown etiology

Risk for compromised **Resilience:** Risk factor: chronic disease

Risk for impaired **Skin Integrity:** Risk factors: chronic inflammation, edema, altered circulation

Risk for decreased **Cardiac** tissue perfusion: Risk factor: altered circulation

LYME DISEASE

Impaired **Comfort** r/t inflammation

Fatigue r/t increased energy requirements

Deficient **Knowledge** r/t lack of information concerning disease, prevention, treatment

Acute **Pain** r/t inflammation of joints, urticaria, rash

Risk for decreased **Cardiac Output:** Risk factor: dysrhythmia

Risk for **Powerlessness:** Risk factor: possible chronic condition

LYMPHEDEMA

Disturbed **Body Image** r/t change in appearance of body part with edema

L

Excess **Fluid Volume** r/t compromised regulatory system; inflammation, obstruction, or removal of lymph glands

Deficient **Knowledge** r/t management of condition

Risk for situational low **Self-Esteem** r/t disturbed body image

LYMPHOMA

See Cancer

M

MACULAR DEGENERATION

Risk-prone **Health Behavior** r/t deteriorating vision

Ineffective **Coping** r/t visual loss

Compromised family **Coping** r/t deteriorating vision of family member

Hopelessness r/t deteriorating vision

Sedentary Lifestyle r/t visual loss

Self-Neglect r/t change in vision

Social Isolation r/t inability to drive because of visual changes

Vision Loss r/t impaired visual function

Risk for **Falls**: Risk factor: visual difficulties

Risk for **Injury**: Risk factor: inability to distinguish traffic lights

Risk for **Powerlessness**: Risk factor: deteriorating vision

Risk for impaired **Religiosity**: Risk factor: possible lack of transportation

Risk for compromised **Resilience**: Risk factor: changing vision

Readiness for enhanced **Self-Health Management**: appropriate choices of daily activities for meeting the goals of a treatment program

MAGNETIC RESONANCE IMAGING (MRI)

See MRI (Magnetic Resonance Imaging)

MAJOR DEPRESSIVE DISORDER

Interrupted **Family Processes** r/t change in health status of family member

Self-Neglect r/t psychological disorder

Risk for ineffective **Activity Planning** r/t compromised ability to process information

Risk for ineffective **Childbearing Process** r/t psychiatric distress

Risk for **Loneliness**: Risk factors: social isolation associated with feelings of sadness, hopelessness

Risk for compromised **Resilience**: Risk factor: psychological disorder

See Depression (Major Depressive Disorder)

MALABSORPTION SYNDROME

Diarrhea r/t lactose intolerance, gluten sensitivity, resection of small bowel

Dysfunctional **Gastrointestinal Motility** r/t disease state

Deficient **Knowledge** r/t lack of information about diet and nutrition

Imbalanced **Nutrition**: less than body requirements r/t inability of body to absorb nutrients because of biological factors

Risk for **Electrolyte Imbalance**: Risk factor: hypovolemia

Risk for imbalanced **Fluid Volume**: Risk factor: diarrhea

Risk for disproportionate **Growth**: Risk factor: malnutrition from malabsorption

See Abdominal Distention

MALADAPTIVE BEHAVIOR

See Crisis; Post-Trauma Syndrome; Suicide Attempt

MALAISE

See Fatigue

MALARIA

Contamination r/t geographic area

Risk for **Contamination**: Risk factors: increased environmental exposure (not wearing protective clothing, not using insecticide or repellant on skin and in room in areas where infected mosquitoes are present); inadequate defense mechanisms (inappropriate use of prophylactic regimen)

Risk for impaired **Liver Function**: Risk factor: complications of disease

Readiness for enhanced community **Coping**: uses resources available for problem solving

Readiness for enhanced **Immunization Status**: expresses desire to enhance immunization status and knowledge of immunization standards

Readiness for enhanced **Resilience**: immunization status

See Anemia

MALE INFERTILITY

See Erectile Dysfunction (ED); Infertility

MALIGNANCY

See Cancer

MALIGNANT HYPERTENSION (ARTERIOLAR NEPHROSCLEROSIS)

Decreased **Cardiac Output** r/t altered afterload, altered contractility

Fatigue r/t disease state, increased blood pressure

Excess **Fluid Volume** r/t decreased renal function

Risk for acute **Confusion**: Risk factors: increased blood urea nitrogen or creatine levels

Risk for imbalanced **Fluid Volume**: Risk factors: hypertension, altered renal function

Risk for ineffective **Renal Perfusion**: Risk factor: hypertension

Risk for ineffective **Cerebral** tissue perfusion: Risk factor: hypertension

Readiness for enhanced **Self-Health Management**: expresses desire to manage the illness, high blood pressure

MALIGNANT HYPERTHERMIA

Hyperthermia r/t anesthesia reaction associated with inherited condition

Risk for ineffective **Renal Perfusion**: Risk factor: hyperthermia

Readiness for enhanced **Self-Health Management**: knowledge of risk factors

MALNUTRITION

Insufficient **Breast Milk** r/t to inadequate nutrition

Adult **Failure to Thrive** r/t undetected malnutrition

Deficient **Knowledge** r/t misinformation about normal nutrition, social isolation, lack of food preparation facilities

Imbalanced **Nutrition**: less than body requirements r/t inability to ingest food, digest food, or absorb nutrients because of biological, psychological, or economic factors; institutionalization (i.e., lack of menu choices)

Ineffective **Protection** r/t inadequate nutrition

Ineffective **Self-Health Management** r/t inadequate nutrition

Self-Neglect r/t inadequate nutrition

Risk for disproportionate **Growth**: Risk factor: malnutrition

Risk for **Powerlessness**: Risk factor: possible inability to provide adequate nutrition

MAMMOGRAPHY

Readiness for enhanced **Resilience**: responsibility for self-care

Readiness for enhanced **Self-Health Management**: follows guidelines for screening

M

MANIC DISORDER, BIPOLAR I

Anxiety r/t change in role function

Ineffective **Coping** r/t situational crisis

Ineffective **Denial** r/t fear of inability to control behavior

Interrupted **Family Processes** r/t family member's illness

Risk-prone **Health Behavior** r/t low self-efficacy

Impaired **Home Maintenance** r/t altered psychological state, inability to concentrate

Disturbed personal **Identity** r/t manic state

Insomnia r/t constant anxious thoughts

Self-Neglect r/t manic state

Noncompliance r/t denial of illness

Imbalanced **Nutrition:** less than body requirements r/t lack of time and motivation to eat, constant movement

Impaired individual **Resilience** r/t psychological disorder

Ineffective **Role Performance** r/t impaired social interactions

Ineffective **Self-Health Management** r/t unpredictability of client, excessive demands on family, chronic illness, social support deficit

Sleep deprivation r/t hyperagitated state

Risk for ineffective **Activity Planning** r/t inability to process information

Risk for **Caregiver Role Strain:** Risk factor: unpredictability of condition

Risk for imbalanced **Fluid Volume:** Risk factor: hypovolemia

Risk for **Powerlessness:** Risk factor: inability to control changes in mood

Risk for impaired **Religiosity:** Risk factor: depression

Risk for **Spiritual Distress:** Risk factor: depression

Risk for **Suicide:** Risk factor: bipolar disorder

Risk for self- or other-directed **Violence:** Risk factors: hallucinations, delusions

Readiness for enhanced **Hope:** expresses desire to enhance problem-solving goals

MANIPULATION OF ORGANS, SURGICAL INCISION

Impaired **Comfort** r/t incision; surgery

Deficient **Knowledge** r/t lack of exposure to information regarding care after surgery and at home

Urinary Retention r/t swelling of urinary meatus

Risk for **Infection:** Risk factor: presence of urinary catheter

MANIPULATIVE BEHAVIOR

Defensive **Coping** r/t superior attitude toward others

Ineffective **Coping** r/t inappropriate use of defense mechanisms

Self-Mutilation r/t use of manipulation to obtain nurturing relationship with others

Self-Neglect r/t maintaining control

Impaired **Social Interaction** r/t self-concept disturbance

Risk for **Loneliness:** Risk factor: inability to interact appropriately with others

Risk for situational low **Self-Esteem:** Risk factor: history of learned helplessness

Risk for **Self-Mutilation:** Risk factor: inability to cope with increased psychological or physiological tension in healthy manner

MARASMUS

See Failure to Thrive, Nonorganic

MARFAN SYNDROME

Decreased **Cardiac Output** r/t dilation of the aortic root, dissection or rupture of the aorta

Risk for decreased **Cardiac** tissue perfusion: Risk factor: heart-related complications from Marfan syndrome

Readiness for enhanced **Self-Health Management:** describes reduction of risk factors

See Mitral Valve Prolapse; Scoliosis

MARSHALL-MARCHETTI-KRANTZ OPERATION

Preoperative

Stress urinary **Incontinence** r/t weak pelvic muscles and pelvic supports

Postoperative

Impaired **Comfort** r/t surgical procedure

Deficient **Knowledge** r/t lack of exposure to information regarding care after surgery and at home

Acute **Pain** r/t manipulation of organs, surgical incision

Urinary Retention r/t swelling of urinary meatus

Risk for **Bleeding:** Risk factor: surgical procedure

Risk for **Infection:** Risk factor: presence of urinary catheter

MASTECTOMY

Disturbed **Body Image** r/t loss of sexually significant body part

Impaired **Comfort** r/t altered body image; difficult diagnosis

Death **Anxiety** r/t threat of mortality associated with breast cancer

Fear r/t change in body image, prognosis

Deficient **Knowledge** r/t self-care activities

Nausea r/t chemotherapy

Acute **Pain** r/t surgical procedure

Sexual Dysfunction r/t change in body image, fear of loss of femininity

Chronic **Sorrow** r/t disturbed body image, unknown long-term health status

Spiritual Distress r/t change in body image

Risk for **Infection:** Risk factors: surgical procedure; broken skin

Risk for impaired physical **Mobility:** Risk factors: nerve or muscle damage, pain

Risk for **Post-Trauma Syndrome:** Risk factors: loss of body part, surgical wounds

Risk for **Powerlessness:** Risk factor: fear of unknown outcome of procedure

Risk for compromised **Resilience:** Risk factor: altered body image

See Cancer; Modified Radical Mastectomy; Surgery, Perioperative; Surgery, Postoperative; Surgery, Preoperative

MASTITIS

Anxiety r/t threat to self, concern over safety of milk for infant

Ineffective **Breastfeeding** r/t breast pain, conflicting advice from health care providers

Deficient **Knowledge** r/t antibiotic regimen, comfort measures

Acute **Pain** r/t infectious disease process, swelling of breast tissue

Ineffective **Role Performance** r/t change in capacity to function in expected role

Risk for disturbed **Maternal/Fetal Dyad:** Risk factors: interrupted/ineffective breastfeeding

MATERNAL INFECTION

Ineffective **Protection** r/t invasive procedures, traumatized tissue

See Postpartum, Normal Care

MATURATIONAL ISSUES, ADOLESCENT

Ineffective **Childbearing Process** r/t unwanted pregnancy/lack of support system

Ineffective **Coping** r/t maturational crises

Risk-prone **Health Behavior** r/t inadequate comprehension, negative attitude toward health care

Interrupted **Family Processes** r/t developmental crises of adolescence

M

resulting from challenge of parental authority and values, situational crises from change in parental marital status

Deficient **Knowledge**: potential for enhanced health maintenance r/t information misinterpretation, lack of education regarding age-related factors

Impaired **Social Interaction** r/t ineffective, unsuccessful, or dysfunctional interaction with peers

Social Isolation r/t perceived alteration in physical appearance, social values not accepted by dominant peer group

Risk for Ineffective **Activity Planning** r/t unrealistic perception of personal competencies

Risk for **Injury/Trauma**: Risk factor: thrill-seeking behaviors

Risk for disturbed personal **Identity** r/t maturational issues

Risk for chronic low **Self-Esteem** r/t lack of sense of belonging in peer group

Risk for situational low **Self-Esteem**: Risk factor: developmental changes

Readiness for enhanced **Communication**: expressing willingness to communicate with parental figures

Readiness for enhanced **Relationship**: expresses desire to enhance communication with parental figures

See Sexuality, Adolescent; Substance Abuse (if relevant)

MAZE III PROCEDURE

See Dysrhythmia; Open Heart Surgery

MD (MUSCULAR DYSTROPHY)

See Muscular Dystrophy (MD)

MEASLES (RUBEOLA)

See Communicable Diseases, Childhood

MECONIUM ASPIRATION

See Respiratory Conditions of the Neonate

MECONIUM DELAYED

Risk for neonatal **Jaundice** r/t inadequate breast milk intake

MELANOMA

Disturbed **Body Image** r/t altered pigmentation, surgical incision

Fear r/t threat to well-being

Ineffective **Health Maintenance** r/t deficient knowledge regarding self-care and treatment of melanoma

Acute **Pain** r/t surgical incision

Readiness for enhanced **Self-Health Management**: describes reduction of risk factors; protection from sunlight's ultraviolet rays

See Cancer

MELENA

Fear r/t presence of blood in feces

Risk for imbalanced **Fluid Volume**: Risk factor: hemorrhage

See GI Bleed (Gastrointestinal Bleeding)

MEMORY DEFICIT

Impaired **Memory** (See **Memory**, impaired, Section II)

MÉNIÈRE'S DISEASE

Risk for **Injury**: Risk factor: symptoms from disease

Readiness for enhanced **Self-Health Management**: expresses desire to manage illness

See Dizziness; Nausea; Vertigo

MENINGITIS/ENCEPHALITIS

Ineffective **Airway Clearance** r/t seizure activity

Impaired **Comfort** r/t altered health status

Excess **Fluid Volume** r/t increased intracranial pressure, syndrome of inappropriate secretion of antidiuretic hormone

Delayed **Growth and Development** r/t effects of physical disability

Decreased **Intracranial Adaptive Capacity** r/t sustained increase in intracranial pressure of 10 to 15 mm Hg

Impaired **Mobility** r/t neuromuscular or central nervous system insult

Acute **Pain** r/t biological injury

Risk for **Aspiration:** Risk factor: seizure activity

Risk for acute **Confusion:** Risk factor: infection of brain

Risk for **Falls:** Risk factor: neuromuscular dysfunction

Risk for **Injury:** Risk factor: seizure activity

Risk for compromised **Resilience:** Risk factor: illness

Risk for **Shock:** Risk factor: infection

Risk for ineffective **Cerebral** tissue perfusion: Risk factors: Inflamed cerebral tissues and meninges, increased intracranial pressure; infection

Readiness for enhanced **Immunization Status:** expresses desire to enhance immunization status and knowledge of immunization standards

See Hospitalized Child

MENINGOCELE

See Neural Tube Defects

MENOPAUSE

Impaired **Comfort** r/t symptoms associated with menopause

Insomnia r/t hormonal shifts

Impaired **Memory** r/t change in hormonal levels

Sexual Dysfunction r/t menopausal changes

Ineffective **Sexuality Pattern** r/t altered body structure, lack of physiological lubrication, lack of knowledge of artificial lubrication

Ineffective **Thermoregulation** r/t changes in hormonal levels

Risk for urge urinary **Incontinence:** Risk factor: changes in hormonal levels affecting bladder function

Risk for imbalanced **Nutrition:** more than body requirements: Risk factor: change in metabolic rate caused by fluctuating hormone levels

Risk for **Powerlessness:** Risk factor: changes associated with menopause

Risk for compromised **Resilience:** Risk factor: menopause

Risk for situational low **Self-Esteem:** Risk factors: developmental changes, menopause

Readiness for enhanced **Self-Care:** expresses satisfaction with body image

Readiness for enhanced **Self-Health Management:** verbalized desire to manage menopause

Readiness for enhanced **Spiritual Well-Being:** desire for harmony of mind, body, and spirit

M

MENORRHAGIA

Fear r/t loss of large amounts of blood

Risk for deficient **Fluid Volume:** Risk factor: excessive loss of menstrual blood

MENTAL ILLNESS

Compromised family **Coping** r/t lack of available support from client

Defensive **Coping** r/t psychological impairment, substance abuse

Disabled family **Coping** r/t chronically unexpressed feelings of guilt, anxiety, hostility, or despair

Ineffective **Coping** r/t situational crisis, coping with mental illness

Ineffective **Denial** r/t refusal to acknowledge abuse problem, fear of the social stigma of disease

Risk-prone **Health Behavior** r/t low self-efficacy

Disturbed personal **Identity** r/t psychoses

Ineffective **Relationship** r/t effects of mental illness in partner relationship

Chronic **Sorrow** r/t presence of mental illness

Stress overload r/t multiple coexisting stressors

Ineffective family **Therapeutic Regimen Management** r/t chronicity of condition, unpredictability of client, unknown prognosis

Risk for **Loneliness:** Risk factor: social isolation

Risk for **Powerlessness:** Risk factor: lifestyle of helplessness

Risk for compromised **Resilience:** Risk factor: chronic illness

Risk for chronic low **Self-Esteem** r/t presence of mental illness/repeated negative reinforcement

MENTAL RETARDATION

Impaired verbal **Communication** r/t developmental delay

Interrupted **Family Processes** r/t crisis of diagnosis and situational transition

Grieving r/t loss of perfect child, birth of child with congenital defect or subsequent head injury

Delayed **Growth and Development** r/t cognitive or perceptual impairment, developmental delay

Deficient community **Health** r/t lack of programs to address developmental deficiencies

Impaired **Home Maintenance** r/t insufficient support systems

Self-Neglect r/t learning disability

Self-Care deficit: bathing, dressing, feeding, toileting r/t perceptual or cognitive impairment

Self-Mutilation r/t inability to express tension verbally

Social Isolation r/t delay in accomplishing developmental tasks

Spiritual Distress r/t chronic condition of child with special needs

Stress overload r/t intense, repeated stressor (chronic condition)

Impaired **Swallowing** r/t neuromuscular impairment

Risk for ineffective **Activity Planning** r/t inability to process information

Risk for delayed **Development:** Risk factor: cognitive or perceptual impairment

Risk for disproportionate **Growth:** Risk factor: mental retardation

Risk for impaired **Religiosity:** Risk factor: social isolation

Risk for **Self-Mutilation:** Risk factors: separation anxiety, depersonalization

Readiness for enhanced family **Coping:** adaptation and acceptance of child's condition and needs

See Child with Chronic Condition; Safety, Childhood

METABOLIC ACIDOSIS

See Ketoacidosis, Alcoholic; Ketoacidosis, Diabetic

METABOLIC ALKALOSIS

Deficient **Fluid Volume** r/t fluid volume loss, vomiting, gastric suctioning, failure of regulatory mechanisms

METASTASIS

See Cancer

METHICILLIN-RESISTANT *STAPHYLOCOCCUS AUREUS* (MRSA)

See MRSA (Methicillin-Resistant Staphylococcus aureus*)*

MI (MYOCARDIAL INFARCTION)

Anxiety r/t threat of death, possible change in role status

Decreased **Cardiac Output** r/t ventricular damage, ischemia, dysrhythmias

Constipation r/t decreased peristalsis from decreased physical activity, medication effect, change in diet

Ineffective family **Coping** r/t spouse or significant other's fear of partner loss

Death **Anxiety** r/t seriousness of medical condition

Ineffective **Denial** r/t fear, deficient knowledge about heart disease

Interrupted **Family Processes** r/t crisis, role change

Fear r/t threat to well-being

Ineffective **Health Maintenance** r/t deficient knowledge regarding self-care and treatment

Acute **Pain** r/t myocardial tissue damage from inadequate blood supply

Situational low **Self-Esteem** r/t crisis of MI

Ineffective **Sexuality Pattern** r/t fear of chest pain, possibility of heart damage

Risk for **Powerlessness**: Risk factor: acute illness

Risk for **Shock**: Risk factors: hypotension, hypoxia

Risk for **Spiritual Distress**: Risk factors: physical illness: MI

Risk for decreased **Cardiac** tissue perfusion: Risk factors: coronary artery spasm, hypertension, hypoxia

Readiness for enhanced **Knowledge**: expresses an interest in learning about condition

See Angioplasty (Coronary); Coronary Artery Bypass Grafting (CABG)

MIDCAB (MINIMALLY INVASIVE DIRECT CORONARY ARTERY BYPASS)

Risk for **Bleeding**: Risk factor: surgery

Risk for **Infection**: Risk factor: large breasts on incision line

Readiness for enhanced **Self-Health Management**: pre- and postoperative care associated with the surgery

See Angioplasty, Coronary; Coronary Artery Bypass Grafting (CABG)

MIDLIFE CRISIS

Ineffective **Coping** r/t inability to deal with changes associated with aging

Powerlessness r/t lack of control over life situation

Spiritual Distress r/t questioning beliefs or value system

Risk for disturbed personal **Identity** r/t social role change

Risk for chronic low **Self-Esteem**

Readiness for enhanced **Relationship**: meets goals for lifestyle change

Readiness for enhanced **Spiritual Well-Being**: desire to find purpose and meaning to life

MIGRAINE HEADACHE

Impaired **Comfort** r/t altered health status

Disturbed **Energy Field** r/t pain, disruption of normal flow of energy

Ineffective **Health Maintenance** r/t deficient knowledge regarding prevention and treatment of headaches

Acute **Pain**: headache r/t vasodilation of cerebral and extracerebral vessels

Risk for compromised **Resilience**: Risk factors: chronic illness, impaired comfort

Readiness for enhanced **Self-Health Management**: expressed desire to manage the illness

MILK INTOLERANCE

See Lactose Intolerance

MINIMALLY INVASIVE DIRECT CORONARY ARTERY BYPASS (MIDCAB)

See MIDCAB (Minimally Invasive Direct Coronary Artery Bypass)

MISCARRIAGE

See Pregnancy Loss

M

MITRAL STENOSIS

Activity Intolerance r/t imbalance between oxygen supply and demand

Anxiety r/t possible worsening of symptoms, activity intolerance, fatigue

Decreased **Cardiac Output** r/t incompetent heart valves, abnormal forward or backward blood flow, flow into a dilated chamber, flow through an abnormal passage between chambers

Fatigue r/t reduced cardiac output

Ineffective **Health Maintenance** r/t deficient knowledge regarding self-care with disorder

Risk for **Infection:** Risk factors: invasive procedure, risk for endocarditis

Risk for decreased **Cardiac** tissue perfusion: Risk factor: incompetent heart valve

MITRAL VALVE PROLAPSE

Anxiety r/t symptoms of condition: palpitations, chest pain

Fatigue r/t abnormal catecholamine regulation, decreased intravascular volume

Fear r/t lack of knowledge about mitral valve prolapse, feelings of having a heart attack

Ineffective **Health Maintenance** r/t deficient knowledge regarding methods to relieve pain and treat dysrhythmia and shortness of breath, need for prophylactic antibiotics before invasive procedures

Acute **Pain** r/t mitral valve regurgitation

Risk for **Infection:** Risk factor: invasive procedures

Risk for **Powerlessness:** Risk factor: unpredictability of onset of symptoms

Risk for ineffective **Cerebral** tissue perfusion: Risk factor: postural hypotension

Readiness for enhanced **Knowledge:** expresses an interest in learning about condition

MOBILITY, IMPAIRED BED

Impaired bed **Mobility** (See **Mobility,** bed, impaired, Section II)

MOBILITY, IMPAIRED PHYSICAL

Impaired physical **Mobility** (See **Mobility,** physical, impaired, Section II)

Risk for **Falls:** Risk factor: impaired physical mobility

MOBILITY, IMPAIRED WHEELCHAIR

Impaired wheelchair **Mobility** (See **Mobility,** wheelchair, impaired, Section II)

MODIFIED RADICAL MASTECTOMY

Decisional Conflict r/t treatment of choice

Readiness for enhanced **Communication:** willingness to enhance communication

See Mastectomy

MONONUCLEOSIS

Activity Intolerance r/t generalized weakness

Impaired **Comfort** r/t sore throat, muscle aches

Fatigue r/t disease state, stress

Ineffective **Health Maintenance** r/t deficient knowledge concerning transmission and treatment of disease

Hyperthermia r/t infectious process

Acute **Pain** r/t enlargement of lymph nodes, oropharyngeal edema

Impaired **Swallowing** r/t enlargement of lymph nodes, oropharyngeal edema

Risk for **Injury:** Risk factor: possible rupture of spleen

Risk for **Loneliness:** Risk factor: social isolation

M

MOOD DISORDERS

Risk-prone **Health Behavior** r/t hopelessness, altered locus of control

Caregiver Role Strain r/t symptoms associated with disorder of care receiver

Self-Neglect r/t depression

Social Isolation r/t alterations in mental status

Risk for situational low **Self-Esteem:** Risk factor: unpredictable changes in mood

Readiness for enhanced **Communication:** expresses feelings

See specific disorder: Depression (Major Depressive Disorder); Dysthymic Disorder; Hypomania; Manic Disorder, Bipolar I

MOON FACE

Disturbed **Body Image** r/t change in appearance from disease and medication

Risk for situational low **Self-Esteem:** Risk factor: change in body image

See Cushing's Syndrome

MORAL/ETHICAL DILEMMAS

Decisional Conflict r/t questioning personal values and belief, which alter decision

Moral Distress r/t conflicting information guiding moral or ethical decision-making

Risk for **Powerlessness:** Risk factor: lack of knowledge to make a decision

Risk for **Spiritual Distress:** Risk factor: moral or ethical crisis

Readiness for enhanced **Decision-Making:** expresses desire to enhance congruency of decisions with personal values and goals

Readiness for enhanced **Religiosity:** requests assistance in expanding religious options

Readiness for enhanced **Resilience:** vulnerable state

Readiness for enhanced **Spiritual Well-Being:** request for interaction with others regarding difficult decisions

MORNING SICKNESS

See Hyperemesis Gravidarum; Pregnancy, Normal

MOTION SICKNESS

See Labyrinthitis

MOTTLING OF PERIPHERAL SKIN

Ineffective peripheral **Tissue Perfusion** r/t interruption of arterial flow, decreased circulating blood volume

Risk for **Vascular Trauma:** Risk factor: nature of solution

MOURNING

See Grieving

MOUTH LESIONS

See Mucous Membrane, Impaired Oral

MRI (MAGNETIC RESONANCE IMAGING)

Anxiety r/t fear of being in closed spaces

Deficient **Knowledge** r/t unfamiliarity with information resources; exam information

Readiness for enhanced **Knowledge:** expresses interest in learning about exam

Readiness for enhanced **Self-Health Management:** describes reduction of risk factors associated with exam

MRSA (METHICILLIN-RESISTANT *STAPHYLOCOCCUS AUREUS*)

Hyperthermia r/t infection

Impaired **Skin Integrity** r/t infection

Delayed **Surgical Recovery** r/t infection

Impaired **Tissue Integrity** r/t wound, infection

Risk for **Loneliness:** Risk factor: physical isolation

M

Risk for compromised **Resilience**: Risk factor: illness

Risk for **Shock**: Risk factor: sepsis

MUCOCUTANEOUS LYMPH NODE SYNDROME

See Kawasaki Disease

MUCOUS MEMBRANE, IMPAIRED ORAL

Impaired **Oral Mucous Membrane** (See **Oral Mucous Membrane**, impaired, Section II)

MULTIINFARCT DEMENTIA

See Dementia

MULTIPLE GESTATION

Anxiety r/t uncertain outcome of pregnancy

Insufficient **Breast Milk** r/t multiple births

Ineffective **Childbearing Process** r/t unavailable support system

Death **Anxiety** r/t maternal complications associated with multiple gestation

Fatigue r/t physiological demands of a multifetal pregnancy and/or care of more than one infant

Impaired **Home Maintenance** r/t fatigue

Stress urinary **Incontinence** r/t increased pelvic pressure

Insomnia r/t impairment of normal sleep pattern; parental responsibilities

Neonatal Jaundice r/t feeding pattern not well established

Deficient **Knowledge** r/t caring for more than one infant

Impaired physical **Mobility** r/t increased uterine size

Imbalanced **Nutrition**: less than body requirements r/t physiological demands of a multifetal pregnancy

Stress overload r/t multiple coexisting stressors, family demands

Impaired **Transfer Ability** r/t enlarged uterus

Risk for ineffective **Breastfeeding**: Risk factors: lack of support, physical demands of feeding more than one infant

Risk for **Constipation**: Risk factor: enlarged uterus

Risk for delayed **Development**: fetus: Risk factor: multiple gestation

Risk for disproportionate **Growth**: fetus: Risk factor: multiple gestation

Risk for neonatal **Jaundice** r/t feeding pattern not well-established

Readiness for enhanced **Childbearing Process**: demonstrates appropriate care for infant and mother

Readiness for enhanced **Family Processes**: family adapting to change with more than one infant

MULTIPLE PERSONALITY DISORDER (DISSOCIATIVE IDENTITY DISORDER)

Anxiety r/t loss of control of behavior and feelings

Disturbed **Body Image** r/t psychosocial changes

Defensive **Coping** r/t unresolved past traumatic events, severe anxiety

Ineffective **Coping** r/t history of abuse

Hopelessness r/t long-term stress

Disturbed personal **Identity** r/t severe child abuse

Chronic low **Self-Esteem** r/t rejection, failure

Risk for **Self-Mutilation**: Risk factor: need to act out to relieve stress

Readiness for enhanced **Communication**: willingness to discuss problems associated with condition

See Dissociative Identity Disorder (Not Otherwise Specified)

MULTIPLE SCLEROSIS (MS)

Ineffective **Activity Planning** r/t unrealistic perception of personal competence

Ineffective **Airway Clearance** r/t decreased energy or fatigue

Disturbed **Energy Field** r/t disruption in energy flow resulting from disharmony between mind and body

Impaired physical **Mobility** r/t neuromuscular impairment

Self-Neglect r/t functional impairment

Powerlessness r/t progressive nature of disease

Self-Care deficit: specify r/t neuromuscular impairment

Sexual Dysfunction r/t biopsychosocial alteration of sexuality

Chronic **Sorrow** r/t loss of physical ability

Spiritual Distress r/t perceived hopelessness of diagnosis

Urinary Retention r/t inhibition of the reflex arc

Risk for **Latex Allergy Response**: Risk factor: possible repeated exposures to latex associated with intermittent catheterizations

Risk for **Disuse Syndrome**: Risk factor: physical immobility

Risk for **Injury**: Risk factors: altered mobility, sensory dysfunction

Risk for imbalanced **Nutrition**: less than body requirements: Risk factors: impaired swallowing, depression

Risk for **Powerlessness**: Risk factor: chronic illness

Risk for impaired **Religiosity**: Risk factor: illness

Risk for **Thermal Injury** r/t neuromuscular impairment

Readiness for enhanced **Self-Care**: expresses desire to enhance knowledge of strategies and responsibility for self-care

Readiness for enhanced **Self-Health Management**: expresses a desire to manage condition

Readiness for enhanced **Spiritual Well-Being**: struggling with chronic debilitating condition

See Neurologic Disorders

MUMPS

See Communicable Diseases, Childhood

MURMURS

Decreased **Cardiac Output** r/t altered preload/afterload

Risk for decreased **Cardiac** tissue perfusion: Risk factor: incompetent valve

MUSCULAR ATROPHY/ WEAKNESS

Risk for **Disuse Syndrome**: Risk factor: impaired physical mobility

Risk for **Falls**: Risk factor: impaired physical mobility

MUSCULAR DYSTROPHY (MD)

Activity Intolerance r/t fatigue

Ineffective **Activity Planning** r/t unrealistic perception of personal competence

Ineffective **Airway Clearance** r/t muscle weakness and decreased ability to cough

Constipation r/t immobility

Disturbed **Energy Field** r/t illness

Fatigue r/t increased energy requirements to perform activities of daily living

Impaired **Mobility** r/t muscle weakness and development of contractures

Imbalanced **Nutrition**: less than body requirements r/t impaired swallowing or chewing

Imbalanced **Nutrition**: more than body requirements r/t inactivity

Self-Care deficit: feeding, bathing, dressing, toileting r/t muscle weakness and fatigue

Self-Neglect r/t functional impairment

M

Impaired **Transfer Ability** r/t muscle weakness

Impaired **Walking** r/t muscle weakness

Risk for **Aspiration**: Risk factor: impaired swallowing

Risk for ineffective **Breathing Pattern**: Risk factor: muscle weakness

Risk for **Disuse Syndrome**: Risk factor: complications of immobility

Risk for **Falls**: Risk factor: muscle weakness

Risk for impaired **Gas Exchange**: Risk factors: ineffective airway clearance and ineffective breathing pattern caused by muscle weakness

Risk for **Infection**: Risk factor: pooling of pulmonary secretions as a result of immobility and muscle weakness

Risk for **Injury**: Risk factors: muscle weakness and unsteady gait

Risk for **Powerlessness**: Risk factor: chronic condition

Risk for impaired **Religiosity**: Risk factor: illness

Risk for compromised **Resilience**: Risk factor: chronic illness

Risk for impaired **Skin Integrity**: Risk factors: immobility, braces, or adaptive devices

Risk for situational low **Self-Esteem**: Risk factor: presence of chronic condition

Risk for decreased **Cardiac** tissue perfusion: Risk factor: hypoxia associated with cardiomyopathy

Readiness for enhanced **Self-Concept**: acceptance of strength and abilities

See Child with Chronic Condition; Hospitalized Child

MVA (MOTOR VEHICLE ACCIDENT)

See Fracture; Head Injury; Injury; Pneumothorax

MYASTHENIA GRAVIS

Ineffective **Airway Clearance** r/t decreased ability to cough and swallow

Interrupted **Family Processes** r/t crisis of dealing with diagnosis

Fatigue r/t paresthesia, aching muscles

Impaired physical **Mobility** r/t defective transmission of nerve impulses at the neuromuscular junction

Imbalanced **Nutrition**: less than body requirements r/t difficulty eating and swallowing

Impaired **Swallowing** r/t neuromuscular impairment

Risk for **Caregiver Role Strain**: Risk factor: severity of illness of client

Risk for impaired **Religiosity**: Risk factor: illness

Risk for compromised **Resilience**: Risk factor: new diagnosis of chronic, serious illness

Readiness for enhanced **Spiritual Well-Being**: heightened coping with serious illness

See Neurologic Disorders

MYCOPLASMA PNEUMONIA

See Pneumonia

MYELOCELE

See Neural Tube Defects

MYELOGRAM, CONTRAST

Acute **Pain** r/t irritation of nerve roots

Urinary Retention r/t pressure on spinal nerve roots

Risk for deficient **Fluid Volume**: Risk factor: possible dehydration

Risk for ineffective **Cerebral** tissue perfusion: Risk factors: hypotension, loss of cerebrospinal fluid

MYELOMENINGOCELE

See Neural Tube Defects

MYOCARDIAL INFARCTION (MI)

See MI (Myocardial Infarction)

MYOCARDITIS

Activity Intolerance r/t reduced cardiac reserve and prescribed bed rest

Decreased **Cardiac Output** r/t altered preload/afterload

Deficient **Knowledge** r/t treatment of disease

Risk for decreased **Cardiac** tissue perfusion: Risk factors: hypoxia, hypovolemia, cardiac tamponade

Readiness for enhanced **Knowledge:** treatment of disease

See CHF (Congestive Heart Failure), if appropriate

MYRINGOTOMY

Fear r/t hospitalization, surgical procedure

Ineffective **Health Maintenance** r/t deficient knowledge regarding care after surgery

Acute **Pain** r/t surgical procedure

Risk for **Infection:** Risk factor: invasive procedure

See Ear Surgery

MYXEDEMA

See Hypothyroidism

N

NARCISSISTIC PERSONALITY DISORDER

Decisional Conflict r/t lack of realistic problem-solving skills

Defensive **Coping** r/t grandiose sense of self

Interrupted **Family Processes** r/t taking advantage of others to achieve own goals

Disturbed personal **Identity** r/t psychological impairment

Ineffective **Relationship** r/t lack of mutual support/respect between partners

Impaired individual **Resilience** r/t psychological disorders

Impaired **Social Interaction** r/t self-concept disturbance

Risk-prone **Health** behavior r/t low self-efficacy

Risk for **Loneliness** r/t inability to interact appropriately with others

Risk for **Self-Mutilation:** Risk factor: inadequate coping

NARCOLEPSY

Anxiety r/t fear of lack of control over falling asleep

Disturbed **Sleep Pattern** r/t uncontrollable desire to sleep

Risk for **Trauma:** Risk factor: falling asleep during potentially dangerous activity

Readiness for enhanced **Sleep:** expression of willingness to enhance sleep

NARCOTIC USE

Risk for **Constipation:** Risk factor: effects of opioids on peristalsis

See Substance Abuse (if relevant)

NASOGASTRIC SUCTION

Impaired **Oral Mucous Membrane** r/t presence of nasogastric tube

Risk for imbalanced **Fluid Volume:** Risk factor: loss of gastrointestinal fluids without adequate replacement

Risk for dysfunctional **Gastrointestinal Motility:** Risk factor: blockage in the intestines

NAUSEA

Nausea: biophysical, situational, treatment-related (See **Nausea,** Section II)

NEAR-DROWNING

Ineffective **Airway Clearance** r/t aspiration, impaired gas exchange

Aspiration r/t aspiration of fluid into the lungs

Fear: parental r/t possible death of child, possible permanent and debilitating sequelae

Impaired **Gas Exchange** r/t laryngospasm, holding breath, aspiration

Grieving r/t potential death of child, unknown sequelae, guilt about accident

Ineffective **Health Maintenance** r/t parental deficient knowledge regarding safety measures appropriate for age

Hypothermia r/t central nervous system injury, prolonged submersion in cold water

Risk for delayed **Development/** disproportionate **Growth:** Risk factors: hypoxemia, cerebral anoxia

Risk for complicated **Grieving:** Risk factors: potential death of child, unknown sequelae, guilt about accident

Risk for **Infection:** Risk factors: aspiration, invasive monitoring

Risk for ineffective **Cerebral** tissue perfusion: Risk factor: hypoxia

Readiness for enhanced **Spiritual Well-Being:** struggle with survival of life-threatening situation

See Child with Chronic Condition; Hospitalized Child; Safety, Childhood; Terminally Ill Child/Death of Child, Parent

NEARSIGHTEDNESS

Readiness for enhanced **Self-Health Management:** early diagnosis and appropriate referral for eyeglasses or contact lenses when nearsightedness is suspected; signs that may indicate a vision problem, including sitting close to television, holding books very close when reading, or having difficulty reading the blackboard in school or signs on a wall

NEARSIGHTEDNESS; CORNEAL SURGERY

See LASIK Eye Surgery (Laser-Assisted in Situ Keratomileusis)

NECK VEIN DISTENTION

Decreased **Cardiac Output** r/t decreased contractility of heart resulting in increased preload

Excess **Fluid Volume** r/t excess fluid intake, compromised regulatory mechanisms

See CHF (Congestive Heart Failure)

NECROSIS, RENAL TUBULAR; ATN (ACUTE TUBULAR NECROSIS); NECROSIS, ACUTE TUBULAR

See Renal Failure

NECROTIZING ENTEROCOLITIS (NEC)

Ineffective **Breathing Pattern** r/t abdominal distention, hypoxia

Diarrhea r/t infection

Disturbed **Energy Field** r/t illness

Deficient **Fluid Volume** r/t vomiting, gastrointestinal bleeding

Neonatal **Jaundice** r/t feeding pattern not well-established

Imbalanced **Nutrition:** less than body requirements r/t decreased ability to absorb nutrients, decreased perfusion to gastrointestinal tract

Risk for **Infection:** Risk factors: bacterial invasion of gastrointestinal tract, invasive procedures

Risk for dysfunctional **Gastrointestinal Motility:** Risk factor: infection

Risk for ineffective **Gastrointestinal Perfusion:** Risk factors: shunting of blood away from mesenteric circulation and toward vital organs as a result of perinatal stress, hypoxia

See Hospitalized Child; Premature Infant (Child)

N

NECROTIZING FASCIITIS (FLESH-EATING BACTERIA)

Decreased **Cardiac Output** r/t tachycardia and hypotension

Fear r/t possible fatal outcome of disease

Grieving r/t poor prognosis associated with disease

Hyperthermia r/t presence of infection

Acute **Pain** r/t toxins interfering with blood flow

Ineffective peripheral **Tissue Perfusion** r/t thrombosis of the subcutaneous blood vessels, leading to necrosis of nerve fibers

Ineffective **Protection** r/t cellulites resistant to treatment

Risk for **Shock:** Risk factors: infection; sepsis

See Renal Failure; Septicemia; Shock, Septic

NEGATIVE FEELINGS ABOUT SELF

Self-Neglect r/t negative feelings

Chronic low **Self-esteem** r/t long-standing negative self-evaluation

Situational low **Self-esteem** r/t inappropriate learned negative feelings about self

Readiness for enhanced **Self-Concept:** expresses willingness to enhance self-concept

NEGLECT, UNILATERAL

Unilateral Neglect (See **Unilateral Neglect,** Section II)

NEGLECTFUL CARE OF FAMILY MEMBER

Caregiver Role Strain r/t care demands of family member, lack of social or financial support

Disabled family **Coping** r/t highly ambivalent family relationships, lack of respite care

Interrupted **Family Processes** r/t situational transition or crisis

Deficient **Knowledge** r/t care needs

Impaired individual **Resilience** r/t vulnerability from neglect

Risk for compromised **Human Dignity:** Risk factor: inadequate participation in decision-making

NEONATAL JAUNDICE

Neonatal **Jaundice** (See Neonatal **Jaundice,** Section II)

NEONATE

Readiness for enhanced **Childbearing Process:** appropriate care of newborn

See Newborn, Normal; Newborn, Postmature; Newborn, Small for Gestational Age (SGA)

NEOPLASM

Fear r/t possible malignancy

See Cancer

NEPHRECTOMY

Anxiety r/t surgical recovery, prognosis

Ineffective **Breathing Pattern** r/t location of surgical incision

Constipation r/t lack of return of peristalsis

Acute **Pain** r/t incisional discomfort

Spiritual Distress r/t chronic illness

Impaired **Urinary Elimination** r/t loss of kidney

Risk for **Bleeding:** Risk factor: surgery

Risk for **Electrolyte Imbalance:** Risk factor: renal dysfunction

Risk for imbalanced **Fluid Volume:** Risk factors: vascular losses, decreased intake

Risk for **Infection:** Risk factors: invasive procedure, lack of deep breathing because of location of surgical incision

Risk for ineffective **Renal Perfusion:** Risk factor: renal disease

N

NEPHROSTOMY, PERCUTANEOUS

Acute **Pain** r/t invasive procedure

Impaired **Urinary Elimination** r/t nephrostomy tube

Risk for **Infection:** Risk factor: invasive procedure

NEPHROTIC SYNDROME

Activity Intolerance r/t generalized edema

Disturbed **Body Image** r/t edematous appearance and side effects of steroid therapy

Excess **Fluid Volume** r/t edema resulting from oncotic fluid shift caused by serum protein loss and renal retention of salt and water

Imbalanced **Nutrition:** less than body requirements r/t anorexia, protein loss

Imbalanced **Nutrition:** more than body requirements r/t increased appetite attributable to steroid therapy

Social Isolation r/t edematous appearance

Risk for **Infection:** Risk factor: altered immune mechanisms caused by disease and effects of steroids

Risk for ineffective **Renal Perfusion:** Risk factor: renal disease

Risk for impaired **Skin Integrity:** Risk factor: edema

See Child with Chronic Condition; Hospitalized Child

NERVE ENTRAPMENT

See Carpal Tunnel Syndrome

NEURAL TUBE DEFECTS (MENINGOCELE, MYELOMENINGOCELE, SPINA BIFIDA, ANENCEPHALY)

Constipation r/t immobility or less than adequate mobility

Grieving r/t loss of perfect child, birth of child with congenital defect

Delayed **Growth and Development** r/t physical impairments, possible cognitive impairment

Reflex urinary **Incontinence** r/t neurogenic impairment

Total urinary **Incontinence** r/t neurogenic impairment

Urge urinary **Incontinence** r/t neurogenic impairment

Impaired **Mobility** r/t neuromuscular impairment

Chronic low **Self-Esteem** r/t perceived differences, decreased ability to participate in physical and social activities at school

Impaired **Skin Integrity** r/t incontinence

Risk for **Latex Allergy Response:** Risk factor: multiple exposures to latex products

Risk for imbalanced **Nutrition:** more than body requirements: Risk factors: diminished, limited, or impaired physical activity

Risk for **Powerlessness:** Risk factor: debilitating disease

Risk for impaired **Skin Integrity:** lower extremities: Risk factor: decreased sensory perception

Readiness for enhanced family **Coping:** effective adaptive response by family members

Readiness for enhanced **Family Processes:** family supports each other

See Child with Chronic Condition; Premature Infant (Child)

NEURALGIA

See Trigeminal Neuralgia

NEURITIS (PERIPHERAL NEUROPATHY)

Activity Intolerance r/t pain with movement

Ineffective **Health Maintenance** r/t deficient knowledge regarding self-care with neuritis

Acute **Pain** r/t stimulation of affected nerve endings, inflammation of sensory nerves

See Neuropathy, Peripheral

NEUROFIBROMATOSIS

Disturbed **Energy Field** r/t disease

Compromised **Family** coping r/t cost and emotional needs of disease

Impaired **Skin Integrity** r/t café-au-lait spots

Risk for delayed **Development:** learning disorders including attention deficit hyperactivity disorder, low intelligent quotient scores, and developmental delay: Risk factor: genetic disorder

Risk for disproportionate **Growth:** short stature, precocious puberty, delayed maturation, thyroid disorders: Risk factor: genetic disorder

Risk for **Injury:** Risk factor: possible problems with balance

Risk for decreased **Cardiac** tissue perfusion: Risk factor: hypertension

Risk for compromised **Resilience:** Risk factor: presence of chronic disease

Risk for **Spiritual Distress:** Risk factor: possible severity of disease

Readiness for enhanced **Decision-Making:** expresses desire to enhance understanding of choices and meaning of choices, genetic counseling

Readiness for enhanced **Self-Health Management:** seeks cancer screening, education and genetic counseling

See Abdominal Distention; Surgery, Perioperative; Surgery, Postoperative; Surgery, Preoperative

NEUROGENIC BLADDER

Overflow urinary **Incontinence** r/t detrusor external sphincter dyssynergia

Reflex urinary **Incontinence** r/t neurological impairment

Urinary Retention r/t interruption in the lateral spinal tracts

Risk for **Latex Allergy** response: Risk factors: repeated exposures to latex associated with possible repeated catheterizations

NEUROLOGIC DISORDERS

Ineffective **Airway Clearance** r/t perceptual or cognitive impairment, decreased energy, fatigue

Acute **Confusion** r/t dementia, alcohol abuse, drug abuse, delirium

Ineffective **Coping** r/t disability requiring change in lifestyle

Risk for dry **Eye** r/t lagophthalmos (lack of spontaneous blink reflex)

Disturbed **Energy Field** r/t illness

Interrupted **Family Processes** r/t situational crisis, illness, or disability of family member

Grieving r/t loss of usual body functioning

Impaired **Home Maintenance** r/t client's or family member's disease

Impaired **Memory** r/t neurological disturbance

Impaired physical **Mobility** r/t neuromuscular impairment

Imbalanced **Nutrition:** less than body requirements r/t impaired swallowing, depression, difficulty feeding self

Powerlessness r/t progressive nature of disease

Self-Care deficit: specify r/t neuromuscular dysfunction

Sexual Dysfunction r/t biopsychosocial alteration of sexuality

Social Isolation r/t altered state of wellness

Impaired **Swallowing** r/t neuromuscular dysfunction

N

Wandering r/t cognitive impairment

Risk for Disuse Syndrome: Risk factors: physical immobility, neuromuscular dysfunction

Risk for Injury: Risk factors: altered mobility, sensory dysfunction, cognitive impairment

Risk for ineffective Cerebral tissue perfusion: Risk factor: cerebral disease/injury

Risk for impaired Religiosity: Risk factor: life transition

Risk for impaired Skin Integrity: Risk factors: altered sensation, altered mental status, paralysis

See specific condition: Alcohol Withdrawal; Amyotrophic Lateral Sclerosis (ALS); CVA (Cerebrovascular Accident); Delirium; Dementia; Guillain-Barré Syndrome; Head Injury; Huntington's Disease; Multiple Sclerosis (MS); Myasthenia Gravis; Muscular Dystrophy; Parkinson's Disease

NEUROPATHY, PERIPHERAL

Chronic Pain r/t damage to nerves in the peripheral nervous system as a result of medication side effects, vitamin deficiency, or diabetes

Ineffective Thermoregulation r/t decreased ability to regulate body temperature

Risk for Injury: Risk factors: lack of muscle control, decreased sensation

Risk for Thermal Injury r/t nerve damage

See Peripheral Vascular Disease (PVD)

NEUROSURGERY

See Craniectomy/Craniotomy

NEWBORN, NORMAL

Breastfeeding r/t normal oral structure and gestational age greater than 34 weeks

Ineffective Protection r/t immature immune system

Ineffective Thermoregulation r/t immaturity of neuroendocrine system

Risk for Sudden Infant Death Syndrome: Risk factors: lack of knowledge regarding infant sleeping in prone or side-lying position, prenatal or postnatal infant smoke exposure, infant overheating or overwrapping, loose articles in the sleep environment

Risk for Infection: Risk factor: open umbilical stump

Risk for Injury: Risk factors: immaturity, need for caretaking

Readiness for enhanced Childbearing Process: appropriate care of newborn

Readiness for enhanced organized Infant behavior: demonstrates adaptive response to pain

Readiness for enhanced Parenting: providing emotional and physical needs of infant

NEWBORN, POSTMATURE

Hypothermia r/t depleted stores of subcutaneous fat

Impaired Skin Integrity r/t cracked and peeling skin as a result of decreased vernix

Risk for ineffective Airway Clearance: Risk factor: meconium aspiration

Risk for unstable blood Glucose level: Risk factor: depleted glycogen stores

Risk for Injury: Risk factor: hypoglycemia caused by depleted glycogen stores

NEWBORN, SMALL FOR GESTATIONAL AGE (SGA)

Neonatal Jaundice r/t neonate age and difficulty feeding

Imbalanced Nutrition: less than body requirements r/t history of placental insufficiency

Ineffective Thermoregulation r/t decreased brown fat, subcutaneous fat

Risk for Sudden Infant Death Syndrome: Risk factor: low birth weight

Risk for delayed **Development**: Risk factor: history of placental insufficiency

Risk for disproportionate **Growth**: Risk factor: history of placental insufficiency

Risk for **Injury**: Risk factors: hypoglycemia, perinatal asphyxia, meconium aspiration

NICOTINE ADDICTION

Risk-prone **Health Behavior** r/t smoking

Ineffective **Health Maintenance** r/t lack of ability to make a judgment about smoking cessation

Powerlessness r/t perceived lack of control over ability to give up nicotine

Readiness for enhanced **Decision-Making**: expresses desire to enhance understanding and meaning of choices

Readiness for enhanced **Self-Health Management**: expresses desire to learn measures to stop smoking

NIDDM (NON–INSULIN-DEPENDENT DIABETES MELLITUS)

Readiness for enhanced **Self-Health Management**: expresses desire for information on exercise and diet to manage diabetes

See Diabetes Mellitus

NIGHTMARES

Disturbed **Energy Field** r/t disharmony of body and mind

Post-Trauma Syndrome r/t disaster, war, epidemic, rape, assault, torture, catastrophic illness, or accident

NIPPLE SORENESS

Impaired **Comfort** r/t physical condition

See Painful Breasts, Sore Nipples

NOCTURIA

Urge urinary **Incontinence** r/t decreased bladder capacity, irritation of bladder stretch receptors causing spasm, alcohol, caffeine, increased fluids, increased urine concentration, overdistention of bladder

Impaired **Urinary Elimination** r/t sensory motor impairment, urinary tract infection

Risk for **Powerlessness**: Risk factor: inability to control nighttime voiding

NOCTURNAL MYOCLONUS

See Restless Leg Syndrome; Stress

NOCTURNAL PAROXYSMAL DYSPNEA

See PND (Paroxysmal Nocturnal Dyspnea)

NONCOMPLIANCE

Noncompliance (See **Noncompliance**, Section II)

NON-INSULIN-DEPENDENT DIABETES MELLITUS (NIDDM)

See Diabetes Mellitus

NORMAL PRESSURE HYDROCEPHALUS (NPH)

Impaired verbal **Communication** r/t obstruction of flow of cerebrospinal fluid

Acute **Confusion** r/t dementia caused by obstruction to flow of cerebrospinal fluid

Impaired **Memory** r/t neurological disturbance

Risk for **Falls**: Risk factor: unsteady gait as a result of obstruction of cerebrospinal fluid

Risk for ineffective **Cerebral** tissue perfusion: Risk factor: fluid pressing on the brain

NORWALK VIRUS

See Viral Gastroenteritis

NSTEMI (NON–ST-ELEVATION MYOCARDIAL INFARCTION)

See MI (Myocardial Infarction)

N

NURSING

*See Breastfeeding, Effective;
Breastfeeding, Ineffective;
Breastfeeding, Interrupted*

NUTRITION

Readiness for enhanced **Nutrition** (See
Nutrition, readiness for enhanced,
Section II)

NUTRITION, IMBALANCED

Imbalanced **Nutrition:** less than body
requirements (See **Nutrition:** less
than body requirements, imbalanced,
Section II)

Imbalanced **Nutrition:** more than body
requirements (See **Nutrition:** more
than body requirements, imbalanced,
Section II)

Risk for imbalanced **Nutrition:** more than
body requirements (See **Nutrition:** more
than body requirements, imbalanced,
risk for, Section II)

OBESITY

Disturbed **Body Image** r/t eating
disorder, excess weight

Risk-prone **Health Behavior:** r/t negative
attitude toward health care

Imbalanced **Nutrition:** more than body
requirements r/t caloric intake exceeding
energy expenditure

Chronic low **Self-Esteem** r/t ineffective
coping, overeating

Risk for ineffective peripheral **Tissue
Perfusion** r/t sedentary lifestyle or
concurrent illnesses: hypertension/
diabetes mellitus

Readiness for enhanced **Nutrition:**
expresses willingness to enhance nutrition

OBS (ORGANIC BRAIN SYNDROME)

See Organic Mental Disorders

OBSESSIVE-COMPULSIVE DISORDER (OCD)

*See OCD (Obsessive-Compulsive
Disorder)*

OBSTRUCTION, BOWEL

See Bowel Obstruction

OBSTRUCTIVE SLEEP APNEA

Insomnia r/t blocked airway

Imbalanced **Nutrition:** more than body
requirements r/t excessive intake related
to metabolic need

*See PND (Paroxysmal Nocturnal
Dyspnea)*

OCD (OBSESSIVE-COMPULSIVE DISORDER)

Ineffective Activity planning r/t
unrealistic perception of events

Anxiety r/t threat to self-concept, unmet
needs

Decisional Conflict r/t inability to make
a decision for fear of reprisal

Disabled family **Coping** r/t family process
being disrupted by client's ritualistic
activities

Ineffective **Coping** r/t expression
of feelings in an unacceptable way,
ritualistic behavior

Risk-prone **Health Behavior** r/t
inadequate comprehension associated
with repetitive thoughts

Powerlessness r/t unrelenting
repetitive thoughts to perform irrational
activities

Impaired individual **Resilience** r/t
psychological disorder

Risk for situational low **Self-Esteem:**
Risk factor: inability to control repetitive
thoughts and actions

ODD (OPPOSITIONAL DEFIANT DISORDER)

Anxiety r/t feelings of anger and hostility
toward authority figures

Ineffective **Coping** r/t lack of self-control or perceived lack of self-control

Disabled **Family** coping r/t feelings of anger, hostility; defiant behavior toward authority figures

Risk-prone **Health Behavior** r/t multiple stressors associated with condition

Ineffective **Impulse Control** r/t anger/compunction to engage in disruptive behaviors

Chronic or situational low **Self-Esteem** r/t poor self-control and disruptive behaviors

Impaired **Social Interaction** r/t being touchy or easily annoyed, blaming others for own mistakes, constant trouble in school

Social Isolation r/t unaccepted social behavior

Ineffective family **Therapeutic Regimen Management** r/t difficulty in limit setting and managing oppositional behaviors

Risk for ineffective **Activity Planning** r/t unrealistic perception of events/hedonism

Risk for Impaired **Parenting:** Risk factors: children's difficult behaviors and inability to set limits

Risk for **Powerlessness:** Risk factor: inability to deal with difficulty behaviors

Risk for **Spiritual Distress:** Risk factors: anxiety and stress in dealing with difficulty behaviors

Risk for other-directed **Violence:** Risk factors: history of violence, threats of violence against others; history of antisocial behavior; history of indirect violence

OLDER ADULT

See Aging

OLIGURIA

Deficient **Fluid Volume** r/t active fluid loss, failure of regulatory mechanism

See Cardiac Output, Decreased; Renal Failure; Shock, Hypovolemic

OMPHALOCELE

See Gastroschisis/Omphalocele

OOPHORECTOMY

Risk for ineffective **Sexuality Pattern:** Risk factor: altered body function

See Surgery, Perioperative; Surgery, Postoperative; Surgery, Preoperative

OPCAB (OFF-PUMP CORONARY ARTERY BYPASS)

See Angioplasty, Coronary; Coronary Artery Bypass Grafting (CABG)

OPEN HEART SURGERY

Risk for decreased **Cardiac** tissue perfusion: Risk factor: cardiac surgery

See Coronary Artery Bypass Grafting (CABG); Dysrhythmia

OPEN REDUCTION OF FRACTURE WITH INTERNAL FIXATION (FEMUR)

Anxiety r/t outcome of corrective procedure

Impaired physical **Mobility** r/t postoperative position, abduction of leg, avoidance of acute flexion

Powerlessness r/t loss of control, unanticipated change in lifestyle

Risk for **Perioperative Positioning Injury:** Risk factor: immobilization

Risk for **Peripheral Neurovascular Dysfunction:** Risk factors: mechanical compression, orthopedic surgery, immobilization

See Surgery, Postoperative Care

OPIATE USE

Risk for **Constipation:** Risk factor: effects of opiates on peristalsis

See Drug Abuse; Drug Withdrawal

OPPORTUNISTIC INFECTION

Delayed **Surgical Recovery** r/t abnormal blood profiles, impaired healing

O

Risk for **Infection**: Risk factor: abnormal blood profiles

See AIDS (Acquired Immunodeficiency Syndrome); HIV (Human Immunodeficiency Virus)

OPPOSITIONAL DEFIANT DISORDER (ODD)

See ODD (Oppositional Defiant Disorder)

ORAL MUCOUS MEMBRANE, IMPAIRED

Impaired **Oral Mucous Membrane** (See **Oral Mucous Membrane**, impaired, Section II)

ORAL THRUSH

See Candidiasis, Oral

ORCHITIS

Readiness for enhanced **Self-Health Management**: follows recommendations for mumps vaccination

See Epididymitis

ORGANIC MENTAL DISORDERS

Adult **Failure to Thrive** r/t undetected organic mental disorder

Impaired **Social Interaction** r/t disturbed thought processes

Risk for **Injury**: Risk factors: disorientation to time, place, person

Risk for disturbed personal **Identity** r/t delusions/fluctuating perceptions of stimuli

See Dementia

ORTHOPEDIC TRACTION

Ineffective **Role Performance** r/t limited physical mobility

Impaired **Social Interaction** r/t limited physical mobility

Impaired **Transfer Ability** r/t limited physical mobility

Risk for impaired **Religiosity**: Risk factor: immobility

See Traction and Casts

ORTHOPNEA

Ineffective **Breathing Pattern** r/t inability to breathe with head of bed flat

Decreased **Cardiac Output** r/t inability of heart to meet demands of body

ORTHOSTATIC HYPOTENSION

See Dizziness

OSTEOARTHRITIS

Activity Intolerance r/t pain after exercise or use of joint

Acute **Pain** r/t movement

Impaired **Transfer Ability** r/t pain

See Arthritis

OSTEOMYELITIS

Deficient **Diversional Activity** r/t prolonged immobilization, hospitalization

Fear: parental r/t concern regarding possible growth plate damage caused by infection, concern that infection may become chronic

Ineffective **Health Maintenance** r/t continued immobility at home, possible extensive casts, continued antibiotics

Hyperthermia r/t infectious process

Impaired physical **Mobility** r/t imposed immobility as a result of infected area

Acute **Pain** r/t inflammation in affected extremity

Risk for **Constipation**: Risk factor: immobility

Risk for **Infection**: Risk factor: inadequate primary and secondary defenses

Risk for impaired **Skin Integrity**: Risk factor: irritation from splint or cast

See Hospitalized Child

OSTEOPOROSIS

Deficient **Knowledge** r/t diet, exercise, need to abstain from alcohol and nicotine

Impaired physical **Mobility** r/t pain, skeletal changes

Imbalanced **Nutrition**: less than body requirements r/t inadequate intake of calcium and vitamin D

Acute **Pain** r/t fracture, muscle spasms

Risk for **Injury**: fracture: Risk factors: lack of activity, risk of falling resulting from environmental hazards, neuromuscular disorders, diminished senses, cardiovascular responses, responses to drugs

Risk for **Powerlessness**: Risk factor: debilitating disease

Readiness for enhanced **Self-Health Management**: expresses desire to manage the treatment of illness and prevent complications

OSTOMY

See Child with Chronic Condition; Colostomy; Ileal Conduit; Ileostomy

OTITIS MEDIA

Acute **Pain** r/t inflammation, infectious process

Risk for delayed **Development**: speech and language: Risk factor: frequent otitis media

Risk for **Infection**: Risk factors: eustachian tube obstruction, traumatic eardrum perforation, infectious disease process

Readiness for enhanced **Knowledge**: information on treatment and prevention of disease

OVARIAN CARCINOMA

Death **Anxiety** r/t unknown outcome, possible poor prognosis

Fear r/t unknown outcome, possible poor prognosis

Ineffective **Health Maintenance** r/t deficient knowledge regarding self-care, treatment of condition

Readiness for enhanced **Family Processes**: family functioning meets needs of client

Readiness for enhanced **Resilience**: participates in support groups

See Chemotherapy; Hysterectomy; Radiation Therapy

P

PACEMAKER

Anxiety r/t change in health status, presence of pacemaker

Death **Anxiety** r/t worry over possible malfunction of pacemaker

Deficient **Knowledge** r/t self-care program, when to seek medical attention

Acute **Pain** r/t surgical procedure

Risk for **Bleeding**: Risk factor: surgery

Risk for **Infection**: Risk factors: invasive procedure, presence of foreign body (catheter and generator)

Risk for decreased **Cardiac** tissue perfusion: Risk factor: pacemaker malfunction

Risk for **Powerlessness**: Risk factor: presence of electronic device to stimulate heart

Readiness for enhanced **Self-Health Management**: appropriate health care management of pacemaker

PAGET'S DISEASE

Disturbed **Body Image** r/t possible enlarged head, bowed tibias, kyphosis

Deficient **Knowledge** r/t appropriate diet high in protein and calcium, mild exercise

Chronic **Sorrow** r/t chronic condition with altered body image

Risk for **Trauma**: fracture: Risk factor: excessive bone destruction

P

PAIN, ACUTE

Disturbed **Energy Field** r/t unbalanced energy field

Acute **Pain** (See **Pain,** acute, Section II)

PAIN, CHRONIC

Impaired **Comfort** r/t altered health status

Disturbed **Energy Field** r/t unbalanced energy field

Chronic **Pain** (See **Pain,** chronic, Section II)

PAINFUL BREASTS, ENGORGEMENT

Impaired **Comfort** r/t physical condition

Acute **Pain** r/t distention of breast tissue

Ineffective **Role Performance** r/t change in physical capacity to assume role of breastfeeding mother

Impaired **Tissue Integrity** r/t excessive fluid in breast tissues

Risk for ineffective **Breastfeeding**: Risk factors: pain, infant's inability to latch on to engorged breast

Risk for **Infection**: Risk factor: milk stasis

Risk for disturbed **Maternal/Fetal Dyad**: Risk factor: discomfort

PAINFUL BREASTS, SORE NIPPLES

Ineffective **Breastfeeding** r/t pain

Insufficient **Breast Milk** r/t long breastfeeding time/pain response

Impaired **Comfort** r/t physical condition

Acute **Pain** r/t cracked nipples

Ineffective **Role Performance** r/t change in physical capacity to assume role of breastfeeding mother

Impaired **Skin Integrity** r/t mechanical factors involved in suckling, breastfeeding management

Risk for **Infection**: Risk factor: break in skin

PALLOR OF EXTREMITIES

Ineffective peripheral **Tissue Perfusion** r/t interruption of vascular flow

PALPITATIONS (HEART PALPITATIONS)

See Dysrhythmia

PANCREATIC CANCER

Death **Anxiety** r/t possible poor prognosis of disease process

Ineffective family **Coping** r/t poor prognosis

Fear r/t poor prognosis of the disease

Grieving r/t shortened life span

Deficient **Knowledge** r/t disease-induced diabetes, home management

Spiritual Distress r/t poor prognosis

Risk for impaired **Liver Function**: Risk factor: complications from underlying disease

See Cancer; Chemotherapy; Radiation Therapy; Surgery, Perioperative; Surgery, Postoperative; Surgery, Preoperative

PANCREATITIS

Ineffective **Breathing Pattern** r/t splinting from severe pain

Ineffective **Denial** r/t ineffective coping, alcohol use

Diarrhea r/t decrease in pancreatic secretions resulting in steatorrhea

Adult **Failure to Thrive** r/t pain

Deficient **Fluid Volume** r/t vomiting, decreased fluid intake, fever, diaphoresis, fluid shifts

Ineffective **Health Maintenance** r/t deficient knowledge concerning diet, alcohol use, medication

Nausea r/t irritation of gastrointestinal system

Imbalanced **Nutrition**: less than body requirements r/t inadequate dietary intake, increased nutritional needs as a result of acute illness, increased metabolic needs caused by increased body temperature

Acute **Pain** r/t irritation and edema of the inflamed pancreas

Chronic **Sorrow** r/t chronic illness

Readiness for enhanced **Comfort**: expresses desire to enhance comfort

PANIC DISORDER (PANIC ATTACKS)

Ineffective **Activity Planning** r/t unrealistic perception of events

Anxiety r/t situational crisis

Risk-prone **Health Behavior** r/t low self-efficacy

Ineffective **Coping** r/t personal vulnerability

Disturbed personal **Identity** r/t situational crisis

Post-Trauma Syndrome r/t previous catastrophic event

Social Isolation r/t fear of lack of control

Risk for **Loneliness**: Risk factor: inability to socially interact because of fear of losing control

Risk for **Post-Trauma Syndrome**: Risk factors: perception of the event, diminished ego strength

Risk for **Powerlessness**: Risk factor: ineffective coping skills

Readiness for enhanced **Coping**: seeks problem-oriented and emotion-oriented strategies to manage condition

See Anxiety; Anxiety Disorder

PARALYSIS

Disturbed **Body Image** r/t biophysical changes, loss of movement, immobility

Impaired **Comfort** r/t prolonged immobility

Constipation r/t effects of spinal cord disruption, inadequate fiber in diet

Ineffective **Health Maintenance** r/t deficient knowledge regarding self-care with paralysis

Impaired **Home Maintenance** r/t physical disability

Reflex urinary **Incontinence** r/t neurological impairment

Impaired physical **Mobility** r/t neuromuscular impairment

Impaired wheelchair **Mobility** r/t neuromuscular impairment

Self-Neglect r/t functional impairment

Powerlessness r/t illness-related regimen

Self-Care deficit: specify r/t neuromuscular impairment

Sexual Dysfunction r/t loss of sensation, biopsychosocial alteration

Chronic **Sorrow** r/t loss of physical mobility

Impaired **Transfer Ability** r/t paralysis

Risk for **Autonomic Dysreflexia** r/t cause of paralysis

Risk for **Latex Allergy Response**: Risk factor: possible repeated urinary catheterizations

Risk for **Disuse Syndrome**: Risk factor: paralysis

Risk for **Falls**: Risk factor: paralysis

Risk for **Injury**: Risk factors: altered mobility, sensory dysfunction

Risk for **Post-Trauma Syndrome**: Risk factor: event causing paralysis

Risk for impaired **Religiosity**: Risk factors: immobility, possible lack of transportation

Risk for compromised **Resilience**: Risk factor: chronic disability

Risk for situational low **Self-Esteem**: Risk factor: change in body image and function

Risk for impaired **Skin Integrity**: Risk factors: altered circulation, altered sensation, immobility

P

Risk for **Thermal Injury**

Readiness for enhanced **Self-Care:** expresses desire to enhance knowledge and responsibility for strategies for self-care

See Child with Chronic Condition; Hemiplegia; Hospitalized Child; Neural Tube Defects; Spinal Cord Injury

PARALYTIC ILEUS

Constipation r/t decreased gastric motility

Deficient **Fluid Volume** r/t loss of fluids from vomiting, retention of fluid in bowel

Dysfunctional **Gastrointestinal Motility** r/t bowel obstruction

Nausea r/t gastrointestinal irritation

Impaired **Oral Mucous Membrane** r/t presence of nasogastric tube

Acute **Pain** r/t pressure, abdominal distention

See Bowel Obstruction

PARANOID PERSONALITY DISORDER

Ineffective **Activity Planning** r/t unrealistic perception of events

Anxiety r/t uncontrollable intrusive, suspicious thoughts

Risk-prone **Health Behavior** r/t intense emotional state

Disturbed personal **Identity** r/t difficulty with reality testing

Impaired individual **Resilience** r/t psychological disorder

Chronic low **Self-Esteem** r/t inability to trust others

Social Isolation r/t inappropriate social skills

Risk for **Loneliness:** Risk factor: social isolation

Risk for **Post-Trauma Syndrome:** Risk factor: exaggerated sense of responsibility

Risk for **Suicide:** Risk factor: psychiatric illness

Risk for other-directed **Violence:** Risk factor: being suspicious of others and others' actions

PARAPLEGIA

See Spinal Cord Injury

PARATHYROIDECTOMY

Anxiety r/t surgery

Risk for ineffective **Airway Clearance:** Risk factors: edema or hematoma formation, airway obstruction

Risk for **Bleeding:** Risk factor: surgery

Risk for impaired verbal **Communication:** Risk factors: possible laryngeal damage, edema

Risk for **Infection:** Risk factor: surgical procedure

See Hypocalcemia

PARENT ATTACHMENT

Risk for impaired **Attachment** (See **Attachment,** impaired, risk for, Section II)

Readiness for enhanced **Childbearing Process:** demonstrates appropriate care of newborn

See Parental Role Conflict

PARENTAL ROLE CONFLICT

Parental **Role Conflict** (See **Role Conflict,** parental, Section II)

Ineffective **Relationship** r/t unrealistic expectations

Chronic **Sorrow** r/t difficult parent-child relationship

Risk for **Spiritual Distress:** Risk factor: altered relationships

Readiness for enhanced **Parenting:** willingness to enhance parenting

PARENTING

Readiness for enhanced **Parenting** (See **Parenting,** readiness for enhanced, Section II)

PARENTING, IMPAIRED

Impaired **Parenting** (See **Parenting,** impaired, Section II)

Chronic **Sorrow** r/t difficult parent-child relationship

Risk for **Spiritual Distress:** Risk factor: altered relationships

PARENTING, RISK FOR IMPAIRED

Risk for impaired **Parenting** (See **Parenting,** impaired, risk for, Section II)

See Parenting, Impaired

PARESTHESIA

Risk for **Injury** r/t inability to feel temperature changes, pain

Risk for impaired **Skin Integrity** r/t impaired sensation

Risk for **Thermal Injury** r/t neuromuscular impairment

PARKINSON'S DISEASE

Impaired verbal **Communication** r/t decreased speech volume, slowness of speech, impaired facial muscles

Constipation r/t weakness of defecation muscles, lack of exercise, inadequate fluid intake, decreased autonomic nervous system activity

Adult **Failure to Thrive** r/t depression associated with chronic progressive disease

Imbalanced **Nutrition:** less than body requirements r/t tremor, slowness in eating, difficulty in chewing and swallowing

Chronic **Sorrow** r/t loss of physical capacity

Risk for **Injury:** Risk factors: tremors, slow reactions, altered gait

See Neurologic Disorders

PAROXYSMAL NOCTURNAL DYSPNEA (PND)

See PND (Paroxysmal Nocturnal Dyspnea)

PATENT DUCTUS ARTERIOSUS (PDA)

See Congenital Heart Disease/Cardiac Anomalies

PATIENT-CONTROLLED ANALGESIA (PCA)

See PCA (Patient-Controlled Analgesia)

PATIENT EDUCATION

Deficient **Knowledge** r/t lack of exposure to information misinterpretation, unfamiliarity with information resources to manage illness

Readiness for enhanced **Decision-Making:** expresses desire to enhance understanding of choices for decision-making

Deficient **Knowledge** r/t lack of exposure to information, information misinterpretation

Readiness for enhanced **Knowledge** (specify): interest in learning

Readiness for enhanced **Self-Health Management:** expresses desire for information to manage the illness

Readiness for enhanced **Spiritual Well-Being:** desires to reach harmony with self, others, higher power/God

PCA (PATIENT-CONTROLLED ANALGESIA)

Impaired **Comfort** r/t condition requiring PCA, pruritus from medication side effects

Deficient **Knowledge** r/t self-care of pain control

Nausea r/t side effects of medication

Risk for **Injury:** Risk factors: possible complications associated with PCA

Risk for **Vascular Trauma:** Risk factor: insertion site and length of insertion time

Readiness for enhanced **Knowledge:** appropriate management of PCA

P

PECTUS EXCAVATUM

See Marfan Syndrome

PEDICULOSIS

See Lice

PEG (PERCUTANEOUS ENDOSCOPIC GASTROSTOMY)

See Tube Feeding

PELVIC INFLAMMATORY DISEASE (PID)

See PID (Pelvic Inflammatory Disease)

PENILE PROSTHESIS

Ineffective **Sexuality Pattern** r/t use of penile prosthesis

Risk for **Infection**: Risk factor: invasive surgical procedure

Risk for situational low **Self-Esteem**: Risk factors: ineffective sexuality pattern

Readiness for enhanced **Self-Health Management**: seeks information regarding care and use of prosthesis

See Erectile Dysfunction (ED); Impotence

PEPTIC ULCER

See Ulcer, Peptic (Duodenal or Gastric)

PERCUTANEOUS TRANSLUMINAL CORONARY ANGIOPLASTY (PTCA)

See Angioplasty, Coronary

PERICARDIAL FRICTION RUB

Decreased **Cardiac Output**

Acute **Pain** r/t inflammation, effusion

Delayed **Surgical Recovery** r/t complications associated with cardiac problems

Risk for decreased **Cardiac** tissue perfusion: Risk factors: inflammation in pericardial sac, fluid accumulation compressing heart

PERICARDITIS

Activity Intolerance r/t reduced cardiac reserve, prescribed bed rest

Decreased **Cardiac Output**

Deficient **Knowledge** r/t unfamiliarity with information sources

Acute **Pain** r/t biological injury, inflammation

Delayed **Surgical Recovery** r/t complications associated with cardiac problems

Risk for imbalanced **Nutrition**: less than body requirements r/t fever, hypermetabolic state associated with fever

Risk for decreased **Cardiac** tissue perfusion: Risk factor: inflammation in pericardial sac

PERIOPERATIVE POSITIONING

Risk for **Perioperative Positioning Injury** (See **Perioperative Positioning Injury**, risk for, Section II)

PERIPHERAL NEUROPATHY

See Neuropathy, Peripheral

PERIPHERAL NEUROVASCULAR DYSFUNCTION

Risk for **Peripheral Neurovascular Dysfunction** (See **Peripheral Neurovascular Dysfunction**, risk for, Section II)

See Neuropathy, Peripheral; Peripheral Vascular Disease (PVD)

PERIPHERAL VASCULAR DISEASE (PVD)

Activity Intolerance r/t imbalance between peripheral oxygen supply and demand

Ineffective **Health Maintenance** r/t deficient knowledge regarding self-care and treatment of disease

P

Chronic **Pain:** intermittent claudication r/t ischemia

Ineffective peripheral **Tissue Perfusion** r/t disease process

Risk for **Falls:** Risk factor: altered mobility

Risk for **Injury:** Risk factors: tissue hypoxia, altered mobility, altered sensation

Risk for **Peripheral Neurovascular Dysfunction:** Risk factor: possible vascular obstruction

Risk for impaired **Skin Integrity:** Risk factor: altered circulation or sensation

Readiness for enhanced **Self-Health Management:** self-care and treatment of disease

See Neuropathy, Peripheral; Peripheral Neurovascular Dysfunction

PERITONEAL DIALYSIS

Ineffective **Breathing Pattern** r/t pressure from dialysate

Impaired **Home Maintenance** r/t complex home treatment of client

Deficient **Knowledge** r/t treatment procedure, self-care with peritoneal dialysis

Acute **Pain** r/t instillation of dialysate, temperature of dialysate

Chronic **Sorrow** r/t chronic disability

Risk for unstable blood **Glucose** level r/t increased concentrations of glucose dialysate

Risk for ineffective **Coping:** Risk factor: disability requiring change in lifestyle

Risk for imbalanced **Fluid Volume:** Risk factor: medical procedure

Risk for **Infection:** peritoneal: Risk factor: invasive procedure, presence of catheter, dialysate

Risk for **Powerlessness:** Risk factor: chronic condition and care involved

See Child with Chronic Condition; Hemodialysis; Hospitalized Child; Renal Failure; Renal Failure, Acute/Chronic, Child

PERITONITIS

Ineffective **Breathing Pattern** r/t pain, increased abdominal pressure

Constipation r/t decreased oral intake, decrease of peristalsis

Deficient **Fluid Volume** r/t retention of fluid in bowel with loss of circulating blood volume

Nausea r/t gastrointestinal irritation

Imbalanced **Nutrition:** less than body requirements r/t nausea, vomiting

Acute **Pain** r/t inflammation, stimulation of somatic nerves

Risk for dysfunctional **Gastrointestinal Motility:** Risk factor: gastrointestinal disease

PERNICIOUS ANEMIA

Diarrhea r/t malabsorption of nutrients

Fatigue r/t imbalanced nutrition: less than body requirements

Impaired **Memory** r/t anemia; lack of adequate red blood cells

Nausea r/t altered oral mucous membrane; sore tongue, bleeding gums

Imbalanced **Nutrition:** less than body requirements r/t lack of appetite associated with nausea and altered oral mucous membrane

Impaired **Oral Mucous Membrane** r/t vitamin deficiency; inability to absorb vitamin B_{12} associated with lack of intrinsic factor

Risk for **Falls:** Risk factors: dizziness, lightheadedness

Risk for **Peripheral Neurovascular Dysfunction:** Risk factor: anemia

PERSISTENT FETAL CIRCULATION

See Congenital Heart Disease/Cardiac Anomalies

P

PERSONAL IDENTITY PROBLEMS

Disturbed personal **Identity** (See **Identity**, personal, disturbed, Section II)

Risk for disturbed personal **Identity**

PERSONALITY DISORDER

Ineffective **Activity Planning** r/t unrealistic perception of events

Impaired individual **Resilience** r/t psychological disorder

See specific disorder: Antisocial Personality Disorder; Borderline Personality Disorder; OCD (Obsessive-Compulsive Disorder); Paranoid Personality Disorder

PERTUSSIS (WHOOPING COUGH)

See Respiratory Infections, Acute Childhood

PESTICIDE CONTAMINATION

Contamination r/t use of environmental contaminants; pesticides

Risk for **Allergy Response** r/t repeated exposure to pesticides

Risk for disproportionate **Growth**: Risk factor: environmental contamination

PETECHIAE

See Anticoagulant Therapy; Clotting Disorder; DIC (Disseminated Intravascular Coagulation); Hemophilia

PETIT MAL SEIZURE

Readiness for enhanced **Self-Health Management**: wears medical alert bracelet; limits hazardous activities such as driving, swimming, working at heights, operating equipment

See Epilepsy

PHARYNGITIS

See Sore Throat

PHENYLKETONURIA (PKU)

See PKU (Phenylketonuria)

PHEOCHROMOCYTOMA

Anxiety r/t symptoms from increased catecholamines—headache, palpitations, sweating, nervousness, nausea, vomiting, syncope

Ineffective **Health Maintenance** r/t deficient knowledge regarding treatment and self-care

Insomnia r/t high levels of catecholamines

Nausea r/t increased catecholamines

Risk for adverse reaction to iodinated **Contrast** media r/t pheochromocytoma

Risk for decreased **Cardiac** tissue perfusion: Risk factor: hypertension

See Surgery, Perioperative; Surgery, Postoperative; Surgery, Preoperative

PHLEBITIS

See Thrombophlebitis

PHOBIA (SPECIFIC)

Fear r/t presence or anticipation of specific object or situation

Powerlessness r/t anxiety about encountering unknown or known entity

Impaired individual **Resilience** r/t psychological disorder

Readiness for enhanced **Power**: expresses readiness to enhance identification of choices that can be made for change

See Anxiety; Anxiety Disorder; Panic Disorder (Panic Attacks)

PHOTOSENSITIVITY

Ineffective **Health Maintenance** r/t deficient knowledge regarding medications inducing photosensitivity

Risk for dry **Eye** r/t pharmaceutical agents/sunlight exposure

Risk for impaired **Skin Integrity:** Risk factor: exposure to sun

PHYSICAL ABUSE

See Abuse, Child; Abuse, Spouse, Parent, or Significant Other

PICA

Anxiety r/t stress from urge to eat nonnutritive substances

Imbalanced **Nutrition:** less than body requirements r/t eating nonnutritive substances

Impaired **Parenting** r/t lack of supervision, food deprivation

Risk for **Constipation:** Risk factor: presence of undigestible materials in gastrointestinal tract

Risk for **Infection:** Risk factor: ingestion of infectious agents via contaminated substances

Risk for **Gastrointestinal Motility:** Risk factor: abnormal eating behavior

Risk for **Poisoning:** Risk factor: ingestion of substances containing lead

See Anemia

PID (PELVIC INFLAMMATORY DISEASE)

Ineffective **Health Maintenance** r/t deficient knowledge regarding self-care, treatment of disease

Acute **Pain** r/t biological injury; inflammation, edema, congestion of pelvic tissues

Ineffective **Sexuality Pattern** r/t medically imposed abstinence from sexual activities until acute infection subsides, change in reproductive potential

Risk for urge urinary **Incontinence:** Risk factors: inflammation, edema, congestion of pelvic tissues

Risk for **Infection:** Risk factors: insufficient knowledge to avoid exposure to pathogens; proper hygiene, nutrition, other health habits

See Maturational Issues, Adolescent; STD (Sexually Transmitted Disease)

PIH (PREGNANCY-INDUCED HYPERTENSION/PREECLAMPSIA)

Anxiety r/t fear of the unknown, threat to self and infant, change in role functioning

Death **Anxiety** r/t threat of preeclampsia

Deficient **Diversional Activity** r/t bed rest

Interrupted **Family Processes** r/t situational crisis

Impaired **Home Maintenance** r/t bed rest

Deficient **Knowledge** r/t lack of experience with situation

Impaired physical **Mobility** r/t medically prescribed limitations

Impaired **Parenting** r/t bed rest

Powerlessness r/t complication threatening pregnancy, medically prescribed limitations

Ineffective **Role Performance** r/t change in physical capacity to assume role of pregnant woman or resume other roles

Situational low **Self-Esteem** r/t loss of idealized pregnancy

Impaired **Social Interaction** r/t imposed bed rest

Risk for imbalanced **Fluid Volume:** Risk factors: hypertension, altered renal function

Risk for **Injury:** fetal: Risk factors: decreased uteroplacental perfusion, seizures

Risk for **Injury:** maternal: Risk factors: vasospasm, high blood pressure

Readiness for enhanced **Knowledge:** desire for information on managing condition

See Malignant Hypertension (Arteriolar Nephrosclerosis)

PILOERECTION

Hypothermia r/t exposure to cold environment

P

PIMPLES

See Acne

PINK EYE

See Conjunctivitis

PINWORMS

Impaired **Comfort** r/t itching

Impaired **Home Maintenance** r/t inadequate cleaning of bed linen and toilet seats

Insomnia r/t discomfort

Readiness for enhanced **Self-Health Management:** proper handwashing; short, clean fingernails; avoiding hand, mouth, nose contact with unwashed hands; appropriate cleaning of bed linen and toilet seats

PITUITARY CUSHING'S

See Cushing's Syndrome

PKU (PHENYLKETONURIA)

Risk for delayed **Development:** Risk factors: not following strict dietary program; eating foods extremely low in phenylalanine; avoiding eggs, milk, any foods containing aspartame (NutraSweet)

Readiness for enhanced **Self-Health Management:** testing for PKU and following prescribed dietary regimen

PLACENTA ABRUPTIO

Death **Anxiety** r/t threat of mortality associated with bleeding

Fear r/t threat to self and fetus

Ineffective **Health Maintenance** r/t deficient knowledge regarding treatment and control of hypertension associated with placenta abruptio

Acute **Pain:** abdominal/back r/t premature separation of placenta before delivery

Risk for **Bleeding:** Risk factor: placenta abruptio

Risk for deficient **Fluid Volume:** Risk factor: maternal blood loss

Risk for disturbed **Maternal/Fetal Dyad:** Risk factor: complication of pregnancy

Risk for **Powerlessness:** Risk factors: complications of pregnancy and unknown outcome

Risk for **Shock:** Risk factor: hypovolemia

Risk for **Spiritual Distress:** Risk factor: fear from unknown outcome of pregnancy

PLACENTA PREVIA

Death **Anxiety** r/t threat of mortality associated with bleeding

Disturbed **Body Image** r/t negative feelings about body and reproductive ability, feelings of helplessness

Ineffective **Coping** r/t threat to self and fetus

Deficient **Diversional Activity** r/t long-term hospitalization

Interrupted **Family Processes** r/t maternal bed rest, hospitalization

Fear r/t threat to self and fetus, unknown future

Impaired **Home Maintenance** r/t maternal bed rest, hospitalization

Impaired physical **Mobility** r/t medical protocol, maternal bed rest

Ineffective **Role Performance** r/t maternal bed rest, hospitalization

Situational low **Self-Esteem** r/t situational crisis

Spiritual Distress r/t inability to participate in usual religious rituals, situational crisis

Risk for **Bleeding:** Risk factor: placenta previa

Risk for **Constipation:** Risk factor: bed rest, pregnancy

Risk for deficient **Fluid Volume:** Risk factor: maternal blood loss

Risk for imbalanced **Fluid Volume:** Risk factor: maternal blood loss

Risk for **Injury:** fetal and maternal: Risk factors: threat to uteroplacental perfusion, hemorrhage

Risk for disturbed **Maternal/Fetal Dyad:** Risk factor: complication of pregnancy

Risk for impaired **Parenting:** Risk factors: maternal bed rest, hospitalization

Risk for ineffective peripheral **Tissue Perfusion:** placental: Risk factors: dilation of cervix, loss of placental implantation site

Risk for **Powerlessness:** Risk factors: complications of pregnancy and unknown outcome

Risk for **Shock:** Risk factor: hypovolemia

PLANTAR FASCIITIS

Impaired **Comfort** r/t pain

Impaired physical **Mobility** r/t discomfort

Acute **Pain** r/t inflammation

Chronic **Pain** r/t inflammation

PLEURAL EFFUSION

Ineffective **Breathing Pattern** r/t pain

Excess **Fluid Volume** r/t compromised regulatory mechanisms; heart, liver, or kidney failure

Hyperthermia r/t increased metabolic rate secondary to infection

Acute **Pain** r/t inflammation, fluid accumulation

PLEURAL FRICTION RUB

Ineffective **Breathing Pattern** r/t pain

Acute **Pain** r/t inflammation, fluid accumulation

See cause of Pleural Friction Rub

PLEURAL TAP

See Pleural Effusion

PLEURISY

Ineffective **Breathing Pattern** r/t pain

Impaired **Gas Exchange** r/t ventilation-perfusion imbalance

Acute **Pain** r/t pressure on pleural nerve endings associated with fluid accumulation or inflammation

Risk for ineffective **Airway Clearance:** Risk factors: increased secretions, ineffective cough because of pain

Risk for **Infection:** Risk factor: exposure to pathogens

Risk for impaired physical **Mobility:** Risk factors: activity intolerance, inability to "catch breath"

PMS (PREMENSTRUAL TENSION SYNDROME)

Fatigue r/t hormonal changes

Excess **Fluid Volume** r/t alterations of hormonal levels inducing fluid retention

Deficient **Knowledge** r/t methods to deal with and prevent syndrome

Acute **Pain** r/t hormonal stimulation of gastrointestinal structures

Risk for **Powerlessness:** Risk factors: lack of knowledge and ability to deal with symptoms

Risk for compromised **Resilience:** Risk factor: PMS symptoms

Readiness for enhanced **Communication:** willingness to express thoughts and feelings about PMS

Readiness for enhanced **Self-Health Management:** desire for information to manage and prevent symptoms

PND (PAROXYSMAL NOCTURNAL DYSPNEA)

Anxiety r/t inability to breathe during sleep

Ineffective **Breathing Pattern** r/t increase in carbon dioxide levels, decrease in oxygen levels

Insomnia r/t suffocating feeling from fluid in lungs on awakening from sleep

Sleep deprivation r/t inability to breathe during sleep

Risk for decreased **Cardiac** tissue perfusion: Risk factor: hypoxia

P

Risk for **Powerlessness**: Risk factor: inability to control nocturnal dyspnea

Readiness for enhanced **Sleep**: expresses willingness to learn measures to enhance sleep

PNEUMONECTOMY

See Thoracotomy

PNEUMONIA

Activity Intolerance r/t imbalance between oxygen supply and demand

Ineffective **Airway Clearance** r/t inflammation and presence of secretions

Impaired **Gas Exchange** r/t decreased functional lung tissue

Ineffective **Self-Health Management** r/t deficient knowledge regarding self-care and treatment of disease

Hyperthermia r/t dehydration, increased metabolic rate, illness

Deficient **Knowledge** r/t risk factors predisposing person to pneumonia, treatment

Imbalanced **Nutrition**: less than body requirements r/t loss of appetite

Impaired **Oral Mucous Membrane** r/t dry mouth from mouth breathing, decreased fluid intake

Risk for acute **Confusion**: Risk factor: underlying illness

Risk for deficient **Fluid Volume**: Risk factor: inadequate intake of fluids

Risk for **Vascular Trauma**: Risk factor: irritation from IV antibiotics

Readiness for enhanced **Immunization Status**: expresses desire to increase immunization status

See Respiratory Infections, Acute Childhood

PNEUMOTHORAX

Fear r/t threat to own well-being, difficulty breathing

Impaired **Gas Exchange** r/t ventilation-perfusion imbalance

Acute **Pain** r/t recent injury, coughing, deep breathing

Risk for **Injury**: Risk factor: possible complications associated with closed chest drainage system

See Chest Tubes

POISONING, RISK FOR

Risk for **Poisoning** (See **Poisoning,** risk for, Section II)

POLIOMYELITIS

Readiness for enhanced **Immunization Status**: expresses desire to increase immunization status

See Paralysis

POLYDIPSIA

Readiness for enhanced **Fluid Balance**: no excessive thirst when diabetes is controlled

See Diabetes Mellitus

POLYPHAGIA

Readiness for enhanced **Nutrition**: knowledge of appropriate diet for diabetes

See Diabetes Mellitus

POLYURIA

Readiness for enhanced **Urinary Elimination**: willingness to learn measures to enhance urinary elimination

See Diabetes Mellitus

POSTOPERATIVE CARE

See Surgery, Postoperative

POSTPARTUM DEPRESSION

Anxiety r/t new responsibilities of parenting

Disturbed **Body Image** r/t normal postpartum recovery

Ineffective **Childbearing Process** r/t depression/lack of support system

Ineffective **Coping** r/t hormonal changes, maturational crisis

Fatigue r/t childbirth, postpartum state

Risk-prone Health Behavior r/t lack of support systems

Impaired Home Maintenance r/t fatigue, care of newborn

Deficient Knowledge r/t lifestyle changes

Impaired Parenting r/t hormone-induced depression

Ineffective Role Performance r/t new responsibilities of parenting

Sexual Dysfunction r/t fear of another pregnancy, postpartum pain, lochia flow

Sleep deprivation r/t environmental stimulation of newborn

Impaired Social Interaction r/t change in role functioning

Risk for disturbed personal Identity r/t role change/depression/inability to cope

Risk for Post-Trauma Syndrome: Risk factors: trauma or violence associated with labor and birth process, medical/surgical interventions, history of sexual abuse

Risk for situational low Self-Esteem: Risk factor: decreased power over feelings of sadness

Risk for Spiritual Distress: Risk factors: altered relationships, social isolation

Readiness for enhanced Hope: expresses desire to enhance hope and interconnectedness with others

See Depression (Major Depressive Disorder)

POSTPARTUM HEMORRHAGE

Activity intolerance r/t anemia from loss of blood

Death Anxiety r/t threat of mortality associated with bleeding

Disturbed Body Image r/t loss of ideal childbirth

Interrupted Breastfeeding r/t separation from infant for medical treatment

Insufficient Breast Milk r/t fluid volume depletion

Decreased Cardiac Output r/t hypovolemia

Fear r/t threat to self, unknown future

Deficient Fluid Volume r/t uterine atony, loss of blood

Impaired Home Maintenance r/t lack of stamina

Deficient Knowledge r/t lack of exposure to situation

Acute Pain r/t nursing and medical interventions to control bleeding

Ineffective peripheral Tissue Perfusion r/t hypovolemia

Risk for Bleeding: Risk factor: postpartum complications

Risk for imbalanced Fluid Volume: Risk factor: maternal blood loss

Risk for Infection: Risk factors: loss of blood, depressed immunity

Risk for disturbed Maternal/Fetal Dyad. Risk factor: complication of pregnancy

Risk for impaired Parenting: Risk factor: weakened maternal condition

Risk for Powerlessness: Risk factor: acute illness

Risk for Shock: Risk factor: hypovolemia

POSTPARTUM, NORMAL CARE

Anxiety r/t change in role functioning, parenting

Effective Breastfeeding r/t basic breastfeeding knowledge, support of partner and health care provider

Constipation r/t hormonal effects on smooth muscles, fear of straining with defecation, effects of anesthesia

Fatigue r/t childbirth, new responsibilities of parenting, body changes

Acute Pain r/t episiotomy, lacerations, bruising, breast engorgement, headache, sore nipples, epidural or intravenous (IV) site, hemorrhoids

Sexual Dysfunction r/t recent childbirth

P

Impaired **Skin Integrity** r/t episiotomy, lacerations

Sleep deprivation r/t care of infant

Impaired **Urinary Elimination** r/t effects of anesthesia, tissue trauma

Risk for **Constipation:** Risk factors: hormonal effects on smooth muscles, fear of straining with defecation, effects of anesthesia

Risk for imbalanced **Fluid Volume:** Risk factors: shift in blood volume, edema

Risk for urge urinary **Incontinence:** Risk factors: effects of anesthesia or tissue trauma

Risk for **Infection:** Risk factors: tissue trauma, blood loss

Readiness for enhanced family **Coping:** adaptation to new family member

Readiness for enhanced **Hope:** desire to increase hope

Readiness for enhanced **Parenting:** expressing willingness to enhance parenting skills

POST-TRAUMA SYNDROME

Post-Trauma Syndrome (See **Post-Trauma Syndrome,** Section II)

POST-TRAUMA SYNDROME, RISK FOR

Risk for **Post-Trauma Syndrome** (See **Post-Trauma Syndrome,** risk for, Section II)

POST-TRAUMATIC STRESS DISORDER (PTSD)

See PTSD (Post-Traumatic Stress Disorder)

POTASSIUM, INCREASE/ DECREASE

See Hyperkalemia; Hypokalemia

POWER/POWERLESSNESS

Powerlessness (See **Powerlessness,** Section II)

Risk for ineffective **Childbearing Process** r/t maternal powerlessness

Risk for **Powerlessness** (See **Powerlessness,** risk for, Section II)

Readiness for enhanced **Power** (See **Power,** readiness for enhanced, Section II)

PREECLAMPSIA

See PIH (Pregnancy-Induced Hypertension/Preeclampsia)

PREGNANCY, CARDIAC DISORDERS

See Cardiac Disorders in Pregnancy

PREGNANCY-INDUCED HYPERTENSION/ PREECLAMPSIA (PIH)

See PIH (Pregnancy-Induced Hypertension/Preeclampsia)

PREGNANCY LOSS

Anxiety r/t threat to role functioning, health status, situational crisis

Compromised family **Coping** r/t lack of support by significant other because of personal suffering

Ineffective **Coping** r/t situational crisis

Grieving r/t loss of pregnancy, fetus, or child

Complicated **Grieving** r/t sudden loss of pregnancy, fetus, or child

Acute **Pain** r/t surgical intervention

Ineffective **Role Performance** r/t inability to assume parenting role

Ineffective **Sexuality Pattern** r/t self-esteem disturbance resulting from pregnancy loss and anxiety about future pregnancies

Chronic **Sorrow** r/t loss of a fetus or child

Spiritual Distress r/t intense suffering

Risk for **Bleeding:** Risk factor: pregnancy complication

Risk for deficient **Fluid Volume**: Risk factor: blood loss

Risk for complicated **Grieving**: Risk factor: loss of pregnancy

Risk for **Infection**: Risk factor: retained products of conception

Risk for **Powerlessness**: Risk factor: situational crisis

Risk for **Ineffective Relationship** r/t poor communication skills in dealing with the loss

Risk for **Spiritual Distress**: Risk factor: intense suffering

Readiness for enhanced **Communication**: willingness to express feelings and thoughts about loss

Readiness for enhanced **Hope**: expresses desire to enhance hope

Readiness for enhanced **Spiritual Well-Being**: desire for acceptance of loss

PREGNANCY, NORMAL

Anxiety r/t unknown future, threat to self secondary to pain of labor

Disturbed **Body Image** r/t altered body function and appearance

Interrupted **Family Processes** r/t developmental transition of pregnancy

Fatigue r/t increased energy demands

Fear r/t labor and delivery

Deficient **Knowledge** r/t primiparity

Nausea r/t hormonal changes of pregnancy

Imbalanced **Nutrition**: less than body requirements r/t growing fetus, nausea

Imbalanced **Nutrition**: more than body requirements r/t deficient knowledge regarding nutritional needs of pregnancy

Sleep deprivation r/t uncomfortable pregnancy state

Impaired **Urinary Elimination** r/t frequency caused by increased pelvic pressure and hormonal stimulation

Risk for **Constipation**: Risk factor: pregnancy

Risk for **Sexual Dysfunction**: Risk factors: altered body function, self-concept, body image with pregnancy

Readiness for enhanced **Childbearing Process**: appropriate prenatal care

Readiness for enhanced family **Coping**: satisfying partner relationship, attention to gratification of needs, effective adaptation to developmental tasks of pregnancy

Readiness for enhanced **Family Processes**: family adapts to change

Readiness for enhanced **Nutrition**: desire for knowledge of appropriate nutrition during pregnancy

Readiness for enhanced **Parenting**: expresses willingness to enhance parenting skills

Readiness for enhanced **Relationship**: meeting developmental goals associated with pregnancy

Readiness for enhanced **Self-Health Management**: seeks information for prenatal self-care

Readiness for enhanced **Spiritual Well-Being**: new role as parent

See Discomforts of Pregnancy

PREMATURE DILATION OF THE CERVIX (INCOMPETENT CERVIX)

Ineffective **Activity Planning** r/t unrealistic perception of events

Ineffective **Coping** r/t bed rest, threat to fetus

Deficient **Diversional Activity** r/t bed rest

Fear r/t potential loss of infant

Grieving r/t potential loss of infant

Deficient **Knowledge** r/t treatment regimen, prognosis for pregnancy

Impaired physical **Mobility** r/t imposed bed rest to prevent preterm birth

Powerlessness r/t inability to control outcome of pregnancy

P

Ineffective **Role Performance** r/t inability to continue usual patterns of responsibility

Situational low **Self-Esteem** r/t inability to complete normal pregnancy

Sexual Dysfunction r/t fear of harm to fetus

Impaired **Social Interaction** r/t bed rest

Risk for **Infection:** Risk factors: invasive procedures to prevent preterm birth

Risk for **Injury:** fetal: Risk factors: preterm birth, use of anesthetics

Risk for **Injury:** maternal: Risk factors: surgical procedures to prevent preterm birth (e.g., cerclage)

Risk for compromised **Resilience:** Risk factor: complication of pregnancy

Risk for **Spiritual Distress:** Risk factors: physical/psychological stress

PREMATURE INFANT (CHILD)

Insufficient **Breast Milk** r/t ineffective sucking, latching on of the infant

Impaired **Gas Exchange** r/t effects of cardiopulmonary insufficiency

Delayed **Growth and Development:** developmental lag r/t prematurity, environmental and stimulation deficiencies, multiple caretakers

Disorganized **Infant** behavior r/t prematurity

Insomnia r/t noisy and noxious intensive care environment

Neonatal **Jaundice** r/t infant experiences difficulty making transition to extrauterine life

Imbalanced **Nutrition:** less than body requirements r/t delayed or understimulated rooting reflex, easy fatigue during feeding, diminished endurance

Impaired **Swallowing** r/t decreased or absent gag reflex, fatigue

Ineffective **Thermoregulation** r/t large body surface/weight ratio, immaturity of thermal regulation, state of prematurity

Risk for delayed **Development:** Risk factor: prematurity

Risk for disproportionate **Growth:** Risk factor: prematurity

Risk for **Infection:** Risk factors: inadequate, immature, or undeveloped acquired immune response

Risk for **Injury:** Risk factor: prolonged mechanical ventilation, retinopathy of prematurity (ROP) secondary to 100% oxygen environment

Risk for neonatal **Jaundice** r/t to late preterm birth

Readiness for enhanced organized **Infant** behavior: use of some self-regulatory measures

PREMATURE INFANT (PARENT)

Ineffective **Breastfeeding** r/t disrupted establishment of effective pattern secondary to prematurity or insufficient opportunities

Decisional Conflict r/t support system deficit, multiple sources of information

Parental **Role Conflict** r/t expressed concerns, expressed inability to care for child's physical, emotional, or developmental needs

Compromised family **Coping** r/t disrupted family roles and disorganization, prolonged condition exhausting supportive capacity of significant persons

Grieving r/t loss of perfect child possibly leading to complicated grieving

Complicated **Grieving** (prolonged) r/t unresolved conflicts

Chronic **Sorrow** r/t threat of loss of a child, prolonged hospitalization

Spiritual Distress r/t challenged belief or value systems regarding moral or ethical implications of treatment plans

Risk for impaired **Attachment:** Risk factors: separation, physical barriers, lack of privacy

Risk for disturbed **Maternal/Fetal Dyad**: Risk factor: complication of pregnancy

Risk for **Powerlessness**: Risk factor: inability to control situation

Risk for compromised **Resilience**: Risk factor: premature infant

Risk for **Spiritual Distress**: Risk factors: challenged belief or value systems regarding moral or ethical implications of treatment plans

Readiness for enhanced **Family Process**: adaptation to change associated with premature infant

See Child with Chronic Condition; Hospitalized Child

PREMATURE RUPTURE OF MEMBRANES

Anxiety r/t threat to infant's health status

Disturbed **Body Image** r/t inability to carry pregnancy to term

Ineffective **Coping** r/t situational crisis

Grieving r/t potential loss of infant

Situational low **Self-Esteem** r/t inability to carry pregnancy to term

Risk for **Infection**: Risk factor: rupture of membranes

Risk for **Injury**: fetal: Risk factor: risk of premature birth

Risk for disturbed **Maternal/Fetal Dyad**: Risk factor: complication of pregnancy

PREMENSTRUAL TENSION SYNDROME (PMS)

See PMS (Premenstrual Tension Syndrome)

PRENATAL CARE, NORMAL

Readiness for enhanced **Childbearing Process**: appropriate prenatal lifestyle

Readiness for enhanced **Knowledge**: appropriate prenatal care

Readiness for enhanced **Spiritual Well-Being**: new role as parent

See Pregnancy, Normal

PRENATAL TESTING

Anxiety r/t unknown outcome, delayed test results

Acute **Pain** r/t invasive procedures

Risk for **Infection** r/t invasive procedures during amniocentesis or chorionic villus sampling

Risk for **Injury**: fetal r/t invasive procedures

PREOPERATIVE TEACHING

See Surgery, Preoperative Care

PRESSURE ULCER

Impaired **Comfort** r/t pressure ulcer

Impaired bed **Mobility** r/t intolerance to activity, pain, cognitive impairment, depression, severe anxiety

Imbalanced **Nutrition**: less than body requirements r/t limited access to food, inability to absorb nutrients because of biological factors, anorexia

Acute **Pain** r/t tissue destruction, exposure of nerves

Impaired **Skin Integrity**: stage I or II pressure ulcer r/t physical immobility, mechanical factors, altered circulation, skin irritants

Impaired **Tissue Integrity**: stage III or IV pressure ulcer r/t altered circulation, impaired physical mobility

Risk for **Infection**: Risk factors: physical immobility, mechanical factors (shearing forces, pressure, restraint, altered circulation, skin irritants)

PRETERM LABOR

Anxiety r/t threat to fetus, change in role functioning, change in environment and interaction patterns, use of tocolytic drugs

Ineffective **Coping** r/t situational crisis, preterm labor

Deficient **Diversional Activity** r/t long-term hospitalization

P

Grieving r/t loss of idealized pregnancy, potential loss of fetus

Impaired **Home Maintenance** r/t medical restrictions

Impaired physical **Mobility** r/t medically imposed restrictions

Ineffective **Role Performance** r/t inability to carry out normal roles secondary to bed rest or hospitalization, change in expected course of pregnancy

Situational low **Self-Esteem** r/t threatened ability to carry pregnancy to term

Sexual Dysfunction r/t actual or perceived limitation imposed by preterm labor and/or prescribed treatment, separation from partner because of hospitalization

Sleep deprivation r/t change in usual pattern secondary to contractions, hospitalization, treatment regimen

Impaired **Social Interaction** r/t prolonged bed rest or hospitalization

Risk for **Injury**: fetal: Risk factors: premature birth, immature body systems

Risk for **Injury**: maternal: Risk factor: use of tocolytic drugs

Risk for **Powerlessness**: Risk factor: lack of control over preterm labor

Risk for **Vascular Trauma**: Risk factor: IV medication

Readiness for enhanced **Childbearing Process**: appropriate prenatal lifestyle

Readiness for enhanced **Comfort**: expresses desire to enhance relaxation

Readiness for enhanced **Communication**: willingness to discuss thoughts and feelings about situation

PROBLEM-SOLVING ABILITY

Defensive **Coping** r/t situational crisis

Risk for chronic low **Self-Esteem** r/t repeated failures

Readiness for enhanced **Communication**: willing to share ideas with others

Readiness for enhanced **Relationship**: shares information and ideas between partners

Readiness for enhanced **Resilience**: identifies available resources

Readiness for enhanced **Spiritual Well-Being**: desires to draw on inner strength and find meaning and purpose to life

PROJECTION

Anxiety r/t threat to self-concept

Defensive **Coping** r/t inability to acknowledge that own behavior may be a problem, blaming others

Chronic low **Self-Esteem** r/t failure

Impaired **Social Interaction** r/t self-concept disturbance, confrontational communication style

Risk for **Loneliness**: Risk factor: blaming others for problems

Risk for **Post-Trauma Syndrome**: Risk factor: diminished ego strength

See Paranoid Personality Disorder

PROLAPSED UMBILICAL CORD

Fear r/t threat to fetus, impending surgery

Ineffective peripheral **Tissue Perfusion**: fetal r/t interruption in umbilical blood flow

Risk for **Injury**: fetal: Risk factors: cord compression, ineffective tissue perfusion

Risk for **Injury**: maternal: Risk factor: emergency surgery

PROSTATECTOMY

See TURP (Transurethral Resection of the Prostate)

PROSTATIC HYPERTROPHY

Ineffective **Health Maintenance** r/t deficient knowledge regarding self-care and prevention of complications

Insomnia r/t nocturia

Urinary **Retention** r/t obstruction

Risk for urge urinary **Incontinence**: Risk factor: small bladder capacity

Risk for **Infection**: Risk factors: urinary residual after voiding, bacterial invasion of bladder

See BPH (Benign Prostatic Hypertrophy)

PROSTATITIS

Impaired **Comfort** r/t inflammation

Ineffective **Health Maintenance** r/t deficient knowledge regarding treatment

Urge urinary **Incontinence** r/t irritation of bladder

Ineffective **Protection** r/t depressed immune system

PROTECTION, ALTERED

Ineffective **Protection** (See **Protection**, ineffective, Section II)

PRURITUS

Impaired **Comfort** r/t itching

Deficient **Knowledge** r/t methods to treat and prevent itching

Risk for impaired **Skin Integrity**: Risk factor: scratching from pruritus

PSORIASIS

Disturbed **Body Image** r/t lesions on body

Impaired **Comfort** r/t irritated skin

Ineffective **Health Maintenance** r/t deficient knowledge regarding treatment modalities

Powerlessness r/t lack of control over condition with frequent exacerbations and remissions

Impaired **Skin Integrity** r/t lesions on body

PSYCHOSIS

Ineffective **Activity Planning** r/t compromised ability to process information

Ineffective **Health Maintenance** r/t cognitive impairment, ineffective individual and family coping

Self-Neglect r/t mental disorder

Impaired individual **Resilience** r/t psychological disorder

Situational low **Self-Esteem** r/t excessive use of defense mechanisms (e.g., projection, denial, rationalization)

Risk for disturbed personal **Identity** r/t psychosis

Risk for **Post-Trauma Syndrome**: Risk factor: diminished ego strength

See Schizophrenia

PTCA (PERCUTANEOUS TRANSLUMINAL CORONARY ANGIOPLASTY)

See Angioplasty, Coronary

PTSD (POST-TRAUMATIC STRESS DISORDER)

P

Anxiety r/t exposure to internal or external cues that symbolize or resemble an aspect of the traumatic event

Death **Anxiety** r/t psychological stress associated with traumatic event

Ineffective **Breathing Pattern** r/t hyperventilation associated with anxiety

Ineffective **Coping** r/t extreme anxiety

Disturbed **Energy Field** r/t disharmony of mind, body, spirit

Ineffective **Impulse Control** r/t re-experience of initial trauma

Insomnia r/t recurring nightmares

Post-Trauma Syndrome r/t exposure to a traumatic event

Sleep deprivation r/t nightmares associated with traumatic event

Spiritual Distress r/t feelings of detachment or estrangement from others

Risk for **Powerlessness**: Risk factors: flashbacks, reliving event

Risk for ineffective **Relationship** r/t stressful life events

Risk for self- or other-directed **Violence**: Risk factors: fear of self or others

Readiness for enhanced **Comfort**: expresses desire to enhance relaxation

Readiness for enhanced **Communication**: willingness to express feelings and thoughts

Readiness for enhanced **Spiritual Well-Being**: desire for harmony after stressful event

PULMONARY EDEMA

Anxiety r/t fear of suffocation

Ineffective **Breathing Pattern** r/t presence of tracheobronchial secretions

Impaired **Gas Exchange** r/t extravasation of extravascular fluid in lung tissues and alveoli

Ineffective **Health Maintenance** r/t deficient knowledge regarding treatment regimen

Sleep deprivation r/t inability to breathe

Risk for decreased **Cardiac** tissue perfusion: Risk factor: heart failure

See CHF (Congestive Heart Failure)

PULMONARY EMBOLISM

Decreased **Cardiac Output** r/t right ventricular failure secondary to obstructed pulmonary artery

Fear r/t severe pain, possible death

Impaired **Gas Exchange** r/t altered blood flow to alveoli secondary to lodged embolus

Deficient **Knowledge** r/t activities to prevent embolism, self-care after diagnosis of embolism

Acute **Pain** r/t biological injury, lack of oxygen to cells

Ineffective peripheral **Tissue Perfusion**: r/t deep vein thrombus formation

Delayed **Surgical Recovery** r/t complications associated with respiratory difficulty

See Anticoagulant Therapy

PULMONARY STENOSIS

See Congenital Heart Disease/Cardiac Anomalies

PULSE DEFICIT

Decreased **Cardiac Output** r/t dysrhythmia

See Dysrhythmia

PULSE OXIMETRY

Readiness for enhanced **Knowledge**: information associated with treatment regimen

See Hypoxia

PULSE PRESSURE, INCREASED

See Intracranial Pressure, Increased

PULSE PRESSURE, NARROWED

See Shock, Hypovolemic

PULSES, ABSENT OR DIMINISHED PERIPHERAL

Ineffective peripheral **Tissue Perfusion** r/t interruption of arterial flow

Risk for **Peripheral Neurovascular Dysfunction**: Risk factors: fractures, mechanical compression, orthopedic surgery trauma, immobilization, burns, vascular obstruction

See cause of Absent or Diminished Peripheral Pulses

PURPURA

See Clotting Disorder

PYELONEPHRITIS

Ineffective **Health Maintenance** r/t deficient knowledge regarding self-care, treatment of disease, prevention of further urinary tract infections

Insomnia r/t urinary frequency

Acute **Pain** r/t inflammation and irritation of urinary tract

Impaired **Urinary Elimination** r/t irritation of urinary tract

Risk for urge urinary **Incontinence**: Risk factor: irritation of urinary tract

Risk for ineffective **Renal Perfusion**: Risk factor: infection

PYLORIC STENOSIS

Imbalanced **Nutrition**: less than body requirements r/t vomiting secondary to pyloric sphincter obstruction

Acute **Pain** r/t abdominal fullness

Risk for imbalanced **Fluid Volume**: Risk factors: vomiting, dehydration

See Hospitalized Child

PYLOROMYOTOMY (PYLORIC STENOSIS REPAIR)

See Surgery Preoperative, Perioperative, Postoperative

R

RA (RHEUMATOID ARTHRITIS)

See Rheumatoid Arthritis (RA)

RABIES

Ineffective **Health Maintenance** r/t deficient knowledge regarding care of wound, isolation, and observation of infected animal

Acute **Pain** r/t multiple immunization injections

Risk for ineffective **Cerebral** tissue perfusion: Risk factor: rabies virus

Readiness for enhanced **Immunization Status**: desires to enhance immunization status

RADIAL NERVE DYSFUNCTION

Acute **Pain** r/t trauma to hand or arm
See Neuropathy, Peripheral

RADIATION THERAPY

Activity Intolerance r/t fatigue from possible anemia

Disturbed **Body Image** r/t change in appearance, hair loss

Diarrhea r/t irradiation effects

Fatigue r/t malnutrition from lack of appetite, nausea, and vomiting

Deficient **Knowledge** r/t what to expect with radiation therapy

Nausea r/t side effects of radiation

Imbalanced **Nutrition**: less than body requirements r/t anorexia, nausea, vomiting, irradiation of areas of pharynx and esophagus

Impaired **Oral Mucous Membrane** r/t irradiation effects

Ineffective **Protection** r/t suppression of bone marrow

Risk for **Powerlessness**: Risk factors: medical treatment and possible side effects

Risk for compromised **Resilience**: Risk factor: radiation treatment

Risk for impaired **Skin Integrity**: Risk factor: irradiation effects

Risk for **Spiritual Distress**: Risk factors: radiation treatment, prognosis

RADICAL NECK DISSECTION

See Laryngectomy

RAGE

Risk-prone **Health Behavior** r/t multiple stressors

Impaired individual **Resilience** r/t poor impulse control

Stress overload r/t multiple coexisting stressors

Risk for **Self-Mutilation**: Risk factor: command hallucinations

Risk for **Suicide**: Risk factor: desire to kill self

R

Risk for other-directed **Violence**: Risk factors: panic state, manic excitement, organic brain syndrome

RAPE-TRAUMA SYNDROME

Rape-Trauma Syndrome (See **Rape-Trauma Syndrome**, Section II)

Chronic **Sorrow** r/t forced loss of virginity

Risk for ineffective **Childbearing Process** r/t to trauma and violence

Risk for chronic low **Self-Esteem** r/t perceived lack of respect from others/ feeling violated

Risk for ineffective **Relationship** r/t to trauma and violence

Risk for **Post-Trauma Syndrome**: Risk factors: trauma or violence associated with rape

Risk for **Powerlessness**: Risk factor: inability to control thoughts about incident

Risk for **Spiritual Distress**: Risk factor: forced loss of virginity

RASH

Impaired **Comfort** r/t pruritus

Impaired **Skin Integrity** r/t mechanical trauma

Risk for **Latex Allergy Response**: Risk factor: allergy to products associated with latex

Risk for **Infection**: Risk factors: traumatized tissue, broken skin

Readiness for enhanced **Immunization Status**: desire to prevent infectious disease

RATIONALIZATION

Defensive **Coping** r/t situational crisis, inability to accept blame for consequences of own behavior

Ineffective **Denial** r/t fear of consequences, actual or perceived loss

Impaired individual **Resilience** r/t psychological disturbance

Risk for **Post-Trauma Syndrome**: Risk factor: survivor's role in event

Readiness for enhanced **Communication**: expressing desire to share thoughts and feelings

Readiness for enhanced **Spiritual Well-Being**: possibility of seeking harmony with self, others, higher power, God

RATS, RODENTS IN THE HOME

Impaired **Home Maintenance** r/t lack of knowledge, insufficient finances

Risk for **Allergy Response** r/t repeated exposure to environmental contamination

See Filthy Home Environment

RAYNAUD'S DISEASE

Deficient **Knowledge** r/t lack of information about disease process, possible complications, self-care needs regarding disease process and medication

Ineffective peripheral **Tissue Perfusion** r/t transient reduction of blood flow

RDS (RESPIRATORY DISTRESS SYNDROME)

See Respiratory Conditions of the Neonate

RECTAL FULLNESS

Constipation r/t decreased activity level, decreased fluid intake, inadequate fiber in diet, decreased peristalsis, side effects from antidepressant or antipsychotic therapy

Risk for **Constipation**: Risk factor: habitual denial or ignoring of urge to defecate

RECTAL LUMP

See Hemorrhoids

RECTAL PAIN/BLEEDING

Constipation r/t pain on defecation

Deficient **Knowledge** r/t possible causes of rectal bleeding, pain, treatment modalities

Acute **Pain** r/t pressure of defecation

Risk for **Bleeding**: Risk factor: rectal disease

RECTAL SURGERY

See Hemorrhoidectomy

RECTOCELE REPAIR

Constipation r/t painful defecation

Ineffective **Health Maintenance** r/t deficient knowledge of postoperative care of surgical site, dietary measures, exercise to prevent constipation

Acute **Pain** r/t surgical procedure

Urinary Retention r/t edema from surgery

Risk for **Bleeding**: Risk factor: surgery

Risk for urge urinary **Incontinence**: Risk factor: edema from surgery

Risk for **Infection**: Risk factors: surgical procedure, possible contamination of site with feces

REFLEX INCONTINENCE

Reflex urinary **Incontinence** (See **Incontinence**, urinary, reflex, Section II)

REGRESSION

Anxiety r/t threat to or change in health status

Defensive **Coping** r/t denial of obvious problems, weaknesses

Self-Neglect r/t functional impairment

Powerlessness r/t health care environment

Impaired individual **Resilience** r/t psychological disturbance

Ineffective **Role Performance** r/t powerlessness over health status

See Hospitalized Child; Separation Anxiety

REGRETFUL

Anxiety r/t situational or maturational crises

Death **Anxiety** r/t feelings of not having accomplished goals in life

Risk for **Spiritual Distress**: Risk factor: inability to forgive

REHABILITATION

Ineffective **Coping** r/t loss of normal function

Impaired physical **Mobility** r/t injury, surgery, psychosocial condition warranting rehabilitation

Self-Care deficit: specify r/t impaired physical mobility

Readiness for enhanced **Comfort**: expresses desire to enhance feeling of comfort

Readiness for enhanced **Self-Concept**: accepts strengths and limitations

Readiness for enhanced **Self-Health Management**: expression of desire to manage rehabilitation

RELATIONSHIP

Ineffective **Relationship**

Risk for ineffective **Relationship** (see Section II)

RELAXATION TECHNIQUES

Anxiety r/t disturbed energy field

Readiness for enhanced **Comfort**: expresses desire to enhance relaxation

Readiness for enhanced **Religiosity**: requests religious materials or experiences

Readiness for enhanced **Resilience**: desire to enhance resilience

Readiness for enhanced **Self-Concept**: willingness to enhance self-concept

Readiness for enhanced **Self-Health Management**: desire to manage illness

Readiness for enhanced **Spiritual Well-Being**: seeking comfort from higher power

R

RELIGIOSITY

Impaired **Religiosity** (See **Religiosity,** impaired, Section II)

Risk for impaired **Religiosity** (See **Religiosity,** impaired, risk for, Section II)

Readiness for enhanced **Religiosity** (See **Religiosity,** readiness for enhanced, Section II)

RELIGIOUS CONCERNS

Spiritual Distress r/t separation from religious or cultural ties

Risk for impaired **Religiosity:** Risk factors: ineffective support, coping, caregiving

Risk for **Spiritual Distress:** Risk factors: physical or psychological stress

Readiness for enhanced **Spiritual Well-Being:** desire for increased spirituality

RELOCATION STRESS SYNDROME

Relocation Stress Syndrome (See **Relocation Stress Syndrome,** Section II)

Risk for **Relocation Stress Syndrome** (See **Relocation Stress Syndrome,** risk for, Section II)

RENAL FAILURE

Activity Intolerance r/t effects of anemia, congestive heart failure

Death **Anxiety** r/t unknown outcome of disease

Decreased **Cardiac Output** r/t effects of congestive heart failure, elevated potassium levels interfering with conduction system

Impaired **Comfort** r/t pruritus

Ineffective **Coping** r/t depression resulting from chronic disease

Fatigue r/t effects of chronic uremia and anemia

Excess **Fluid Volume** r/t decreased urine output, sodium retention, inappropriate fluid intake

Noncompliance r/t complex medical therapy

Imbalanced **Nutrition:** less than body requirements r/t anorexia, nausea, vomiting, altered taste sensation, dietary restrictions

Impaired **Oral Mucous Membrane** r/t irritation from nitrogenous waste products

Chronic **Sorrow** r/t chronic illness

Spiritual Distress r/t dealing with chronic illness

Impaired **Urinary Elimination** r/t effects of disease, need for dialysis

Risk for **Electrolyte Imbalance:** Risk factor: renal dysfunction

Risk for **Infection:** Risk factor: altered immune functioning

Risk for **Injury:** Risk factors: bone changes, neuropathy, muscle weakness

Risk for impaired **Oral Mucous Membrane:** Risk factors: dehydration, effects of uremia

Risk for ineffective **Renal Perfusion:** Risk factor: renal disease

Risk for **Powerlessness:** Risk factor: chronic illness

Risk for **Shock:** Risk factor: infection

RENAL FAILURE, ACUTE/ CHRONIC, CHILD

Disturbed **Body Image** r/t growth retardation, bone changes, visibility of dialysis access devices (shunt, fistula), edema

Deficient **Diversional Activity** r/t immobility during dialysis

See Child with Chronic Condition; Hospitalized Child; Renal Failure

RENAL FAILURE, NONOLIGURIC

Anxiety r/t change in health status

Risk for deficient **Fluid Volume:** Risk factor: loss of large volumes of urine

See Renal Failure

RENAL TRANSPLANTATION, DONOR

Decisional Conflict r/t harvesting of kidney from traumatized donor

Moral Distress r/t conflict among decision makers, end-of-life decisions, time constraints for decision-making

Spiritual Distress r/t grieving from loss of significant person

Readiness for enhanced **Communication:** expressing thoughts and feelings about situation

Readiness for enhanced family **Coping:** decision to allow organ donation

Readiness for enhanced **Decision-Making:** expresses desire to enhance understanding and meaning of choices

Readiness for enhanced **Resilience:** decision to donate organs

Readiness for enhanced **Spirituality:** inner peace resulting from allowance of organ donation

See Nephrectomy

RENAL TRANSPLANTATION, RECIPIENT

Anxiety r/t possible rejection, procedure

Impaired Health Maintenance r/t long-term home treatment after transplantation, diet, signs of rejection, use of medications

Deficient Knowledge r/t specific nutritional needs, possible paralytic ileus, fluid or sodium restrictions

Ineffective Protection r/t immunosuppression therapy

Impaired Urinary Elimination r/t possible impaired renal function

Risk for Bleeding: Risk factor: surgical procedure

Risk for Infection: Risk factor: use of immunosuppressive therapy to control rejection

Risk for ineffective Renal Perfusion: Risk factor: transplanted kidney

Risk for Shock: Risk factor: possible hypovolemia

Risk for Spiritual Distress: Risk factor: obtaining transplanted kidney from someone's traumatic loss

Readiness for enhanced **Spiritual Well-Being:** acceptance of situation

See Kidney Transplant

RESPIRATORY ACIDOSIS

See Acidosis, Respiratory

RESPIRATORY CONDITIONS OF THE NEONATE (RESPIRATORY DISTRESS SYNDROME [RDS], MECONIUM ASPIRATION, DIAPHRAGMATIC HERNIA)

Ineffective Airway Clearance r/t sequelae of attempts to breathe in utero resulting in meconium aspiration

Ineffective Breathing Pattern r/t prolonged ventilator dependence

Fatigue r/t increased energy requirements and metabolic demands

Impaired Gas Exchange r/t decreased surfactant, immature lung tissue

Risk for Infection: Risk factors: tissue destruction or irritation as a result of aspiration of meconium fluid

See Bronchopulmonary Dysplasia; Hospitalized Child; Premature Infant, Child

RESPIRATORY DISTRESS

See Dyspnea

RESPIRATORY DISTRESS SYNDROME (RDS)

See Respiratory Conditions of the Neonate

RESPIRATORY INFECTIONS, ACUTE CHILDHOOD (CROUP, EPIGLOTTITIS, PERTUSSIS, PNEUMONIA, RESPIRATORY SYNCYTIAL VIRUS)

Activity Intolerance r/t generalized weakness, dyspnea, fatigue, poor oxygenation

R

Ineffective **Airway Clearance** r/t excess tracheobronchial secretions

Anxiety/Fear r/t oxygen deprivation, difficulty breathing

Ineffective **Breathing Pattern** r/t inflamed bronchial passages, coughing

Deficient **Fluid Volume** r/t insensible losses (fever, diaphoresis), inadequate oral fluid intake

Impaired **Gas Exchange** r/t insufficient oxygenation as a result of inflammation or edema of epiglottis, larynx, bronchial passages

Hyperthermia r/t infectious process

Imbalanced **Nutrition:** less than body requirements r/t anorexia, fatigue, generalized weakness, poor sucking and breathing coordination, dyspnea

Risk for **Aspiration:** Risk factors: inability to coordinate breathing, coughing, sucking

Risk for **Infection:** transmission to others: Risk factor: virulent infectious organisms

Risk for **Injury** (to pregnant others): Risk factors: exposure to aerosolized medications (e.g., ribavirin, pentamidine), resultant potential fetal toxicity

Risk for **Suffocation:** Risk factors: inflammation of larynx, epiglottis

See Hospitalized Child

RESPIRATORY SYNCYTIAL VIRUS

See Respiratory Infections, Acute Childhood

RESTLESS LEG SYNDROME

Insomnia r/t leg discomfort during sleep relieved by frequent leg movement

Sleep deprivation r/t frequent leg movements

See Stress

RETARDED GROWTH AND DEVELOPMENT

See Growth and Development Lag

RETCHING

Nausea r/t chemotherapy, postsurgical anesthesia, irritation to gastrointestinal system, stimulation of neuropharmacological mechanisms

Imbalanced **Nutrition:** less than body requirements r/t inability to ingest food

RETINAL DETACHMENT

Anxiety r/t change in vision, threat of loss of vision

Deficient **Knowledge** r/t symptoms, need for early intervention to prevent permanent damage

Vision Loss r/t impaired visual impairment

Risk for impaired **Home Maintenance:** Risk factors: postoperative care, activity limitations, care of affected eye

Risk for compromised **Resilience:** Risk factor: possible loss of vision

See Vision Impairment

RETINOPATHY, DIABETIC

See Diabetic Retinopathy

RETINOPATHY OF PREMATURITY (ROP)

Risk for **Injury:** Risk factors: prolonged mechanical ventilation, ROP secondary to 100% oxygen environment

See Retinal Detachment

REYE'S SYNDROME

Ineffective **Breathing Pattern** r/t neuromuscular impairment

Compromised family **Coping** r/t acute situational crisis

Deficient **Fluid Volume** r/t vomiting, hyperventilation

Excess **Fluid Volume:** cerebral r/t cerebral edema

Impaired **Gas Exchange** r/t hyperventilation, sequelae of increased intracranial pressure

Grieving r/t uncertain prognosis and sequelae

Ineffective **Health Maintenance** r/t deficient knowledge regarding use of salicylates during viral illness of child

Imbalanced **Nutrition:** less than body requirements r/t effects of liver dysfunction, vomiting

Situational low **Self-Esteem:** family r/t negative perceptions of self, perceived inability to manage family situation, expressions of guilt

Impaired **Skin Integrity** r/t effects of decorticate or decerebrate posturing, seizure activity

Risk for **Injury:** Risk factors: combative behavior, seizure activity

Risk for impaired **Liver Function:** Risk factor: infection

Risk for ineffective **Cerebral** tissue perfusion: Risk factor: infection

See Hospitalized Child

RH FACTOR INCOMPATIBILITY

Anxiety r/t unknown outcome of pregnancy

Neonatal Jaundice r/t Rh factor incompatibility

Deficient **Knowledge** r/t treatment regimen from lack of experience with situation

Powerlessness r/t perceived lack of control over outcome of pregnancy

Risk for **Injury:** fetal: Risk factors: intrauterine destruction of red blood cells, transfusions

Risk for neonatal **Jaundice** r/t Rh factor incompatibility

Readiness for enhanced **Self-Health Management:** prenatal care, compliance with diagnostic and treatment regimen

RHABDOMYOLYSIS

Ineffective **Coping** r/t seriousness of condition

Impaired physical **Mobility** r/t myalgia and muscle weakness

Impaired **Urinary Elimination** r/t presence of myoglobin in the kidneys

Risk for deficient **Fluid Volume:** Risk factor: reduced blood flow to kidneys

Risk for ineffective **Renal Perfusion:** Risk factor: possible renal failure

Risk for **Shock:** Risk factor: hypovolemia

Readiness for enhanced **Self-Health Management:** seeks information to avoid condition

See Renal Failure

RHEUMATIC FEVER

See Endocarditis

RHEUMATOID ARTHRITIS (RA)

Imbalanced **Nutrition:** less than body requirements r/t loss of appetite

Risk for compromised **Resilience:** Risk factor: chronic, painful, progressive disease

See Arthritis; JRA (Juvenile Rheumatoid Arthritis)

RIB FRACTURE

Ineffective **Breathing Pattern** r/t fractured ribs

Acute **Pain** r/t movement, deep breathing

See Ventilator Client (if relevant)

RIDICULE OF OTHERS

Defensive **Coping** r/t situational crisis, psychological impairment, substance abuse

Risk for **Post-Trauma Syndrome:** Risk factor: perception of the event

RINGWORM OF BODY

Impaired **Comfort** r/t pruritus

Impaired **Skin Integrity** r/t presence of macules associated with fungus

See Itching; Pruritus

R

RINGWORM OF NAILS

Disturbed **Body Image** r/t appearance of nails, removed nails

RINGWORM OF SCALP

Disturbed **Body Image** r/t possible hair loss (alopecia)

See Itching; Pruritus

RISK FOR RELOCATION STRESS SYNDROME

Risk for **Relocation Stress Syndrome** (See **Relocation Stress Syndrome**, risk for, Section II)

ROACHES, INVASION OF HOME WITH

Impaired **Home Maintenance** r/t lack of knowledge, insufficient finances

See Filthy Home Environment

ROLE PERFORMANCE, ALTERED

Ineffective **Role Performance** (See **Role Performance**, ineffective, Section II)

ROP (RETINOPATHY OF PREMATURITY)

See Retinopathy of Prematurity (ROP)

Risk for dry **Eye** r/t mechanical ventilation

RSV (RESPIRATORY SYNCYTIAL VIRUS)

See Respiratory Infection, Acute Childhood

RUBELLA

See Communicable Diseases, Childhood

RUBOR OF EXTREMITIES

Ineffective peripheral **Tissue Perfusion** r/t interruption of arterial flow

See Peripheral Vascular Disease (PVD)

RUPTURED DISK

See Low Back Pain

S

SAD (SEASONAL AFFECTIVE DISORDER)

Readiness for enhanced **Resilience**: uses SAD lights during winter months

See Depression (Major Depressive Disorder)

SADNESS

Complicated **Grieving** r/t actual or perceived loss

Spiritual Distress r/t intense suffering

Risk for **Powerlessness**: Risk factor: actual or perceived loss

Risk for **Spiritual Distress**: Risk factor: loss of loved one

Readiness for enhanced **Communication**: willingness to share feelings and thoughts

Readiness for enhanced **Spiritual Well-Being**: desire for harmony after actual or perceived loss

See Depression (Major Depressive Disorder); Major Depressive Disorder

SAFE SEX

Readiness for enhanced **Self-Health Management**: taking appropriate precautions during sexual activity to keep from contacting a sexually transmitted disease

See Sexuality, Adolescent; STD (Sexually Transmitted Disease)

SAFETY, CHILDHOOD

Deficient **Knowledge**: potential for enhanced health maintenance r/t parental knowledge and skill acquisition regarding appropriate safety measures

Risk for **Aspiration** (See **Aspiration**, risk for, Section II)

Risk for **Injury/Trauma**: Risk factors: developmental age, altered home maintenance

S

Risk for impaired **Parenting:** Risk factors: lack of available and effective role model, lack of knowledge, misinformation from other family members (old wives' tales)

Risk for **Poisoning:** Risk factors: use of lead-based paint; presence of asbestos or radon gas; drugs not locked in cabinet; household products left in accessible area (bleach, detergent, drain cleaners, household cleaners); alcohol and perfume within reach of child; presence of poisonous plants; atmospheric pollutants

Risk for **Thermal Injury** r/t inadequate supervision

Readiness for enhanced **Childbearing Process:** appropriate knowledge for care of child

Readiness for enhanced **Immunization Status:** expresses desire to enhance immunization status

SALMONELLA

Impaired **Home Maintenance** r/t improper preparation or storage of food, lack of safety measures when caring for pet reptile

Risk for **Electrolyte Imbalance:** Risk factor: diarrhea

Readiness for enhanced **Self-Health Management:** avoiding improperly prepared or stored food, wearing gloves when handling pet reptiles or their feces

See Gastroenteritis; Gastroenteritis, Child

SALPINGECTOMY

Decisional Conflict r/t sterilization procedure

Grieving r/t possible loss from tubal pregnancy

Risk for impaired **Urinary Elimination:** Risk factor: trauma to ureter during surgery

See Hysterectomy; Surgery, Perioperative Care; Surgery,

Postoperative Care; Surgery, Preoperative Care

SARCOIDOSIS

Anxiety r/t change in health status

Impaired **Gas Exchange** r/t ventilation-perfusion imbalance

Ineffective **Health Maintenance** r/t deficient knowledge regarding home care and medication regimen

Acute **Pain** r/t possible disease affecting joints

Ineffective **Protection** r/t immune disorder

Risk for decreased **Cardiac** tissue perfusion: Risk factor: dysrhythmias

Risk for impaired **Skin Integrity:** Risk factor: immunological disorder

SARS (SEVERE ACUTE RESPIRATORY SYNDROME)

Risk for **Infection:** Risk factor: increased environmental exposure (travelers in close proximity to infected persons, traveling when a fever is present)

Readiness for enhanced **Knowledge:** information regarding travel and precautions to avoid exposure to SARS

See Pneumonia

SBE (SELF-BREAST EXAMINATION)

Readiness for enhanced **Knowledge:** self-breast examination

Readiness for enhanced **Self-Health Management:** desires to have information about SBE

SCABIES

See Communicable Diseases, Childhood

SCARED

Anxiety r/t threat of death, threat to or change in health status

Death **Anxiety** r/t unresolved issues surrounding end-of-life decisions

Fear r/t hospitalization, real or imagined threat to own well-being

Impaired individual **Resilience** r/t violence

Readiness for enhanced **Communication:** willingness to share thoughts and feelings

Ineffective **Activity Planning** r/t compromised ability to process information

Anxiety r/t unconscious conflict with reality

Impaired verbal **Communication** r/t psychosis, disorientation, inaccurate perception, hallucinations, delusions

Ineffective **Coping** r/t inadequate support systems, unrealistic perceptions, inadequate coping skills, disturbed thought processes, impaired communication

Deficient **Diversional Activity** r/t social isolation, possible regression

Interrupted **Family Processes** r/t inability to express feelings, impaired communication

Fear r/t altered contact with reality

Ineffective **Health Maintenance** r/t cognitive impairment, ineffective individual and family coping, lack of material resources

Impaired **Home Maintenance** r/t impaired cognitive or emotional functioning, insufficient finances, inadequate support systems

Hopelessness r/t long-term stress from chronic mental illness

Disturbed personal **Identity** r/t psychiatric disorder

Insomnia r/t sensory alterations contributing to fear and anxiety

Impaired **Memory** r/t psychosocial condition

Self-Neglect r/t psychosis

Imbalanced **Nutrition:** less than body requirements r/t fear of eating, lack of awareness of hunger, disinterest toward food

Impaired individual **Resilience** r/t psychological disorder

Self-Care deficit: specify r/t loss of contact with reality, impairment of perception

Sleep deprivation r/t intrusive thoughts, nightmares

Impaired **Social Interaction** r/t impaired communication patterns, self-concept disturbance, disturbed thought processes

Social Isolation r/t lack of trust, regression, delusional thinking, repressed fears

Chronic **Sorrow** r/t chronic mental illness

Spiritual Distress r/t loneliness, social alienation

Ineffective family **Therapeutic Regimen Management** r/t chronicity and unpredictability of condition

Risk for **Caregiver Role Strain:** Risk factors: bizarre behavior of client, chronicity of condition

Risk for compromised **Human Dignity:** Risk factor: stigmatizing label

Risk for **Loneliness:** Risk factor: inability to interact socially

Risk for **Post-Trauma Syndrome:** Risk factor: diminished ego strength

Risk for **Powerlessness:** Risk factor: intrusive, distorted thinking

Risk for impaired **Religiosity:** Risk factors: ineffective coping, lack of security

Risk for **Suicide:** Risk factor: psychiatric illness

Risk for self- and other-directed **Violence:** Risk factors: lack of trust, panic, hallucinations, delusional thinking

Readiness for enhanced **Hope:** expresses desire to enhance interconnectedness with others and problem-solve to meet goals

Readiness for enhanced **Power:** expresses willingness to enhance participation in choices for daily living and health and enhance knowledge for participation in change

SCIATICA

See Neuropathy, Peripheral

SCOLIOSIS

Risk-prone **Health Behavior** r/t lack of developmental maturity to comprehend long-term consequences of noncompliance with treatment procedures

Disturbed **Body Image** r/t use of therapeutic braces, postsurgery scars, restricted physical activity

Ineffective **Breathing Pattern** r/t restricted lung expansion caused by severe curvature of spine

Impaired **Comfort** r/t altered health status and body image

Impaired **Gas Exchange** r/t restricted lung expansion as a result of severe presurgery curvature of spine, immobilization

Impaired physical **Mobility** r/t restricted movement, dyspnea caused by severe curvature of spine

Acute **Pain** r/t musculoskeletal restrictions, surgery, reambulation with cast or spinal rod

Impaired **Skin Integrity** r/t braces, casts, surgical correction

Chronic **Sorrow** r/t chronic disability

Ineffective **Health Maintenance** r/t deficient knowledge regarding treatment modalities, restrictions, home care, postoperative activities

Risk for **Infection:** Risk factor: surgical incision

Risk for **Perioperative Positioning Injury:** Risk factor: prone position

Risk for compromised **Resilience:** Risk factor: chronic condition

Readiness for enhanced **Self-Health Management:** desires knowledge regarding treatment for condition

See Hospitalized Child; Maturational Issues, Adolescent

SEDENTARY LIFESTYLE

Activity Intolerance r/t sedentary lifestyle

Sedentary lifestyle (See **Sedentary** lifestyle, Section II)

Risk for ineffective peripheral **Tissue Perfusion** r/t lack of exercise/movement

Readiness for enhanced **Coping:** seeking knowledge of new strategies to adjust to sedentary lifestyle

SEIZURE DISORDERS, ADULT

Acute **Confusion** r/t postseizure state

Social Isolation r/t unpredictability of seizures, community-imposed stigma

Risk for ineffective **Airway Clearance:** Risk factor: accumulation of secretions during seizure

Risk for **Falls:** Risk factor: uncontrolled seizure activity

Risk for unstable blood **Glucose** Level (hypoglycemia)

Risk for **Powerlessness:** Risk factor: possible seizure

Risk for compromised **Resilience:** Risk factor: chronic illness

Readiness for enhanced **Knowledge:** anticonvulsive therapy

Readiness for enhanced **Self-Care:** expresses desire to enhance knowledge and responsibility for self-care

See Epilepsy

SEIZURE DISORDERS, CHILDHOOD (EPILEPSY, FEBRILE SEIZURES, INFANTILE SPASMS)

Ineffective **Health Maintenance** r/t lack of knowledge regarding anticonvulsive therapy, fever reduction (febrile seizures)

S

Social Isolation r/t unpredictability of seizures, community-imposed stigma

Risk for ineffective **Airway Clearance:** Risk factor: accumulation of secretions during seizure

Risk for delayed **Development** and disproportionate **Growth:** Risk factors: effects of seizure disorder, parental overprotection

Risk for **Falls:** Risk factor: possible seizure

Risk for **Injury:** Risk factors: uncontrolled movements during seizure, falls, drowsiness caused by anticonvulsants

See Epilepsy

SELF-BREAST EXAMINATION (SBE)

See SBE (Self-Breast Examination)

SELF-CARE

Readiness for enhanced **Self-Care** (See **Self-Care,** readiness for enhanced, Section II)

SELF-CARE DEFICIT, BATHING

Bathing **Self-Care** deficit (See **Self-Care** deficit, bathing, Section II)

SELF-CARE DEFICIT, DRESSING

Dressing **Self-Care** deficit (See **Self-Care** deficit, dressing, Section II)

SELF-CARE DEFICIT, FEEDING

Feeding **Self-Care** deficit (See **Self-Care** deficit, feeding, Section II)

SELF-CARE DEFICIT, TOILETING

Toileting **Self-Care** deficit (See **Self-Care** deficit, toileting, Section II)

SELF-CONCEPT

Readiness for enhanced **Self-Concept** (See **Self-Concept,** readiness for enhanced, Section II)

SELF-DESTRUCTIVE BEHAVIOR

Post-Trauma Syndrome r/t unresolved feelings from traumatic event

Risk for **Self-Mutilation:** Risk factors: feelings of depression, rejection, self-hatred, depersonalization; command hallucinations

Risk for **Suicide:** Risk factor: history of self-destructive behavior

Risk for self-directed **Violence:** Risk factors: panic state, history of child abuse, toxic reaction to medication

SELF-ESTEEM, CHRONIC LOW

Chronic low **Self-Esteem** (See **Self-Esteem,** low, chronic, Section II)

Risk for disturbed personal **Identity** r/t chronic low self-esteem

SELF-ESTEEM, SITUATIONAL LOW

Situational low **Self-Esteem** (See **Self-Esteem,** low, situational, Section II)

Risk for situational low **Self-Esteem** (See **Self-Esteem,** low, situational, risk for, Section II)

SELF-HEALTH MANAGEMENT, INEFFECTIVE

Ineffective **Self-Health Management** (See **Self-Health Management,** ineffective, Section II)

SELF-HEALTH MANAGEMENT, READINESS FOR ENHANCED

Readiness for enhanced **Self-Health Management** (See **Self-Health Management,** readiness for enhanced, Section II)

SELF-MUTILATION, RISK FOR

Self-Mutilation (See **Self-Mutilation,** Section II)

Ineffective **Impulse Control** r/t ineffective management of anxiety

Risk for **Self-Mutilation** (See **Self-Mutilation,** risk for, Section II)

SENILE DEMENTIA

Sedentary lifestyle r/t lack of interest

Ineffective **Relationship** r/t cognitive changes in one partner

See Dementia

SEPARATION ANXIETY

Ineffective **Coping** r/t maturational and situational crises, vulnerability related to developmental age, hospitalization, separation from family and familiar surroundings, multiple caregivers

Insomnia r/t separation for significant others

Risk for impaired **Attachment:** Risk factor: separation

See Hospitalized Child

SEPSIS, CHILD

Imbalanced **Nutrition:** less than body requirements r/t anorexia, generalized weakness, poor sucking reflex

Ineffective peripheral **Tissue Perfusion:** r/t arterial or venous blood flow exchange problems, septic shock

Delayed **Surgical Recovery** r/t presence of infection

Ineffective **Thermoregulation** r/t infectious process, septic shock

Risk for impaired **Skin Integrity:** Risk factors: desquamation caused by disseminated intravascular coagulation

See Hospitalized Child; Premature Infant, Child

SEPTICEMIA

Imbalanced **Nutrition:** less than body requirements r/t anorexia, generalized weakness

Ineffective peripheral **Tissue Perfusion** r/t decreased systemic vascular resistance

Risk for imbalanced **Fluid Volume** r/t vasodilation of peripheral vessels, leaking of capillaries

Risk for **Shock:** Risk factors: hypotension, hypovolemia

See Sepsis, Child; Shock, Septic

SEVERE ACUTE RESPIRATORY SYNDROME (SARS)

See SARS (Severe Acute Respiratory Syndrome); Pneumonia

SEXUAL DYSFUNCTION

Sexual Dysfunction (See **Sexual Dysfunction,** Section III)

Ineffective **Relationship** r/t reported sexual dissatisfaction between partners

Chronic **Sorrow** r/t loss of ideal sexual experience, altered relationships

Risk for chronic low **Self-Esteem**

See Erectile Dysfunction (ED)

SEXUALITY, ADOLESCENT

Disturbed **Body Image** r/t anxiety caused by unachieved developmental milestone (puberty) or deficient knowledge regarding reproductive maturation as manifested by amenorrhea or expressed concerns regarding lack of growth of secondary sex characteristics

Decisional Conflict: sexual activity r/t undefined personal values or beliefs, multiple or divergent sources of information, lack of relevant information

Ineffective **Impulse Control** r/t denial of consequences of actions

Deficient **Knowledge:** potential for enhanced health maintenance r/t multiple or divergent sources of information or lack of relevant information regarding sexual transmission of disease, contraception, prevention of toxic shock syndrome

See Maturational Issues, Adolescent

S

SEXUALITY PATTERN, INEFFECTIVE

Ineffective **Sexuality Pattern** (See **Sexuality Pattern,** ineffective, Section II)

SEXUALLY TRANSMITTED DISEASE (STD)

See STD (Sexually Transmitted Disease)

SHAKEN BABY SYNDROME

Decreased **Intracranial Adaptive Capacity** r/t brain injury

Impaired **Parenting** r/t stress, history of being abusive

Impaired individual **Resilience** r/t poor impulse control

Stress overload r/t intense repeated family stressors, family violence

Risk for other-directed **Violence:** Risk factors: history of violence against others, perinatal complications

See Child Abuse; Suspected Child Abuse and Neglect (SCAN), Child; Suspected Child Abuse and Neglect (SCAN), Parent

SHAKINESS

Anxiety r/t situational or maturational crisis, threat of death

SHAME

Situational low **Self-Esteem** r/t inability to deal with past traumatic events, blaming of self for events not under one's control

SHINGLES

Impaired **Comfort** r/t inflammation

Acute **Pain** r/t vesicular eruption along the nerves

Ineffective **Protection** r/t abnormal blood profiles

Social Isolation r/t altered state of wellness, contagiousness of disease

Risk for **Infection:** Risk factor: tissue destruction

Readiness for enhanced **Immunization Status:** expresses desire to enhance immunization status

See Itching

SHIVERING

Impaired **Comfort** r/t altered health status

Fear r/t serious threat to health status

Hypothermia r/t exposure to cool environment

Risk for **Injury:** Risk factor: prolonged shock resulting in multiple organ failure or death

Risk for decreased **Cardiac** tissue perfusion: Risk factor: hypotension, hypovolemia

Risk for ineffective **Renal Perfusion:** Risk factor: hypovolemia

Risk for **Shock** (See **Shock,** risk for, Section II)

See Shock, Cardiogenic; Shock, Hypovolemic; Shock, Septic

SHOCK, CARDIOGENIC

Decreased **Cardiac Output** r/t decreased myocardial contractility, dysrhythmia

SHOCK, HYPOVOLEMIC

Deficient **Fluid Volume** r/t abnormal loss of fluid, trauma, third spacing

SHOCK, SEPTIC

Deficient **Fluid Volume** r/t abnormal loss of fluid through capillaries, pooling of blood in peripheral circulation

Ineffective **Protection** r/t inadequately functioning immune system

See Sepsis, Child; Septicemia

SHOULDER REPAIR

Self-Care deficit: bathing, dressing, feeding r/t immobilization of affected shoulder

Risk for **Perioperative Positioning Injury:** Risk factor: immobility

S

See Surgery, Preoperative; Surgery, Perioperative; Surgery, Postoperative; Total Joint Replacement (Total Hip/Total Knee/Shoulder)

SICKLE CELL ANEMIA/CRISIS

Activity Intolerance r/t fatigue, effects of chronic anemia

Impaired **Comfort** r/t altered health status

Deficient **Fluid Volume** r/t decreased intake, increased fluid requirements during sickle cell crisis, decreased ability of kidneys to concentrate urine

Impaired physical **Mobility** r/t pain, fatigue

Acute **Pain** r/t viscous blood, tissue hypoxia

Ineffective peripheral **Tissue Perfusion** r/t effects of red cell sickling, infarction of tissues

Risk for disproportionate **Growth**: Risk factor: chronic illness

Risk for **Infection**: Risk factor: alterations in splenic function

Risk for decreased **Cardiac** tissue perfusion: Risk factors: effects of red cell sickling, infarction of tissues

Risk for ineffective cerebral, gastrointestinal, renal **Tissue Perfusion**: Risk factors: effects of red cell sickling, infarction of tissues

Risk for compromised **Resilience**: Risk factor: chronic illness

Readiness for enhanced **Immunization Status**: receives appropriate immunizations to prevent disease

See Child with Chronic Condition; Hospitalized Child

SIDS (SUDDEN INFANT DEATH SYNDROME)

Anxiety/Fear: parental r/t life-threatening event

Interrupted **Family Processes** r/t stress as a result of special care needs of infant with apnea

Grieving r/t potential loss of infant

Insomnia: parental/infant r/t home apnea monitoring

Deficient **Knowledge:** potential for enhanced health maintenance r/t knowledge or skill acquisition of cardiopulmonary resuscitation and home apnea monitoring

Impaired **Resilience** r/t sudden loss

Risk for **Sudden Infant Death Syndrome** (See **Sudden Infant Death Syndrome,** risk for, Section II)

Risk for **Powerlessness**: Risk factor: unanticipated life-threatening event

See Terminally Ill Child/Death of Child, Parent

SITUATIONAL CRISIS

Ineffective **Coping** r/t situational crisis

Interrupted **Family Processes** r/t situational crisis

Risk for ineffective **Activity Planning** r/t inability to process information

Risk for disturbed personal **Identity** r/t situational crisis

Readiness for enhanced **Communication**: willingness to share feelings and thoughts

Readiness for enhanced **Religiosity**: requests religious material and/or experiences

Readiness for enhanced **Resilience**: desire to enhance resilience

Readiness for enhanced **Spiritual Well-Being**: desire for harmony following crisis

SJS (STEVENS-JOHNSON SYNDROME)

See Stevens-Johnson Syndrome (SJS)

SKIN CANCER

Ineffective **Health Maintenance** r/t deficient knowledge regarding self-care with skin cancer

Ineffective **Protection** r/t weakened immune system

S

Impaired **Skin Integrity** r/t abnormal cell growth in skin, treatment of skin cancer

Readiness for enhanced **Knowledge:** self-care to prevent and treat skin cancer

Readiness for enhanced **Self-Health Management:** follows preventive measures

SKIN DISORDERS

Impaired **Skin Integrity** (See **Skin Integrity,** impaired, Section II)

SKIN INTEGRITY, RISK FOR IMPAIRED

Risk for impaired **Skin Integrity** (See **Skin Integrity,** impaired, risk for, Section II)

SKIN TURGOR, CHANGE IN ELASTICITY

Deficient **Fluid Volume** r/t active fluid loss

SLEEP

Readiness for enhanced **Sleep** (See **Sleep,** readiness for enhanced, Section II)

SLEEP APNEA

See PND (Paroxysmal Nocturnal Dyspnea)

SLEEP DEPRIVATION

Fatigue r/t lack of sleep

Sleep deprivation (See **Sleep** deprivation, Section II)

SLEEP PATTERN DISORDERS

Insomnia (See **Insomnia,** Section II)

SLEEP PATTERN, DISTURBED, PARENT/CHILD

Insomnia: child r/t anxiety or fear

Insomnia: parent r/t parental responsibilities, stress

See Suspected Child Abuse and Neglect (SCAN), Child and Parent

SLURRING OF SPEECH

Impaired verbal **Communication** r/t decrease in circulation to brain, brain tumor, anatomical defect, cleft palate

Situational low **Self-Esteem** r/t speech impairment

See Communication Problems

SMALL BOWEL RESECTION

See Abdominal Surgery

SMELL, LOSS OF ABILITY TO

Risk for **Injury:** Risk factors: inability to detect gas fumes, smoke smells

See Anosmia

SMOKE INHALATION

Ineffective **Airway Clearance** r/t smoke inhalation

Impaired **Gas Exchange** r/t ventilation-perfusion imbalance

Risk for acute **Confusion:** Risk factor: decreased oxygen supply

Risk for **Poisoning:** Risk factor: exposure to carbon monoxide

Readiness for enhanced **Self-Health Management:** functioning smoke detectors and carbon monoxide detectors in home and work, plan for escape route worked out and reviewed

See Atelectasis; Burns; Pneumonia

SMOKING BEHAVIOR

Insufficient **Breast Milk** r/t smoking

Risk-prone **Health Behavior** r/t smoking

Altered **Health Maintenance** r/t denial of effects of smoking, lack of effective support for smoking withdrawal

Readiness for enhanced **Knowledge:** expresses interest in smoking cessation

Risk for dry **Eye** r/t smoking

Risk for ineffective peripheral **Tissue Perfusion** r/t effect of nicotine

Risk for **Thermal Injury** r/t unsafe smoking behavior

S

SOCIAL INTERACTION, IMPAIRED

Impaired **Social Interaction** (See **Social Interaction**, impaired, Section II)

SOCIAL ISOLATION

Social Isolation (See **Social Isolation**, Section II)

SOCIOPATHIC PERSONALITY

See Antisocial Personality Disorder

SODIUM, DECREASE/ INCREASE

See Hyponatremia; Hypernatremia

SOMATIZATION DISORDER

Anxiety r/t unresolved conflicts channeled into physical complaints or conditions

Ineffective **Coping** r/t lack of insight into underlying conflicts

Ineffective **Denial** r/t displaces psychological stress to physical symptoms

Nausea r/t anxiety

Chronic **Pain** r/t unexpressed anger, multiple physical disorders, depression

Impaired individual **Resilience** r/t possible psychological disorders

SORE NIPPLES, BREASTFEEDING

Ineffective **Breastfeeding** r/t deficient knowledge regarding correct feeding procedure

See Painful Breasts, Sore Nipples

SORE THROAT

Impaired **Comfort** r/t sore throat

Deficient **Knowledge** r/t treatment, relief of discomfort

Impaired **Oral Mucous Membrane** r/t inflammation or infection of oral cavity

Impaired **Swallowing** r/t irritation of oropharyngeal cavity

SORROW

Grieving r/t loss of significant person, object, or role

Chronic **Sorrow** (See **Sorrow**, chronic, Section II)

Readiness for enhanced **Communication**: expresses thoughts and feelings

Readiness for enhanced **Spiritual Well-Being**: desire to find purpose and meaning of loss

SPASTIC COLON

See IBS (Irritable Bowel Syndrome)

SPEECH DISORDERS

Anxiety r/t difficulty with communication

Impaired verbal **Communication** r/t anatomical defect, cleft palate, psychological barriers, decrease in circulation to brain

Delayed **Growth and Development** r/t effects of physical or mental disability

SPINA BIFIDA

See Neural Tube Defects

SPINAL CORD INJURY

Deficient **Diversional Activity** r/t long-term hospitalization, frequent lengthy treatments

Fear r/t powerlessness over loss of body function

Complicated **Grieving** r/t loss of usual body function

Sedentary Lifestyle r/t lack of resources or interest

Impaired wheelchair **Mobility** r/t neuromuscular impairment

Urinary Retention r/t inhibition of reflex arc

Risk for **Latex Allergy Response**: Risk factor: continuous or intermittent catheterization

Risk for **Autonomic Dysreflexia**: Risk factors: bladder or bowel distention, skin

S

irritation, deficient knowledge of patient and caregiver

Risk for ineffective **Breathing Pattern:** Risk factor: neuromuscular impairment

Risk for **Infection:** Risk factors: chronic disease, stasis of body fluids

Risk for **Loneliness:** Risk factor: physical immobility

Risk for **Powerlessness:** Risk factor: loss of function

See Child with Chronic Condition; Hospitalized Child; Neural Tube Defects; Paralysis

SPINAL FUSION

Impaired bed **Mobility** r/t impaired ability to turn side to side while keeping spine in proper alignment

Impaired physical **Mobility** r/t musculoskeletal impairment associated with surgery, possible back brace

Readiness for enhanced **Knowledge:** expresses interest in information associated with surgery

See Acute Back; Back Pain; Scoliosis; Surgery, Preoperative Care; Surgery, Perioperative Care; Surgery, Postoperative Care

SPIRITUAL DISTRESS

Spiritual Distress (See **Spiritual Distress,** Section II)

Risk for chronic low **Self-Esteem** r/t unresolved spiritual issues

Risk for **Spiritual Distress** (See **Spiritual Distress,** risk for, Section II)

SPIRITUAL WELL-BEING

Readiness for enhanced **Spiritual Well-Being** (See **Spiritual Well-Being,** readiness for enhanced, Section II)

SPLENECTOMY

See Abdominal Surgery

SPRAINS

Acute **Pain** r/t physical injury

Impaired physical **Mobility** r/t injury

STAPEDECTOMY

Acute **Pain** r/t headache

Hearing Loss caused by edema from surgery

Risk for **Falls:** Risk factor: dizziness

Risk for **Infection:** Risk factor: invasive procedure

STASIS ULCER

Impaired **Tissue Integrity** r/t chronic venous congestion

See CHF (Congestive Heart Failure); Varicose Veins

STD (SEXUALLY TRANSMITTED DISEASE)

Impaired **Comfort** r/t infection

Fear r/t altered body function, risk for social isolation, fear of incurable illness

Ineffective **Health Maintenance** r/t deficient knowledge regarding transmission, symptoms, treatment of STD

Ineffective **Sexuality Pattern** r/t illness, altered body function

Social Isolation r/t fear of contracting or spreading disease

Risk for **Infection:** spread of infection: Risk factor: lack of knowledge concerning transmission of disease

Readiness for enhanced **Knowledge:** seeks information regarding prevention and treatment of STDs

See Maturational Issues, Adolescent; PID (Pelvic Inflammatory Disease)

STEMI (ST-ELEVATION MYOCARDIAL INFARCTION)

See MI (Myocardial Infarction)

STENT (CORONARY ARTERY STENT)

Risk for **Injury**: Risk factor: complications associated with stent placement

Risk for decreased **Cardiac** tissue perfusion: Risk factor: possible restenosis

Risk for **Vascular Trauma**: Risk factor: insertion site, catheter width

Readiness for enhanced **Decision-Making**: expresses desire to enhance risk-benefit analysis, understanding and meaning of choices, and decisions regarding treatment

See Angioplasty, Coronary; Cardiac Catheterization

STERILIZATION SURGERY

Decisional Conflict r/t multiple or divergent sources of information, unclear personal values or beliefs

See Surgery, Preoperative Care; Surgery, Perioperative Care; Surgery, Postoperative Care; Tubal Ligation; Vasectomy

STERTOROUS RESPIRATIONS

Ineffective **Airway Clearance** r/t pharyngeal obstruction

STEVENS-JOHNSON SYNDROME (SJS)

Impaired **Oral Mucous Membrane** r/t immunocompromised condition associated with allergic medication reaction

Acute **Pain** r/t painful skin lesions and painful oral mucosa lesions

Impaired **Skin Integrity** r/t allergic medication reaction

Risk for acute **Confusion**: Risk factors: dehydration, electrolyte disturbances

Risk for imbalanced **Fluid Volume**: Risk factors: factors affecting fluid needs (hypermetabolic state, hyperthermia), excessive losses through normal routes (vomiting and diarrhea)

Risk for **Infection**: Risk factor: broken skin

Risk for impaired **Liver Function**: Risk factor: infection

STILLBIRTH

See Pregnancy Loss

STOMA

See Colostomy; Ileostomy

STOMATITIS

Impaired **Oral Mucous Membrane** r/t pathological conditions of oral cavity

STONE, KIDNEY

See Kidney Stone

STOOL, HARD/DRY

Constipation r/t inadequate fluid intake, inadequate fiber intake, decreased activity level, decreased gastric motility

STRAINING WITH DEFECATION

Decreased **Cardiac Output** r/t vagal stimulation with dysrhythmia resulting from Valsalva maneuver

Constipation r/t less than adequate fluid intake, less than adequate dietary intake

STREP THROAT

Risk for **Infection**: Risk factor: exposure to pathogen

See Sore Throat

STRESS

Anxiety r/t feelings of helplessness, feelings of being threatened

Ineffective **Coping** r/t ineffective use of problem-solving process, feelings of apprehension or helplessness

Disturbed **Energy Field** r/t low energy level, feelings of hopelessness

Fear r/t powerlessness over feelings

Stress overload r/t intense or multiple stressors

S

Risk for **Post-Trauma Syndrome**: Risk factors: perception of event, survivor's role in event

Readiness for enhanced **Communication**: shows willingness to share thoughts and feelings

Readiness for enhanced **Spiritual Well-Being**: expresses desire for harmony and peace in stressful situation

See Anxiety

STRESS OVERLOAD

Stress overload (See **Stress** overload, Section II)

STRESS URINARY INCONTINENCE

Stress urinary **Incontinence** r/t degenerative change in pelvic muscles

Risk for urge urinary **Incontinence**: Risk factor: involuntary sphincter relaxation

See Incontinence of Urine

STRIDOR

Ineffective **Airway Clearance** r/t obstruction, tracheobronchial infection, trauma

STROKE

See CVA (Cerebrovascular Accident)

STUTTERING

Anxiety r/t impaired verbal communication

Impaired verbal **Communication** r/t anxiety, psychological problems

SUBARACHNOID HEMORRHAGE

Acute **Pain**: headache r/t irritation of meninges from blood, increased intracranial pressure

Risk for ineffective **Cerebral** tissue perfusion: Risk factor: bleeding from cerebral vessel

See Intracranial Pressure, Increased

SUBSTANCE ABUSE

Compromised/disabled family **Coping** r/t codependency issues

Defensive **Coping** r/t substance abuse

Ineffective **Coping** r/t use of substances to cope with life events

Ineffective **Denial** r/t refusal to acknowledge substance abuse problem

Dysfunctional **Family Processes** r/t substance abuse

Deficient community **Health** r/t prevention and control of illegal substances in community

Ineffective **Impulse Control** r/t addictive process

Ineffective **Relationship** r/t inability for well-balanced collaboration between partners

Insomnia r/t irritability, nightmares, tremors

Risk for impaired **Attachment**: Risk factor: substance abuse

Risk for disturbed personal **Identity** r/t ingestion/inhalation of toxic chemicals

Risk for chronic low **Self-Esteem**

Risk for **Thermal Injury**

Risk for **Vascular Trauma**: Risk factor: chemical irritant

Risk for self- or other-directed **Violence**: Risk factors: reactions to substances used, impulsive behavior, disorientation, impaired judgment

Readiness for enhanced **Coping**: seeking social support and knowledge of new strategies

Readiness for enhanced **Self-Concept**: accepting strengths and limitations

See Alcoholism; Drug Abuse; Maturational Issues, Adolescent

SUBSTANCE ABUSE, ADOLESCENT

See Alcohol Withdrawal; Maturational Issues, Adolescent; Substance Abuse

SUBSTANCE ABUSE IN PREGNANCY

Ineffective **Childbearing Process** r/t use of substance abuse

Defensive **Coping** r/t denial of situation, differing value system

Ineffective **Health Maintenance** r/t addiction

Deficient **Knowledge** r/t lack of exposure to information regarding effects of substance abuse in pregnancy

Noncompliance r/t differing value system, cultural influences, addiction

Risk for impaired **Attachment**: Risk factors: substance abuse, inability of parent to meet infant's or own personal needs

Risk for **Infection**: Risk factors: intravenous drug use, lifestyle

Risk for **Injury**: fetal: Risk factor: effects of drugs on fetal growth and development

Risk for **Injury**: maternal: Risk factor: drug use

Risk for impaired **Parenting**: Risk factor: lack of ability to meet infant's needs

See Alcoholism; Drug Abuse; Substance Abuse

SUCKING REFLEX

Effective **Breastfeeding** r/t regular and sustained sucking and swallowing at breast

SUDDEN INFANT DEATH SYNDROME (SIDS)

See SIDS (Sudden Infant Death Syndrome)

SUFFOCATION, RISK FOR

Risk for **Suffocation** (See **Suffocation**, risk for, Section II)

SUICIDE ATTEMPT

Risk-prone **Health Behavior** r/t low self-efficacy

Ineffective **Coping** r/t anger, complicated grieving

Hopelessness r/t perceived or actual loss, substance abuse, low self-concept, inadequate support systems

Ineffective **Impulse Control** r/t inability to modulate stress/anxiety

Post-Trauma Syndrome r/t history of traumatic events, abuse, rape, incest, war, torture

Impaired individual **Resilience** r/t poor impulse control

Situational low **Self-Esteem** r/t guilt, inability to trust, feelings of worthlessness or rejection

Social Isolation r/t inability to engage in satisfying personal relationships

Spiritual Distress r/t hopelessness, despair

Risk for **Post-Trauma Syndrome**: Risk factor: survivor's role in suicide attempt

Risk for **Suicide** (See **Suicide**, risk for, Section II)

Readiness for enhanced **Communication**: willingness to share thoughts and feelings

Readiness for enhanced **Spiritual Well-Being**: desire for harmony and inner strength to help redefine purpose for life

See Violent Behavior

SUPPORT SYSTEM

Readiness for enhanced family **Coping**: ability to adapt to tasks associated with care, support of significant other during health crisis

Readiness for enhanced **Family Processes**: activities support the growth of family members

Readiness for enhanced **Parenting**: children or other dependent person(s) expressing satisfaction with home environment

SUPPRESSION OF LABOR

See Preterm Labor; Tocolytic Therapy

S

SURGERY, PERIOPERATIVE CARE

Risk for imbalanced **Fluid Volume:** Risk factor: surgery

Risk for **Perioperative Positioning Injury:** Risk factors: predisposing condition, prolonged surgery

SURGERY, POSTOPERATIVE CARE

Activity Intolerance r/t pain, surgical procedure

Anxiety r/t change in health status, hospital environment

Deficient **Knowledge** r/t postoperative expectations, lifestyle changes

Nausea r/t manipulation of gastrointestinal tract, postsurgical anesthesia

Imbalanced **Nutrition:** less than body requirements r/t anorexia, nausea, vomiting, decreased peristalsis

Ineffective peripheral **Tissue Perfusion** r/t hypovolemia, circulatory stasis, obesity, prolonged immobility, decreased coughing, decreased deep breathing

Acute **Pain** r/t inflammation or injury in surgical area

Delayed **Surgical Recovery** r/t extensive surgical procedure, postoperative surgical infection

Urinary Retention r/t anesthesia, pain, fear, unfamiliar surroundings, client's position

Risk for **Bleeding:** Risk factor: surgical procedure

Risk for ineffective **Breathing Pattern:** Risk factors: pain, location of incision, effects of anesthesia or opioids

Risk for **Constipation:** Risk factors: decreased activity, decreased food or fluid intake, anesthesia, pain medication

Risk for imbalanced **Fluid Volume:** Risk factors: hypermetabolic state, fluid loss

during surgery, presence of indwelling tubes

Risk for **Infection:** Risk factors: invasive procedure, pain, anesthesia, location of incision, weakened cough as a result of aging

SURGERY, PREOPERATIVE CARE

Anxiety r/t threat to or change in health status, situational crisis, fear of the unknown

Insomnia r/t anxiety about upcoming surgery

Deficient **Knowledge** r/t preoperative procedures, postoperative expectations

Readiness for enhanced **Knowledge:** shows understanding of preoperative and postoperative expectations for self-care

SURGICAL RECOVERY, DELAYED

Delayed **Surgical Recovery** (See **Surgical Recovery,** delayed, Section II)

SUSPECTED CHILD ABUSE AND NEGLECT (SCAN), CHILD

Ineffective **Activity Planning** r/t lack of family support

Anxiety/Fear: child r/t threat of punishment for perceived wrongdoing

Deficient community **Health** r/t inadequate reporting and follow-up of SCAN

Disturbed personal **Identity** r/t dysfunctional family processes

Rape-Trauma Syndrome r/t altered lifestyle because of abuse, changes in residence

Risk for compromised **Resilience:** Risk factor: adverse situation

Readiness for enhanced community **Coping:** obtaining resources to prevent child abuse, neglect

See Child Abuse; Hospitalized Child; Maturational Issues, Adolescent

SUSPECTED CHILD ABUSE AND NEGLECT (SCAN), PARENT

Disabled family **Coping** r/t dysfunctional family, underdeveloped nurturing parental role, lack of parental support systems or role models

Dysfunctional **Family Processes** r/t inadequate coping skills

Ineffective **Health Maintenance** r/t deficient knowledge of parenting skills as a result of unachieved developmental tasks

Impaired **Home Maintenance** r/t disorganization, parental dysfunction, neglect of safe and nurturing environment

Ineffective **Impulse Control** r/t projection of anger/frustration onto the child

Impaired **Parenting** r/t unrealistic expectations of child; lack of effective role model; unmet social, emotional, or maturational needs of parents; interruption in bonding process

Powerlessness r/t inability to perform parental role responsibilities

Impaired individual **Resilience** r/t poor impulse control

Chronic low **Self-Esteem** r/t lack of successful parenting experiences

Risk for other-directed **Violence:** parent to child: Risk factors: inadequate coping mechanisms, unresolved stressors, unachieved maturational level by parent

SUSPICION

Disturbed personal **Identity** r/t psychiatric disorder

Powerlessness r/t repetitive paranoid thinking

Impaired **Social Interaction** r/t disturbed thought processes, paranoid delusions, hallucinations

Risk for self- or other-directed **Violence:** Risk factor: inability to trust

SWALLOWING DIFFICULTIES

Impaired **Swallowing** (See **Swallowing**, impaired, Section III)

SWINE FLU (H1N1)

See Influenza

SYNCOPE

Anxiety r/t fear of falling

Decreased **Cardiac Output** r/t dysrhythmia

Impaired physical **Mobility** r/t fear of falling

Social Isolation r/t fear of falling

Risk for **Falls:** Risk factor: syncope

Risk for **Injury:** Risk factors: altered sensory perception, transient loss of consciousness, risk for falls

Risk for ineffective **Cerebral** tissue perfusion: Risk factor: interruption of blood flow

SYPHILIS

See STD (Sexually Transmitted Disease)

SYSTEMIC LUPUS ERYTHEMATOSUS

See Lupus Erythematosus

T

T & A (TONSILLECTOMY AND ADENOIDECTOMY)

Ineffective **Airway Clearance** r/t hesitation or reluctance to cough because of pain

Deficient **Knowledge:** potential for enhanced health maintenance r/t insufficient knowledge regarding postoperative nutritional and rest requirements, signs and symptoms of complications, positioning

Nausea r/t gastric irritation, pharmaceuticals, anesthesia

Acute **Pain** r/t surgical incision

Risk for **Aspiration/Suffocation**: Risk factors: postoperative drainage and impaired swallowing

Risk for deficient **Fluid Volume**: Risk factors: decreased intake because of painful swallowing, effects of anesthesia (nausea, vomiting), hemorrhage

Risk for imbalanced **Nutrition**: less than body requirements: Risk factors: hesitation or reluctance to swallow

TACHYCARDIA

See Dysrhythmia

TACHYPNEA

Ineffective **Breathing Pattern** r/t pain, anxiety

See cause of Tachypnea

TARDIVE DYSKINESIA

Ineffective **Self-Health Management** r/t complexity of therapeutic regimen or medication

Deficient **Knowledge** r/t cognitive limitation in assimilating information relating to side effects associated with neuroleptic medications

Risk for **Injury**: Risk factor: drug-induced abnormal body movements

TASTE ABNORMALITY

Adult **Failure to Thrive** r/t imbalanced nutrition: less than body requirements associated with taste abnormality

TB (PULMONARY TUBERCULOSIS)

Ineffective **Airway Clearance** r/t increased secretions, excessive mucus

Ineffective **Breathing Pattern** r/t decreased energy, fatigue

Fatigue r/t disease state

Impaired **Gas Exchange** r/t disease process

Ineffective **Self-Health Management** r/t deficient knowledge of prevention and treatment regimen

Impaired **Home Maintenance** management r/t client or family member with disease

Hyperthermia r/t infection

Risk for **Infection**: Risk factors: insufficient knowledge regarding avoidance of exposure to pathogens

Readiness for enhanced **Self-Health Management**: takes medications according to prescribed protocol for prevention and treatment

TBI (TRAUMATIC BRAIN INJURY)

Interrupted **Family Processes** r/t traumatic injury to family member

Chronic **Sorrow** r/t change in health status and functional ability

Risk for **Post-Trauma Syndrome**: Risk factor: perception of event causing TBI

Risk for impaired **Religiosity**: Risk factor: impaired physical mobility

Risk for compromised **Resilience**: Risk factor: crisis of injury

See Head Injury; Neurologic Disorders

TD (TRAVELER'S DIARRHEA)

Diarrhea r/t travel

Risk for deficient **Fluid Volume**: Risk factors: excessive loss of fluids, diarrhea

Risk for **Infection**: Risk factors: insufficient knowledge regarding avoidance of exposure to pathogens (water supply, iced drinks, local cheeses, ice cream, undercooked meat, fish and shellfish, uncooked vegetables, unclean eating utensils, improper handwashing)

TEMPERATURE, DECREASED

Hypothermia r/t exposure to cold environment

Hyperthermia r/t dehydration, illness, trauma

Ineffective **Thermoregulation** r/t trauma, illness

See Toxic Epidermal Necrolysis (TEN)

Anxiety r/t threat to or change in health status, situational crisis

Disturbed **Energy Field** r/t change in health status, discouragement, pain

Readiness for enhanced **Communication:** expresses willingness to share feelings and thoughts

See Stress

Death **Anxiety** r/t unresolved issues relating to death and dying

Disturbed **Energy Field** r/t impending disharmony of mind, body, spirit

Risk for **Spiritual Distress:** Risk factor: impending death

Readiness for enhanced **Religiosity:** requests religious material and/or experiences

Readiness for enhanced **Spiritual Well-Being:** desire to achieve harmony of mind, body, spirit

See Terminally Ill Child/Death of Child, Parent

Disturbed **Body Image** r/t effects of terminal disease, already critical feelings of group identity and self-image

Ineffective **Coping** r/t inability to establish personal and peer identity because of the threat of being different or not being healthy, inability to achieve maturational tasks

Impaired **Social Interaction/Social Isolation** r/t forced separation from peers

See Child with Chronic Condition; Hospitalized Child, Terminally Ill Child/Death of Child, Parent

Ineffective **Coping** r/t separation from parents and familiar environment attributable to inability to understand dying process

See Child with Chronic Condition, Terminally Ill Child/Death of Child, Parent

Fear r/t perceived punishment, bodily harm, feelings of guilt caused by magical thinking (i.e., believing that thoughts cause events)

See Child with Chronic Condition, Terminally Ill Child/Death of Child, Parent

Fear r/t perceived punishment, body mutilation, feelings of guilt

See Child with Chronic Condition, Terminally Ill Child/Death of Child, Parent

Compromised family **Coping** r/t inability or unwillingness to discuss impending death and feelings with child or support child through terminal stages of illness

Decisional Conflict r/t continuation or discontinuation of treatment,

T

do-not-resuscitate decision, ethical issues regarding organ donation

Ineffective **Denial** r/t complicated grieving

Interrupted **Family Processes** r/t situational crisis

Grieving r/t death of child

Hopelessness r/t overwhelming stresses caused by terminal illness

Insomnia r/t grieving process

Impaired **Parenting** r/t risk for overprotection of surviving siblings

Powerlessness r/t inability to alter course of events

Impaired **Social Interaction** r/t complicated grieving

Social Isolation: imposed by others r/t feelings of inadequacy in providing support to grieving parents

Social Isolation: self-imposed r/t unresolved grief, perceived inadequate parenting skills

Spiritual Distress r/t sudden and unexpected death, prolonged suffering before death, questioning the death of youth, questioning the meaning of one's own existence

Risk for complicated **Grieving:** Risk factors: prolonged, unresolved, obstructed progression through stages of grief and mourning

Risk for compromised **Resilience:** Risk factor: impending death

Readiness for enhanced family **Coping:** impact of crisis on family values, priorities, goals, or relationships; expressed interest or desire to attach meaning to child's life and death

TETRALOGY OF FALLOT

See Congenital Heart Disease/Cardiac Anomalies

TETRAPLEGIA

Autonomic Dysreflexia r/t spinal cord injury

Grieving r/t loss of previous functioning

Risk for **Aspiration**

Risk for imbalance in body **Temperature,** hyperthermia/hypothermia

Risk for **Infection** r/t stasis

Powerlessness r/t inability to perform previous activities

Risk for impaired **Skin Integrity** r/t physical immobilization

THERAPEUTIC REGIMEN MANAGEMENT, INEFFECTIVE: FAMILY

Ineffective family **Therapeutic Regimen Management** (See **Therapeutic Regimen Management,** family, ineffective, Section II)

THERAPEUTIC TOUCH

Disturbed **Energy Field** r/t low energy levels, disturbance in energy fields, pain, depression, fatigue

THERMAL INJURY, RISK FOR

(See **Thermal Injury,** Risk for, Section II)

THERMOREGULATION, INEFFECTIVE

Ineffective **Thermoregulation** (See **Thermoregulation,** ineffective, Section II)

THORACENTESIS

See Pleural Effusion

THORACOTOMY

Activity Intolerance r/t pain, imbalance between oxygen supply and demand, presence of chest tubes

Ineffective **Airway Clearance** r/t drowsiness, pain with breathing and coughing

Ineffective **Breathing** pattern r/t decreased energy, fatigue, pain

Deficient **Knowledge** r/t self-care, effective breathing exercises, pain relief

Acute **Pain** r/t surgical procedure, coughing, deep breathing

Risk for **Bleeding:** Risk factor: surgery

Risk for **Infection:** Risk factor: invasive procedure

Risk for **Injury:** Risk factor: disruption of closed-chest drainage system

Risk for **Perioperative Positioning Injury:** Risk factor: lateral positioning, immobility

Risk for **Vascular Trauma:** Risk factor: chemical irritant; antibiotics

THOUGHT DISORDERS

See Schizophrenia

THROMBOCYTOPENIC PURPURA

See ITP (Idiopathic Thrombocytopenic Purpura)

THROMBOPHLEBITIS

Constipation r/t inactivity, bed rest

Deficient **Diversional Activity** r/t bed rest

Deficient **Knowledge** r/t pathophysiology of condition, self-care needs, treatment regimen and outcome

Sedentary **Lifestyle** r/t deficient knowledge of benefits of physical exercise

Impaired physical **Mobility** r/t pain in extremity, forced bed rest

Acute **Pain** r/t vascular inflammation, edema

Ineffective peripheral **Tissue Perfusion** r/t interruption of venous blood flow

Delayed **Surgical Recovery** r/t complication associated with inactivity

Risk for **Bleeding:** Risk factors: treatment; anticoagulants

Risk for **Injury:** Risk factor: possible embolus

Risk for **Vascular Trauma:** Risk factor: anticoagulant therapy

See Anticoagulant Therapy

THYROIDECTOMY

Risk for ineffective **Airway Clearance** r/t edema or hematoma formation, airway obstruction

Risk for impaired verbal **Communication:** Risk factors: edema, pain, vocal cord or laryngeal nerve damage

Risk for **Injury:** Risk factor: possible parathyroid damage or removal

See Surgery, Preoperative Care; Surgery, Perioperative Care; Surgery, Postoperative Care

TIA (TRANSIENT ISCHEMIC ATTACK)

Acute **Confusion** r/t hypoxia

Readiness for enhanced **Self-Health Management:** obtains knowledge regarding treatment prevention of inadequate oxygenation

See Syncope

TIC DISORDER

See Tourette's Syndrome (TS)

TINEA CAPITIS

Impaired **Comfort** r/t inflammation from pruritus

See Ringworm of Scalp

TINEA CORPORIS

See Ringworm of Body

TINEA CRURIS

See Jock Itch; Itching; Pruritus

TINEA PEDIS

See Athlete's Foot; Itching; Pruritus

TINEA UNGUIUM (ONYCHOMYCOSIS)

See Ringworm of Nails

T

TINNITUS

Ineffective **Health Maintenance** r/t deficient knowledge regarding self-care with tinnitus

TISSUE DAMAGE, CORNEAL, INTEGUMENTARY, OR SUBCUTANEOUS

Impaired **Tissue Integrity** (See **Tissue Integrity,** impaired, Section II)

TISSUE PERFUSION, INEFFECTIVE PERIPHERAL

Ineffective peripheral **Tissue Perfusion** (See **Tissue Perfusion,** peripheral, ineffective, Section III)

Risk for ineffective peripheral **Tissue Perfusion**

TOILETING PROBLEMS

Toileting **Self-Care** deficit r/t impaired transfer ability, impaired mobility status, intolerance of activity, neuromuscular impairment, cognitive impairment

Impaired **Transfer Ability** r/t neuromuscular deficits

TOILET TRAINING

Deficient **Knowledge:** parent r/t signs of child's readiness for training

Risk for **Constipation:** Risk factor: withholding stool

Risk for **Infection:** Risk factor: withholding urination

TONSILLECTOMY AND ADENOIDECTOMY (T & A)

See T & A (Tonsillectomy and Adenoidectomy)

TOOTHACHE

Impaired **Dentition** r/t ineffective oral hygiene, barriers to self-care, economic barriers to professional care, nutritional deficits, lack of knowledge regarding dental health

Acute **Pain** r/t inflammation, infection

TOTAL ANOMALOUS PULMONARY VENOUS RETURN

See Congenital Heart Disease/Cardiac Anomalies

TOTAL JOINT REPLACEMENT (TOTAL HIP/TOTAL KNEE/ SHOULDER)

Disturbed **Body Image** r/t large scar, presence of prosthesis

Impaired physical **Mobility** r/t musculo-skeletal impairment, surgery, prosthesis

Risk for **Injury:** neurovascular: Risk factors: altered peripheral tissue perfusion, altered mobility, prosthesis

Risk for **Peripheral Neurovascular Dysfunction** r/t immobilization

Ineffective peripheral **Tissue Perfusion** r/t surgery

See Surgery, Preoperative Care; Surgery, Perioperative Care; Surgery, Postoperative Care

TOTAL PARENTERAL NUTRITION (TPN)

See TPN (Total Parenteral Nutrition)

TOURETTE'S SYNDROME (TS)

Hopelessness r/t inability to control behavior

Impaired individual **Resilience** r/t uncontrollable behavior

Risk for situational low **Self-Esteem:** Risk factors: uncontrollable behavior, motor and phonic tics

See Attention Deficit Disorder

TOXEMIA

See PIH (Pregnancy-Induced Hypertension/Preeclampsia)

TOXIC EPIDERMAL NECROLYSIS (TEN) (ERYTHEMA MULTIFORME)

Death **Anxiety** r/t uncertainty of prognosis

See Stevens-Johnson Syndrome (SJS)

T

TPN (TOTAL PARENTERAL NUTRITION)

Imbalanced **Nutrition**: less than body requirements r/t inability to ingest or digest food or absorb nutrients as a result of biological or psychological factors

Risk for unstable blood **Glucose** level

Risk for **Electrolyte Imbalance**

Risk for excess **Fluid Volume**: Risk factor: rapid administration of TPN

Risk for **Infection**: Risk factors: concentrated glucose solution, invasive administration of fluids

Risk for **Vascular Trauma**: Risk factors: insertion site, length of treatment time

TRACHEOESOPHAGEAL FISTULA

Ineffective **Airway Clearance** r/t aspiration of feeding because of inability to swallow

Imbalanced **Nutrition**: less than body requirements r/t difficulties in swallowing

Risk for **Aspiration**: Risk factors: common passage of air and food

Risk for **Vascular Trauma**: Risk factors: venous medications and site

See Respiratory Conditions of the Neonate; Hospitalized Child

TRACHEOSTOMY

Ineffective **Airway Clearance** r/t increased secretions, mucous plugs

Anxiety r/t impaired verbal communication, ineffective airway clearance

Disturbed **Body Image** r/t abnormal opening in neck

Impaired verbal **Communication** r/t presence of mechanical airway

Deficient **Knowledge** r/t self-care, home maintenance management

Acute **Pain** r/t edema, surgical procedure

Risk for **Aspiration**: Risk factor: presence of tracheostomy

Risk for **Bleeding**: Risk factor: surgical incision

Risk for **Infection**: Risk factors: invasive procedure, pooling of secretions

TRACTION AND CASTS

Constipation r/t immobility

Deficient **Diversional Activity** r/t immobility

Impaired physical **Mobility** r/t imposed restrictions on activity because of bone or joint disease injury

Acute **Pain** r/t immobility, injury, or disease

Self-Care deficit: feeding, dressing, bathing, toileting r/t degree of impaired physical mobility, body area affected by traction or cast

Impaired **Transfer Ability** r/t presence of traction, casts

Risk for **Disuse Syndrome**: Risk factor: mechanical immobilization

See Casts

TRANSFER ABILITY

Impaired **Transfer Ability** (See Transfer Ability, impaired, Section II)

TRANSIENT ISCHEMIC ATTACK (TIA)

See TIA (Transient Ischemic Attack)

TRANSPOSITION OF GREAT VESSELS

See Congenital Heart Disease/Cardiac Anomalies

TRANSURETHRAL RESECTION OF THE PROSTATE (TURP)

See TURP (Transurethral Resection of the Prostate)

TRAUMA IN PREGNANCY

Anxiety r/t threat to self or fetus, unknown outcome

T

Deficient **Knowledge** r/t lack of exposure to situation

Acute **Pain** r/t trauma

Impaired **Skin Integrity** r/t trauma

Risk for **Bleeding**: Risk factor: trauma

Risk for imbalanced **Fluid Volume**: Risk factor: fluid loss

Risk for **Infection**: Risk factor: traumatized tissue

Risk for **Injury**: fetal: Risk factor: premature separation of placenta

Risk for disturbed **Maternal/Fetal Dyad**: Risk factor: complication of pregnancy

TRAUMA, RISK FOR

Risk for **Trauma** (See **Trauma,** risk for, Section II)

TRAUMATIC BRAIN INJURY (TBI)

See TBI (Traumatic Brain Injury); Intracranial Pressure, Increased

Ineffective **Impulse Control** r/t brain disorder

TRAUMATIC EVENT

Post-Trauma Syndrome r/t previously experienced trauma

TRAVELER'S DIARRHEA (TD)

See TD (Traveler's Diarrhea)

TREMBLING OF HANDS

Anxiety/Fear r/t threat to or change in health status, threat of death, situational crisis

TRICUSPID ATRESIA

See Congenital Heart Disease/Cardiac Anomalies

TRIGEMINAL NEURALGIA

Ineffective **Self-Health Management** r/t deficient knowledge regarding prevention of stimuli that trigger pain

Imbalanced **Nutrition**: less than body requirements r/t pain when chewing

Acute **Pain** r/t irritation of trigeminal nerve

Risk for **Injury** (eye): Risk factor: possible decreased corneal sensation

TRUNCUS ARTERIOSUS

See Congenital Heart Disease/Cardiac Anomalies

TS (TOURETTE'S SYNDROME)

See Tourette's Syndrome (TS)

TSE (TESTICULAR SELF-EXAMINATION)

Readiness for enhanced **Self-Health Management**: seeks information regarding self-examination

TUBAL LIGATION

Decisional Conflict r/t tubal sterilization

See Laparoscopy

TUBE FEEDING

Risk for **Aspiration**: Risk factors: improperly administered feeding, improper placement of tube, improper positioning of client during and after feeding, excessive residual feeding or lack of digestion, altered gag reflex

Risk for imbalanced **Fluid Volume**: Risk factor: inadequate water administration with concentrated feeding

Risk for imbalanced **Nutrition**: less than body requirements: Risk factors: intolerance to tube feeding, inadequate calorie replacement to meet metabolic needs

TUBERCULOSIS (TB)

See TB (Pulmonary Tuberculosis)

TURP (TRANSURETHRAL RESECTION OF THE PROSTATE)

Deficient Knowledge r/t postoperative self-care, home maintenance management

Acute **Pain** r/t incision, irritation from catheter, bladder spasms, kidney infection

Urinary Retention r/t obstruction of urethra or catheter with clots

Risk for **Bleeding:** Risk factor: surgery

Risk for deficient **Fluid Volume:** Risk factors: fluid loss, possible bleeding

Risk for urge urinary **Incontinence:** Risk factor: edema from surgical procedure

Risk for **Infection:** Risk factors: invasive procedure, route for bacteria entry

Risk for ineffective **Renal Perfusion:** Risk factor: hypovolemia

ULCER, PEPTIC (DUODENAL OR GASTRIC)

Fatigue r/t loss of blood, chronic illness

Ineffective **Health Maintenance** r/t lack of knowledge regarding health practices to prevent ulcer formation

Nausea r/t gastrointestinal irritation

Acute **Pain** r/t irritated mucosa from acid secretion

Risk for ineffective **Gastrointestinal Perfusion:** Risk factor: ulcer

See GI Bleed (Gastrointestinal Bleeding)

ULCERATIVE COLITIS

See Inflammatory Bowel Disease (Child and Adult)

ULCERS, STASIS

See Stasis Ulcer

UNILATERAL NEGLECT OF ONE SIDE OF BODY

Unilateral Neglect (See Unilateral Neglect, Section II)

UNSANITARY LIVING CONDITIONS

Impaired Home Maintenance r/t impaired cognitive or emotional functioning, lack of knowledge, insufficient finances

Risk for **Allergy Response** r/t to exposure to environmental contaminants

URGENCY TO URINATE

Urge urinary Incontinence (See **Incontinence,** urinary, urge, Section II)

Risk for urge urinary **Incontinence** (See **Incontinence,** urinary, urge, risk for, Section II)

URINARY DIVERSION

See Ileal Conduit

URINARY ELIMINATION, IMPAIRED

Impaired Urinary Elimination (See **Urinary Elimination,** impaired, Section II)

URINARY INCONTINENCE

See Incontinence of Urine

URINARY READINESS

Readiness for enhanced Urinary Elimination (See **Urinary Elimination,** readiness for enhanced, Section II)

URINARY RETENTION

Urinary Retention (See **Urinary Retention,** Section II)

URINARY TRACT INFECTION (UTI)

See UTI (Urinary Tract Infection)

UROLITHIASIS

See Kidney Stone

UTERINE ATONY IN LABOR

See Dystocia

UTERINE ATONY IN POSTPARTUM

See Postpartum Hemorrhage

U

UTERINE BLEEDING

See Hemorrhage; Postpartum Hemorrhage; Shock, Hypovolemic

UTI (URINARY TRACT INFECTION)

Ineffective **Health Maintenance** r/t deficient knowledge regarding methods to treat and prevent UTIs

Acute **Pain**: dysuria r/t inflammatory process in bladder

Impaired **Urinary Elimination**: frequency r/t urinary tract infection

Risk for urge urinary **Incontinence**: Risk factor: hyperreflexia from cystitis

Risk for ineffective **Renal Perfusion**: Risk factor: infection

VAD (VENTRICULAR ASSIST DEVICE)

See Ventricular Assist Device (VAD)

VAGINAL HYSTERECTOMY

Urinary Retention r/t edema at surgical site

Risk for urge urinary **Incontinence**: Risk factors: edema, congestion of pelvic tissues

Risk for **Infection**: Risk factor: surgical site

Risk for **Perioperative Positioning Injury**: Risk factor: lithotomy position

See Postpartum Hemorrhage

VAGINITIS

Impaired **Comfort** r/t pruritus, itching

Ineffective **Health Maintenance** r/t deficient knowledge regarding self-care with vaginitis

Ineffective **Sexuality Pattern** r/t abstinence during acute stage, pain

VAGOTOMY

See Abdominal Surgery

VALUE SYSTEM CONFLICT

Decisional Conflict r/t unclear personal values or beliefs

Spiritual Distress r/t challenged value system

Readiness for enhanced **Spiritual Well-Being**: desire for harmony with self, others, higher power, God

VARICOSE VEINS

Ineffective **Health Maintenance** r/t deficient knowledge regarding health care practices, prevention, treatment regimen

Chronic **Pain** r/t impaired circulation

Ineffective peripheral **Tissue Perfusion** r/t venous stasis

Risk for impaired **Skin Integrity**: Risk factor: altered peripheral tissue perfusion

VASCULAR DEMENTIA (FORMERLY CALLED MULTIINFARCT DEMENTIA)

See Dementia

VASCULAR OBSTRUCTION, PERIPHERAL

Anxiety r/t lack of circulation to body part

Acute **Pain** r/t vascular obstruction

Ineffective peripheral **Tissue Perfusion** r/t interruption of circulatory flow

Risk for **Peripheral Neurovascular Dysfunction**: Risk factor: vascular obstruction

VASECTOMY

Decisional Conflict r/t surgery as method of permanent sterilization

VASOCOGNOPATHY

See Alzheimer's Disease; Dementia

VENEREAL DISEASE

See STD (Sexually Transmitted Disease)

VENTILATION, IMPAIRED SPONTANEOUS

Impaired **Spontaneous Ventilation** (See **Spontaneous Ventilation**, impaired, Section II)

VENTILATOR CLIENT

Ineffective **Airway Clearance** r/t increased secretions, decreased cough and gag reflex

Ineffective **Breathing Pattern** r/t decreased energy and fatigue as a result of possible altered nutrition: less than body requirements

Impaired verbal **Communication** r/t presence of endotracheal tube, decreased mentation

Fear r/t inability to breathe on own, difficulty communicating

Impaired **Gas Exchange** r/t ventilation-perfusion imbalance

Powerlessness r/t health treatment regimen

Social Isolation r/t impaired mobility, ventilator dependence

Impaired **Spontaneous Ventilation** r/t metabolic factors, respiratory muscle fatigue

Dysfunctional **Ventilatory Weaning Response** r/t psychological, situational, physiological factors

Risk for **Latex Allergy Response**: Risk factor: repeated exposure to latex products

Risk for **Infection**: Risk factors: presence of endotracheal tube, pooled secretions

Risk for compromised **Resilience**: Risk factor: illness

See Child with Chronic Condition; Hospitalized Child; Respiratory Conditions of the Neonate

VENTILATORY WEANING RESPONSE, DYSFUNCTIONAL (DVWR)

Dysfunctional **Ventilatory Weaning Response** (See **Ventilatory Weaning Response**, dysfunctional, Section II)

VENTRICULAR ASSIST DEVICE (VAD)

Risk for **Vascular Trauma**: Risk factor: insertion site

Readiness for enhanced **Decision-Making**: expresses desire to enhance the understanding of the meaning of choices regarding implanting a ventricular assist device

See Open Heart Surgery

VENTRICULAR FIBRILLATION

See Dysrhythmia

VERTIGO

See Syncope

VIOLENT BEHAVIOR

Risk for other-directed **Violence** (See **Violence**, other-directed, risk for, Section II)

Risk for self-directed **Violence** (See **Violence**, self-directed, risk for, Section II)

VIRAL GASTROENTERITIS

Diarrhea r/t infectious process, rotavirus, Norwalk virus

Ineffective **Self-Health Management** r/t inadequate handwashing

Risk for dysfunctional **Gastrointestinal Motility**: Risk factor: infection

See Gastroenteritis, Child

VISION IMPAIRMENT

Fear r/t loss of sight

Social Isolation r/t altered state of wellness, inability to see

Vision Loss r/t impaired visual function; integration; reception; and or transmission

Risk for compromised **Resilience**: Risk factor: presence of new crisis

See Blindness; Cataracts; Glaucoma

V

VOMITING

Nausea r/t chemotherapy, postsurgical anesthesia, irritation to the gastrointestinal system, stimulation of neuropharmacological mechanisms

Risk for **Electrolyte Imbalance**: Risk factor: vomiting

Risk for imbalanced **Fluid Volume**: Risk factors: decreased intake, loss of fluids with vomiting

Risk for imbalanced **Nutrition**: less than body requirements: Risk factor: inability to ingest food

VON RECKLINGHAUSEN'S DISEASE

See Neurofibromatosis

WALKING IMPAIRMENT

Impaired Walking (See **Walking,** impaired, Section II)

WANDERING

Wandering (See **Wandering,** Section II)

WEAKNESS

Fatigue r/t decreased or increased metabolic energy production

Risk for **Falls**: Risk factor: weakness

WEIGHT GAIN

Imbalanced Nutrition: more than body requirements r/t excessive intake in relation to metabolic need

WEIGHT LOSS

Imbalanced Nutrition: less than body requirements r/t inability to ingest food because of biological, psychological, economic factors

WELLNESS-SEEKING BEHAVIOR

Readiness for enhanced **Self-Health Management**: expresses desire for increased control of health practice

WERNICKE-KORSAKOFF SYNDROME

See Korsakoff's Syndrome

WEST NILE VIRUS

See Meningitis/Encephalitis

WHEELCHAIR USE PROBLEMS

Impaired wheelchair **Mobility** (See **Mobility,** wheelchair, impaired, Section II)

WHEEZING

Ineffective Airway Clearance r/t tracheobronchial obstructions, secretions

WILMS' TUMOR

Constipation r/t obstruction associated with presence of tumor

Acute **Pain** r/t pressure from tumor

See Chemotherapy; Hospitalized Child; Radiation Therapy; Surgery, Preoperative Care; Surgery, Perioperative Care; Surgery, Postoperative Care

WITHDRAWAL FROM ALCOHOL

See Alcohol Withdrawal

WITHDRAWAL FROM DRUGS

See Drug Withdrawal

WOUND DEBRIDEMENT

Acute **Pain** r/t debridement of wound

Impaired **Tissue Integrity** r/t debridement, open wound

Risk for **Infection**: Risk factors: open wound, presence of bacteria

W

WOUND DEHISCENCE, EVISCERATION

Fear r/t client fear of body parts "falling out," surgical procedure not going as planned

Imbalanced **Nutrition:** less than body requirements r/t inability to digest nutrients, need for increased protein for healing

Risk for deficient **Fluid Volume:** Risk factors: inability to ingest nutrients, obstruction, fluid loss

Risk for **Injury:** Risk factor: exposed abdominal contents

Risk for delayed **Surgical Recovery:** Risk factors: separation of wound, exposure of abdominal contents

WOUND INFECTION

Disturbed **Body Image** r/t dysfunctional open wound

Hyperthermia r/t increased metabolic rate, illness, infection

Imbalanced **Nutrition:** less than body requirements r/t biological factors, infection, hyperthermia

Impaired **Tissue Integrity** r/t wound, presence of infection

Risk for imbalanced **Fluid Volume:** Risk factor: increased metabolic rate

Risk for **Infection:** spread of: Risk factor: imbalanced nutrition: less than body requirements

Risk for delayed **Surgical Recovery:** Risk factor: presence of infection

WOUNDS (OPEN)

See Lacerations

W

A

Activity Intolerance

NANDA-I Definition

Insufficient physiological or psychological energy to endure or complete required or desired daily activities

Defining Characteristics

Abnormal blood pressure response to activity; abnormal heart rate response to activity; EKG changes reflecting arrhythmias; EKG changes reflecting ischemia; exertional discomfort; exertional dyspnea; verbal report of fatigue; verbal report of weakness

Related Factors (r/t)

Bed rest; generalized weakness; imbalance between oxygen supply/demand; immobility; sedentary lifestyle

Client Outcomes

Client Will (Specify Time Frame):

- Participate in prescribed physical activity with appropriate changes in heart rate, blood pressure, and breathing rate; maintain monitor patterns (rhythm and ST segment) within normal limits
- State symptoms of adverse effects of exercise and report onset of symptoms immediately
- Maintain normal skin color, and skin is warm and dry with activity
- Verbalize an understanding of the need to gradually increase activity based on testing, tolerance, and symptoms
- Demonstrate increased tolerance to activity

Nursing Interventions

- Determine cause of activity intolerance (see Related Factors) and determine whether cause is physical, psychological, or motivational.
- If mainly on bed rest, minimize cardiovascular deconditioning by positioning the client in an upright position several times daily if possible.

● = Independent   ▲ = Collaborative

- Assess the client daily for appropriateness of activity and bed rest orders. Mobilize the client as soon as it is possible.
- If client is mostly immobile, consider use of a transfer chair: a chair that becomes a stretcher.
- When appropriate, gradually increase activity, allowing the client to assist with positioning, transferring, and self-care as possible. Progress from sitting in bed to dangling, to standing, to ambulation. Always have the client dangle at the bedside before trying standing to evaluate for postural hypotension.
- When getting a client up, observe for symptoms of intolerance such as nausea, pallor, dizziness, visual dimming, and impaired consciousness, as well as changes in vital signs; manual blood pressure monitoring is best.
- If the client experiences symptoms of postural hypotension, take precautions when getting the client out of bed. Put graduated compression stockings on client or use lower limb compression bandaging, if ordered, to return blood to the heart and brain. Have the client dangle at the side of the bed with legs hanging over the edge of the bed, flex and extend feet several times after sitting up, then stand up slowly with someone holding the client. If client becomes lightheaded or dizzy, return client to bed immediately.
- Perform range-of-motion (ROM) exercises if the client is unable to tolerate activity or is mostly immobile. See care plan for **Risk for Disuse Syndrome.**
- Monitor and record the client's ability to tolerate activity: note pulse rate, blood pressure, monitor pattern, dyspnea, use of accessory muscles, and skin color before, during, and after the activity. If the following signs and symptoms of cardiac decompensation develop, activity should be stopped immediately:
  - Onset of chest discomfort or pain
  - Dyspnea
  - Palpitations
  - Excessive fatigue
  - Lightheadedness, confusion, ataxia, pallor, cyanosis, nausea, or any peripheral circulatory insufficiency
  - Dysrhythmia

- Exercise hypotension
- Excessive rise in blood pressure
- Inappropriate bradycardia
- Increased heart rate

▲ Instruct the client to stop the activity immediately and report to the physician if the client is experiencing the following symptoms: new or worsened intensity or increased frequency of discomfort; tightness or pressure in chest, back, neck, jaw, shoulders, and/or arms; palpitations; dizziness; weakness; unusual and extreme fatigue; excessive air hunger.

- Observe and document skin integrity several times a day. Refer to the care plan **Risk for impaired Skin Integrity.**

- Assess for constipation. If present, refer to care plan for **Constipation.**

▲ Refer the client to physical therapy to help increase activity levels and strength.

▲ Consider a dietitian referral to assess nutritional needs related to activity intolerance; provide nutrition as needed. If client is unable to eat food, use enteral or parenteral feedings as needed.

- Recognize that malnutrition causes significant morbidity due to the loss of lean body mass.

- Provide emotional support and encouragement to the client to gradually increase activity. Work with the client to set mutual goals that increase activity levels. Fear of breathlessness, pain, or falling may decrease willingness to increase activity.

▲ Observe for pain before activity. If possible, treat pain before activity and ensure that the client is not heavily sedated.

▲ Obtain any necessary assistive devices or equipment needed before ambulating the client (e.g., walkers, canes, crutches, portable oxygen).

▲ Use a gait walking belt when ambulating the client.

Activity Intolerance Due to Respiratory Disease

- If the client is able to walk and has chronic obstructive pulmonary disease (COPD), use the traditional 6-minute walk distance to evaluate ability to walk.

▲ Ensure that the chronic pulmonary client has oxygen saturation testing with exercise. Use supplemental oxygen to keep oxygen saturation 90% or above or as prescribed with activity.

- Instruct and assist a COPD client in using conscious, controlled breathing techniques during exercise, including pursed-lip breathing, and inspiratory muscle use.
- ▲ Evaluate the client's nutritional status. Refer to a dietitian if needed. Use nutritional supplements to increase nutritional level if needed.
- ▲ For the client in the intensive care unit, consider mobilizing the client in a four-phase method if there is sufficient knowledgeable staff available to protect the client from harm.
- ▲ Refer the COPD client to a pulmonary rehabilitation program.

Activity Intolerance Due to Cardiovascular Disease

- If the client is able to walk and has heart failure, consider use of the 6-minute walk test to determine physical ability.
- Allow for periods of rest before and after planned exertion periods such as meals, baths, treatments, and physical activity.
- ▲ Refer to a heart failure program or cardiac rehabilitation program for education, evaluation, and guided support to increase activity and rebuild life.
- See care plan for **Decreased Cardiac Output** for further interventions.

Geriatric

- Slow the pace of care. Allow the client extra time to carry out physical activities.
- Encourage families to help/allow an elderly client to be independent in whatever activities possible.
- ▲ Assess for swaying, poor balance, weakness, and fear of falling while elders stand/walk. If present, refer to physical therapy. Refer to the care plan for **Risk for Falls** and **Impaired Walking.**
- ▲ Evaluate medications the client is taking to see if they could be causing activity intolerance. Medications such as beta-blockers; lipid lowering agents, which can damage muscle; antipsychotics, which have a common side effect of orthostatic hypotension; some antihypertensives; and lowering the blood pressure to normal in the elderly can result in decreased functioning.

● = Independent ▲ = Collaborative

A

▲ If the client has heart disease causing activity intolerance, refer for cardiac rehabilitation.

▲ Refer the disabled elderly client to physical therapy for functional training including gait training, stepping, and sit-to-stand exercises, or for strength training.

• When mobilizing the elderly client, watch for orthostatic hypotension accompanied by dizziness and fainting.

Home Care

▲ Begin discharge planning as soon as possible with case manager or social worker to assess need for home support systems and the need for community or home health services.

▲ Assess the home environment for factors that contribute to decreased activity tolerance such as stairs or distance to the bathroom. Refer to occupational therapy, if needed, to assist the client in restructuring the home and ADL patterns.

▲ Refer to physical therapy for strength training and possible weight training, to regain strength, increase endurance, and improve balance. If the client is homebound, the physical therapist can also initiate cardiac rehabilitation.

• Encourage progress with positive feedback.

• Teach the client/family the importance of and methods for setting priorities for activities, especially those having a high energy demand (e.g., home/family events). Instruct in realistic expectations.

• Encourage routine low-level exercise periods such as a daily short walk or chair exercises. Provide the client/family with resources such as senior centers, exercise classes, educational and recreational programs, and volunteer opportunities that can aid in promoting socialization and appropriate activity.

▲ Refer to medical social services as necessary to assist the family in adjusting to major changes in patterns of living because of activity intolerance.

▲ Assess the need for long-term supports for optimal activity tolerance of priority activities (e.g., assistive devices, oxygen, medication, catheters, massage), especially for a hospice client. Evaluate intermittently.

• = Independent   ▲ = Collaborative

▲ Refer to home health aide services to support the client and family through changing levels of activity tolerance. Introduce aide support early. Instruct the aide to promote independence in activity as tolerated.

• Allow terminally ill clients and their families to guide care.

• Provide increased attention to comfort and dignity of the terminally ill client in care planning.

▲ Institute case management of frail elderly to support continued independent living.

Client/Family Teaching and Discharge Planning

• Instruct the client on techniques to utilize for avoiding activity intolerance, such as controlled breathing techniques.

• Teach the client techniques to decrease dizziness from postural hypotension when standing up.

• Help client with energy conservation and work simplification techniques in ADLs.

• Describe to the client the symptoms of activity intolerance, including which symptoms to report to the physician.

• Explain to the client how to use assistive devices, oxygen, or medications before or during activity.

• Help client set up an activity log to record exercise and exercise tolerance.

Risk for Activity Intolerance

NANDA-I Definition

At risk for experiencing insufficient physiological or psychological energy to endure or complete required or desired daily activities

Risk Factors

Circulatory problems, deconditioned status, history of previous intolerance, inexperience with activity, respiratory problems

Client Outcomes, Nursing Interventions, and Client/Family Teaching

Refer to care plan for **Activity Intolerance.**

• = Independent   ▲ = Collaborative

Ineffective Activity Planning   A

NANDA-I Definition

Inability to prepare for a set of actions fixed in time and under certain conditions

Defining Characteristics

Failure pattern of behavior; history of procrastination; lack of plan; lack of resources; lack of sequential organization; reports excessive anxieties about a task to be undertaken; reports fear toward a task to be undertaken; reports worries toward a task to be undertaken; unmet goals for chosen activity

Related Factors (r/t)

Compromised ability to process information; defensive flight behavior when faced with proposed solution; hedonism; lack of family support; lack of friend support; unrealistic perception of events; unrealistic perception of personal competence

Client Outcomes

Client Will (Specify Time Frame):

- State fear(s) and worry of task to be undertaken
- Identify and verbalize symptoms of anxiety toward task to be undertaken
- State a plan/resources/goal/organization and time frame for task to be undertaken

Nursing Interventions

- Establish a contract.
  - Before the first conference/meeting with the client, begin by establishing an agenda and get the assurance that the client will participate. Record the information. Give precise information on the upcoming session. At each session identify precisely the tasks to be accomplished for each session and the upcoming tasks for subsequent session.
  - Ask the client how he perceives the situation in order to gather his personal vision of the problem and how he envisages his self-involvement. Specify the goals.

• = Independent   ▲ = Collaborative

A

- Assess the client's actual level of function (functionality) (at work, in school, at the hospital) by identifying actual dysfunctional behaviors.
▲ Refer the client for cognitive-behavioral therapy. The work for the client begins with the understanding that his thoughts affect his emotions and reactions and therefore the success of meeting his objectives. Suggest that the client change his self-concept, for example, "Stop thinking of yourself as powerless."
▲ Confront and restructure the following unrealistic idea: "Running away is a better reaction when confronted with a dangerous object." The true syllogism is "running away is the reaction when confronted with an object that is 'imagined' to be dangerous." Instruct the client to practice and repeat the following statement: "I have the power to change by changing my ideas."
- Lower the anxiety level tied to the client's fear of not succeeding.
▲ Research the client's rising anxiety behaviors and show evidence of the client's "catastrophic" thoughts by repeating what negative thoughts the client has expressed, for example, "It would be dreadful if I would not succeed," "I can never do. . . ."
  - Verify if the lack of success of the project would lower the client's self-image.
▲ Determine as fairly as possible the success factors needed for the planning and success of the project: financial resources; the family situation; prior medical, psychiatric, and psychosocial conditions; material resources; and the ability to manage stress.
  - Identify the informational needs of the person: understanding of their state of health, supervision of their treatment if they are receiving treatment, diet, and important telephone numbers.
  - Identify and reinforce the elements of the client's personality that may help him to succeed with his plan. Have the client drill and repeat: "I can change my goals (dreams) with a plan."
- Assist the client to plan in a realistic way for work, studies, or the choice not to continue a project *(determination des objectifs)*.

● = Independent   ▲ = Collaborative

A

- Carry out the general objective by using secondary objectives in successive stages and in a logical progression. Remember that the attainment of these objectives may imply a modification of the schedule. Use a schedule, calendar, or agenda to write down the dates. For realistic planning: choose simple tasks, limit long hours of work, protect biopsychosocial well-being, improve techniques (of relaxation, of study, of concentration, of memory, aptitude of reading, writing, the way of taking notes).
- Anticipate the obstacles the client may encounter.
  - Establish a safeguard that will be helpful in pursuing the goal. It should be nonpunitive, but help the client to remember the importance of the instrument's use to attain the micro-objectives, the base of success. It could be written down like this: "I am going to take a 30-minute walk for 2 days. If I do it I will let myself watch TV for 1 hour, otherwise I will take a 1-hour walk for the next 2 days." Drill and repeat: "I will realize my goals no matter what."
  - Ask yourself the following questions: is the person alone, is he capable of attaining his objective in a day or would it be better to get something going with a support team? What is the proof that this person can realistically attain his objectives?
- ▲ Discuss the resources that the person has already used in order to verify if the changes assert themselves. Identify the potentially pivotal helping people.
- ▲ Clarify and coordinate the project in collaboration with a multidisciplinary team in the field and with other specialists (doctor, employment center, teacher, technician, etc.).
  - If necessary, coordinate the orientation of the person toward other structures or treatments that have not been used, for example: individual or group therapy, an educational support person, a financial aid person.
  - Tackle the client's fears and worries and encourage him to make a cognitive reconstruction. Use "desire thinking." Drill and repeat: "I can change false ideas that make me believe that I am unable to carry out (achieve) my plan."

● = Independent   ▲ = Collaborative

NOTE: The above interventions may be adapted for the geriatric and multicultural client, and for home care and client/family teaching and discharge planning.

Refer to care plans **Anxiety, Readiness for enhanced family Coping, Readiness for enhanced Decision-Making, Fear, Readiness for enhanced Hope, Readiness for enhanced Power, Readiness for enhanced Spiritual Well-Being, Readiness for enhanced Self-Health Management** for additional interventions.

Risk for Ineffective Activity Planning

NANDA-I Definition

At risk for an inability to prepare for a set of actions fixed in time and under certain conditions

Risk Factors

Compromised ability to process information; defensive flight behavior when faced with proposed solution; hedonism; history of procrastination; ineffective support systems; insufficient support systems; unrealistic perception of events; unrealistic perception of personal competence.

Client Outcomes, Nursing Interventions, Client/Family Teaching and Discharge Planning

Refer to **Ineffective Activity Planning.**

Ineffective Airway Clearance

NANDA-I Definition

Inability to clear secretions or obstructions from the respiratory tract to maintain a clear airway

Defining Characteristics

Absent cough; adventitious breath sounds (rales, crackles, rhonchi, wheezes); changes in respiratory rate and rhythm; cyanosis; difficulty vocalizing; diminished breath sounds; dyspnea; excessive sputum; orthopnea; restlessness; wide-eyed

Related Factors (r/t)

Environmental

Secondhand smoke; smoke inhalation; smoking

• = Independent   ▲ = Collaborative

A

Obstructed Airway
Airway spasm; excessive mucus; exudate in the alveoli; foreign body in airway; presence of artificial airway; retained secretions; secretions in the bronchi

Physiological
Allergic airways; asthma; COPD; hyperplasia of the bronchial walls; infection; neuromuscular dysfunction

Client Outcomes

Client Will (Specify Time Frame):
- Demonstrate effective coughing and clear breath sounds
- Maintain a patent airway at all times
- Explain methods useful to enhance secretion removal
- Explain the significance of changes in sputum to include color, character, amount, and odor
- Identify and avoid specific factors that inhibit effective airway clearance

Nursing Interventions
- Auscultate breath sounds q 1 to 4 hours.
- Monitor respiratory patterns, including rate, depth, and effort.
- Monitor blood gas values and pulse oxygen saturation levels as available.
- ▲ Administer oxygen as ordered.
- Position the client to optimize respiration (e.g., head of bed elevated 30-45 degrees and repositioned at least every 2 hours).
- Help the client deep breathe and perform controlled coughing. Have the client inhale deeply, hold breath for several seconds, and cough two or three times with mouth open while tightening the upper abdominal muscles.
- If the client has obstructive lung disease, such as COPD, cystic fibrosis, or bronchiectasis, consider helping the client use the forced expiratory technique, the "huff cough." The client does a series of coughs while saying the word "huff."
- ▲ Encourage the client to use an incentive spirometer if ordered. Recognize that controlled coughing and deep breathing may be just as effective.

• = Independent   ▲ = Collaborative

A

- Encourage activity and ambulation as tolerated. If unable to ambulate the client, turn the client from side to side at least every 2 hours. (See interventions for **Impaired Gas Exchange** for further information on positioning a respiratory client.)
- Encourage fluid intake of up to 2500 mL/day within cardiac or renal reserve.
▲ Administer medications such as bronchodilators or inhaled steroids as ordered. Watch for side effects such as tachycardia or anxiety with bronchodilators, or inflamed pharynx with inhaled steroids.
▲ Provide percussion, vibration, and oscillation as appropriate.
- Observe sputum, noting color, odor, and volume.

Critical Care

▲ If the client is intubated and is stable, consider getting the client up to sit at the edge of the bed, transfer to a chair, or walk as appropriate, if an effective interdisciplinary team is developed to keep the client safe.
▲ If the client is intubated, consider use of kinetic therapy, using a kinetic bed that slowly moves the client with 40-degree turns.
- Reposition the client as needed. Use rotational or kinetic bed therapy as above in clients for whom side-to-side turning is contraindicated or difficult.
- When suctioning an endotracheal tube or tracheostomy tube for a client on a ventilator, do the following:
  - Explain the process of suctioning beforehand and ensure the client is not in pain or overly anxious.
  - Hyperoxygenate before and between endotracheal suction sessions.
  - Suction for less than 15 seconds.
  - Use a closed, in-line suction system.
  - Avoid saline instillation before suctioning.
  - With a subglottic suctioning drainage tube in place, be sure to irrigate per manufacturer's instructions if it becomes clogged.
  - Document results of coughing and suctioning, particularly client tolerance and secretion characteristics such as color, odor, and volume.

● = Independent   ▲ = Collaborative

Pediatric

- Educate parents about the risk factors for ineffective airway clearance such as foreign body ingestion and passive smoke exposure.
- See the care plan **Risk for Suffocation** for more interventions on choking.
- Educate children and parents on the importance of adherence to peak expiratory flow (PEF) monitoring for asthma self-management.
- Educate parents and other caregivers that cough and cold medications bought over the counter are not safe for a child under 2 unless specifically ordered by a health care provider.

Geriatric

- Encourage ambulation as tolerated without causing exhaustion.
- Actively encourage the elderly to deep breathe and cough.
- Ensure adequate hydration within cardiac and renal reserves.

Home Care

- Some of the above interventions may be adapted for home care use.
- ▲ Begin discharge planning as soon as possible with case manager or social worker to assess need for home support systems, assistive devices, and community or home health services.
- Assess home environment for factors that exacerbate airway clearance problems (e.g., presence of allergens, lack of adequate humidity in air, poor air flow, stressful family relationships).
- Assess affective climate within family and family support system. Refer to care plan for **Caregiver Role Strain.**
- Refer to GOLD guidelines for management of home care and indications of hospital admission criteria.
- When respiratory procedures are being implemented, explain equipment and procedures to family members, and provide needed emotional support.

● = Independent   ▲ = Collaborative

- When electrically based equipment for respiratory support is being implemented, evaluate home environment for electrical safety, proper grounding, and so on. Ensure that notification is sent to the local utility company, the emergency medical team, and police and fire departments.
- Provide family with support for care of a client with chronic or terminal illness.
- Refer to care plan for **Anxiety.** Refer to care plan for **Powerlessness.**
- Instruct the client to avoid exposure to persons with upper respiratory infections, to avoid crowds of people, and wash hands after each exposure to groups of people, or public places.
▲ Determine client adherence to medical regimen. Instruct the client and family in importance of reporting effectiveness of current medications to physician.
- Teach the client when and how to use inhalant or nebulizer treatments at home.
- Teach the client/family importance of maintaining regimen and having PRN drugs easily accessible at all times.
- Instruct the client and family in the importance of maintaining proper nutrition, adequate fluids, rest, and behavioral pacing for energy conservation and rehabilitation.
- Instruct in use of dietary supplements as indicated.
- Identify an emergency plan, including criteria for use.
▲ Refer for home health aide services for assistance with ADLs.
▲ Assess family for role changes and coping skills. Refer to medical social services as necessary.
▲ For the client dying at home with a terminal illness, if the "death rattle" is present with gurgling, rattling, or crackling sounds in the airway with each breath, recognize that anticholinergic medications can often help control symptoms, if given early in the process.
▲ For the client with a "death rattle," nursing care includes turning to mobilize secretions, keeping the head of the bed elevated for postural drainage of secretions, and avoiding suctioning.

• = Independent   ▲ = Collaborative

A

Client/Family Teaching and Discharge Planning

▲ Teach the importance of not smoking. Refer to a smoking cessation program, and encourage clients who relapse to keep trying to quit. Consider using the Motivational Interviewing technique to increase motivation for smoking cessation. Ensure that client receives appropriate medications to support smoking cessation from the primary health care provider.

▲ Teach the client how to use a flutter clearance device if ordered, which vibrates to loosen mucus and gives positive pressure to keep airways open.

▲ Teach the client how to use peak expiratory flow rate (PEFR) meter if ordered and when to seek medical attention if PEFR reading drops. Also teach how to use metered dose inhalers and self-administer inhaled corticosteroids as ordered following precautions to decrease side effects.

• Teach the client how to deep breathe and cough effectively.

• Teach the client/family to identify and avoid specific factors that exacerbate ineffective airway clearance, including known allergens and especially smoking (if relevant) or exposure to secondhand smoke.

• Educate the client and family about the significance of changes in sputum characteristics, including color, character, amount, and odor.

• Teach the client/family about the need to take ordered antibiotics until the prescription has run out.

• Teach the family of the dying client in hospice with a "death rattle," that rarely are clients aware of the fluid that has accumulated, and help them find evidence of comfort in the client's nonverbal behavior.

Risk for Allergy Response

NANDA-I Definition

Risk of an exaggerated immune response or reaction to substances

Risk Factors

Chemical products (e.g., bleach, cosmetics); dander; environmental substances (e.g., mold, dust, pollen); foods (e.g., peanuts, shellfish,

• = Independent   ▲ = Collaborative

mushrooms); insect stings; pharmaceutical agents (e.g., penicillins); repeated exposure to environmental substances

Client Outcomes

Client Will (Specify Time Frame):
• State risk factors for allergies
• Demonstrate knowledge of plan to treat allergic reaction

Nursing Interventions

• A careful history is important in detecting allergens and avoidance of allergen.
▲ Carefully assess the client for allergies. Below is information that is important for clients with allergies. Refer for immediate treatment if anaphylaxis is suspected.

Causes

Common allergens include: animal dander, bee stings or stings from other insects, foods, especially nuts, fish, and shellfish, insect bites, medications, plants, pollens

Symptoms

Common symptoms of a mild allergic reaction include: Hives (especially over the neck and face), itching, nasal congestion, rashes, watery, red eyes

Symptoms of a moderate or severe reaction include: Cramps or pain in the abdomen, chest discomfort or tightness, diarrhea, difficulty breathing, difficulty swallowing, dizziness or lightheadedness, fear or feeling of apprehension or anxiety, flushing or redness of the face, nausea and vomiting, palpitations, swelling of the face, eyes, or tongue, weakness, wheezing, unconsciousness

First Aid

For a mild to moderate reaction: Calm and reassure the person having the reaction, as anxiety can worsen symptoms.
1. Try to identify the allergen and have the person avoid further contact with it. If the allergic reaction is from a bee sting, scrape the stinger off the skin with something firm (such as a fingernail or plastic credit card). Do not use tweezers; squeezing the stinger will release more venom.

• = Independent   ▲ = Collaborative

2. If the person develops an itchy rash, apply cool compresses and over-the-counter hydrocortisone cream.
3. Watch the person for signs of increasing distress.
4. Get medical help. For a mild reaction, a physician may recommend over-the-counter medications (such as antihistamines).

For a severe allergic reaction (anaphylaxis):

1. Check the person's airway, breathing, and circulation (the ABCs of Basic Life Support). A warning sign of dangerous throat swelling is a very hoarse or whispered voice, or coarse sounds when the person is breathing in air. If necessary, begin rescue breathing and CPR.
2. Call 911.
3. Calm and reassure the person.
4. If the allergic reaction is from a bee sting, scrape the stinger off the skin with something firm (such as a fingernail or plastic credit card). Do not use tweezers—squeezing the stinger will release more venom.
5. If the person has emergency allergy medication on hand, help the person take or inject the medication. Avoid oral medication if the person is having difficulty breathing.
6. Take steps to prevent *shock*. Have the person lie flat, raise the person's feet about 12 inches, and cover him or her with a coat or blanket. Do NOT place the person in this position if a head, neck, back, or leg injury is suspected or if it causes discomfort.

Do Not

- Do NOT assume that any allergy shots the person has already received will provide complete protection.
- Do NOT place a pillow under the person's head if he or she is having trouble breathing. This can block the airways.
- Do NOT give the person anything by mouth if the person is having trouble breathing.

When to Contact a Medical Professional

Call for immediate medical emergency assistance if:

- The person is having a severe allergic reaction—always call 911. Do not wait to see if the reaction is getting worse.
- The person has a history of severe allergic reactions (check for a medical ID tag).

• = Independent   ▲ = Collaborative

Prevention

- Avoid triggers such as foods and medications that have caused an allergic reaction (even a mild one) in the past. Ask detailed questions about ingredients when you are eating away from home. Carefully examine ingredient labels.
- If you have a child who is allergic to certain foods, introduce one new food at a time in small amounts so you can recognize an allergic reaction.
- People who know that they have had serious allergic reactions should wear a medical ID tag.
- If you have a history of serious allergic reactions, carry emergency medications (such as a chewable form of diphenhydramine and injectable epinephrine or a bee sting kit) according to your health care provider's instructions.
- Do not use your injectable epinephrine on anyone else. They may have a condition (such as a heart problem) that could be negatively affected by this drug.
- ▲ Refer for skin testing to confirm IgE-mediated allergic response.

  Note: Do not use serum-specific IgG testing in the diagnosis of food allergy.

  See care plans for **Latex Allergy Response** and **Risk for Latex Allergy Response.**

Pediatric

- ▲ Teach parents and children with allergies to peanuts and tree nuts to avoid them and to identify them.
- ▲ Suspect FPIES (food protein-induced enterocolitis syndrome) in formula-fed infants with repetitive emesis, diarrhea, dehydration, and lethargy 1 to 5 hours after ingesting the offending food (the most common are cow's milk, soy, and rice). Remove the offending food.
- ▲ Children should be screened for seafood allergies and avoid seafood and any foods containing seafood if an allergy is detected.

Anxiety

NANDA-I Definition

A vague uneasy feeling of discomfort or dread accompanied by an autonomic response (the source often nonspecific or unknown to the individual); a feeling of apprehension caused by anticipation of danger. It is an alerting signal that warns of impending danger and enables the individual to take measures to deal with threat

Defining Characteristics

Behavioral

Diminished productivity; expressed concerns due to change in life events; extraneous movement; fidgeting; glancing about; insomnia; poor eye contact; restlessness; scanning; vigilance

Affective

Apprehensive; anguish; distressed; fearful; feelings of inadequacy; focus on self; increased wariness; irritability; jittery; overexcited; painful increased helplessness; persistent increased helplessness; rattled; regretful; uncertainty; worried

Physiological

Facial tension; hand tremors; increased perspiration; increased tension; shakiness; trembling; voice quivering

Sympathetic

Anorexia; cardiovascular excitation; diarrhea; dry mouth; facial flushing; heart pounding; increased blood pressure; increased pulse; increased reflexes; increased respiration; pupil dilation; respiratory difficulties; superficial vasoconstriction; twitching; weakness

Parasympathetic

Abdominal pain; decreased blood pressure; decreased pulse; diarrhea; faintness; fatigue; nausea; sleep disturbance; tingling in extremities; urinary frequency; urinary hesitancy; urinary urgency

Cognitive

Awareness of physiological symptoms; blocking of thought; confusion; decreased perceptual field; difficulty concentrating; diminished ability

● = Independent　　　　　▲ = Collaborative

A

to learn; diminished ability to problem solve; fear of unspecified consequences; forgetfulness; impaired attention; preoccupation; rumination; tendency to blame others

Related Factors (r/t)

Change in: economic status, environment, health status, interaction patterns, role function, role status; exposure to toxins; familial association; heredity; interpersonal contagion; interpersonal transmission; maturational crises; situational crises; stress; substance abuse; threat of death; threat to: economic status, environment, health status, interaction patterns, role function, role status; self-concept; unconscious conflict about essential goals of life; unconscious conflict about essential values; unmet needs

Client Outcomes

Client Will (Specify Time Frame):
- Identify and verbalize symptoms of anxiety
- Identify, verbalize, and demonstrate techniques to control anxiety
- Verbalize absence of or decrease in subjective distress
- Have vital signs that reflect baseline or decreased sympathetic stimulation
- Have posture, facial expressions, gestures, and activity levels that reflect decreased distress
- Demonstrate improved concentration and accuracy of thoughts
- Demonstrate return of basic problem-solving skills
- Demonstrate increased external focus
- Demonstrate some ability to reassure self

Nursing Interventions

- Assess the client's level of anxiety and physical reactions to anxiety (e.g., tachycardia, tachypnea, nonverbal expressions of anxiety). Consider using the Hamilton Anxiety Scale, which grades 14 symptoms on a scale of 0 (not present) to 4 (very severe). Symptoms evaluated are mood, tension, fear, insomnia, concentration, worry, depressed mood, somatic complaints, and cardiovascular, respiratory, gastrointestinal, genitourinary, autonomic, and behavioral symptoms.
- Rule out withdrawal from alcohol, sedatives, or smoking as the cause of anxiety.

• = Independent ▲ = Collaborative

A

- Use empathy to encourage the client to interpret the anxiety symptoms as normal.
- If irrational thoughts or fears are present, offer the client accurate information and encourage him or her to talk about the meaning of the events contributing to the anxiety.
- Encourage the client to use positive self-talk.
- Intervene when possible to remove sources of anxiety.
- Explain all activities, procedures, and issues that involve the client; use nonmedical terms and calm, slow speech. Do this in advance of procedures when possible, and validate the client's understanding.
- Provide backrubs/massage for the client to decrease anxiety.
- Use therapeutic touch and healing touch techniques.
- Guided imagery can be used to decrease anxiety.
- Suggest yoga to the client.
- Provide clients with a means to listen to music of their choice or audiotapes.

Pediatric

- The above interventions may be adapted for the pediatric client.

Geriatric

- ▲ Monitor the client for depression. Use appropriate interventions and referrals.
- Older adults report less worry than younger adults.
- Observe for adverse changes if antianxiety drugs are taken.
- Provide a quiet environment with diversion.

Multicultural

- Assess for the presence of culture-bound anxiety states.
- Identify how anxiety is manifested in the culturally diverse client.
- For diverse clients experiencing preoperative anxiety, provide music of their choice.

Home Care

- The above interventions may be adapted for home care use.
- ▲ Assess for suicidal ideation. Implement emergency plan as indicated. Suicidal ideation may occur in response to

● = Independent   ▲ = Collaborative

A

co-occurring depression or a sense of hopelessness over severe anxiety symptoms or once antidepressant medications have been started. See care plan for **Risk for Suicide.**

- Assess for influence of anxiety on medical regimen.
- Assess for presence of depression.
- Assist family to be supportive of the client in the face of anxiety symptoms.
▲ Consider referral for the prescription of antianxiety or antidepressant medications for clients who have panic disorder (PD) or other anxiety-related psychiatric disorders.
▲ Assist the client/family to institute medication regimen appropriately. Instruct in side effects, importance of taking medications as ordered, and effects to report immediately to nurse or physician.
▲ Refer for psychiatric home health care services for client reassurance and implementation of a therapeutic regimen.

Client/Family Teaching and Discharge Planning

▲ Teach use of appropriate community resources in emergency situations (e.g., suicidal thoughts), such as hotlines, emergency departments, law enforcement, and judicial systems.
- Teach the client/family the symptoms of anxiety.
- Teach the client techniques to self-manage anxiety.
- Teach the client to visualize or fantasize about the absence of anxiety or pain, successful experience of the situation, resolution of conflict, or outcome of procedure.
- Teach relationship between a healthy physical and emotional lifestyle and a realistic mental attitude.

Death Anxiety

NANDA-I Definition

Vague uneasy feeling of discomfort or dread generated by perceptions of a real or imagined threat to one's existence

Defining Characteristics

Reports concerns of overworking the caregiver; reports deep sadness; reports fear of developing terminal illness; reports fear of loss of mental

• = Independent   ▲ = Collaborative

abilities when dying; reports fear of pain related to dying; reports fear of premature death; reports fear of the process of dying; reports fear of prolonged dying; reports fear of suffering related to dying; reports feeling powerless over dying; reports negative thoughts related to death and dying; reports worry about the impact of one's own death on significant others

Related Factors (r/t)

Anticipating adverse consequences of general anesthesia; anticipating impact of death on others; anticipating pain; anticipating suffering; confronting reality of terminal disease; discussions on topic of death; experiencing dying process; near-death experience; nonacceptance of own mortality; observations related to death; perceived proximity of death; uncertainty about an encounter with a higher power; uncertainty about the existence of a higher power; uncertainty about life after death; uncertainty of prognosis

Client Outcomes

Client Will (Specify Time Frame):

- State concerns about impact of death on others
- Express feelings associated with dying
- Seek help in dealing with feelings
- Discuss realistic goals
- Use prayer or other religious practice for comfort

Nursing Interventions

- Assess the psychosocial maturity of the individual.
- ▲ Assess clients for pain and provide pain relief measures.
- Assess client for fears related to death.
- Assist clients with life planning: consider and redefine main life goals, focus on areas of strength and/or goals that will provide satisfaction, adopt realistic goals, and recognize those that are impossible to achieve.
- Assist clients with life review and reminiscence.
- Provide music of a client's choosing.
- Provide social support for families, understanding what is most important to families who are caring for clients at the end of life.
- Encourage clients to pray.

Geriatric

- Carefully assess older adults for issues regarding death anxiety.
- Provide back massage for clients who have anxiety regarding issues such as death.
- Refer to care plan for **Grieving.**

Multicultural

- Assist clients to identify with their culture and its values.
- Refer to care plans for **Anxiety** and **Grieving.**

Home Care

- The above interventions may be adapted for home care.
- Identify times and places when anxiety is greatest. Provide for psychological support at those times, using such strategies as personal contact, telephone contact, diversionary activities, or therapeutic self.
- Support religious beliefs; encourage client to participate in services and activities of choice.
- ▲ Refer to medical social services or mental health services, including support groups as appropriate (e.g., anticipatory grieving groups from hospice, visiting volunteers of hospice).
- Encourage the client to verbalize feelings to family/caregivers, counselors, and self.
- Identify client's preferences for end-of-life care; provide assistance in honoring preferences as much as practicable.
- ▲ Assist the client in making contact with death-related planning organizations, if appropriate, such as the Cremation Society and funeral homes.
- ▲ Refer for psychiatric home health care services for client reassurance and implementation of a therapeutic regimen.
- Refer to care plan for **Powerlessness.**

Client/Family Teaching and Discharge Planning

- Promote more effective communication to family members engaged in the caregiving role. Encourage them to talk to their loved one about areas of concern. Both caregivers and care receivers avoid discussing.

A

- Allow family members to be physically close to their dying loved one, giving them permission, instruction, and opportunities to touch. Keep family members informed.
- To increase clients' knowledge about end-of-life issues, teach them and their family members about options for care, such as advance directives.

Risk for Aspiration

NANDA-I Definition

At risk for entry of gastrointestinal secretions, oropharyngeal secretions, solids, or fluids into the tracheobronchial passages

Risk Factors

Decreased gastrointestinal motility; delayed gastric emptying; depressed cough; depressed gag reflex; facial surgery; facial trauma; gastrointestinal tubes; incompetent lower esophageal sphincter; increased gastric residual; increased intragastric pressure; impaired swallowing; medication administration; neck trauma; neck surgery; oral surgery; oral trauma; presence of endotracheal tube; presence of tracheostomy tube; reduced level of consciousness; situations hindering elevation of upper body; tube feedings; wired jaws

Client Outcomes

Client Will (Specify Time Frame):
- Maintain patent airway and clear lung sounds
- Swallow and digest oral, nasogastric, or gastric feeding without aspiration

Nursing Interventions

- Monitor respiratory rate, depth, and effort. Note any signs of aspiration such as dyspnea, cough, cyanosis, wheezing, hoarseness, foul-smelling sputum, or fever. If new onset of symptoms, perform oral suction and notify provider immediately.
- Auscultate lung sounds frequently and before and after feedings; note any new onset of crackles or wheezing.
- Take vital signs frequently, noting onset of a temperature, increased respiratory rate.

● = Independent   ▲ = Collaborative

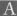

- Before initiating oral feeding, check client's gag reflex and ability to swallow by feeling the laryngeal prominence as the client attempts to swallow. If client is having problems swallowing, see nursing interventions for **Impaired Swallowing.**
- If client needs to be fed, feed slowly and allow adequate time for chewing and swallowing.
- When feeding client, watch for signs of impaired swallowing or aspiration, including coughing, choking, and spitting food.
- Have suction machine available when feeding high-risk clients. If aspiration does occur, suction immediately.
- Keep the head of bed elevated at 30 to 45 degrees, preferably sitting up in a chair at 90 degrees when feeding. Keep head elevated for an hour afterward.
▲ Note presence of any nausea, vomiting, or diarrhea. Treat nausea promptly with antiemetics.
- If the client shows symptoms of nausea and vomiting, position on side.
- Listen to bowel sounds frequently, noting if they are decreased, absent, or hyperactive.
- Note new onset of abdominal distention or increased rigidity of abdomen.
▲ If client has a tracheostomy, ask for referral to speech pathologist for swallowing studies before attempting to feed. After the evaluation, the decision should be made to have cuff either inflated or deflated when client eats.
- Provide meticulous oral care including brushing of teeth at least two times per day.

Enteral Feedings

▲ Insert nasogastric feeding tube using the internal nares to distal-lower esophageal-sphincter distance, an updated version of the Hanson method.
▲ Tape the feeding tube securely to the nose using a skin protectant under the tape.
▲ Check to make sure the initial nasogastric feeding tube placement was confirmed by x-ray, with the openings of the tube in the stomach, not the esophagus, or lungs. This is especially important if a small-bore feeding tube is used, although larger

● = Independent   ▲ = Collaborative

A

tubes used for feedings or medication administration should be verified by x-ray also.

- After x-ray verification of correct placement of the tube or the intestines, mark the tube's exit site clearly with tape or a permanent marker.
- Measure and record the length of the tube that is outside of the body at defined intervals to help ensure correct placement.
- Note the placement of the tube on any chest or abdominal x-rays that are done on the client.
- Check the pH of the aspirate. If the pH reading is 4 or less, the tube is probably in the stomach.
- Utilize a number of determinants of correct placement for verification of correct placement before each feeding or every 4 hours if client is on continuous feeding. Measure length of tube outside of body, any recent x-ray results, pH of aspirate if relevant, and characteristic appearance of aspirate. If findings do not ensure correct placement of the tube, obtain an x-ray to verify placement. Do not rely on the air insufflation method.
▲ Follow unit policy regarding checking for gastric residual volume during continuous feedings or before feedings, and holding feedings if increased residual feeding is present.
- Follow unit protocol regarding returning or discarding gastric residual volume.
- Do not use glucose testing to determine correct placement of enteral tube, and to identify aspirated enteral feeding.
- Do not use blue dye to tint enteral feedings.
- During enteral feedings, position client with head of bed elevated 30 to 45 degrees.
- Take actions to prevent inadvertent misconnections with enteral feeding tubes into IV lines, and other harmful places. Safety actions that should be taken to prevent misconnections include:
  - Trace tubing back to origin. Recheck connections at time of client transfer and at change of shift
  - Label all tubing
  - Use oral syringes for medications through the enteral feeding; **do not use IV syringes**

● = Independent   ▲ = Collaborative

- Teach nonprofessional personnel "Do Not Reconnect." If a line becomes dislodged, find the nurse instead of taking the chance of plugging it into the wrong place.

Critical Care

- Recognize that critically ill clients are at an increased risk for aspiration because of severe illness and interventions that compromise the gag reflex.
- Recognize that intolerance to feeding as defined by increased gastric residual is more common early in the feeding process.

Geriatric

- Carefully check elderly client's gag reflex and ability to swallow before feeding.
- Watch for signs of aspiration pneumonia in the elderly with cerebrovascular accidents, even if there are no apparent signs of difficulty swallowing or of aspiration.
- ▲ Recognize that the elderly with aspiration pneumonia have fewer symptoms than younger people; repeat cases of pneumonia in the elderly are generally associated with aspiration.
- ▲ Use central nervous system depressants cautiously; elderly clients may have an increased incidence of aspiration with altered levels of consciousness.
- Keep an elderly, mostly bedridden client sitting upright for 45 minutes to 1 hour following meals.
- Recommend to families that enteral feedings may or may not be indicated for clients with advanced dementia. Instead if possible use hand-feeding assistance, modified food consistency as needed, and feeding favorite foods for comfort.

Home Care

- The above interventions may be adapted for home care use.
- For clients at high risk for aspiration, obtain complete information from the discharging institution regarding institutional management.
- Assess the client and family for willingness and cognitive ability to learn and cope with swallowing, feeding, and related disorders.

● = Independent   ▲ = Collaborative

- Assess caregiver understanding and reinforce teaching regarding positioning and assessment of the client for possible aspiration.
- Provide the client with emotional support in dealing with fears of aspiration. Refer to care plan for **Anxiety.**
- Establish emergency and contingency plans for care of client.
▲ Have a speech and occupational therapist assess client's swallowing ability and other physiological factors and recommend strategies for working with client in the home (e.g., pureeing foods served to client; providing adaptive equipment for independence in eating).
- Obtain suction equipment for the home as necessary.
- Teach caregivers safe, effective use of suctioning devices. Inform client and family that only individuals instructed in suctioning should perform the procedure.
▲ Institute case management of frail elderly to support continued independent living.

Client/Family Teaching and Discharge Planning

- Teach the client and family signs of aspiration and precautions to prevent aspiration.
- Teach the client and family how to safely administer tube feeding.

Risk for impaired Attachment

NANDA-I Definition

At risk for disruption of the interactive process between parent/significant other and child that fosters the development of a protective and nurturing reciprocal relationship

Risk Factors

Anxiety associated with the parent role; disorganized infant behavior; ill child who is unable effectively to initiate parental contact; inability of parent(s) to meet personal needs; lack of privacy; parental conflict resulting from disorganized infant behavior; parent-child separation; physical barriers; premature infant; substance abuse

• = Independent   ▲ = Collaborative

A

Client Outcomes

Parent(s)/Caregiver(s) Will (Specify Time Frame):

- Be willing to consider pumping breast milk (and storing appropriately) or breastfeeding, if feasible
- Demonstrate behaviors that indicate secure attachment to infant/child
- Provide a safe environment, free of physical hazards
- Provide nurturing environment sensitive to infant/child's need for nutrition/feeding, sleeping, comfort, and social play
- Read and respond contingently to infant/child's distress
- Support infant's self-regulation capabilities, intervening when needed
- Engage in mutually satisfying interactions that provide opportunities for attachment
- Give infant nurturing sensory experiences (e.g., holding, cuddling, stroking, rocking)
- Demonstrate an awareness of developmentally appropriate activities that are pleasurable, emotionally supportive, and growth fostering
- Avoid physical and emotional abuse and/or neglect as retribution for parent's perception of infant/child's misbehavior
- State appropriate community resources and support services

Nursing Interventions

- Establish a trusting relationship with parent/caregiver.
- Encourage mothers to breastfeed their infants and provide support.
- Support mothers of preterm infants in providing pumped breast milk to their babies until they are ready for oral feedings and transitioning from gavage to breast.
- Identify factors related to postpartum depression (PPD)/major depression and offer appropriate interventions/referrals.
- Identify eating disorders/comorbid factors related to depression and offer appropriate interventions/referrals.
- Nurture parents so that they in turn can nurture their infant/child.
- Offer parents opportunities to verbalize their childhood fears associated with attachment.
- Suggest journaling or scrapbooking as a way for parents of hospitalized infants to cope with stress and emotions.

● = Independent   ▲ = Collaborative

A

- Offer parent-to-parent support to parents of NICU infants.
- Encourage parents of hospitalized infants to "personalize the baby" by bringing in clothing, pictures of themselves, toys, and tapes of their voices.
- Encourage physical closeness using skin-to-skin experiences as appropriate.
- Plan ways for parents to interact/assist with infant/child caregiving.
- Educate parents about the importance of the infant-caregiver relationship as a foundation for the development of the infant's self-regulation capacities.
- Assist parents in developing new caregiving competencies and/or revising/extending old ones.
- Educate parents in reading/responding sensitively to their infant's unique "body language" (behavior cues) that communicate approach ("I'm ready to play"), avoidance/stress ("I'm unhappy. I need a change."), and self-calming ("I'm helping myself").
- Educate and support parent's ability to relieve infant/child's stress/distress.
- Guide parents in adapting their behaviors/activities with infant/child cues and changing needs.
- Attend to both parents and infant/child to strengthen high-quality interactions.
- Assist parents with providing pleasurable sensory learning experiences (i.e., sight, sound, movement, touch, and body awareness).
- Encourage parents and caregivers to massage their infants and children.
- Identify mothers who may need assistance in enhancing maternal role attainment (MRA).
- Recognize that fathers, compared to mothers, may have different starting points in the attachment process in the NICU as nurses encourage parents to have early skin-to-skin contact.

Pediatric

- Recognize and support infant/child's capacity for self-regulation and intervene when appropriate.
- Provide lyrical, soothing music in nursery and home that is age-appropriate (i.e., corrected, in the case of premature infants) and contingent with state/behavioral cues.

• = Independent ▲ = Collaborative

- Recognize and support infant/child's attention capabilities.
- Encourage opportunities for mutually satisfying interactions between infant and parent.
- Encourage opportunities for physical closeness.

Multicultural

- Provide culturally sensitive parent support to non–English-speaking mothers and families.
- Discuss cultural norms with families to provide care that is appropriate for enhancing attachment with the infant/child.
- Promote the attachment process in women who have abused substances by providing a culturally based, women-centered treatment environment.
- Promote attachment process/development of maternal sensitivity in incarcerated women.
- Empower family members to draw on personal strengths in which multiple worldviews/values are recognized, incorporated, and negotiated.
- Encourage positive involvement and relationship development between children and noncustodial fathers to enhance health and development.

Home Care

- The above interventions may be adapted for home care use.
- Assess quality of interaction between parent and infant/child.
- Use "interaction coaching" (i.e., teaching mother to let the infant lead) so that the mother will match her interaction style to the baby's cues.
- Identify community resources/supportive network systems for mothers showing depressive symptoms.
- Provide supportive care for infants and children whose parents have been deployed during wartime.
- Provide support to custodial grandparents.

Autonomic Dysreflexia

NANDA-I Definition

Life-threatening, uninhibited sympathetic response of the nervous system to a noxious stimulus after a spinal cord injury at T7 or above

Defining Characteristics

Blurred vision; bradycardia; chest pain; chilling; conjunctival congestion; diaphoresis (above the injury); headache (a diffuse pain in different portions of the head and not confined to any nerve distribution area); Horner's syndrome; metallic taste in mouth; nasal congestion; pallor (below the injury); paresthesia; paroxysmal hypertension; pilomotor reflex; red splotches on skin (above the injury); tachycardia

Related Factors (r/t)

Bladder distention; bowel distention; deficient caregiver knowledge; deficient client knowledge; skin irritation

Client Outcomes/Goals

Client Will (Specify Time Frame):

- Maintain normal vital signs
- Remain free of dysreflexia symptoms
- Explain symptoms, prevention, and treatment of dysreflexia

Nursing Interventions

- Monitor the client for symptoms of dysreflexia, particularly those with high-level and more extensive spinal cord injuries. See Defining Characteristics.
- ▲ Collaborate with health care practitioners to identify the cause of dysreflexia (e.g., distended bladder, impaction, pressure ulcer, urinary calculi, bladder infection, acute condition in the abdomen, penile pressure, ingrown toenail, or other source of noxious stimuli).
- ▲ If symptoms of dysreflexia are present, place client in high Fowler's position, remove all support hoses or binders, and immediately determine the noxious stimuli causing the response. If blood pressure cannot be decreased within 1 minute, notify the physician STAT.

• = Independent   ▲ = Collaborative

A

- ▲ To determine the stimulus for dysreflexia:
  - First, assess bladder function. Check for distention, and if present catheterize using an anesthetic jelly as a lubricant. Do not use Valsalva maneuver or Crede's method to empty the bladder. Ensure existing catheter patency. Also note signs of urinary tract infection.
  - Second, assess bowel function. Numb the bowel area with a topical anesthetic as ordered, and once agent is effective (5 minutes), check for impaction.
  - Third, assess the skin, looking for any points of pressure.
- ▲ Initiate antihypertensive therapy as soon as ordered and monitor for cardiac dysrhythmias.
- ▲ Be careful not to increase noxious sensory stimuli. If numbing agent is ordered, use it on anus and 1 inch of rectum before attempting to remove a fecal impaction. Also spray pressure ulcer with it. If necessary to replace an obstructed catheter, use an anesthetic jelly as ordered.
- • Monitor vital signs every 3 to 5 minutes during acute event; continue to monitor vital signs after event is resolved (symptoms resolve and vital signs return to baseline).
- • Watch for complications of dysreflexia, including signs of cerebral hemorrhage, seizures, MI, or intraocular hemorrhage.
- • Accurately and completely record any incidences of dysreflexia; especially note the precipitating stimuli.
- • Use the following interventions to prevent dysreflexia:
  - Ensure that drainage from an indwelling catheter is good and that bladder is not distended.
  - Ensure a regular pattern of defecation to prevent fecal impaction.
  - Frequently change position of client to relieve pressure and prevent the formation of pressure ulcers.
- ▲ If ordered, apply an anesthetic agent to any wound below level of injury before performing wound care.
- ▲ Because episodes can recur, notify all health care team members of the possibility of a dysreflexia episode.
- ▲ For female clients with spinal cord injury who become pregnant, collaborate with obstetrical health care practitioners to monitor for signs and symptoms of dysreflexia.

• = Independent   ▲ = Collaborative

Home Care

A

- The above interventions may be adapted for home care use.
- Instruct the client with any known proclivity toward dysreflexia to wear a medical alert bracelet and carry a medical alert wallet card when not in a safe environment (i.e., not with someone who knows client has the condition and can respond appropriately).
- ▲ Establish an emergency plan: obtain provider/physician orders for medications to be used in situations in which first aid does not work and plans to identify potential stimuli.
- ▲ If orders have not been obtained or client does not have medications, use emergency medical services.
- When episode of dysreflexia is resolved, monitor blood pressure every 30 to 60 minutes for next 5 hours or admit to institution for observation.

Client/Family Teaching and Discharge Planning

- Teach recognition of the earliest symptoms of dysreflexia, the actions that should be taken when they occur, and the need to summon help immediately. Give client a written card that contains this information.
- Teach steps to prevent dysreflexia episodes: care of bladder, bowel, and skin and prevention of other forms of noxious stimuli (i.e., not wearing clothing that is too tight).
- Discuss the potential impact of sexual intercourse and pregnancy on autonomic dysreflexia.

Risk for Autonomic Dysreflexia

NANDA-I

Definition

At risk for life-threatening, uninhibited response of the sympathetic nervous system; post-spinal shock; in an individual with spinal cord injury or lesion at T6 or above (has been demonstrated in clients with injuries at T7 and T8)

● = Independent ▲ = Collaborative

B

Risk Factors

An injury/lesion at T6 or above and at least one of the following noxious stimuli:

- **Cardiac/pulmonary problems:** pulmonary emboli, deep vein thrombosis
- **Gastrointestinal stimuli:** bowel distention, constipation, difficult passage of stool, digital stimulation, enemas, esophageal reflux, fecal impaction, gallstones, gastric ulcers, GI system pathology, hemorrhoids, suppositories
- **Musculoskeletal:** cutaneous stimulations (e.g., pressure ulcer, ingrown toenail, dressings, burns, rash); fractures, heterotrophic bone; pressure over bony prominences or genitalia; range-of-motion exercises, spasm; sunburns, wounds
- **Neurological stimuli:** painful/irritating stimuli below the level of injury
- **Regulatory stimuli:** extreme environmental temperatures, temperature fluctuations
- **Reproductive stimuli:** ejaculation, labor and delivery, menstruation, ovarian cyst, pregnancy, sexual intercourse
- **Situational stimuli:** constrictive clothing (e.g., straps, stockings, shoes); reactions to pharmaceutical agents (e.g., decongestants, sympathomimetics, vasoconstrictors), opioid withdrawal, positioning, surgical procedures
- **Urological stimuli:** bladder distention, bladder spasms, calculi, catheterization, cystitis, detrusor sphincter dyssynergia, epididymitis, instrumentation, surgery, urethritis, urinary tract infection

Client Outcomes, Nursing Interventions, and Client/Family Teaching

Refer to care plan for **Autonomic Dysreflexia.**

Risk for Bleeding

NANDA-I Definition

At risk for a decrease in blood volume that may compromise health

Risk Factors

Aneurysm; circumcision; deficient knowledge; disseminated intravascular coagulopathy; history of falls; gastrointestinal disorders; impaired liver function; inherent coagulopathies; postpartum complications; pregnancy-related complications; trauma; treatment-related side effects.

B

Client Outcomes

Client Will (Specify Time Frame):

- Discuss precautions to prevent bleeding complications
- Explain actions that should be taken if bleeding happens
- Maintain adherence to agreed upon anticoagulant medication and lab work regimens
- Monitor for signs and symptoms of bleeding
- Maintain a mean arterial pressure above 70 mm Hg, a heart rate between 60 and 100 with a normal rhythm, and urine output greater than 0.5 mL/kg/hr
- Maintain warm, dry skin

Nursing Interventions

- Perform admission risk assessment for falls and for signs of bleeding.
- Monitor the client closely for hemorrhage especially in those at increased risk for bleeding. Watch for any signs of bleeding including: bleeding of the gums, blood in sputum, emesis, urine or stool, bleeding from a wound, bleeding into the skin with petechiae, and purpura.
- If bleeding develops, apply pressure over the site as needed or appropriate, on the appropriate pressure site over an artery, and use pressure dressings as needed.
- ▲ Monitor coagulation studies, including prothrombin time (PT), international normalized ratio (INR), activated partial thromboplastin time (aPTT), fibrinogen, fibrin degradation/split products, and platelet counts as appropriate.
- ▲ Assess vital signs at frequent intervals to assess for physiological evidence of bleeding such as tachycardia, tachypnea, and hypotension. Symptoms may include dizziness, shortness of breath, and fatigue.
- ▲ Monitor all medications for the potential to increase bleeding including aspirin, NSAIDs, SSRIs, and complementary and alternative therapies such as coenzyme Q (10) and ginger.

• = Independent   ▲ = Collaborative

Safety Guidelines: Joint Commission National Patient Safety Goals 2011: Safety Guidelines for Anticoagulant Administration

Follow approved protocol for anticoagulant administration:

- Use prepackaged medications and prefilled or premixed parenteral therapy as ordered
- Check laboratory tests (i.e., INR) before administration
- Use programmable pumps when using parenteral administration
- Ensure appropriate education for client/family and all staff concerning anticoagulants used
- Notify dietary services when warfarin prescribed (to reduce vitamin K in diet)
- Monitor for any symptoms of bleeding prior to administration.
▲ Before administering anticoagulants, assess the clotting profile of the client. If the client is on warfarin, assess the INR. Hold the medication if the INR is outside of the recommended parameters and notify the physician or advanced practice nurse.
▲ Recognize that vitamin K may be given orally or intravenously as ordered for INR levels greater than 5.0. In some circumstances fresh frozen plasma (FFP), prothrombin complex concentrate (PCC), and/or recombinant factor VIIa (rVIIa) may be administered if serious or life-threatening bleeding occurs.
▲ Manage fluid resuscitation and volume expansion as ordered.
▲ Consider discussing the co-administration of a proton-pump inhibitor alongside traditional NSAIDs, or with the use of a cyclo-oxygenase 2 inhibitor with the prescriber.
- Ensure adequate nurse staffing in order to be able to provide a high level of surveillance capability.

Pediatric

▲ Recognize that prophylactic vitamin K administration should be used in neonates for vitamin K deficiency bleeding (VKDB).
▲ Recognize warning signs of VKDB including minimal bleeds, evidence of cholestasis (icteric sclera, dark urine, irritability), and failure to thrive.
▲ Use caution in administering NSAIDs in children.

● = Independent   ▲ = Collaborative

▲ Monitor children and adolescents for potential bleeding.

▲ Closely monitor post-cardiotomy clients requiring extra-corporeal life support when cardiopulmonary bypass (CPB) duration is prolonged.

Client/Family Teaching and Discharge Planning

• Teach client and family or significant others about any anticoag-ulant medications prescribed including when to take, how often to have lab tests done, signs of bleeding to report, dietary restric-tions needed, and precautions to be followed. Instruct the client to report any adverse side effects to his/her health care provider.

• Instruct the client and family on disease process and rationale for care.

• Provide client and family or significant others with both oral and written educational materials that meet the standards of cli-ent education and health literacy.

Disturbed Body Image

NANDA-I Definition

Confusion in mental picture of one's physical self

Defining Characteristics

Behaviors of acknowledgment of one's body; behaviors of avoidance of one's body; behaviors of monitoring one's body; nonverbal response to actual change in body (e.g., appearance, structure, function); nonverbal response to perceived change in body (e.g., appearance, structure, func-tion); reports feelings that reflect an altered view of one's body (e.g., appearance, structure, function); reports perceptions that reflect an altered view of one's body in appearance

Objective

Actual change in function; actual change in structure; behaviors of acknowledging one's body; behaviors of monitoring one's body; change in ability to estimate spatial relationship of body to environment; change in social involvement; extension of body boundary to incorpo-rate environmental objects; intentional hiding of body part; intentional overexposure of body part; missing body part; not looking at body part;

• = Independent   ▲ = Collaborative

B

not touching body part; trauma to nonfunctioning part; unintentional hiding of body part; unintentional overexposing of body part

Subjective

Depersonalization of loss by use of impersonal pronouns; depersonalization of part by use of impersonal pronouns; emphasis on remaining strengths; focus on past appearance; focus on past function; focus on past strength; heightened achievement; personalization of loss by name; personalization of body part by name; preoccupation with chance; preoccupation with loss; refusal to verify actual change; reports change in lifestyle; reports fear of reaction by others; reports negative feelings about body (e.g., feelings of helplessness, hopelessness, powerlessness)

Related Factors (r/t)

Biophysical; cognitive; cultural; developmental changes; illness; injury; perceptual; psychosocial; spiritual; surgery; trauma; treatment regimen

Client Outcomes

Client Will (Specify Time Frame):

- Demonstrate adaptation to changes in physical appearance or body function as evidenced by adjustment to lifestyle change
- Identify and change irrational beliefs and expectations regarding body size or function
- Recognize health-destructive behaviors and demonstrate willingness to adhere to treatments or methods that will promote health
- Verbalize congruence between body reality and body perception
- Describe, touch, or observe affected body part
- Demonstrate social involvement rather than avoidance and utilize adaptive coping and/or social skills
- Utilize cognitive strategies or other coping skills to improve perception of body image and enhance functioning
- Utilize strategies to enhance appearance (e.g., wig, clothing)

Nursing Interventions

- Incorporate psychosocial questions related to body image as part of nursing assessment to identify clients at risk for body image disturbance (e.g., body builders; cancer survivors; clients with eating disorders, burns, skin disorders, polycystic ovary disease; or those with stomas/ostomies/colostomies or other disfiguring conditions).

● = Independent   ▲ = Collaborative

- If client is at risk for body image disturbance, consider using a tool such as the Body Image Quality of Life Inventory (BIQLI) or Body Areas Satisfaction Scale (BASS), which quantifies both the positive and negative effects of body image on one's psychosocial quality of life.
▲ Assess for history of childhood maltreatment in clients suffering from body dissatisfaction, anorexia, or other eating disorders and make appropriate psychosocial referrals if indicated.
▲ Assess for body dysmorphic disorder (BDD) (pathological preoccupation with muscularity and leanness; occurs more often in males than in females) and refer to psychiatry or other appropriate provider.
▲ Assess for steroid use, if BDD is identified.
- Assess for lipodystrophy (an abnormal redistribution of adipose tissue) in clients receiving antiretroviral therapy as a treatment for HIV/AIDS. This condition is common and can be a source of distress to clients.
▲ If client is at risk for anorexia nervosa, consider investigation of emotional qualifiers, using a tool to assess emotional intelligence such as the EQ-1.
- Discuss expectations for weight loss and anticipated body changes with clients planning to undergo bariatric surgery for morbid obesity. Assist the client in identifying realistic goals.
▲ Use cognitive-behavioral therapy (CBT) to assist the client to express his emotions and feelings.
- Help client describe ideal self, identify self-criticisms, and give suggestions to support acceptance of self.
- Discuss spirituality as an adjunct to improving body satisfaction.
- Provide education and support for clients receiving treatments or medications that have the potential to alter body image. Discuss alternatives if available.
- Encourage clients to write a narrative description of their changes.
- Take cues from clients regarding readiness to look at wound (may ask if client has seen wound yet) and utilize clients' questions or comments as way to teach about wound care and healing.

B

▲ Encourage client to participate in regular aerobic and/or non-aerobic exercise when feasible.

▲ Provide client with a list of appropriate community support groups (e.g., Reach to Recovery, Ostomy Association).

Pediatric

NOTE: Many of the above interventions are appropriate for the pediatric client.

▲ Refer parents of children with eating disorders to a support group.

▲ Refer children and families with severe facial burns for psychosocial support.

▲ Assess family dynamics and refer parents of adolescents with anorexia or other eating disorders to professional family counseling if indicated.

• Discuss with parents the potentially negative influence media has on younger children as a source of unrealistic ideals of body image.

▲ Consider using a measurement tool such as the Children's Body Image Scale (CBIS) if a child is at risk for body image disturbance.

Geriatric

• Focus on remaining abilities. Have client make a list of strengths.

• Encourage regular exercise for the elderly.

Multicultural

• Assess for the influence of cultural beliefs, regional norms, and values on the client's body image.

• Acknowledge that body image disturbances can affect all individuals regardless of culture, race, or ethnicity.

Home Care

• Assess client's level of social support as it is one of the determinants of client's recovery and emotional health.

• Assess family/caregiver level of acceptance of client's body changes.

• = Independent   ▲ = Collaborative

B

- Encourage client to discuss concerns related to sexuality and provide support or information as indicated. Many conditions that affect body image also affect sexuality.
- Teach all aspects of care. Involve client and caregivers in self-care as soon as possible. Do this in stages if client still has difficulty looking at or touching changed body part.

Client/Family Teaching and Discharge Planning

- Teach appropriate care of surgical site (e.g., mastectomy site, amputation site, ostomy site, etc.).
- Inform client of available community support groups, such as Internet discussion boards.
- Encourage significant others to offer support.
▲ Refer clients who are having difficulty with personal acceptance, personal and social body image disruption, sexual concerns, reduced self-care skills, and the management of surgical complications to an interdisciplinary team or specialist (e.g., ostomy nurse) if available.

Insufficient Breast Milk

NANDA-I Definition

Low production of maternal breast milk

Defining Characteristics

Infant

Constipation; does not seem satisfied after sucking time; frequent crying; long breastfeeding time; refuses to suck; voids small amounts of concentrated urine (less than four to six times a day); wants to suck very frequently; weight gain is lower than 500 g in a month (comparing two measures)

• = Independent   ▲ = Collaborative

Mother

B

Milk production does not progress; no milk appears when mother's nipple is pressed; volume of expressed breast milk is less than prescribed volume

Related Factors

Infant

Ineffective latching on; ineffective sucking; insufficient opportunity to suckle; rejection of breast; short sucking time

Mother

Alcohol intake; fluid volume depletion (e.g., dehydration, hemorrhage); malnutrition; medication side effects (e.g., contraceptives, diuretics); pregnancy; tobacco smoking

Client Outcomes

Client Will (Specify Time Frame):
- State knowledge of indicators of adequate milk supply
- State and demonstrate measures to ensure adequate milk supply

Nursing Interventions

- Initiate skin-to-skin contact at birth and undisturbed contact for the first hour following birth; the mother should be encouraged to watch the baby, not the clock.
- Encourage postpartum women to start breastfeeding based on infant need as early as possible and reduce formula use to increase breastfeeding frequency. Use nonnarcotic analgesics as early as possible.
- Provide suggestions for mothers on how to increase milk production and how to determine if there is insufficient milk supply.
- Instruct mothers that breastfeeding frequency, sucking times, and amounts are variable and normal. Assist mothers in optimal milk removal frequency.
- ▲ Consider the use of medication for mothers of preterm infants with insufficient expressed breast milk.

Pediatric

- Provide individualized follow-up with extra home visits or outpatient visits for teen mothers within the first few days

● = Independent   ▲ = Collaborative

after hospital discharge and encourage schools to be more compatible with breastfeeding.

Multicultural

- Provide information and support to mothers on benefits of breastfeeding at antenatal visits.

Refer to care plans **Interrupted Breastfeeding, Readiness for enhanced Breastfeeding** for additional interventions.

Ineffective Breastfeeding

NANDA-I Definition

Dissatisfaction or difficulty a mother, infant, or child experiences with the breastfeeding process

Defining Characteristics

Inadequate milk supply; infant arching at the breast; infant crying at the breast; infant inability to latch on to maternal breast correctly; infant exhibiting crying within the first hour after breastfeeding; infant exhibiting fussiness within the first hour after breastfeeding; insufficient emptying of each breast per feeding; insufficient opportunity for suckling at the breast; no observable signs of oxytocin release; nonsustained suckling at the breast; observable signs of inadequate infant intake; perceived inadequate milk supply; persistence of sore nipples beyond first week of breastfeeding; resisting latching on; unresponsive to other comfort measures; unsatisfactory breastfeeding process

Related Factors (r/t)

Infant anomaly; infant receiving supplemental feedings with artificial nipple; interruption in breastfeeding; knowledge deficit; maternal ambivalence; maternal anxiety; maternal breast anomaly; nonsupportive family; nonsupportive partner; poor infant sucking reflex; prematurity; previous breast surgery; previous history of breastfeeding failure

Client Outcomes

Client Will (Specify Time Frame):

- Achieve effective breastfeeding (dyad)
- Verbalize/demonstrate techniques to manage breastfeeding problems (mother)

● = Independent   ▲ = Collaborative

B

- Manifest signs of adequate intake at the breast (infant)
- Manifest positive self-esteem in relation to the infant feeding process (mother)
- Explain alternative method of infant feeding if unable to continue exclusive breastfeeding (mother)

Nursing Interventions

- Identify women with risk factors for lower breastfeeding initiation and continuation rates (age less than 20 years, low socioeconomic status) as well as factors contributing to ineffective breastfeeding as early as possible in the perinatal experience.
- Provide time for clients to express expectations and concerns and give emotional support.
- Use valid and reliable tools to measure breastfeeding performance and to predict early discontinuance of breastfeeding whenever possible/feasible.
- Promote comfort and relaxation to reduce pain and anxiety.
- Avoid supplemental feedings.
- Monitor infant behavioral cues and responses to breastfeeding.
- Provide necessary equipment/instruction/assistance for milk expression as needed.
- ▲ Provide referrals and resources: lactation consultants, nurse and peer support programs, community organizations, and written and electronic sources of information.
- See care plan for **Readiness for enhanced Breastfeeding.**

Multicultural

- Assess whether the client's concerns about the amount of milk taken during breastfeeding is contributing to dissatisfaction with the breastfeeding process.
- Assess the influence of family support on the decision to continue or discontinue breastfeeding.
- Provide traditional ethnic foods for breastfeeding mothers.
- See care plan for **Readiness for enhanced Breastfeeding.**

Home Care

- The above interventions may be adapted for home care use.
- Provide anticipatory guidance in relation to home management of breastfeeding.

● = Independent   ▲ = Collaborative

B

- Investigate availability/refer to public health department, hospital home follow-up breastfeeding program, or other postdischarge support.
- Refer to care plan for **Risk for impaired Attachment.**

Client/Family Teaching and Discharge Planning

- Instruct the client on maternal breastfeeding behaviors/techniques (preparation for, positioning, initiation of/promoting latch-on, burping, completion of session, and frequency of feeding). Consider use of a video.
- Teach the client self-care measures for the breastfeeding woman (e.g., breast care, management of breast/nipple discomfort, nutrition/fluid, rest/activity).
- Provide information regarding infant cues and behaviors related to breastfeeding and appropriate maternal responses (e.g., cues that infant is ready to feed, behaviors during feeding that contribute to effective breastfeeding, measures of infant feeding adequacy).
- Provide education to father/family/significant others as needed.

Interrupted Breastfeeding

NANDA-I Definition

Break in the continuity of the breastfeeding process as a result of inability or inadvisability to put baby to breast for feeding

Defining Characteristics

Infant receives no nourishment at the breast for some or all feedings; lack of knowledge about expression of breast milk; lack of knowledge about storage of breast milk; maternal desire to eventually provide breast milk for child's nutritional needs; maternal desire to maintain breastfeeding for child's nutritional needs; maternal desire to provide breast milk for child's nutritional needs; separation of mother and child

Related Factors (r/t)

Contraindications to breastfeeding; infant illness; maternal employment; maternal illness; need to abruptly wean infant; prematurity

• = Independent ▲ = Collaborative

Client Outcomes

B

Client Will (Specify Time Frame):

Infant
* Receive mother's breast milk if not contraindicated by maternal conditions (e.g., certain drugs, infections) or infant conditions (e.g., true breast milk jaundice)

Maternal
* Maintain lactation
* Achieve effective breastfeeding or satisfaction with the breast-feeding experience
* Demonstrate effective methods of breast milk collection and storage

Nursing Interventions

* Discuss mother's desire/intention to begin or resume breastfeeding.
* Provide anticipatory guidance to the mother/family regarding potential duration of the interruption when possible/feasible.
* Reassure mother/family that early measures to sustain lactation and promote parent-infant attachment can make it possible to resume breastfeeding when the condition/situation requiring interruption is resolved.
* Reassure the mother/family that the infant will benefit from any amount of breast milk provided.
▲ Collaborate with the mother/family/health care providers/ employers (as needed) to develop a plan for expression of breast milk/infant feeding/kangaroo care/skin-to-skin contact (SSC).
* Monitor for signs indicating infant's ability to breastfeed and interest in breastfeeding.
* Observe mother performing psychomotor skills (expression, storage, alternative feeding, kangaroo care, and/or breastfeeding) and assist as needed.
▲ Use supplementation only as medically indicated.
* Provide anticipatory guidance for common problems associated with interrupted breastfeeding (e.g., incomplete emptying of milk glands, diminishing milk supply, infant difficulty with resuming breastfeeding, or infant refusal of alternative feeding method).
▲ Initiate follow-up and make appropriate referrals.

● = Independent ▲ = Collaborative

- Assist the client to accept and learn an alternative method of infant feeding if effective breastfeeding is not achieved.
- See care plans for **Readiness for enhanced Breastfeeding** and **Ineffective Breastfeeding**.

Multicultural

- Teach culturally appropriate techniques for maintaining lactation.
- Validate the client's feelings with regard to the difficulty of or her dissatisfaction with breastfeeding.
- See care plans for **Readiness for enhanced Breastfeeding** and **Ineffective Breastfeeding**.

Home Care

- The above interventions may be adapted for home care use.

Client/Family Teaching and Discharge Planning

- Teach mother effective methods to express breast milk.
- Teach mother/parents about kangaroo care.
- Instruct mother on safe breast milk handling techniques.
- See care plans for **Readiness for enhanced Breastfeeding** and **Ineffective Breastfeeding**.

Readiness for enhanced Breastfeeding*

NANDA-I Definition

A pattern of proficiency and satisfaction of the mother-infant dyad that is sufficient to support the breastfeeding process and can be strengthened

Defining Characteristics

Adequate infant elimination patterns for age; appropriate infant weight pattern for age; eagerness of infant to nurse; effective mother-infant communication patterns; infant content after feeding; mother reports satisfaction with the breastfeeding process; mother able to position infant at breast to promote a successful latching-on response; regular suckling at the breast; regular swallowing at the breast; signs of oxytocin

---

*Formerly effective breastfeeding.

release; sustained suckling at the breast; sustained swallowing at the breast; symptoms of oxytocin release are present

B

Client Outcomes

Client Will (Specify Time Frame):
- Maintain effective breastfeeding
- Maintain normal growth patterns (infant)
- Verbalize satisfaction with breastfeeding process (mother)

Nursing Interventions

- Encourage expectant mothers to learn about breastfeeding during pregnancy.
- Encourage and facilitate early skin-to-skin contact (SSC) (position includes contact of the naked baby with the mother's bare chest within 2 hours after birth).
- Encourage rooming-in and breastfeeding on demand.
- Monitor the breastfeeding process and identify opportunities to enhance knowledge and experience regarding breastfeeding.
- Give encouragement/positive feedback related to breastfeeding mother-infant interactions.
- Monitor for signs and symptoms of nipple pain and/or trauma.
- Discuss prevention and treatment of common breastfeeding problems.
- Monitor infant responses to breastfeeding.
- Identify current support-person network and opportunities for continued breastfeeding support.
- Avoid supplemental bottle feedings and pacifiers and do not provide samples of formula on discharge.
- ▲ Provide follow-up contact; as available provide home visits and/or peer counseling.

Multicultural

- Assess for the influence of cultural beliefs, norms, and values on current breastfeeding practices.
- Assess mothers' timing preference to begin breastfeeding.

Home Care

- The above interventions may be adapted for home care use.

• = Independent   ▲ = Collaborative

Client/Family Teaching and Discharge Planning

- Include the father and other family members in education about breastfeeding.
- Teach the client the importance of maternal nutrition.
- Reinforce the infant's subtle hunger cues (e.g., quiet-alert state, rooting, sucking, mouthing, hand-to-mouth, hand-to-hand activity) and encourage the client to nurse whenever signs are apparent.
- Review guidelines for frequency (every 2 to 3 hours, or 8 to 12 feedings per 24 hours) and duration (until suckling and swallowing slow down and satiety is reached) of feeding times.
- Provide anticipatory guidance about common infant behaviors.
- Provide information about additional breastfeeding resources.

Ineffective Breathing Pattern

NANDA-I Definition

Inspiration and/or expiration that does not provide adequate ventilation

Defining Characteristics

Alterations in depth of breathing; altered chest excursion; assumption of three-point position; bradypnea; decreased expiratory pressure; decreased inspiratory pressure; decreased minute ventilation; decreased vital capacity; dyspnea; increased anterior-posterior diameter; nasal flaring; orthopnea; prolonged expiration phase; pursed-lip breathing; tachypnea; use of accessory muscles to breathe

Related Factors (r/t)

Anxiety; body position; bony deformity; chest wall deformity; cognitive impairment; fatigue; hyperventilation; hypoventilation syndrome; musculoskeletal impairment; neurological immaturity; neuromuscular dysfunction; obesity; pain; perception impairment; respiratory muscle fatigue; spinal cord injury

Client Outcomes

Client Will (Specify Time Frame):

- Demonstrate a breathing pattern that supports blood gas results within the client's normal parameters

• = Independent   ▲ = Collaborative

B

- Report ability to breathe comfortably
- Demonstrate ability to perform pursed-lip breathing and controlled breathing
- Identify and avoid specific factors that exacerbate episodes of ineffective breathing patterns

Nursing Interventions

- Monitor respiratory rate, depth, and ease of respiration. Normal respiratory rate is 10 to 20 breaths/min in the adult.
- Note pattern of respiration. If client is dyspneic, note what seems to cause the dyspnea, the way in which the client deals with the condition, and how the dyspnea resolves or gets worse.
- Note amount of anxiety associated with the dyspnea.
- Attempt to determine if client's dyspnea is physiological or psychological in cause.

Psychological Dyspnea—Hyperventilation

- Monitor for symptoms of hyperventilation including rapid respiratory rate, sighing breaths, lightheadedness, numbness and tingling of hands and feet, palpitations, and sometimes chest pain.
- Assess cause of hyperventilation by asking client about current emotions and psychological state.
- Ask the client to breathe with you to slow down respiratory rate.
- ▲ Consider having the client breathe in and out of a paper bag as tolerated.
- ▲ If client has chronic problems with hyperventilation, numbness and tingling in extremities, dizziness, and other signs of panic attacks, refer for counseling.

Physiological Dyspnea

- ▲ Ensure that client in acute dyspneic state has received any ordered medications, oxygen, and any other treatment needed.
- Determine severity of dyspnea using a rating scale such as the modified Borg scale, rating dyspnea 0 (best) to 10 (worst) in severity. An alternative scale is the Visual Analogue Scale (VAS) with dyspnea rated as 0 (best) to 100 (worst).
- Note use of accessory muscles, nasal flaring, retractions, irritability, confusion, or lethargy.
- Observe color of tongue, oral mucosa, and skin for signs of cyanosis.

● = Independent   ▲ = Collaborative

- Auscultate breath sounds, noting decreased or absent sounds, crackles, or wheezes.
▲ Monitor oxygen saturation continuously using pulse oximetry. Note blood gas results as available.
- Using touch on the shoulder, coach the client to slow respiratory rate, demonstrating slower respirations; making eye contact with the client; and communicating in a calm, supportive fashion.
- Support the client in using pursed-lip and controlled breathing techniques.
- If the client is acutely dyspneic, consider having the client lean forward over a bedside table, resting elbows on the table if tolerated.
- Position the client in an upright position. *An upright position facilitates lung expansion.* See Nursing Interventions for **Impaired Gas Exchange** for further information on positioning.
▲ Administer oxygen as ordered.
- Increase client's activity to walking three times per day as tolerated. Assist the client to use oxygen during activity as needed. See Nursing Interventions and Rationales for **Activity Intolerance.**
- Schedule rest periods before and after activity.
▲ Evaluate the client's nutritional status. Refer to a dietitian if needed. Use nutritional supplements to increase nutritional level if needed.
- Provide small, frequent feedings.
- Offer a fan to move the air in the environment.
- Encourage the client to take deep breaths at prescribed intervals and do controlled coughing.
- Help the client with chronic respiratory disease to evaluate dyspnea experience to determine if similar to previous incidences of dyspnea and to recognize that he or she made it through those incidences. Encourage the client to be self-reliant if possible, use problem-solving skills, and maximize use of social support.
- See **Ineffective Airway Clearance** if client has a problem with increased respiratory secretions.
▲ Refer the COPD client for pulmonary rehabilitation.

• = Independent   ▲ = Collaborative

B

Geriatric

- Encourage ambulation as tolerated.
- Encourage elderly clients to sit upright or stand and to avoid lying down for prolonged periods during the day.

Home Care

- The above interventions may be adapted for home care use.
- Work with the client to determine what strategies are most helpful during times of dyspnea. Educate and empower the client to self-manage the disease associated with impaired gas exchange.
- Assist the client and family with identifying other factors that precipitate or exacerbate episodes of ineffective breathing patterns (i.e., stress, allergens, stairs, activities that have high energy requirements).
- Assess client knowledge of and compliance with medication regimen.
▲ Refer the client for telemonitoring with a pulmonologist as appropriate, with use of an electronic spirometer, or an electronic peak flowmeter.
- Teach the client and family the importance of maintaining the therapeutic regimen and having PRN drugs easily accessible at all times.
- Provide the client with emotional support in dealing with symptoms of respiratory difficulty. Provide family with support for care of a client with chronic or terminal illness. Refer to care plan for **Anxiety.**
- When respiratory procedures (e.g., apneic monitoring for an infant) are being implemented, explain equipment and procedures to family members, and provide needed emotional support.
- When electrically based equipment for respiratory support is being implemented, evaluate home environment for electrical safety, proper grounding, and so forth. Ensure that notification is sent to the local utility company, the emergency medical team, police and fire departments.
- Refer to GOLD guidelines for management of home care and indications of hospital admission criteria.
- Support clients' efforts at self-care. Ensure they have all the information they need to participate in care.

● = Independent   ▲ = Collaborative

- Identify an emergency plan including when to call the physician or 911.
▲ Refer to occupational therapy for evaluation and teaching of energy conservation techniques.
▲ Refer to home health aide services as needed to support energy conservation.
▲ Institute case management of frail elderly to support continued independent living.

Client/Family Teaching and Discharge Planning

- Teach pursed-lip and controlled breathing techniques.
- Teach about dosage, actions, and side effects of medications.
- Using a prerecorded CD, teach client progressive muscle relaxation techniques.
- Teach the client to identify and avoid specific factors that exacerbate ineffective breathing patterns, such as exposure to other sources of air pollution, especially smoking. If client smokes, refer to the smoking cessation section in the **Impaired Gas Exchange** care plan.

Decreased Cardiac output

NANDA-I Definition

Inadequate volume of blood pumped by the heart per minute to meet metabolic demands of the body

Defining Characteristics

Altered Heart Rate/Rhythm

Arrhythmias; bradycardia; electrocardiographic changes; palpitations; tachycardia

Altered Preload

Edema; decreased central venous pressure (CVP); decreased pulmonary artery wedge pressure (PAWP); fatigue; increased central venous pressure (CVP); increased pulmonary artery wedge pressure (PAWP); jugular vein distention; murmurs; weight gain

● = Independent   ▲ = Collaborative

C

Altered Afterload

Clammy skin; dyspnea; decreased peripheral pulses; decreased pulmonary vascular resistance (PVR); decreased systemic vascular resistance (SVR); increased pulmonary vascular resistance (PVR); increased systemic vascular resistance (SVR); oliguria, prolonged capillary refill; skin color changes; variations in blood pressure readings

Altered Contractility

Crackles; cough; decreased ejection fraction; decreased left ventricular stroke work index (LVSWI); decreased stroke volume index (SVI); decreased cardiac index; decreased cardiac output; orthopnea; paroxysmal nocturnal dyspnea; S3 sounds; S4 sounds

Behavioral/Emotional

Anxiety; restlessness

Related Factors (r/t)

Altered heart rate; altered heart rhythm; altered stroke volume: altered preload, altered afterload, altered contractility

Client Outcomes

Client Will (Specify Time Frame):

- Demonstrate adequate cardiac output as evidenced by blood pressure, pulse rate and rhythm within normal parameters for client; strong peripheral pulses; maintained level of mentation, lack of chest discomfort or dyspnea, and adequate urinary output; an ability to tolerate activity without symptoms of dyspnea, syncope, or chest pain
- Remain free of side effects from the medications used to achieve adequate cardiac output
- Explain actions and precautions to prevent primary or secondary cardiac disease

Nursing Interventions

- Recognize primary characteristics of decreased cardiac output as fatigue, dyspnea, edema, orthopnea, paroxysmal nocturnal dyspnea, and increased central venous pressure. Recognize secondary characteristics of decreased cardiac output as weight gain, hepatomegaly, jugular venous distention, palpitations,

• = Independent   ▲ = Collaborative

lung crackles, oliguria, coughing, clammy skin, and skin color changes.

- Monitor and report presence and degree of symptoms including dyspnea at rest or with reduced exercise capacity, orthopnea, paroxysmal nocturnal dyspnea, nocturnal cough, distended abdomen, fatigue, or weakness. Monitor and report signs including jugular vein distention, S3 gallop, rales, positive hepatojugular reflux, ascites, laterally displaced or pronounced PMI, heart murmurs, narrow pulse pressure, cool extremities, tachycardia with pulsus alternans, and irregular heartbeat.
- Monitor orthostatic blood pressures and daily weights.
- Recognize that decreased cardiac output can occur in a number of non-cardiac disorders such as septic shock and hypovolemia. Expect variation in orders for differential diagnoses related to the etiology of decreased cardiac output, as orders will be distinct to address primary cause of altered cardiac output.
- ▲ Administer oxygen as needed per physician's order.
- Monitor pulse oximetry regularly, using a forehead sensor if needed.
- Place client in semi-Fowler's or high Fowler's position with legs down or in a position of comfort.
- During acute events, ensure client remains on short-term bed rest or maintains activity level that does not compromise cardiac output.
- Provide a restful environment by minimizing controllable stressors and unnecessary disturbances. Schedule rest periods after meals and activities.
- ▲ Apply graduated compression stockings or intermittent sequential pneumatic compression (ISPC) leg sleeves as ordered. Ensure proper fit by measuring accurately. Remove stocking at least twice a day, then reapply. Assess the condition of the extremities frequently. Graduated compression stockings may be contraindicated in clients with peripheral arterial disease.
- ▲ Check blood pressure, pulse, and condition before administering cardiac medications such as angiotensin-converting enzyme (ACE) inhibitors, angiotensin receptor blockers

C

(ARBs), digoxin, and beta-blockers such as carvedilol. Notify physician if heart rate or blood pressure is low before holding medications.

- Observe for and report chest pain or discomfort; note location, radiation, severity, quality, *duration*, associated manifestations such as nausea, indigestion, and diaphoresis; also note precipitating and relieving factors.
▲ If chest pain is present, refer to the interventions in **Risk for decreased Cardiac tissue perfusion** care plan.
- Recognize the effect of sleep disordered breathing in HF.
▲ Closely monitor fluid intake, including intravenous lines. Maintain fluid restriction if ordered.
- Monitor intake and output. If client is acutely ill, measure hourly urine output and note decreases in output.
▲ Note results of electrocardiography and chest radiography.
▲ Note results of diagnostic imaging studies such as echocardiogram, radionuclide imaging, or dobutamine-stress echocardiography.
▲ Watch laboratory data closely, especially arterial blood gases, CBC, electrolytes including sodium, potassium and magnesium, BUN, creatinine, digoxin level, and B-type natriuretic peptide (BNP assay).
- Gradually increase activity when client's condition is stabilized by encouraging slower paced activities or shorter periods of activity with frequent rest periods following exercise prescription; observe for symptoms of intolerance. Take blood pressure and pulse before and after activity and note changes. *See* **Activity Intolerance.**
▲ Serve small, frequent, sodium-restricted, low saturated fat meals. Sodium-restricted diets help decrease fluid volume excess.
- Serve only small amounts of coffee or caffeine-containing beverages if requested (no more than four cups per 24 hours) if no resulting dysrhythmia.
▲ Monitor bowel function. Provide stool softeners as ordered. Caution client not to strain when defecating.
- Have clients use a commode or urinal for toileting and avoid use of a bedpan.
- Weigh client at same time daily (after voiding).

• = Independent   ▲ = Collaborative

▲ Provide influenza and pneumococcal vaccines prior to discharge for those who have yet to receive them.

• Assess for presence of anxiety and refer for treatment if present. See Nursing Interventions for **Anxiety** to facilitate reduction of anxiety in clients and family.

▲ Refer for treatment when depression is present.

▲ Refer to a cardiac rehabilitation program for education and monitored exercise.

▲ Refer to HF program for education, evaluation, and guided support to increase activity and rebuild quality of life.

Critically Ill

▲ Observe for symptoms of cardiogenic shock, including impaired mentation, hypotension with blood pressure lower than 90 mm Hg, decreased peripheral pulses, cold clammy skin, signs of pulmonary congestion, and decreased organ function. If present, notify physician immediately.

▲ If shock is present, monitor hemodynamic parameters for an increase in pulmonary wedge pressure, an increase in systemic vascular resistance, or a decrease in stroke volume, cardiac output, and cardiac index.

▲ Titrate inotropic and vasoactive medications within defined parameters to maintain contractility, preload, and afterload per physician's order.

▲ When using pulmonary arterial catheter technology, be sure to appropriately level and zero the equipment, use minimal tubing, maintain system patency, perform square wave testing, position the client appropriately, and consider correlation to respiratory and cardiac cycles when assessing waveforms and integrating data into client assessment.

▲ Observe for worsening signs and symptoms of decreased cardiac output when using positive pressure ventilation.

▲ Recognize that clients with cardiogenic pulmonary edema may have noninvasive positive pressure ventilation (NPPV) ordered.

▲ Monitor client for signs and symptoms of fluid and electrolyte imbalance when clients are receiving ultrafiltration or continuous renal replacement therapy (CRRT).

• = Independent ▲ = Collaborative

C

- Recognize that hypoperfusion from low cardiac output can lead to altered mental status and decreased cognition.

Geriatric

- Recognize that elderly clients may demonstrate fatigue and depression as signs of HF and decreased cardiac output.
▲ If client has heart disease causing activity intolerance, refer for cardiac rehabilitation.
- Observe for syncope, dizziness, palpitations, or feelings of weakness associated with an irregular heart rhythm.
▲ Observe for side effects from cardiac medications.
- Design educational interventions specifically for the elderly.

Home Care

- Some of the above interventions may be adapted for home care use. Home care agencies may use specialized staff and methods to care for chronic HF clients.
▲ Continue to monitor client closely for exacerbation of HF when discharged home.
- Assess for signs/symptoms of cognitive impairment.
- Assess for fatigue and weakness frequently. Assess home environment for safety, as well as resources/obstacles to energy conservation. Instruct client and family members on need for behavioral pacing and energy conservation.
- Help family adapt daily living patterns to establish life changes that will maintain improved cardiac functioning in the client. Take the client's perspective into consideration and use a holistic approach in assessing and responding to client planning for the future.
- Assist client to recognize and exercise power in using self-care management to adjust to health change. Refer to care plan for **Powerlessness.**
▲ Explore barriers to medical regimen adherence. Review medications and treatment regularly for needed modifications. Take complaints of side effects seriously and serve as client advocate to address changes as indicated.
▲ Refer for cardiac rehabilitation and strengthening exercises if client is not involved in outpatient cardiac rehabilitation.

• = Independent   ▲ = Collaborative

▲ Refer to medical social services as necessary for counseling about the impact of severe or chronic cardiac disease.

▲ Institute case management of frail elderly to support continued independent living.

▲ As the client chooses, refer to palliative care for care, which can begin earlier in the care of the HF client. Palliative care can be used to increase comfort and quality of life in the HF client before end-of-life care.

▲ If the client's condition warrants, refer to hospice.

• Identify emergency plan in advance, including whether use of cardiopulmonary resuscitation (CPR) is desired. Encourage family members to become certified in cardiopulmonary resuscitation if the client desires.

Client/Family Teaching and Discharge Planning

• Begin discharge planning as soon as possible upon admission to the emergency department (ED) with case manager or social worker to assess home support systems and the need for community or home health services. Consider referral for advanced practice nurse (APN) follow-up.

▲ Refer to case manager or social worker to evaluate client ability to pay for prescriptions.

• Include significant others in client teaching opportunities. Include all six areas of discharge instructions for heart failure hospitalizations: daily weight monitoring/reporting, symptoms recognition/reporting/when to call for help, smoking cessation, low-sodium diet, medication use and adherence, and regular follow-up with providers.

• Teach importance of performing and recording daily weights upon arising for the day, and to report weight gain. Ask if client has a scale at home; if not, assist in getting one.

• Teach types and progression patterns of heart failure symptoms, when to call the physician for help, and when to go to the hospital for urgent care.

• Teach importance of smoking cessation and avoidance of alcohol intake. Help clients who smoke stop by informing them of potential consequences and by helping them find an effective cessation method.

C

- Teach the direct benefits of a low-sodium diet.
▲ Teach the client importance of consistently taking cardio-vascular medications, and include actions, side effects to report.
- Instruct client and family on the importance of regular follow-up care with providers.
- Teach stress reduction (e.g., imagery, controlled breathing, muscle relaxation techniques).
▲ Refer to an outpatient system of care.
- Provide client/family with advance directive information to consider. Allow client to give advance directions about medical care or designate who should make medical decisions if he or she should lose decision-making capacity.

Risk for decreased Cardiac tissue perfusion

NANDA-I Definition

Risk for a decrease in cardiac (coronary) circulation

Risk Factors

Hypertension; hyperlipidemia; cigarette smoking, family history of coronary artery disease; diabetes mellitus; alcohol and drug abuse, obesity, cardiac surgery; hypovolemia; hypoxemia; hypoxia; coronary artery spasm; septic shock, cardiac tamponade; birth control pills, elevated C-reactive protein; lack of knowledge of modifiable risk factors (e.g., smoking, sedentary lifestyle, obesity)

Client Outcomes

Client Will (Specify Time Frame):

- Maintain vital signs within normal range
- Retain a normal cardiac rhythm (have absence of arrhythmias, tachycardia, or bradycardia)
- Be free from chest and radiated discomfort as well as associated symptoms related to acute coronary syndromes
- Deny nausea and be free of vomiting
- Have skin that is dry and of normal temperature

● = Independent   ▲ = Collaborative

Nursing Interventions

- Be aware that the most common cause of acute coronary syndromes (ACS) [unstable angina (UA), non–ST-elevation myocardial infarction (NSTEMI), and ST-elevation myocardial infarction (STEMI)] is reduced myocardial perfusion associated with partially or fully occlusive thrombus development in coronary arteries.
- Assess for symptoms of coronary hypoperfusion and possible ACS including chest discomfort (pressure, tightness, crushing, squeezing, dullness, or achiness), with or without radiation (or originating) in the back, neck, jaw, shoulder, or arm discomfort or numbness; SOB; associated diaphoresis; dizziness, lightheadedness, loss of consciousness; nausea or vomiting with chest discomfort, heartburn or indigestion; associated anxiety.
- Consider atypical presentations for women, and diabetic clients of ACS.
- Review the client's medical, surgical, and social history.
- Perform physical assessments for both CAD and non-coronary findings related to decreased coronary perfusion including vital signs, pulse oximetry, equal blood pressure in both arms, heart rate, respiratory rate, and pulse oximetry. Check bilateral pulses for quality and regularity. Report tachycardia, bradycardia, hypotension or hypertension, pulsus alternans or pulsus paradoxus, tachypnea, or abnormal pulse oximetry reading. Assess cardiac rhythm for arrhythmias; skin and mucous membrane color, temperature and dryness; and capillary refill. Assess neck veins for elevated central venous pressure, cyanosis, and pericardial or pleural friction rub. Examine client for cardiac S4 gallop, new heart murmur, lung crackles, altered mentation, pain to abdominal palpation, decreased bowel sounds, or decreased urinary output.
- ▲ Administer oxygen as ordered and needed for clients presenting with ACS to maintain a PO_2 of at least 90%.
- ▲ Use continuous pulse oximetry as ordered.
- ▲ Insert one or more large-bore intravenous catheters to keep the vein open. Routinely assess saline locks for patency.
- ▲ Observe the cardiac monitor for hemodynamically significant arrhythmias, ST depressions or elevations, T wave inversions and/or q waves as signs of ischemia or injury. Report abnormal findings.

• = Independent   ▲ = Collaborative

C

- Have emergency equipment and defibrillation capability nearby and be prepared to defibrillate immediately if ventricular tachycardia with clinical deterioration or ventricular fibrillation occurs.
▲ Perform a 12-lead ECG as ordered, to be interpreted within 10 minutes of emergency department arrival and during episodes of chest discomfort or angina equivalent.
▲ Administer aspirin as ordered.
▲ Administer nitroglycerin tablets sublingually as ordered, every 5 minutes until the chest pain is resolved while also monitoring the blood pressure for hypotension, for a maximum of three doses as ordered. Administer nitroglycerin paste or intravenous preparations as ordered.
- Do not administer nitroglycerin preparations to clients who have received phosphodiesterase type 5 inhibitors, such as sildenafil, tadalafil, or vardenafil, in the last 24 hours (48 hours for long-acting preparations).
▲ Administer morphine intravenously as ordered every 5 to 30 minutes while monitoring blood pressure when nitroglycerin alone does not relieve chest discomfort.
▲ Assess and report abnormal lab work results of cardiac enzymes, specifically troponin Is, chemistries, hematology, coagulation studies, arterial blood gases, finger stick blood sugar, elevated C-reactive protein, or drug screen.
- Assess for individual risk factors for coronary artery disease, such as hypertension, dyslipidemia, cigarette smoking, diabetes mellitus, or family history of heart disease. Other risk factors including sedentary life style, obesity, or cocaine or amphetamine use. Note age and gender as risk factors.
▲ Administer additional heart medications as ordered including beta blockers, calcium channel blockers, ACE inhibitors, aldosterone antagonists, antiplatelet agents, and anticoagulants. Always check the blood pressure and pulse rate before administering these medications. If the blood pressure or pulse rate is low, contact the physician to see if the medication should be held. Also check platelet counts and coagulation studies as ordered to assess proper effects of these agents.
▲ Administer lipid-lowering therapy as ordered.

• = Independent   ▲ = Collaborative

C

▲ Prepare client with education, withholding meals and/or medications, and intravenous access for cardiac catheterization and possible PCI with door to balloon time of under 90 minutes if STEMI is suspected.

▲ Prepare clients with education, withholding meals and/or medications, and intravenous access for noninvasive cardiac diagnostic procedures such as 2D echocardiogram, exercise or pharmacological stress test, and cardiac CT scan as ordered.

▲ Maintain bed rest or chair rest as ordered by the physician.

▲ Request a referral to a cardiac rehabilitation program.

Geriatric

• Consider atypical presentations for the elderly of possible ACS.

▲ Ask the prescriber about possible reduced dosage of medications for geriatric clients considering weight and creatinine clearance.

• Consider issues such as quality of life, palliative care, end-of-life care, and differences in sociocultural aspects for clients and families when supporting them in decisions regarding aggressiveness of care.

Client/Family Teaching and Discharge Planning

▲ Provide information about provider follow-up.

• Teach the client and family to call 911 for symptoms of new angina, existing angina unresponsive to rest and sublingual nitroglycerin tablets, or heart attack. Do not use friends or family for transportation where 911 is available, unless the delay is expected to be longer than 20 to 30 minutes.

• Upon discharge, instruct clients on symptoms of ischemia, when to cease activity, when to use sublingual nitroglycerin, and when to call 911.

• Upon hospital discharge, educate clients and significant others about discharge medications, including nitroglycerin sublingual tablets or spray, with written, easy to understand, culturally sensitive information.

• Provide client teaching related to risk factors for decreased cardiac tissue perfusion, such as hypertension,

C

hypercholesterolemia, diabetes mellitus, tobacco use, advanced age, and gender (female).
- Instruct the client on antiplatelet and anticoagulation therapy about signs of bleeding, need for ongoing medication compliance, and INR monitoring.
- After discharge, continue education and support for client blood pressure and diabetes control, weight management, and resumption of physical activity.
▲ Provide influenza vaccine prior to discharge.
- Stress the importance of ceasing tobacco use.
- Upon hospital discharge, educate clients about low sodium, low saturated fat diet, with consideration to client education, literacy and health literacy level.
- Teach the importance of exercise.

Caregiver Role Strain

NANDA-I Definition

Difficulty in performing family caregiver role

Defining Characteristics

Caregiving Activities

Apprehension about recipient's care if caregiver unable to provide care; apprehension about the future regarding care recipient's health; apprehension about the future regarding caregiver's ability to provide care; apprehension about possible institutionalization of care recipient; difficulty completing required tasks; difficulty performing required tasks; dysfunctional change in caregiving activities; preoccupation with care routine

Caregiver Health Status
Physical

Cardiovascular disease; diabetes; fatigue; GI upset; headaches; hypertension; rash; weight change

Behavioral

Poor self-care behaviors; increased smoking; increased alcohol consumption; sleep disturbances

● = Independent　　　　　　▲ = Collaborative

Emotional
Anger; anxiety; disturbed sleep; feeling depressed; frustration; impaired individual coping; impatience; increased emotional lability; increased nervousness; lack of time to meet personal needs; somatization; stress

Socioeconomic
Changes in leisure activities; low work productivity; quitting work or refusing career advancement to provide care, withdrawing from social life; financial distress including, but not limited to, poverty and bankruptcy

Caregiver–Care Recipient Relationship
Difficulty watching care recipient go through the illness; grief regarding changed relationship with care recipient; uncertainty regarding changed relationship with care recipient

Family Processes
Concerns about family members; family conflict; family cohesion; family dysfunction

Related Factors (r/t)
Care Recipient Health Status
Addiction; codependence; cognitive problems; dependency; illness chronicity; illness severity; increasing care needs; instability of care recipient's health; problem behaviors; psychological problems; unpredictability of illness course

Caregiver Health Status
Addiction; codependency; cognitive problems; inability to fulfill one's own expectations; inability to fulfill others' expectations; marginal coping patterns; physical problems; psychological problems; unrealistic expectations of self

Caregiver–Care Recipient Relationship
History of poor relationship; mental status of elder inhibiting conversation, presence of abuse or violence; unrealistic expectations of caregiver by care recipient

Caregiving Activities
24-hour care responsibilities; amount of activities (including number of hours and specific activities that are distressful); complexity of

activities; discharge of family members to home with significant care needs; ongoing changes in activities; unpredictability of care situation; years of caregiving

Family Processes
History of family dysfunction; history of marginal family coping

Resources
Caregiver is not developmentally ready for caregiver role; deficient knowledge about community resources; difficulty accessing community resources; emotional strength; formal assistance; formal support; inadequate community resources (e.g., respite services, recreational resources); inadequate equipment for providing care; inadequate physical environment for providing care (e.g., housing, temperature, safety); inadequate transportation; inexperience with caregiving; informal assistance; informal support; insufficient finances; insufficient time; lack of caregiver privacy; lack of support; physical energy

Socioeconomic
Alienation from others; competing role commitments; insufficient recreation; isolation from others; financial distress including potential loss of loss of home and savings

Client Outcomes

Throughout the care situation, the caregiver will:
*   Feel supported by health care professionals, family, and friends
*   Report reduced or acceptable feelings of burden or distress
*   Take part in self-care activities to maintain own physical and psychological/emotional health
*   Identify resources available to help in giving care or to support the caregiver to give care
*   Verbalize mastery of the care situation; feel confident and competent to provide care

Throughout the care situation, the care recipient will:
*   Obtain quality and safe care

• = Independent   ▲ = Collaborative

Nursing Interventions

- Regularly monitor signs of depression, anxiety, burden, and deteriorating physical health in the caregiver throughout the care situation, especially if the marital relationship is poor, the care recipient has cognitive or neuropsychiatric symptoms, there is little social support available, the caregiver becomes enmeshed in the care situation, the caregiver is elderly, female, or has poor preexisting physical or emotional health. Refer to the care plan for **Hopelessness** when appropriate.
- The impact of providing care on the caregiver's emotional health should be assessed at regular intervals using a reliable and valid instrument such as the Caregiver Strain Index, Caregiver Burden Inventory, Caregiver Reaction Assessment, Screen for Caregiver Burden, and the Subjective and Objective Burden Scale.
- Identify potential caregiver resources such as mastery, social support, optimism, and positive aspects of care.
- Screen for caregiver role strain at the onset of the care situation, at regular intervals throughout the care situation, and with changes in care recipient status and care transitions, including institutionalization.
- Watch for caregivers who become enmeshed in the care situation.
- Arrange for intervals of respite care for the caregiver; encourage use if available.
- Regularly monitor social support for the caregiver and help the caregiver to identify and utilize appropriate support systems for varying times in the care situation.
- Encourage the caregiver to grieve over changes in the care recipient's condition and give the caregiver permission to share angry feelings in a safe environment. Refer to nursing interventions for **Grieving.**
- Help the caregiver find personal time to meet his or her needs, learn stress management techniques, schedule regular health screenings, and schedule regular respite time.
- Encourage the caregiver to talk about feelings, concerns, uncertainties, and fears. Support groups can be used to gain mutual and educational support.

• = Independent   ▲ = Collaborative

C

- Observe for any evidence of caregiver or care recipient violence or abuse, particularly verbal abuse; if evidence is present, speak with the caregiver and care recipient separately.
▲ Involve the family in care transitions; use a multidisciplinary team to provide medical and social services for instruction and planning.
▲ Encourage regular communication with the care recipient and with the health care team.
- Help caregiver assess his or her financial resources (services reimbursed by insurance, available support through community and religious organizations) and the impact of providing care on his or her financial status.
- Help the caregiver identify competing occupational demands and potential benefits to maintaining work as a way of providing normalcy. Guide caregivers to seek ways to maintain employment through mechanisms such as job sharing or decreasing hours at work.
- Help the caregiver problem solve to meet the care recipient's needs.

Geriatric

- Monitor the caregiver for psychological distress and signs of depression, especially if caring for a mentally impaired elder or if there was an unsatisfactory marital relationship before caregiving.
- Assess the health of caregivers, particularly their control over chronic diseases, at regular intervals.
- Assess the presence of and use of social support and encourage the use of secondary caregivers with elderly caregivers.
- To improve the ability to provide safe care: provide skills training related to direct care, perform complex monitoring tasks, supervise and interpret client symptoms, assist with decision-making, assist with medication adherence, provide emotional support and comfort, and coordinate care.
- Teach symptom management techniques (assessment, potential causes, aggravating factors, potential alleviating factors, reassessment), particularly for fatigue, constipation, anorexia, and pain.

● = Independent   ▲ = Collaborative

Multicultural

- Assess for the influence of cultural beliefs, norms, and values on the client's ability to modify health behavior.
- Despite the importance of cultural differences in perceptions of caregiver role strain, there are certain characteristics that are distressing to caregivers across multiple cultures.
- Persons with different cultural backgrounds may not perceive the provision of care with equal degrees of distress.
- Recognize that cultures often play a role in identifying who will be recognized as a family caregiver and form partnerships with those groups.
- Encourage spirituality as a source of support for coping.
- Assess for the presence of conflicting values within the culture.
- Recognize that different cultures value and use caregiving resources in different ways.

Home Care

- Assess the client and caregiver at every visit for quality of relationship, and for the quality of caring that exists.
- Assess preexisting strengths and weaknesses the caregiver brings to the situation, as well as current responses, depression, and fatigue levels.
- ▲ Refer the client to home health aide services for assistance with ADLs and light housekeeping. Allow the caregiver to gain confidence in the respite provider.

Client/Family Teaching and Discharge Planning

- Identify client and caregiver factors that necessitate the use of formal home care services, that may affect provision of care, or that need to be addressed before the client can be safely discharged from home care.
- Collaborate with the caregiver and discuss the care needs of the client, disease processes, medications, and what to expect; use a variety of instructional techniques (e.g., explanations, demonstrations, visual aids) until the caregiver is able to express a degree of comfort with care delivery.

• = Independent   ▲ = Collaborative

- Assess family caregiving skill. The identification of caregiver difficulty with any of a core set of processes highlights areas for intervention.
- Discharge care should be individualized to specific caregiver needs and care situations.
- Assess the caregiver's need for information such as information on symptom management, disease progression, specific skills, and available support.
- Teach caregivers warning signs for burnout, depression, and anxiety. Help them identify a resource in case they begin to feel overwhelmed.
- Teach the caregiver methods for managing disruptive behavioral symptoms if present. Refer to the care plan for **Chronic Confusion.**
- Teach the caregiver how to provide the care needed and put a plan in place for monitoring the care provided.
- Provide ongoing support and evaluation of care skills as the care situation and care demands change.
- Provide information regarding the care recipient's diagnosis, treatment regimen, and expected course of illness.
▲ Refer to counseling or support groups to assist in adjusting to the caregiver role and periodically evaluate not only the caregiver's emotional response to care but the safety of the care delivered to the care recipient.

Risk for Caregiver Role Strain

NANDA-I Definition

At risk for caregiver vulnerability for felt difficulty in performing the family caregiver role

Risk Factors

Amount of caregiving tasks; care receiver exhibits bizarre behavior; care receiver exhibits deviant behavior; caregiver health impairment; caregiver is female; caregiver is spouse; caregiver isolation; caregiver not developmentally ready for caregiver role; caregiver's competing role commitments; co-dependency; cognitive problems in care receiver;

● = Independent   ▲ = Collaborative

complexity of caregiving tasks; congenital defect; developmental delay of caregiver; developmental delay of care receiver; discharge of family member with significant home care needs; duration of caregiving required; family dysfunction before the caregiving situation; family isolation; illness severity of the care receiver; inadequate physical environment for providing care (e.g., housing, transportation, community services, equipment); inexperience with caregiving; instability in the care receiver's health; lack of recreation for caregiver; lack of respite for caregiver; marginal caregiver's coping patterns; marginal family adaptation; past history of poor relationship between caregiver and care receiver; premature birth; presence of abuse; presence of situational stressors that normally affect families (e.g., significant loss, disaster or crisis, economic vulnerability, major life events), presence of violence; psychological problems in caregiver; psychological problems in care receiver; substance abuse; unpredictable illness course

Client Outcomes, Nursing Interventions, and Client/Family Teaching

Refer to care plan for **Caregiver Role Strain.**

Risk for ineffective Cerebral tissue perfusion

NANDA-I Definition

Risk for decrease in cerebral tissue circulation

Risk Factors

Abnormal partial thromboplastin time; abnormal prothrombin time; akinetic left ventricular segment; aortic atherosclerosis; arterial dissection; atrial fibrillation; atrial myxoma; brain tumor; carotid stenosis; cerebral aneurysm; coagulopathy (e.g., sickle cell anemia); dilated cardiomyopathy; disseminated intravascular coagulation; embolism; head trauma; hypercholesterolemia; hypertension; infective endocarditis; left atrial appendage thrombosis; mechanical prosthetic valve; mitral stenosis; recent myocardial infarction; sick sinus syndrome; substance abuse; thrombolytic therapy; treatment-related side effects (cardiopulmonary bypass, medications); transient ischemic attack

C

Client Outcomes

Client Will (Specify Time Frame):

- State absence of headache
- Demonstrate appropriate orientation to person, place, time, and situation
- Demonstrate ability to follow simple commands
- Demonstrate equal bilateral motor strength
- Demonstrate adequate swallowing ability

Nursing Interventions

▲ To decrease risk of reduced cerebral perfusion r/t stroke or transient ischemic attack:

■ Obtain a family history of hypertension and stroke to identify persons who may be at increased risk of stroke.

■ Monitor BP regularly, as hypertension is a major risk factor for both ischemic and hemorrhagic stroke.

■ Teach hypertensive clients the importance of taking their physician-ordered antihypertensive agent to prevent stroke.

■ Stress smoking cessation at every encounter with clients, utilizing multimodal techniques to aid in quitting, such as counseling, nicotine replacement, and oral smoking cessation medications.

■ Teach clients who experience a transient ischemic attack (TIA) that they are at increased risk for a stroke.

■ Teach clients with a history of acute coronary syndromes (unstable angina, non-STEMI [non-ST-elevation myocardial infarction], and STEMI [ST-elevation myocardial infarction]) that they are at risk for stroke.

■ Screen clients 65 years of age and older for atrial fibrillation with pulse assessment.

■ Call 911 or activate the rapid response team of a hospital immediately in clients displaying the symptoms of stroke as determined by the Cincinnati Stroke Scale (F: facial drooping, A: arm drift on one side, S: speech slurred), being careful to note the time of symptom appearance. Additional symptoms of stroke include sudden numbness/weakness of face, arm or leg, especially on one side, sudden confusion, trouble speaking or understanding, sudden difficulty seeing in one or both eyes, sudden trouble walking, dizziness, loss of balance or coordination, or sudden severe headache.

• = Independent   ▲ = Collaborative

- Use clinical practice guidelines for glycemic control and BP targets to guide the care of diabetic patients that have had a stroke or TIA.
▲ To decrease risk of reduced cerebral perfusion pressure: Cerebral perfusion pressure = Mean arterial pressure − Intracranial pressure (CPP = MAP − ICP): See care plan for **Decreased Intracranial Adaptive Capacity.**
  - Maintain euvolemia.
  - Maintain head of bed flat or less than 30 degrees in acute stroke clients.

Ineffective Childbearing Process

NANDA-I

Definition

Pregnancy and childbirth process and care of newborn that does not match the environmental context, norms, and expectations

Defining Characteristics

During Pregnancy
- Does not access support systems appropriately
- Does not report appropriate physical preparations
- Does not report appropriate prenatal lifestyle (e.g., diet, elimination, sleep, bodily movement, exercise, personal hygiene)
- Does not report availability of support systems
- Does not report managing unpleasant symptoms in pregnancy
- Does not report a realistic birth plan
- Does not seek necessary knowledge (e.g., of labor and delivery, newborn care)
- Failure to prepare necessary newborn care items
- Inconsistent prenatal health visits
- Lack of prenatal visits
- Lack of respect for unborn baby

During Labor and Delivery
- Does not demonstrate appropriate baby feeding techniques
- Does not demonstrate attachment behavior to the newborn baby

• = Independent ▲ = Collaborative

- Lacks proactivity during labor and delivery
- Does not report lifestyle (e.g., diet, elimination, sleep, bodily movement, personal hygiene) that is appropriate for the stage of labor
- Does not respond appropriately to onset of labor
- Does not report availability of support systems
- Does not access support systems appropriately

After Birth
- Does not demonstrate appropriate baby feeding techniques
- Does not demonstrate appropriate breast care
- Does not demonstrate attachment behavior to the baby
- Does not demonstrate basic baby care techniques
- Does not provide safe environment for the baby
- Does not report appropriate postpartum lifestyle (e.g., diet, elimination, sleep, bodily movement, personal hygiene)
- Does not report availability of support systems
- Does not access support systems appropriately

Related Factors
- Deficient knowledge (e.g., of labor and delivery, newborn care)
- Domestic violence
- Inconsistent prenatal health visits
- Lack of appropriate role models for parenthood
- Lack of cognitive readiness for parenthood
- Lack of maternal confidence
- Lack of prenatal health visits
- Lack of a realistic birth plan
- Lack of sufficient support systems
- Maternal powerlessness
- Maternal psychological distress
- Suboptimal maternal nutrition
- Substance abuse
- Unsafe environment
- Unplanned pregnancy
- Unwanted pregnancy

Client Outcomes

Client Will (Specify Time Frame):
Antepartum
- Obtain early prenatal care in the first trimester and maintain regular visits

• = Independent   ▲ = Collaborative

- Obtain knowledge level needed for appropriate care of oneself during pregnancy including good nutrition and psychological health
- Understand the risks of substance abuse and resources available
- Feel empowered to seek social and spiritual support for emotional well-being during pregnancy
- Utilize support systems for labor and emotional support
- Develop a realistic birth plan taking into account any high-risk pregnancy issues
- Be able to understand the labor and delivery process and comfort measures to manage labor pain

Postpartum
- Utilize a safe environment for self and infant
- Obtain knowledge to provide appropriate newborn care and postpartum care of self
- Obtain knowledge to develop appropriate bonding and parenting skills

Nursing Interventions

- Encourage early prenatal care and regular prenatal visits.
- ▲ Identify any high-risk factors that may require additional surveillance such as preterm labor, hypertensive disorders of pregnancy, diabetes, depression, other chronic medical conditions, presence of fetal anomalies or other high-risk factors.
- ▲ Assess and screen for signs and symptoms of depression during pregnancy and in postpartal period including history of depression or postpartum depression, poor prenatal care, poor weight gain, hygiene issues, sleep problems, substance abuse, and preterm labor. If depression is present, refer for behavioral-cognitive counseling, and/or medication (postpartum period only).
- ▲ Observe for signs of alcohol use and counsel women to stop drinking during pregnancy. Give appropriate referral for treatment if needed.
- ▲ Obtain a smoking history and counsel women to stop smoking for the safety of the baby. Give appropriate referral to smoking cessation program if needed.

● = Independent   ▲ = Collaborative

C

▲ Monitor for substance abuse with recreational drugs. Refer to drug treatment program as needed. Refer opiate-dependent women to methadone clinics to improve maternal and fetal pregnancy outcomes.

▲ Monitor for psychosocial issues including lack of social support system, loneliness, depression, lack of confidence, maternal powerlessness, domestic violence, and socioeconomic problems.

▲ Monitor for signs of domestic violence. Refer to a community program for abused women that provides safe shelter as needed.

• Provide antenatal education to increase the woman's knowledge needed to make informed choices during pregnancy, labor, and birth and to promote a healthy lifestyle.

• Encourage expectant parents to prepare a realistic birth plan in order to prepare for the physical and emotional aspects of the birth process and to plan ahead for how they want various situations handled.

• Encourage good nutritional intake during pregnancy to facilitate proper growth and development of the fetus. Women should consume an additional 300 calories per day during pregnancy and achieve a total weight gain of 25 to 30 lb.

Multicultural

▲ Provide depression screening for clients of all ethnicities.

• Provide obstetrical care that is culturally diverse to ensure a safe and satisfying childbearing experience.

Readiness for enhanced Childbearing Process

NANDA-I Definition

A pattern of preparing for and maintaining a healthy pregnancy, childbirth process, and care of newborn that is sufficient for ensuring well-being and can be strengthened.

Defining Characteristics

During Pregnancy

Attends regular prenatal health visits; demonstrates respect for unborn baby; prepares necessary newborn care items; reports appropriate

• = Independent   ▲ = Collaborative

physical preparations; reports appropriate prenatal lifestyle (e.g., nutrition, elimination, sleep, bodily movement, exercise, personal hygiene); reports availability of support systems; reports realistic birth plan; reports managing unpleasant symptoms in pregnancy; seeks necessary knowledge (e.g., of labor and delivery, newborn care)

During Labor and Delivery

Demonstrates attachment behavior to the newborn baby; is proactive during labor and delivery; reports lifestyle (e.g., diet, elimination, sleep, bodily movement, personal hygiene) that is appropriate for the stage of labor; responds appropriately to onset of labor; uses relaxation techniques appropriate for the stage of labor; utilizes support systems appropriately

After Birth

Demonstrates appropriate baby feeding techniques; demonstrates appropriate breast care; demonstrates attachment behavior to the baby; demonstrates basic baby care techniques; provides safe environment for the baby; reports appropriate postpartum lifestyle (e.g., diet, elimination, sleep, bodily movement, exercise, personal hygiene); utilizes support system appropriately

Client Outcomes

Client Will (Specify Time Frame):
During Pregnancy
- State importance of frequent prenatal care/education
- State knowledge of anatomic, physiological, psychological changes with pregnancy
- Report appropriate lifestyle choices prenatal: activity and exercise/healthy nutritional practices

During Labor and Delivery
- Report appropriate lifestyle choices during labor
- State knowledge of birthing options, signs and symptoms of labor, and effective labor techniques

After Birth
- Report appropriate lifestyle choices postpartum
- State normal physical sensations following delivery
- State knowledge of recommended nutrient intake, strategies to balance activity and rest, appropriate exercise, time frame for resumption of sexual activity, strategies to manage stress

• = Independent   ▲ = Collaborative

- List strategies to bond with infant
- State knowledge of proper handling and positioning of infant/infant safety
- State knowledge of feeding technique and bathing of infant

Nursing Interventions

Refer to care plans **Risk for impaired Attachment; Readiness for enhanced Breastfeeding; Readiness for enhanced family Coping; Readiness for enhanced Family Processes; Risk for disproportionate Growth; Readiness for enhanced Nutrition; Readiness for enhanced Parenting; Ineffective Role performance.**

Prenatal Care

- ▲ Ensure that pregnant clients have an adequate diet and take multimicronutrient supplements during pregnancy.
- Encourage pregnant clients to include enriched cereal grain products in their diets.
- Assess smoking status of pregnant client and offer effective smoking-cessation interventions.
- ▲ Assess for signs of depression and make appropriate referral: inadequate weight gain, underutilization of prenatal care, increased substance use, and premature birth. Past personal or family history of depression, single, poor health functioning, and alcohol use.

Intrapartal Care

- Encourage psychosocial support during labor.
- Consider using aromatherapy during labor.
- Offer immersion bath during labor.
- Provide massage and relaxation techniques during labor.
- Offer the client in labor a light diet and water.

Multicultural

Prenatal

- Provide prenatal care for black and white clients.
- Refer the client to a centering pregnancy group (8 to 10 women of similar gestational age receive group prenatal care after initial obstetrical visit) or group prenatal care.

• = Independent   ▲ = Collaborative

Intrapartal

- Consider the client's culture when assisting in labor and delivery.

Postpartal

- Provide health and nutrition education for Chinese women after childbirth. Provide information and guidance on contemporary postpartum practices and take away common misconceptions about traditional dietary and health behaviors (e.g., fruit and vegetables should be restricted because of cold nature). Encourage a balanced diet and discourage unhealthy hygiene taboos.
- Health and nutrition education should include the Chinese family (particularly the relative who will be staying with the new mother) after the woman gives birth.

Home Care

Prenatal

▲ Involve pregnant drug users in drug treatment programs that include coordinated interventions in several areas: drug use, infectious diseases, mental health, personal and social welfare, and gynecological/obstetric care.

Postpartal

- Provide video conferencing to support new parents.
- Consider reflexology for postpartum women to improve sleep quality.

Client/Family Teaching and Discharge Planning

Prenatal

- Provide dietary and lifestyle counseling as part of prenatal care to pregnant women.
- Provide the following information in parenting classes, via DVD and Internet: support mechanisms, information and antenatal education, breastfeeding, practical baby care, and relationship changes. Include fathers in the parenting classes.
- Provide group prenatal care to families in the military.

• = Independent   ▲ = Collaborative

C

Postpartal

- Encourage physical activity in postpartum women; provide telephone counseling, pedometers, referral to community PA resources, social support, email advice on PA/pedometer goals, and newsletters.
- Teach mothers of young children principles of a healthy lifestyle: substitute high-fat foods with low-fat foods such as fruits and vegetables, increase physical activity, consider a community-based self-management intervention to prevent weight gain.

Risk for ineffective Childbearing Process

NANDA-I Definition

Risk for a pregnancy and childbirth process and care of newborn that does not match the environmental context, norms, and expectations

Risk Factors

Deficient knowledge (e.g., of labor and delivery, newborn care), domestic violence, inconsistent prenatal health visits, lack of appropriate role models for parenthood, lack of cognitive readiness for parenthood, lack of maternal confidence, lack of prenatal health visits, lack of realistic birth plan, lack of sufficient support systems, maternal powerlessness, maternal psychological distress, suboptimal maternal nutrition, substance abuse, unplanned pregnancy, unwanted pregnancy

Client Outcomes, Nursing Interventions, and Client/Family Teaching

Refer to care plan for **Ineffective Childbearing Process.**

Impaired Comfort

NANDA-I Definition

Perceived lack of ease, relief, and transcendence in physical, psychospiritual, environmental, and sociocultural dimensions

• = Independent ▲ = Collaborative

Defining Characteristics

Anxiety; crying; disturbed sleep pattern; fear; illness-related symptoms; inability to relax; insufficient resources (e.g., financial, social support); irritability; moaning; noxious environmental stimuli; reports being uncomfortable; reports being cold; reports being hot; reports distressing symptoms; reports hunger; reports itching; reports lack of ease or contentment in situation; restlessness

Client Outcomes

Client Will (Specify Time Frame):

- Provide evidence for improved comfort compared to baseline
- Identify strategies, with or without significant others, to improve and/or maintain acceptable comfort level
- Perform appropriate interventions, with or without significant others, as needed to improve and/or maintain acceptable comfort level
- Evaluate the effectiveness of strategies to maintain/and or reach an acceptable comfort level
- Maintain an acceptable level of comfort when possible

Nursing Interventions

- Assess client's current level of comfort. This is the first step in helping clients achieve improved comfort.
- Comfort is a holistic state under which pain management is included. Management of discomforts, however, can be better managed, and with fewer analgesics, by also addressing other comfort needs such as anxiety, insufficient information, social isolation, or financial difficulties.
- Assist clients to understand how to rate their current state of holistic comfort, utilizing institution's preferred method of documentation.
- Enhance feelings of trust between the client and the health care provider. To attain the highest comfort level, clients must be able to trust their nurse.
- Manipulate the environment as necessary to improve comfort.
- Encourage early mobilization and provide routine position changes to decrease physical discomforts associated with bed rest.

• = Independent   ▲ = Collaborative

- Provide simple massage.
- Provide healing touch, which is well-suited for clients who cannot tolerate more stimulating interventions such as simple massage.
- Inform the client of options for control of discomfort such as meditation and guided imagery, and provide these interventions if appropriate.
- Utilize empathy as a response to a client's negative emotions.
- Encourage clients to use relaxation techniques to reduce pain, anxiety, depression, and fatigue.

Geriatric

- Utilize hand massage for elders because most respond well to touch and the provider's presence.
- Discomfort from cold can be treated with warmed blankets.
- Use complementary touch therapies such as reflexology on clients with dementia to reduce pain and stress.
- Acknowledge any unmet physical, psychological, emotional, spiritual, and environmental needs when attempting to understand the behavior of an elderly client with dementia.
- Provide simple massage.

Multicultural

- Identify and clarify cultural language used to describe pain and other discomforts.
- Assess skin for ashy or yellow-brown appearance.
- Use soap sparingly if the skin is dry.
- Encourage and allow clients to practice their own cultural beliefs and recognize the impact different cultures have on a client's belief about health care, suffering, and decision-making.
- Assess for cultural and religious beliefs when providing care to clients.

Client/Family Teaching and Discharge Planning

- Teach techniques to use when the client is uncomfortable, including relaxation techniques, guided imagery, hypnosis, and music therapy.

• = Independent   ▲ = Collaborative

- Instruct the client and family on prescribed medications and therapies that improve comfort.
- Teach the client to follow up with the physician or other practitioner if discomfort persists.
- Encourage clients to utilize the Internet as a means of providing education to complement medical care for those who may be homebound or unable to attend face-to-face education.

Mental Health

- Encourage clients to use guided imagery techniques.
- Provide psychospiritual support and a comforting environment in order to enhance comfort.
- Providing music and verbal relaxation therapy can reduce anxiety.
- Caregivers should not hesitate to use humor when caring for their clients.

Readiness for enhanced Comfort

NANDA-I Definition

A pattern of ease, relief and transcendence in physical, psychospiritual, environmental, and/or social dimensions that is sufficient for well-being and can be strengthened

Defining Characteristics

Expresses desire to enhance comfort; expresses desire to enhance feelings of contentment; expresses desire to enhance relaxation; expresses desire to enhance resolution of complaints

Client Outcomes

Client Will (Specify Time Frame):

- Assess current level of comfort as acceptable
- Express the need to achieve an enhanced level of comfort
- Identify strategies to enhance comfort
- Perform appropriate interventions as needed for increased comfort
- Evaluate the effectiveness of interventions at regular intervals
- Maintain an enhanced level of comfort when possible

• = Independent   ▲ = Collaborative

Nursing Interventions

C

- Assess client's current level of comfort.
- Help clients understand that enhanced comfort is a desirable, positive, and achievable goal.
- Enhance feelings of trust between the client and the health care provider.
- Use therapeutic massage for enhancement of comfort.
- Teach and encourage use of guided imagery.
- Use of heat application to enhance pain relief.
- Foster and instill hope in clients whenever possible. See the care plan for **Hopelessness.**
- Provide opportunities for and enhance spiritual care activities.
▲ Enhance social support and family involvement.
▲ Encourage mind-body therapies such as meditation as an enhanced comfort activity.
▲ Promote participation in creative arts and activity programs.
▲ Encourage clients to use health information technology (HIT) as needed. Client services can now include management of medications, symptoms, emotional support, health education, and health information.
- Evaluate the effectiveness of all interventions at regular intervals and adjust therapies as necessary.
▲ Explain all procedures, including sensations likely to be experienced during the procedure.

Pediatric

- Assess and evaluate child's level of comfort at frequent intervals.
- Skin-to-skin contact (SSC) and selection of most effective method improves the comfort of newborns during routine blood draws.
- Adjust the environment as needed to enhance comfort.
- Encourage parental presence whenever possible. The same basic principles for managing pain in adults and children apply to neonates.
- Promote use of alternative comforting strategies such as positioning, presence, massage, spiritual care, music therapy, art therapy, and story-telling to enhance comfort when needed. In addition to oral sucrose, other comfort measures should be

• = Independent   ▲ = Collaborative

used to alleviate pain such as swaddling, skin-to-skin contact with mother, nursing, rocking, and holding.
▲ Support child's spirituality.

Multicultural

- Identify cultural beliefs, values, lifestyles, practices, and problem-solving strategies when assessing clients.
- Enhance cultural knowledge by actively seeking out information regarding different cultural and ethnic groups.
- Recognize the impact of culture on communication styles and techniques.
- Provide culturally competent care to clients from different cultural groups.

Home Care

- The nursing interventions described previously in **Readiness for enhanced Comfort** may be used with clients in the home care setting. When needed, adaptations can be made to meet the needs of specific clients, families, and communities.
- ▲ Make appropriate referrals to other organizations or providers as needed to enhance comfort.
- ▲ Promote an interdisciplinary approach to home care.
- Evaluate regularly if enhanced comfort is attainable in the home care setting.
- Use music therapy at home.

Client/Family Teaching and Discharge Planning

- Teach client how to regularly assess levels of comfort.
- Instruct client that a variety of interventions may be needed at any given time to enhance comfort.
- Help clients to understand that enhanced comfort is an achievable goal.
- Teach techniques to enhance comfort as needed.
- ▲ When needed, empower clients to seek out other health professionals as members of the interdisciplinary team to assist with comforting measures and techniques.
- Encourage self-care activities and continued self-evaluation of achieved comfort levels to ensure enhanced comfort will be maintained.

• = Independent   ▲ = Collaborative

Readiness for enhanced Communication

C NANDA-I Definition

A pattern of exchanging information and ideas with others that is sufficient for meeting one's needs and life's goals and can be strengthened

Defining Characteristics

Able to speak a language; able to write a language; expresses feelings; expresses satisfaction with ability to share ideas with others; expresses satisfaction with ability to share information with others; expresses thoughts; expresses willingness to enhance communication; forms phrases; forms sentences; forms words; interprets nonverbal cues appropriately; uses nonverbal cues appropriately

Client Outcomes

Client Will (Specify Time Frame):

- Express willingness to enhance communication
- Demonstrate ability to speak or write a language
- Form words, phrases, and language
- Express thoughts and feelings
- Use and interpret nonverbal cues appropriately
- Express satisfaction with ability to share information and ideas with others

Nursing Interventions

- Establish a therapeutic nurse-client relationship: provide appropriate education for the client, demonstrate caring by being present to the client.
- Assess the client's readiness to communicate, using an individualized approach. Avoid making assumptions regarding the client's preferred communication method.
- Assess the client's literacy level.
- Listen attentively and provide a comfortable environment for communicating; use these practical guidelines to assist in communication: Slow down and listen to the client's story; use augmentative and alternative communication methods (such as lip-reading, communication boards, writing, body language, and computer/electronic communication devices) as

• = Independent   ▲ = Collaborative

appropriate; repeat instructions if necessary; limit the amount of information given; have the client "teach back" to confirm understanding; avoid asking, "Do you understand?"; be respectful, caring, and sensitive.

▲ Provide communication with specialty nurses such as clinical nurse specialists or nurse practitioners who have knowledge about the client's situation.

▲ Refer couples in maladjusted relationships for psychosocial intervention and social support to strengthen communication; consider nurse specialists.

• Consider using music to enhance communication between client who is dying and his/her family.

• See care plan for **Impaired verbal Communication**.

Pediatric

▲ All individuals involved in the care and everyday life of children with learning difficulties need to have a collaborate approach to communication.

• See care plan for **Impaired verbal Communication**.

Geriatric

▲ Assess for hearing and vision impairments and make appropriate referrals for hearing aids.

• Use touch if culturally acceptable when communicating with older clients and their families.

• Consider singing during caregiving of clients with dementia.

• See care plan for **Impaired verbal Communication**.

Multicultural

• See care plan for **Impaired verbal Communication**.

Home Care

• The interventions described previously may be used in home care.

• See care plan for **Impaired verbal Communication**.

Client/Family Teaching and Discharge Planning

• See care plan for **Impaired verbal Communication**.

• = Independent   ▲ = Collaborative

Impaired verbal Communication

C **NANDA-I Definition**

Decreased, delayed, or absent ability to receive, process, transmit, and/
or use a system of symbols

Defining Characteristics

Absence of eye contact; cannot speak; difficulty expressing thoughts
verbally (e.g., aphasia, dysphasia, apraxia, dyslexia); difficulty forming
sentences; difficulty forming words (e.g., aphonia, dyslalia, dysarthria);
difficulty in comprehending usual communication pattern; difficulty
in maintaining usual communication pattern; difficulty in selective
attending; difficulty in use of body expressions; difficulty in use of facial
expressions; disorientation to person; disorientation to space; disorientation to time; does not speak; dyspnea; inability to speak language of
caregiver; inability to use body expressions; inability to use facial expressions; inappropriate verbalization; partial visual deficit; slurring; speaks
with difficulty; stuttering; total visual deficit; verbalizes with difficulty;
willful refusal to speak

Related Factors (r/t)

Absence of significant others; alteration in self-concept; alteration of
central nervous system; altered perceptions; anatomic defect (e.g., cleft
palate, alteration of the neuromuscular visual system, auditory system,
phonatory apparatus); brain tumor; chronic low self-esteem; cultural
differences; decreased circulation to brain; differences related to developmental; emotional conditions; environmental barriers; lack of information; physical barrier (e.g., tracheostomy, intubation); physiological
conditions; psychological barriers (e.g., psychosis, lack of stimuli); situational low self-esteem; stress; treatment-related side effects (e.g., pharmaceutical agents); weakened musculoskeletal system

Client Outcomes

Client Will (Specify Time Frame):
- Use effective communication techniques
- Use alternative methods of communication effectively
- Demonstrate congruency of verbal and nonverbal behavior
- Demonstrate understanding even if not able to speak
- Express desire for social interactions

• = Independent ▲ = Collaborative

Nursing Interventions

- Assess the language spoken, cultural considerations, literacy level, cognitive level, and use of glasses and/or hearing aids.
- Determine client's own perception of communication difficulties and potential solutions when possible.
- Involve a familiar person when attempting to communicate with a client who has difficulty with communication, if accepted by the client.
- Listen carefully. Validate verbal and nonverbal expressions particularly when dealing with pain and utilize nonverbal scales for pain when appropriate.
- Use therapeutic communication techniques: speak in a well-modulated voice, use simple communication, maintain eye contact at the client's level, get the client's attention before speaking, and show concern for the client.
- Avoid ignoring the client with verbal impairment; be engaged and provide meaningful responses to client concerns.
- Use touch as appropriate.
- Use presence. Spend time with the client, allow time for responses, and make the call light readily available.
- Explain all health care procedures.
- Be persistent in deciphering what the client is saying, and do not pretend to understand when the message is unclear.
- ▲ Utilize an individualized and creative multidisciplinary approach to augmentative and alternative communication assistance and other interventions.
- Use consistent nursing staffing for those with communication impairments.
- ▲ Consult communication specialists as appropriate.
- ▲ When the client is having difficulty communicating, assess and refer for audiology consultation for hearing loss. Suspect hearing loss when:
  - Client frequently complains that people mumble, claims that others' speech is not clear, or client hears only parts of conversations.
  - Client often asks people to repeat what they said.
  - Client's friends or relatives state that client doesn't seem to hear very well, or plays the television or radio too loudly.

• = Independent   ▲ = Collaborative

C

- Client does not laugh at jokes due to missing too much of the story.
- Client needs to ask others about the details of a meeting that the client attended.
- Client cannot hear the doorbell or the telephone.
- Client finds it easier to understand others when facing them, espccially in a noisy environment.
- When communicating with a client with a hearing loss:
  - Obtain client's attention before speaking and face toward his or her unaffected side or better ear while allowing client to see speaker's face at a reasonably close distance.
  - Provide sufficient light and do not stand in front of window.
  - Remove masks if safe to do so, or use see-through masks and reduce background noise whenever possible.
  - Do not raise voice or overenunciate.
  - Avoid making assumptions about the communication choice of those with hearing loss or voice impairments.

Pediatric

- Observe behavioral communication cues in infants.
- Identify and define at least two new forms of socially acceptable communication alternatives that may be used by children with significant disabilities.
- Teach children with severe disabilities functional communication skills.
- ▲ Refer children with primary speech and language delay/disorder for speech and language therapy interventions.

Geriatric

- Carefully assess all clients for hearing difficulty using an audiometer.
- Avoid use of "elderspeak."
- Initiate communication with the client with dementia, and give client time to respond.
- Encourage the client to wear hearing aids, if appropriate.
- Facilitate communication and reminiscing with memory boxes that contain objects, photographs, and writings that have meaning for the client.

- Continue to find means to communicate even with those who are nonverbal.

Multicultural

- Nurses should become more sensitive to the meaning of a culture's nonverbal communication modes, such as eye contact, facial expression, touching, and body language.
- Assess for the influence of cultural beliefs, norms, and values on the client's communication process.
- Assess personal space needs, acceptable communication styles, acceptable body language, interpretation of eye contact, perception of touch, and use of paraverbal modes when communicating with the client.
- Assess for how language barriers contribute to health disparities among ethnic and racial minorities.
- Although touch is generally beneficial, there may be certain instances where it may not be advisable due to cultural considerations.
- Modify and tailor the communication approach in keeping with the client's particular culture.
- Use reminiscence therapy as a language intervention.
- The Office of Minority Health (OMH) of the U.S. Department of Health and Human Services (DHHS) standards on culturally and linguistically appropriate services (CLAS) in health care should be used as needed.

Home Care

The interventions described previously may be adapted for home care use.

Client/Family Teaching and Discharge Planning

- Teach the client and family techniques to increase communication, including the use of communication devices and tactile touch. Incorporate multidisciplinary recommendations.
- ▲ Refer the client to a speech-language pathologist (SLP) or audiologist.

Acute Confusion

C **NANDA-I Definition**

Abrupt onset of reversible disturbances of consciousness attention, cognition, and perception that develop over a short period of time

Defining Characteristics

Fluctuation in cognition, level of consciousness, psychomotor activity; hallucinations; increased agitation; increased restlessness; lack of motivation to follow through with goal-directed behavior or purposeful behavior; lack of motivation to initiate goal-directed behavior or purposeful behavior; misperceptions

Related Factors (r/t)

Alcohol abuse; delirium; dementia; drug abuse; fluctuation in sleep-wake cycle; over 60 years of age; polypharmacy

Client Outcomes

Client Will (Specify Time Frame):
- Demonstrate restoration of cognitive status to baseline
- Be oriented to time, place, and person
- Demonstrate appropriate motor behavior
- Maintain functional capacity

Nursing Interventions

- Assess the client's behavior and cognition systematically and continually throughout the day and night, as appropriate. Utilize a validated tool to assess presence of delirium such as the Confusion Assessment Method (CAM) or Delirium Observation Screening Scale.
- Recognize that delirium may be superimposed on dementia; the nurse must be aware of the client's baseline cognitive function.
- Recognize that there are three distinct types of delirium based on either arousal or motor disturbances:
  - Hyperactive: delirium characterized by restlessness, agitation, hypervigilance, hallucinations and delusions; may be combative

• = Independent ▲ = Collaborative

C

- Hypoactive: delirium characterized by psychomotor retardation, lethargy, sedation, reduced awareness of surroundings and confusion
- Mixture of both hyper- and hypodelirium: the client fluctuates between periods of hyperactivity and agitation and hypoactivity and sedation.
- Identify clients who are at high risk for delirium.
- Identify precipitating factors that may precede the development of delirium: use of restraints, indwelling bladder catheter, metabolic disturbances, polypharmacy, pain, infection, dehydration, constipation, electrolyte imbalances, immobility, general anesthesia, hospital admission for fractures or hip surgery, anticholinergic medications, anxiety, sleep deprivation, and environmental factors.
- Perform an accurate mental status examination that includes the following:
  - Overall appearance, manner, and attitude
  - Behavior characteristics and level of psychomotor behavior (activity may be increased or decreased and may include spastic movements or tremors with delirium)
  - Mood and affect (may be paranoid or fearful with delirium; may have rapid mood swings)
  - Insight and judgment
  - Cognition as evidenced by level of consciousness, orientation to time, place, and person, thought process (thinking may be disorganized, distorted, fragmented, slow or accelerated with delirium), and content (perceptual disturbances such as visual, auditory or tactile delusions or hallucinations)
  - Level of attention (may be decreased with delirium; may be unable to focus, maintain attention or shift attention, or may be hypervigilant)
  - Memory (recent and immediate memory is impaired with delirium; unable to register new information)
  - Arousal (may fluctuate with delirium; sleep-wake cycle may be disturbed)
  - Language (may have rapid, rambling, slurred, incoherent speech)

● = Independent   ▲ = Collaborative

C

▲ Assess for and report possible physiological alterations (e.g., sepsis, hypoglycemia, hypoxia, hypotension, infection, changes in temperature, fluid and electrolyte imbalance, and use of medications with known cognitive and psychotropic side effects).

▲ Treat the underlying risk factors or the causes of delirium in collaboration with the health care team; establish/maintain normal fluid and electrolyte balance; normal body temperature, normal oxygenation (if the client experiences low oxygen saturation, deliver supplemental oxygen), normal blood glucose levels, normal blood pressure.

- Conduct a medication review and eliminate unnecessary medications. Medications that should be minimized or discontinued include anticholinergics, antihistamines, and benzodiazepines; cholinesterase inhibitors should be continued, as should carbidopa and levodopa for clients with parkinsonism.
- Communicate client status, cognition, and behavioral manifestations to all necessary providers.
- Monitor for any trends occurring in these manifestations, including laboratory tests.

• Identify, evaluate, and treat pain quickly and adequately (see care plans for **Acute Pain** or **Chronic Pain**). Around-the-clock acetaminophen may result in less opioid use.
• Promote regulation of bowel and bladder function.
• Ensure adequate nutritional and fluid intake.
• Promote early mobilization and rehabilitation.
• Promote continuity of care; avoid frequent changes in staff and surroundings.
• Plan care that allows for an appropriate sleep-wake cycle. Please refer to the care plan for **Sleep deprivation.**
• Facilitate appropriate sensory input by having clients use aids (e.g., glasses, hearing aids) as needed; check for impacted ear wax.
• Modulate sensory exposure and establish a calm environment.
• Provide reality orientation, including identifying self by name at each contact with the client, calling the client by his/her preferred name, using orientation techniques, providing

• = Independent   ▲ = Collaborative

familiar objects from home such as an afghan, providing clocks and calendars, and gently correcting misperceptions. Facilitate regular visits from family and friends.
- Use gentle, caring communication; provide reassurance of safety; give simple explanations of procedures.
- Provide supportive nursing care, including meeting basic needs such as feeding, toileting, and hydration.
▲ Recognize that delirium is frequently treated with an antipsychotic medication. Administer cautiously as ordered, if there is no other way to keep the client safe. Watch for side effects of the medications.

Critical Care

- Recognize admission risk factors for delirium.
- Monitor for delirium in each client in critical care daily. Utilize the Confusion Assessment Method for the ICU (CAM-ICU) or the Intensive Care Delirium Screening Checklist (ICDSC).
▲ Sedate critical care clients carefully; monitor sedation, analgesia, and delirium scores.
- Awaken the client daily.
- Bundle awakening and breathing coordination, choosing the appropriate sedative, monitoring for delirium, and promotion of exercise and early mobility.
- Initiate mobilization, physical therapy, and occupational therapy early in the ICU stay.
- Encourage visits from families.

Geriatric

- Assess older adults upon hospital admission and routinely for risk factors, precipitating factors, and the presence of delirium.
- Avoid the use of restraints.
▲ Evaluate all medications for potential to cause or exacerbate delirium. Review the Beers Criteria for Potentially Inappropriate Medication Use in Elderly.
- Establish or maintain elimination patterns of urination and defecation.

• = Independent ▲ = Collaborative

▲ Determine if the client is nourished; watch for protein-calorie malnutrition. Consult with physician or dietitian as needed.

• Explain hospital routines and procedures slowly and in simple terms; repeat information as necessary.

• Provide continuity of care when possible, avoid room changes, and encourage visits from family members or significant others.

• If clients know that they are not thinking clearly, acknowledge the concern.

• Keep the client's sleep-wake cycle as normal as possible (e.g., avoid letting the client take daytime naps, avoid waking the client at night, give sedatives but not diuretics at bedtime, provide pain relief and back rubs).

Home Care

• Some of the interventions described previously may be adapted for home care use.

• Assess and monitor for acute changes in cognition and behavior.

• Delirium is reversible but can become chronic if untreated. The client may be discharged from the hospital to home care in a state of undiagnosed delirium.

• Avoid preconceptions about the source of acute confusion; assess each occurrence on the basis of available evidence.

▲ Institute case management of frail elderly clients to support continued independent living if possible once delirium has resolved.

Client/Family Teaching and Discharge Planning

▲ Teach the family to recognize signs of early confusion and seek medical help.

• Counsel the client and family regarding the management of delirium and its sequelae.

Chronic Confusion

NANDA-I Definition

Irreversible, long-standing, and/or progressive deterioration of intellect and personality characterized by decreased ability to interpret environmental

• = Independent   ▲ = Collaborative

stimuli; decreased capacity for intellectual thought processes; and ma
fested by disturbances of memory, orientation, and behavior

Defining Characteristics

Altered interpretation; altered personality; altered response to stimuli;
clinical evidence of organic impairment; impaired long-term memory;
impaired short-term memory; impaired socialization; long-standing
cognitive impairment; no change in level of consciousness; progressive
cognitive impairment

Related Factors (r/t)

Alzheimer's disease; cerebrovascular attack; head injury; Korsakoff's psychosis; multi-infarct dementia

Client Outcomes

Client Will (Specify Time Frame):

- Remain content and free from harm
- Function at maximal cognitive level
- Participate in activities of daily living at the maximum of func-
  tional ability
- Have minimal episodes of agitation (as agitation occurs in up to
  70% of clients with dementia)

Nursing Interventions

- Determine the client's cognitive level using a screening tool
  such as the Mini-Mental State Exam (MMSE), Mini-Cog
  (includes a three-item recall and clock drawing test), or Mon-
  treal Cognitive Assessment.
- ▲ In clients who are complaining of memory loss, assess for
  depression, alcohol use, medication use, sleep, and nutrition.
- ▲ Recognize that pharmacological treatment to slow the progression of Alzheimer's disease is most effective when used
  early in the course of the disease.
- If hospitalized, gather information about the client's preadmission cognitive functioning, daily routines and care, and
  decision-making capacity.
- Assess the client for signs of depression: anxiety, sadness,
  irritability, agitation, somatic complaints, tension, loss of concentration, insomnia, poor appetite, apathy, flat affect, and
  withdrawn behavior.

• = Independent   ▲ = Collaborative

Assess the client for anxiety if he or she reports worry regarding physical or cognitive health, reports feelings of being anxious, shortness of breath, dizziness, or exhibits behaviors such as restlessness, irritability, noise sensitivity, motor tension, fatigue, or sleep disturbances. The Rating Anxiety in Dementia (RAID) Scale may be utilized; this may require caregiver input. Recognize that anxiety is common in dementia, is often undiagnosed, and may significantly impact quality of life.

▲ Recognize that clients with Alzheimer's disease may experience apathy, anxiety and depression, psychomotor agitation, and psychotic or manic syndromes; nonpharmacological interventions for management should be attempted first.

• Determine client's normal routines and attempt to maintain them.

• Obtain information about the client's life history from the family; collaborate with family members to provide optimal care.

• Begin each interaction with the client by gaining and maintaining eye contact, identifying yourself and calling the client by name. Approach the client with a caring, loving, and an accepting attitude, and speak calmly and slowly.

• To enhance communication, use a calm approach, avoid distractions, show interest, keep communication simple, give clear choices, give the client time with word finding, use repetition and rephrasing, and utilize gestures, prompts, and cues or visual aids. Listen attentively to understand nonverbal messages, and engage in topics of interest to the client.

• Promote regular exercise.

• Provide opportunities for contact with nature or nature-based stimuli, such as facilitating time spent outdoors or indoor gardening.

• Provide animal-assisted therapy.

• Break down self-care tasks into simple steps (e.g., instead of saying, "Take a shower," say to the client, "Please follow me. Sit down on the bed. Take off your shoes. Now take off your socks."). Utilize gestures when giving directions; allow for adequate time and model the desired action if needed or possible.

• Promote routines and facilitate success by keeping frequently used items in a visible and consistent location.

● = Independent   ▲ = Collaborative

- Use reminiscence and life review therapeutic interventions for clients in the early to middle stages of dementia; ask questions about the client's past activities, important events and experiences from the past while utilizing photographs, videos, artifacts, music or newspaper clippings, or multimedia technology to stimulate memories.
- For clients in the middle to late stages of dementia, engage them in creative expression through the use of TimeSlips story-telling groups.
- If the client is verbally agitated (repetitive verbalizations, complaints, moaning, muttering, threats, screaming), assess for and address unsatisfied basic needs or environmental factors that may be addressed.
- Utilize music as a nonpharmacological approach to managing anxiety. Identify music preferences of the client; interview family members if necessary. For anxious clients who are having problems relaxing enough to eat, try having them listen to music during meals.
- Assist clients in wayfinding, monitoring them so that they do not get lost in unfamiliar settings.
- For clients who wander, utilize technologies that monitor but do not restrict. Direct the client who is wandering to a more soothing location with lower light levels and less variation in noise if necessary.
- Promote sleep by promoting daytime activity, creating a restful sleep environment, decreasing waking, and promoting quiet.
- Provide structured social and physical activities that are individualized for the client.
- Provide activities for the client, such as folding washcloths and sorting or stacking activities or other hobbies the individual enjoyed prior to the onset of dementia.
- Use cues, such as picture boards denoting day, time, and location, to help client with orientation.
- ▲ If the client becomes increasingly confused and/or agitated, perform the following steps:
  - ■ Assess the client for physiological causes, including acute hypoxia, pain, medication effects, malnutrition, and infections such as urinary tract infection, fatigue, electrolyte disturbances, and constipation.

● = Independent   ▲ = Collaborative

- Assess for psychological causes, including changes in the environment, caregiver, routine, demands to perform beyond capacity, or multiple competing stimuli, including discomfort.
- In clients with agitated behaviors, rather than confronting the client, decrease stimuli in the environment or provide diversional activities such as quiet music, looking through a photo album, or providing the client with textured items to handle.
- If clients with dementia become more agitated, assess for pain.
- Avoid using restraints if at all possible.
▲ Use PRN or low-dose regular dosing of psychotropic or antianxiety drugs only as a last resort; start with the lowest possible dose. They can be effective in managing symptoms of psychosis and aggressive behavior, but have undesirable side effects.
▲ Avoid the use of anticholinergic medications such as diphenhydramine.
- For predictable difficult times, such as during bathing and grooming, try the following:
  - Massage the client's hands or back to relax the client.
  - Approach the client in a client-centered framework: utilize respectful, positive statements, give directions one step at a time, provide short and clear cues, utilize verbal praise for successful task completion.
  - Involve the family in care of the client.
- For care of early dementia clients with primarily symptoms of memory loss, see the care plan for **Impaired Memory.**
- For clients nearing the end of life, consider a hospice referral.
- For care of clients with self-care deficits, see the appropriate care plan **(Feeding Self-Care deficit; Dressing Self-Care deficit; and Toileting Self-Care deficit).**

Geriatric

NOTE: All interventions are appropriate with geriatric clients.

Multicultural

- Assess for the influence of cultural beliefs, norms, and values on the family's or caregiver's understanding of chronic confusion or dementia.
- Inform the client's family or caregiver of the meaning of and reasons for common behavior observed in clients with dementia.
- Assist the family or caregiver in identifying barriers that would prevent the use of social services or other supportive services that could help reduce the impact of caregiving; refer to social services or other supportive services.

Home Care

NOTE: Keeping the client as independent as possible is important. Because community-based care is usually less structured than institutional care, in the home setting the goal of maintaining safety for the client takes on primary importance.

- The interventions described previously may be adapted for home care use.
- Provide information to the family and home care client regarding advance directives.
- Assess the client's memory and executive function deficits before assuming the inability to make any medical decisions; driving capacity and financial capacity should be assessed for clients with mild cognitive impairment.
- Assess the home for safety features and client needs for assistive devices. Refer to the interventions for **Feeding Self-Care deficit, Dressing Self-Care deficit, Bathing Self-Care deficit** as needed.
- Promote cognitive stimulation (conversation, singing, dancing, creative activities, games) and memory training exercises for individuals in the early stages of dementia.
- Provide education and support to the family regarding effective communication and ways to manage cognitive and behavioral changes; be prepared to offer support and information to family members who live at a distance as well.
- Use familiar aspects of the environment (smells, music, foods, pictures) to cue the client, capitalizing on habit to remind the client of activities in which the client can participate.

● = Independent   ▲ = Collaborative

C

- Instruct the caregiver to provide a balanced activity schedule that does not stress the client or deprive him or her of stimulation; avoid sustained low- or high-stimulation activity.
- Encourage the use of preferred music listening to evoke memories and promote relaxation.
▲ If the client will require extensive supervision on an ongoing basis, evaluate the client for day care programs. Refer the family to medical social services to assist with this process if necessary.
- Encourage the family to include the client in family activities when possible. Reinforce the use of therapeutic communication guidelines (see Client/Family Teaching and Discharge Planning) and sensitivity to the number of people present.
- Assess family caregivers for caregiver stress, loneliness, and depression.
- Refer to the care plan for **Caregiver Role Strain.**
▲ Refer the client to medical social services as necessary to evaluate financial resources and initiate benefits or access to providers.
▲ Institute case management for frail elderly clients to support continued independent living.

Client/Family Teaching and Discharge Planning

- In the early stages of dementia, provide the caregiver with information on illness processes, needed care, available services, role changes, and the importance of advance directives discussion; facilitate family cohesion.
- Teach the family how to converse with a memory-impaired person and strategies for handling challenging behaviors.
- Teach the family how to provide physical care for the client (bathing, feeding, and ADLs) as well as coping strategies to deal with the burden of caregiving.
- Discuss with the family what to expect as the dementia progresses.
▲ Counsel the family about resources available regarding end-of-life decisions and legal concerns.
▲ Inform the family that as dementia progresses, hospice care may be available in the home or nursing home in the terminal stages to help the caregiver.
   NOTE: The nursing diagnoses **Impaired Environmental Interpretation Syndrome** and **Chronic Confusion** are very

similar in definition and interventions. **Impaired Environmental Interpretation Syndrome** must be interpreted as a syndrome when other nursing diagnoses would also apply. **Chronic Confusion** may be interpreted as the human response to a situation or situations that require a level of cognition of which the individual is no longer capable.

Risk for acute Confusion

NANDA-I Definition

At risk for reversible disturbances of consciousness, attention, cognition, and perception that develop over a short period of time

Risk Factors

Decreased mobility; decreased restraints; dementia; fluctuation in sleep-wake cycle; history of stroke; impaired cognition; infection; male gender; metabolic abnormalities: azotemia, decreased hemoglobin, dehydration, electrolyte imbalances, increased BUN/creatinine, malnutrition, over 60 years of age, pain; pharmaceutical agents: anesthesia, anticholinergics, diphenhydramine, multiple medications, opioids, psychoactive drugs, sensory deprivation, substance abuse, urinary retention

Client Outcomes, Nursing Interventions, and Client/ Family Teaching

Refer to care plan for **Acute Confusion.**

Constipation

NANDA-I Definition

Decrease in normal frequency of defecation, accompanied by difficult or incomplete passage of stool and/or passage of excessively hard, dry stool

Defining Characteristics

Feeling of rectal fullness; feeling of rectal pressure; straining with defecation; unable to pass stool; abdominal pain; abdominal tenderness; anorexia; atypical presentations in older adults (e.g., change in mental status, urinary incontinence, unexplained falls, elevated body temperature); borborygmi; change in bowel pattern; decreased frequency;

• = Independent   ▲ = Collaborative

decreased volume of stool; distended abdomen; generalized fatigue; hard, formed stool; headache; hyperactive bowel sounds; hypoactive bowel sounds; increased abdominal pressure; indigestion; nausea; oozing liquid stool; palpable abdominal or rectal mass; percussed abdominal dullness; pain with defecation; severe flatus; vomiting

Related Factors (r/t)

Functional
Abdominal muscle weakness; habitual denial; habitual ignoring of urge to defecate; inadequate toileting (e.g., timeliness, positioning for defecation, privacy); irregular defecation habits; insufficient physical activity; recent environmental changes

Psychological
Depression, emotional stress, mental confusion

Pharmacological
Aluminum-containing antacids; anticholinergics, anticonvulsants; antidiarrheal agents, antidepressants, antilipemic agents, bismuth salts, calcium carbonate, calcium channel blockers, diuretics, iron salts, laxative overdose, nonsteroidal antiinflammatory drugs (NSAIDs), opioids, phenothiazines, sedatives, and sympathomimetics

Mechanical
Neurological impairment, electrolyte imbalance, hemorrhoids, Hirschsprung's disease, obesity, postsurgical obstruction, pregnancy, prostate enlargement, rectal abscess, rectal anal fissures, rectal anal stricture, rectal prolapse, rectal ulcer, rectocele, tumors

Physiological
Change in eating patterns; change in usual foods; decreased motility of gastrointestinal tract; defecation disorder; dehydration; inadequate dentition; inadequate oral hygiene; insufficient fiber intake; insufficient fluid intake; poor eating habits

Client Outcomes

Client Will (Specify Time Frame):
- Maintain passage of soft, formed stool every 1 to 3 days without straining
- State relief from discomfort of constipation
- Identify measures that prevent or treat constipation

● = Independent   ▲ = Collaborative

Nursing Interventions

- Assess usual pattern of defecation, including time of day, amount and frequency of stool, consistency of stool; history of bowel habits or laxative use; diet, including fiber and fluid intake; exercise patterns; personal remedies for constipation; obstetrical/gynecological history; surgeries; diseases that affect bowel motility; alterations in perianal sensation; present bowel regimen.
- Consider emotional influences (e.g., depression and anxiety) on defecation.
- Have the client or family keep a 7-day diary of bowel habits, including information such as time of day; usual stimulus; consistency, amount, and frequency of stool; difficulty defecating; fluid consumption; and use of any aids to defecation.
- Use the Bristol Stool Scale to assess stool consistency.
- ▲ Review the client's current medications.
- ▲ If clients are suffering from constipation and are taking constipating medications, consult with the health care provider (with prescriptive powers) about the possibilities of decreasing the medication dosages or finding an alternative medication that is less constipating.
- ▲ Recognize that opioids cause constipation. If the client is receiving temporary opioids (e.g., for acute postoperative pain), request an order for routine stool softeners from the primary care practitioner, monitor bowel movements, and request a laxative if the client develops constipation. If the client is receiving around-the-clock opiates (e.g., for palliative care), request an order for Senokot-S and institute a bowel regimen.
- ▲ If the client is terminally ill and is receiving around-the-clock opioids for palliative care, speak with the prescribing provider about ordering methylnaltrexone, a drug that blocks opioid effects on the gastrointestinal tract without interfering with analgesia.
- If new onset of constipation, determine if the client has recently stopped smoking.
- Palpate for abdominal distention, percuss for dullness, and auscultate bowel sounds.
- ▲ Check for impaction; if present, perform digital removal of stool per provider's order.
- Encourage fiber intake of 20 g/day (for adults) ensuring that the fiber is palatable to the individual and that fluid intake is adequate. Add fiber gradually to decrease bloating and flatus.

• = Independent   ▲ = Collaborative

C

- Use a mixture of bran cereal, applesauce, and prune juice; begin administration in small amounts and gradually increase amount. Keep refrigerated. Always check with the primary care provider before initiating this intervention. It is important that the client also ingest sufficient fluids.
- Provide prune or prune juice daily.
- Encourage a fluid intake of 1.5 to 2 L/day (6 to 8 glasses of liquids per day), unless contraindicated because of other health concerns such as renal or heart disease.
▲ If the client is uncomfortable or in pain due to constipation or has acute or chronic constipation that does not respond to increased fiber, fluid, activity, and appropriate toileting, refer the client to the primary care provider for an evaluation of bowel function and health status.
- Encourage clients to resume walking and activities of daily living as soon as possible if their mobility has been restricted. Encourage turning and changing positions in bed, lifting the hips off the bed, performing range-of-motion exercises, alternately lifting each knee to the chest, doing wheelchair lifts, doing waist twists, stretching the arms away from the body, and pulling in the abdomen while taking deep breaths.
- Ask clients when they normally have a bowel movement and assist them to the bathroom at that same time every day to establish regular elimination.
- Provide privacy for defecation. If not contraindicated, help the client to the bathroom and close the door.
- Help clients onto a bedside commode or toilet so they can either squat or lean forward while sitting. Recognize that it is difficult to impossible to defecate in the lying supine position.
- Teach clients to respond promptly to the defecation urge.
▲ Provide laxatives, suppositories, and enemas only as needed if other more natural interventions are not effective, and as ordered only; establish a client goal of eliminating their use.
▲ When giving large volume enema solutions (e.g., soap-suds or tap-water enemas), measure the amount of fluid given and the amount expelled, especially when giving repeated enemas. Use a low concentration of Castile soap in the soap-suds enema.

• = Independent   ▲ = Collaborative

Geriatric

- Assess older adults for the presence of factors that contribute to constipation, including dietary fiber and fluid intake (less than 1.5 L/day), physical activity, use of constipating medications, and diseases that are associated with constipation.
- Explain the importance of adequate fiber intake, fluid intake, activity, and established toileting routines to ensure soft, formed stool.
- Determine the client's perception of normal bowel elimination and laxative use; promote adherence to a regular schedule.
- Explain why straining (Valsalva maneuver) should be avoided.
- Respond quickly to the client's call for assistance with toileting.
- Offer food, fluids, activity and toileting opportunities to elderly clients who are cognitively impaired.
- Avoid regular use of enemas in the elderly.
▲ Use opioids cautiously.
- Position the client on the toilet or commode and place a small footstool under the feet.

Home Care

- The interventions described previously may be adapted for home care use.
- Take complaints seriously and evaluate claims of constipation in a matter-of-fact manner. Refer to the care plan for **Perceived Constipation.**
- Assess the self-care management activities the client is already using.
- The following treatment recommendations have been offered:
  ▲ Acknowledge the client's life-long experience of bowel function; respect beliefs, attitudes, and preferences, and avoid patronizing responses.
  ▲ Make available comprehensive, useful written information about constipation and possible solutions.
  ▲ Make available empathetic and accessible professional care to provide treatment and advice; a multidisciplinary approach (including physician, nurse, and pharmacist) should be used.

• = Independent   ▲ = Collaborative

▲ Institute a bowel management program.

▲ Consider affordability when suggesting solutions to constipation; discuss cost-effective strategies.

▲ Discuss a range of solutions to constipation and allow the client to choose the preferred options.

▲ Have orders in place for a suppository and enema as the need may occur.

• Although the use of a bedside commode may be necessitated by the client's condition, allow the client to use the toilet in the bathroom when possible and provide assistance.

• In older clients, routinely advise consumption of fluids, fruits, and vegetables as part of the diet, and ambulation if the client is able. Introduce a bowel management program at the first sign of constipation.

▲ Refer for consideration of the use of polyethylene glycol 3350 (PEG-3350) for constipation.

• Advise the client against attempting to remove impacted feces on his or her own.

• When using a bowel program, establish a pattern that is very regular and allows the client to be part of the family unit.

Client/Family Teaching and Discharge Planning

• Instruct the client on normal bowel function and the need for adequate fluid and fiber intake, activity, and a defined toileting pattern in a bowel program.

• Encourage the client to heed defecation warning signs and develop a regular schedule of defecation by using a stimulus such as a warm drink or prune juice.

• Encourage the client to avoid long-term use of laxatives and enemas and to gradually withdraw from their use if they are used regularly.

• If not contraindicated, teach the client how to do bent-leg sit-ups to increase abdominal tone; also encourage the client to contract the abdominal muscles frequently throughout the day. Help the client develop a daily exercise program to increase peristalsis.

• = Independent   ▲ = Collaborative

Perceived Constipation

NANDA-I Definition

Self-diagnosis of constipation and abuse of laxatives, enemas, and suppositories to ensure a daily bowel movement

Defining Characteristics

Expectation of a daily bowel movement that results in overuse of laxatives, enemas, and suppositories; expectation of a passage of stool at same time every day

Related Factors (r/t)

Cultural or family health beliefs, faulty appraisals (long-term expectations/habits); impaired thought processes

Client Outcomes

Client Will (Specify Time Frame):

- Regularly defecate soft, formed stool without use of aids
- Explain the need to decrease or eliminate the use of stimulant laxatives, suppositories, and enemas
- Identify alternatives to stimulant laxatives, enemas, and suppositories for ensuring defecation
- Explain that defecation does not have to occur every day

Nursing Interventions

- Have the client keep a 7-day diary of bowel habits, including information such as time of day; usual stimulus; consistency, amount, and frequency of stool; difficulty defecating; fluid consumption; and use of any aids to defecation.
- Determine the client's perception of an appropriate defecation pattern.
- Recognize the emotional influences (e.g., depression and anxiety) on defecation.
- Monitor the use of laxatives, suppositories, or enemas and suggest replacing them with increased fiber intake along with increased fluids to 2 L/day.
- Encourage fiber intake of 20 g/day (for adults) ensuring that the fiber is palatable to the individual and that fluid intake is adequate. Add fiber gradually to decrease bloating and flatus.

• = Independent ▲ = Collaborative

- Use a mixture of bran cereal, applesauce, and prune juice; begin administration in small amounts and gradually increase amount. Keep refrigerated. Always check with the primary care practitioner before initiating this intervention. It is important that the client also ingest sufficient fluids.
- Teach clients to respond promptly to the defecation urge.
▲ Obtain a referral to a dietitian for analysis of the client's diet and input on how to improve the diet to ensure adequate fiber intake and nutrition.
▲ Assess for signs of depression, other psychological disorders, and a history of physical or sexual abuse.
- Encourage the client to increase activity, walking for at least 30 minutes at least 5 days a week as tolerated.
▲ Observe for the presence of an eating disorder, the use of laxatives to control or decrease weight; refer for counseling if needed.

Home Care

- The interventions described previously may be adapted for home care use.
- Take complaints seriously and evaluate claims of constipation in a matter-of-fact manner.
- Obtain family and client histories of bowel or other patterned behavior problems.
- Observe family cultural patterns related to eating and bowel habits.
- Encourage a mindset and program of self-care management. Elicit from the client the self-talk he or she uses to describe body perceptions; correct fatalistic interpretations.
- Instruct the client in a healthy lifestyle that supports normal bowel function (e.g., activity, fluid intake, diet) and encourage progressive inclusion of these elements into daily activities.
- Discuss the client's self-image. Help the client to reframe the self-concept as capable.
- Instruct the client and family in appropriate expectations for having bowel movements.
- Offer instruction and reassurance regarding explanations for variation from the previous pattern of bowel movements.

● = Independent   ▲ = Collaborative

- Contract with the client and/or a responsible family member regarding the use of laxatives. Have the client maintain a bowel pattern diary. Observe for diarrhea or frequent evacuation.
▲ Teach the family to carry out the bowel program per the physician's orders.
▲ Refer for home health aide services to assist with personal care, including the bowel program, if appropriate.
- Identify a contingency plan for bowel care if the client is dependent on outside persons for such care.

Client/Family Teaching and Discharge Planning

- Explain normal bowel function and the necessary ingredients for a regular bowel regimen (e.g., fluid, fiber, activity, and regular schedule for defecation).
- Work with the client and family to develop a diet that fits the client's lifestyle and includes increased fiber.
- Teach the client that it is not necessary to have daily bowel movements and that the passage of anywhere from three stools each day to three stools each week is considered normal. Explain to the client the harmful effects of the continual use of defecation aids such laxatives and enemas.
- Encourage the client to gradually decrease the use of the usual laxatives and or enemas, and recognize it may take months for the process to do it gradually.
- Determine a method of increasing the client's fluid intake and fit this practice into client's lifestyle.
- Explain what Valsalva maneuver is and why it should be avoided.
- Work with the client and family to design a bowel training routine that is based on previous patterns (before laxative or enema abuse) and incorporates the consumption of warm fluids, increased fiber, and increased fluids; privacy; and a predictable routine.

Additional Nursing Interventions and Rationales, Client/Family Teaching

See care plan for **Constipation.**

• = Independent   ▲ = Collaborative

Risk for Constipation

C **NANDA-I Definition**

At risk for a decrease in normal frequency of defecation accompanied by difficult or incomplete passage of stool and/or passage of excessively hard, dry stool

Risk Factors

Functional

Abdominal weakness; habitual denial/ignoring of urge to defecate; recent environmental changes; inadequate toileting (e.g., timeliness, positioning for defecation, privacy); irregular defecation habits; insufficient physical activity

Psychological

Depression; emotional stress; mental confusion

Physiological

Change in usual eating patterns; change in usual foods; decreased motility of gastrointestinal tract; dehydration; inadequate dentition; inadequate oral hygiene; insufficient fiber intake; insufficient fluid intake; poor eating habits

Pharmacological

Aluminum-containing antacids; anticholinergics; anticonvulsants; antidepressants; antilipemic agents; bismuth salts; calcium carbonate; calcium channel blockers; diuretics; iron salts; laxative overuse; nonsteroidal antiinflammatory drugs; opioids; phenothiazines; sedatives; and sympathomimetics

Mechanical

Electrolyte imbalance; hemorrhoids; Hirschsprung's disease; neurological impairment; obesity; postsurgical obstruction; pregnancy; prostate enlargement; rectal abscess; rectal anal fissures; rectal anal stricture; rectal prolapse; rectal ulcer; rectocele; tumors

Client Outcomes, Nursing Interventions, and Client/Family Teaching

Refer to care plans for Constipation.

• = Independent ▲ = Collaborative

Contamination

NANDA-I Definition

C

Exposure to environmental contaminants in doses sufficient to cause adverse health effects

Defining Characteristics

Pesticides

Dermatological effects of pesticide exposure; gastrointestinal effects of pesticide exposure; neurological effects of pesticide exposure; pulmonary effects of pesticide exposure; renal effects of pesticide exposure; major categories of pesticides: insecticides, herbicides, fungicides, antimicrobials, rodenticides; major pesticides: organophosphates, carbamates, organochlorines, pyrethrum, arsenic, glycophosphates, bipyridyls, chlorophenoxy

Chemicals

Dermatological effects of chemical exposure; gastrointestinal effects of chemical exposure; immunologic effects of chemical exposure; neurological effects of chemical exposure; pulmonary effects of chemical exposure; renal effects of chemical exposure; major chemical agents: petroleum-based agents, anticholinesterase type I agents act on proximal tracheobronchial portion of the respiratory tract, type II agents act on alveoli; type III agents produce systemic effects

Biologicals

Dermatological effects of exposure to biologics; gastrointestinal effects of exposure to biologics; pulmonary effects of exposure to biologics; neurological effects of exposure to biologics; renal effects of exposure to biologics (toxins from organisms [bacteria, viruses, fungi])

Pollution

Neurological effects of pollution exposure; pulmonary effects of pollution exposure (major locations: air, water, soil; major agents: asbestos, radon, tobacco, heavy metal, lead, noise, exhaust)

Waste

Dermatological effects of waste exposure; gastrointestinal effects of waste exposure; hepatic effects of waste exposure; pulmonary effects of waste exposure (categories of waste: trash, raw sewage, industrial waste)

• = Independent   ▲ = Collaborative

Radiation

External exposure through direct contact with radioactive material; genetic effects of radiation exposure; immunologic effects of radiation exposure; neurological effects of radiation exposure; oncological effects of radiation exposure

Related Factors (r/t)

External

Chemical contamination of food; chemical contamination of water; exposure to bioterrorism; exposure to disasters (natural or human-made); exposure to radiation (occupation in radiology; employment in nuclear industries and electrical generating plants; living near nuclear industries and/ or electrical generating plants); exposure through ingestion of radioactive material (e.g., food/water contamination); flaking, peeling paint in presence of young children; flaking, peeling plaster in presence of young children; floor surface (carpeted surfaces hold contaminant residue more than hard floor surfaces); geographic area (living in area where high level of contaminants exist); household hygiene practices; inadequate municipal services (trash removal, sewage treatment facilities); inappropriate use of protective clothing; lack of breakdown of contaminants once indoors (breakdown is inhibited without sun and rain exposure); lack of protective clothing; lacquer in poorly ventilated areas; lacquer without effective protection; living in poverty (increases potential for multiple exposure, lack of access to health care, poor diet); paint in poorly ventilated areas; paint without effective protection; personal hygiene practices; playing in outdoor areas where environmental contaminants are used; presence of atmospheric pollutants; use of environmental contaminants in the home (e.g., pesticides, chemicals, environmental tobacco smoke); unprotected contact with chemicals (e.g., arsenic); unprotected contact with heavy metals (e.g., chromium, lead)

Internal

Age (children <5 years, older adults); concomitant exposures; developmental characteristics of children; female gender; gestational age during exposure; nutritional factors (e.g., obesity, vitamin and mineral deficiencies); preexisting disease states; pregnancy; previous exposures; smoking

Client Outcomes

Client Will (Specify Time Frame):

- Have minimal health effects associated with contamination
- Cooperate with appropriate decontamination protocol
- Participate in appropriate isolation precautions

• = Independent   ▲ = Collaborative

Community Will (Specify Time Frame):

- Utilize health surveillance data system to monitor for contamination incidents
- Utilize disaster plan to evacuate and triage affected members
- Have minimal health effects associated with contamination

Nursing Interventions

▲ Help individuals cope with contamination incident by doing the following:
  - Use groups that have survived terrorist attacks as useful resource for victims
  - Provide accurate information on risks involved, preventive measures, use of antibiotics, and vaccines
  - Assist to deal with feelings of fear, vulnerability, and grief
  - Encourage individuals to talk to others about their fears
  - Assist victims to think positively and to move toward the future

- Triage, stabilize, transport, and treat affected community members.
- Utilize approved procedures for decontamination of persons, clothing, and equipment.
- Utilize appropriate isolation precautions: universal, airborne, droplet, and contact isolation.
- Monitor individual for therapeutic effects, side effects, and compliance with postexposure drug therapy.

▲ Collaborate with other agencies (local health department, emergency medical service [EMS], state and federal agencies).

Geriatric

- Help the client identify age-related factors that may affect response to contamination incidents.
- Encourage family members to acknowledge and validate the client's concerns.
- Advise the elderly to follow public notices related to drinking water.
- Encourage older adults to receive influenza vaccination when it is available beginning as early as late August and continuing through the end of February.

● = Independent   ▲ = Collaborative

Pediatric

- Provide environmental health hazard information.
- Caution families to avoid having children play in streams following heavy rainfall.

Multicultural

- Ask about use of imported or culture-specific products.
- Assess exposure to multiple pollutants, pre-existing disease, poor nutrition, substandard housing, and limited access to health care.

Home Care

- Assess current environmental stressors and identify community resources.
- Residential settings may present household-related hazards that impact health such as spread of nosocomial infections and unsanitary, unsafe conditions.

Client/Family Teaching and Discharge Planning

- Provide truthful information to the person or family affected.
- Discuss signs and symptoms of contamination.
- Explain decontamination protocols.
- Explain need for isolation procedures.
- Emphasize the importance of pre- and postexposure treatment of contamination.

Risk for Contamination

NANDA-I Definition

Accentuated risk of exposure to environmental contaminants in doses sufficient to cause adverse health effects

Risk Factors

See Related Factors in **Contamination** care plan.

● = Independent   ▲ = Collaborative

Client Outcomes

Client Will (Specify Time Frame):
- Remain free of adverse effects of contamination

Community Will (Specify Time Frame):
- Utilize health surveillance data system to monitor for contamination incidents
- Participate in mass casualty and disaster readiness drills
- Remain free of contamination-related health effects
- Minimize exposure to contaminants

Nursing Interventions

▲ Conduct surveillance for environmental contamination. Notify agencies authorized to protect the environment of contaminants in the area.
- Assist individuals to modify the environment to minimize risk or assist in relocating to safer environment.
- Schedule mass casualty and disaster readiness drills.
- Provide accurate information on risks involved, preventive measures, use of antibiotics, and vaccines.
- Assist to deal with feelings of fear and vulnerability.
- For more interventions including Pediatric, Geriatric, Multicultural, and Home Care, see the **Contamination** care plan.

Risk for adverse reaction to iodinated Contrast media

NANDA-I Definition

At risk for any noxious or unintended reaction associated with the use of iodinated contrast media that can occur within 7 days after contrast agent injection

Risk Factors

Anxiety; concurrent use of medications (e.g., beta-blockers, interleukin-2, metformin, nephrotoxic medications); dehydration; extremes of age; fragile veins (e.g., prior or actual chemotherapy treatment or radiation in the limb to be injected, multiple attempts to obtain intravenous

• = Independent   ▲ = Collaborative

C

access, indwelling intravenous lines in place for more than 24 hours, previous axillary lymph node dissection in the limb to be injected, distal intravenous access sites: hand, wrist, foot, ankle); generalized debilitation; history of allergies; history of previous adverse effect from iodinated contrast media; physical and chemical properties of the contrast media (e.g., iodine concentration, viscosity, high osmolality, ion toxicity); unconsciousness; underlying disease (e.g., heart disease, pulmonary disease, blood dyscrasias, endocrine disease, renal disease, pheochromocytoma, autoimmune disease)

Client Outcomes

Client Will (Specify Time Frame):

- Maintain normal blood urea nitrogen and serum creatinine levels
- Maintain urine output of 0.5 mL/kg/hr
- Maintain serum electrolytes (K^+, PO_4, Na^+) within normal limits

Nursing Interventions

Contrast-Induced Nephropathy (CIN)

▲ Protect clients from contrast media-induced nephropathy by taking the following actions:
  - Watching for closely spaced studies using contrast media and consulting with provider for change in scheduling of studies if needed
  - Notifying the provider and the radiology staff if the client has preexisting renal disease
  - Ensuring that clients having diagnostic testing with contrast are well hydrated with IV saline as ordered before and after the examination
  - Recognizing that many clients with decreased renal function are not aware of their health status, and that a questionnaire checklist administered before testing may not be satisfactory to find clients with impaired renal function that should receive contrast media carefully or who are not a candidate for testing utilizing contrast media because of possible increased renal dysfunction.
  - Recognizing that cancer clients are often very vulnerable to contrast induced nephropathy due to frequent imaging examinations.

• = Independent ▲ = Collaborative

▲ Monitor the client carefully for symptoms of hypovolemia following use of contrast media including intake and output, blood pressure measurements, and new onset of postural hypotension with dizziness.

▲ Monitor the client carefully for symptoms of acute failure following use of contrast media including decreased or normal urinary output, and increased creatinine levels.

Allergic Reaction to Contrast Media

• Recognize that both allergic and anaphylactoid reactions can occur. Anaphylaxis occurs rapidly, often within 20 minutes of injection, versus a less serious anaphylactoid reaction, which can occur later after an hour.

• Watch carefully for symptoms of a reaction, which can be either mild, moderate, or severe. Report all symptoms to primary care physician because symptoms can advance from mild to severe rapidly.

  • *Mild Reactions*: Urticaria, pruritus, rhinorrhea, nausea, emesis, diaphoresis, coughing, dizziness

  • *Moderate Reactions*: Persistent emesis, widespread urticaria, headache, edema of the face, laryngeal edema, mild dyspnea, palpitations, tachycardia/bradycardia, hypertension, abdominal cramps

  • *Severe Reactions:* Severe bronchospasm, severe arrhythmias, severe hypotension, pulmonary edema, laryngeal edema, seizures, syncope, death

Vein Damage and Damage to Vascular Access Devices

• After diagnostic testing using contrast media given IV, inspect the IV site used for administration for possible problems such as extravasation, or development of compartment syndrome with excessive amounts of contrast pushed into the tissues under pressure.

• Recognize that a vascular access device utilized for administration of contrast media can rupture from the high pressures utilized to administer the contrast media.

Geriatric

▲ Screen the elderly client thoroughly before diagnostic testing utilizing contrast media.

• = Independent   ▲ = Collaborative

Readiness for enhanced community Coping

C

NANDA-I Definition

Pattern of community activities for adaptation and problem solving that is satisfactory for meeting the demands or needs of the community but that can be improved for management of current and future problems/stressors

Defining Characteristics

One or more characteristics that indicate effective coping:

Active planning by community for predicted stressors; active problem solving by community when faced with issues; agreement that community is responsible for stress management; positive communication among community members; positive communication between community/aggregates and larger community; programs available for recreation; programs available for relaxation; resources sufficient for managing stressors

Community Outcomes

Community Will (Specify Time Frame):

• Develop enhanced coping strategies
• Maintain effective coping strategies for management of stress

Nursing Interventions

NOTE: Interventions depend on the specific aspects of community coping that can be enhanced (e.g., planning for stress management, communication, development of community power, community perceptions of stress, community coping strategies).

• Describe the roles of community/public health nurses in working with healthy communities.
• Help the community to obtain funds for additional programs.
• Encourage positive attitudes toward the community through the media and other sources.
• Help community members to collaborate with one another for power enhancement and coping skills.

• = Independent   ▲ = Collaborative

- Assist community members with cognitive skills and habits of mind for problem solving.
- Demonstrate optimum use of power resources.
- Reduce poverty whenever possible.
▲ Collaborate with community members to improve educational levels within the community.

Multicultural

- Refer to care plan **Ineffective community Coping.**

Client/family Teaching and Discharge Planning

- Review coping skills, power for coping, and the use of power resources.

Defensive Coping

NANDA-I Definition

Repeated projection of falsely positive self-evaluation based on a self-protective pattern that defends against underlying perceived threats to positive self-regard

Defining Characteristics

Denial of obvious problems; denial of obvious weaknesses; difficulty establishing relationships; difficulty in perception of reality testing; difficulty maintaining relationships; grandiosity; hostile laughter; hypersensitivity to criticism; hypersensitivity to slight; lack of follow-through in therapy; lack of follow-through in treatment; lack of participation in therapy; lack of participation in treatment; projection of blame; projection of responsibility; rationalization of failures; reality distortion; ridicule of others; superior attitude toward others

Related Factors (r/t)

Conflict between self-perception and value system; deficient support system; fear of failure; fear of humiliation; fear of repercussions; lack of resilience; low level of confidence in others; low level of self-confidence; uncertainty; unrealistic expectations of self

• = Independent   ▲ = Collaborative

Client Outcomes

Client Will (Specify Time Frame):

C

- Acknowledge need for change in coping style
- Accept responsibility for own behavior
- Establish realistic goals with validation from caregivers
- Solicit caregiver validation in decision-making

Nursing Interventions

- Assess for possible symptoms associated with defensive coping: depressive symptoms, excessive self-focused attention, negativism and anxiety, hypertension, post-traumatic stress disorder (PTSD) (e.g., exposure to terrorism), unjust world beliefs.
- Stimulate cognitive-behavioral stress management (CBSM).
- Ask appropriate questions to assess whether denial (defensive coping) is being used in association with alcoholism.
- Promote interventions with multisensory stimulation environments.
- Empower the client/caregiver's self-knowledge.

Geriatric

- ▲ Identify problems with alcohol in the elderly with the appropriate tools and make suitable referrals.
- Encourage exercise for positive coping.
- Stimulate individual reminiscence therapy.
- Stimulate group reminiscence therapy.

Multicultural

- Acknowledge racial/ethnic differences at the onset of care.
- Assess an individual's sociocultural backgrounds in teaching self-management and self-regulation as a means of supporting hope and coping with a diagnosis of type 2 diabetes.
- Encourage the client to use spiritual coping mechanisms such as faith and prayer.
- Encourage spirituality as a source of support for coping.

• = Independent   ▲ = Collaborative

Home Care

▲ Refer the client for a behavioral program that teaches coping skills via "Lifeskills" workshop and/or video.

Client/Family Teaching and Discharge Planning

• Teach coping skills to family caregivers of cancer clients.
• Teach caregivers the COPE intervention (creativity, optimism, planning, expert information) to assist with symptom management.
• Family-based intervention may prevent anxiety disorders in the offspring of parents with anxiety disorders.

Ineffective Coping

NANDA-I Definition

Inability to form a valid appraisal of the stressors, inadequate choices of practiced responses, and/or inability to use available resources

Defining Characteristics

Change in usual communication patterns; decreased use of social support; destructive behavior toward others; destructive behavior toward self; difficulty organizing information; fatigue; high illness rate; inability to attend to information; inability to meet basic needs; inability to meet role expectations; inadequate problem solving; lack of goal-directed behavior; lack of resolution of problem; poor concentration; reports inability to ask for help; reports inability to cope; risk taking; sleep pattern disturbance; substance abuse; use of forms of coping that impede adaptive behavior

Related Factors (r/t)

Disturbance in pattern of appraisal of threat; disturbance in pattern of tension release; gender differences in coping strategies; high degree of threat; inability to conserve adaptive energies; inadequate level of confidence in ability to cope; inadequate level of perception of control; inadequate opportunity to prepare for stressor; inadequate resources available; inadequate social support created by characteristics of relationships; maturational crisis; situational crisis; uncertainty

• = Independent   ▲ = Collaborative

C

Client Outcomes

Client Will (Specify Time Frame):

• Use effective coping strategies
• Use behaviors to decrease stress
• Remain free of destructive behavior toward self or others
• Report decrease in physical symptoms of stress
• Report increase in psychological comfort
• Seek help from a health care professional as appropriate

Nursing Interventions

• Observe for contributing factors of ineffective coping such as poor self-concept, grief, lack of problem-solving skills, lack of support, recent change in life situation, maturational or situational crises.
• Use verbal and nonverbal therapeutic communication approaches including empathy, active listening, and confrontation to encourage the client and family to express emotions such as sadness, guilt, and anger (within appropriate limits); verbalize fears and concerns; and set goals.
• Collaborate with the client to identify strengths such as the ability to relate the facts and to recognize the source of stressors.
• Encourage the client to describe previous stressors and the coping mechanisms used. Be supportive of coping behaviors; allow the client time to relax.
• Assist the client to set realistic goals and identify personal skills and knowledge.
• Provide information regarding care before care is given.
• Discuss changes with the client before making them.
• Provide mental and physical activities within the client's ability (e.g., reading, television, radio, crafts, outings, movies, dinners out, social gatherings, exercise, sports, games).
• Discuss the client's and family's power to change a situation or the need to accept a situation.
• Offer instruction regarding alternative coping strategies.
• Encourage use of spiritual resources as desired.
• Encourage use of social support resources.
▲ Refer for additional or more intensive therapies as needed.

• = Independent   ▲ = Collaborative

Pediatric

- Monitor the client's risk of harming self or others and intervene appropriately. See care plan for **Risk for Suicide.**
- Support adolescent and children's individual coping styles.
- Encourage moderate aerobic exercise (as appropriate).

Geriatric

- ▲ Assess and report possible physiological alterations (e.g., sepsis, hypoglycemia, hypotension, infection, changes in temperature, fluid and electrolyte imbalances, and use of medications with known cognitive and psychotropic side effects).
- Screen for elder neglect or other forms of elder mistreatment.
- Encourage the client to make choices (as appropriate) and participate in planning care and scheduled activities.
- Target selected coping mechanisms for older persons based on client features, use, and preferences.
- Increase and mobilize support available to older persons by encouraging a variety of mechanisms involving family, friends, peers, and health care providers.
- Actively listen to complaints and concerns.
- Engage the client in reminiscence.

Multicultural

- Assess for the influence of cultural beliefs, norms, and values on the client's perceptions of effective coping.
- Assess the influence of fatalism on the client's coping behavior.
- Assess the influence of cultural conflicts that may affect coping abilities.
- Assess for intergenerational family problems that can overwhelm coping abilities.
- Encourage spirituality as a source of support for coping.
- Negotiate with the client with regard to the aspects of coping behavior that will need to be modified.
- Encourage moderate aerobic exercise (as appropriate).
- Identify which family members the client can count on for support.
- Support the inner resources that clients use for coping.
- Use an empowerment framework to redefine coping strategies.

• = Independent   ▲ = Collaborative

C

Home Care

- The interventions described previously may be adapted for home care use.
- ▲ Assess for suicidal tendencies. Refer for mental health care immediately if indicated.
- Identify an emergency plan should the client become suicidal.
- Observe the family for coping behavior patterns. Obtain family and client history as possible.
- ▲ Assess for effective symptoms after cerebrovascular accident (CVA) in the elderly, particularly emotional lability and depression. Refer for evaluation and treatment as indicated.
- Encourage the client to use self-care management to increase the experience of personal control. Identify with the client all available supports and sense of attachment to others. Refer to the care plan for **Powerlessness.**
- ▲ Refer the client and family to support groups.
- ▲ If monitoring medication use, contract with the client or solicit assistance from a responsible caregiver.
- ▲ Institute case management for frail elderly clients to support continued independent living.
- ▲ If the client is homebound, refer for psychiatric home health care services for client reassurance and implementation of a therapeutic regimen.

Client/Family Teaching and Discharge Planning

- Teach the client to problem solve. Have the client define the problem and cause, and list the advantages and disadvantages of the options.
- Provide the seriously ill client and his or her family with needed information regarding the condition and treatment.
- Teach relaxation techniques.
- Work closely with the client to develop appropriate educational tools that address individualized needs.
- ▲ Teach the client about available community resources (e.g., therapists, ministers, counselors, self-help groups).

● = Independent   ▲ = Collaborative

Readiness for Enhanced Coping

NANDA-I Definition

C

A pattern of cognitive and behavioral efforts to manage demands that is sufficient for well-being and can be strengthened

Defining Characteristics

Acknowledges power; aware of possible environmental changes; defines stressors as manageable; seeks knowledge of new strategies; seeks social support; uses a broad range of emotion-oriented strategies; uses a broad range of problem-oriented strategies; uses spiritual resources

Client Outcomes

Client Will (Specify Time Frame):

- Acknowledge personal power
- State awareness of possible environmental changes that may contribute to decreased coping
- State that stressors are manageable
- Seek new effective coping strategies
- Seek social support for problems associated with coping
- Demonstrate ability to cope, using a broad range of coping strategies
- Use spiritual support of personal choice

Nursing Interventions

- Assess and support positive psychological strengths, that is, hope, optimism, self-efficacy, resiliency, and social support.
- Be physically and emotionally present for the client.
- Empower the client to set realistic goals and to engage in problem solving.
- Encourage expression of positive thoughts and emotions.
- Encourage the client to use spiritual coping mechanisms such as faith and prayer.
- Help the client with serious and chronic conditions such as depression, cancer diagnosis, and chemotherapy treatment to maintain social support networks or assist in building new ones.
- ▲ Refer women facing diagnostic and curative breast cancer surgery for psychosocial support.

● = Independent   ▲ = Collaborative

▲ Refer for cognitive-behavioral therapy (CBT) to enhance coping skills. Refer to the care plans for **Readiness for enhanced Communication** and **Readiness for enhanced Spiritual well-being.**

Pediatric

- Encourage exercise for children and adolescents to promote positive self-esteem, to enhance coping, and to prevent behavioral and psychological problems.
- Suggest that parents with children diagnosed with cancer continue with psychosocial support during and after treatment. They may use computer-mediated support groups to exchange messages with other parents.

Geriatric

- Consider the use of telephone support for caregivers of family members with dementia.
- Use technology for social support and to help elders stay connected to family and friends.
- Support a positive sense of humor and social support.
- Refer the older client to self-help support groups. Suggest the "Red Hat Society" for older women.
- ▲ Refer the client with Alzheimer's disease who is terminally ill to hospice.

Multicultural

- Assess an individual's sociocultural backgrounds in teaching self-management and self-regulation as a means of supporting hope and coping with a diagnosis.
- Encourage spirituality as a source of support for coping.
- Refer to care plan for **Ineffective Coping.**

Home Care

- The interventions described previously may be adapted for home care use.
- Provide an Internet-based health coach to encourage self-management for clients with chronic conditions such as depression, impaired mobility and chronic pain.

● = Independent ▲ = Collaborative

- Refer the client to mutual health support groups.
- Refer prostate cancer clients and their spouses to family programs that include family-based interventions of communication, hope, coping, uncertainty, and symptom management.
▲ Refer combat veterans and service members directly involved in combat as well as those providing support to combatants, including nurses for mental health services.

Client/Family Teaching and Discharge Planning

- Teach the client about available community resources (e.g., therapists, ministers, counselors, self-help groups, family-education groups).
- Teach caregivers the COPE intervention (creativity, optimism, planning, expert information) to assist with symptom management.
- Teach expressive writing and education about emotions.

Ineffective community Coping

NANDA-I Definition

Pattern of community activities for adaptation and problem solving that is unsatisfactory for meeting the demands or needs of the community

Defining Characteristics

Community does not meet its own expectations; deficits in community participation; excessive community conflicts; expressed community powerlessness; expressed vulnerability; high illness rates; increased social problems (e.g., homicides, vandalism, arson, terrorism, robbery, infanticide, abuse, divorce, unemployment, poverty, militancy, mental illness); stressors perceived as excessive

Related Factors (r/t)

Deficits in community social support services; deficits in community social support resources; natural disasters; human-made disasters; inadequate resources for problem solving; ineffective community systems (e.g., lack of emergency medical system, transportation system, or disaster planning systems); nonexistent community systems

● = Independent ▲ = Collaborative

C

Community Outcomes

A Broad Range of Community Members Will (Specify Time Frame):

- Participate in community actions to improve power resources
- Develop improved communication among community members
- Participate in problem solving
- Demonstrate cohesiveness in problem solving
- Develop new strategies for problem solving
- Express power to deal with change and manage problems

Nursing Interventions

NOTE: The diagnosis of **Ineffective Coping** does not apply and should not be used when stress is being imposed by external sources or circumstance. If the community is a victim of circumstances, using the nursing diagnosis **Ineffective Coping** is equivalent to blaming the victim. See the care plan for **Readiness for enhanced community Coping.**

▲ Establish a collaborative partnership with the community (see the care plan for **Readiness for enhanced community Coping** for additional references).

- Assist the community with team building.
- Participate with community members in the identification of stressors and assessment of distress; for example, observe and participate in faith-based organizations that want to improve community stress management.

▲ Identify the health services and information resources that are currently available in the community.

▲ Consult with community mediation services, for example, the National Association of Community Mediation.

- Work with community members to increase awareness of ineffective coping behaviors (e.g., conflicts that prevent community members from working together, anger and hate that paralyze the community, health risk behaviors of adolescents).
- Provide support to the community and help community members to identify and mobilize additional supports.
- Advocate for the community in multiple arenas (e.g., television, newspapers, and governmental agencies).
- Write grant proposals to help community members obtain funds for programs that reduce stress or improve coping.

● = Independent   ▲ = Collaborative

- Work with members of the community to identify and develop coping strategies that promote a sense of power (e.g., obtaining sources for funding, collaborating with other communities).
- Protect children from exposure to community conflicts.

Multicultural

- Acknowledge the stressors unique to racial/ethnic communities.
- Identify community strengths with community members.
- Work with members of the community to prioritize and target health goals specific to the community.
- Establish and sustain partnerships with key individuals within communities when developing and implementing programs.
- Use mentoring strategies for community members.
- Use community church settings as a forum for advocacy, teaching, and program implementation.

Community Teaching

- Teach strategies for stress management.
- Explain the relationship between enhancing power resources and coping.

Compromised family Coping

NANDA-I Definition

A usually supportive primary person (family member, significant other, or close friend) provides insufficient, ineffective, or compromised support, comfort, assistance, or encouragement that may be needed by the client to manage or master adaptive tasks related to his or her health challenge

Defining Characteristics

Objective

Significant person attempts assistive behaviors with unsatisfactory results; significant person attempts supportive behaviors with unsatisfactory results; significant person displays protective behavior disproportionate to client's abilities; significant person displays protective behavior disproportionate to client's need for autonomy; significant

• = Independent   ▲ = Collaborative

person enters into limited personal communication with client; significant person withdraws from client

C Subjective

Client expresses a complaint about significant person's response to health problem; client expresses a concern about significant person's response to health problem; significant person expresses an inadequate knowledge base, which interferes with effective supportive behaviors; significant person reports an inadequate understanding, which interferes with effective supportive behaviors; significant person reports preoccupation with personal reaction (e.g., fear, anticipatory grief, guilt, anxiety) to client's need

Related Factors (r/t)

Coexisting situations affecting the significant person; developmental crises that the significant person may be facing; exhaustion of supportive capacity of significant people; inadequate information by a primary person; inadequate understanding of information by a primary person; incorrect information by a primary person; incorrect understanding of information by a primary person; lack of reciprocal support; little support provided by client, in turn, for primary person; prolonged disease that exhausts supportive capacity of significant people; situational crises that the significant person may be facing; temporary family disorganization; temporary family role changes; temporary preoccupation by a significant person

Client Outcomes

Family/Significant Person Will (Specify Time Frame):

• Verbalize internal resources to help deal with the situation
• Verbalize knowledge and understanding of illness, disability, or disease
• Provide support and assistance as needed
• Identify need for and seek outside support

Nursing Interventions

• Assess the strengths and deficiencies of the family system.
• Assess how family members interact with each other; observe verbal and nonverbal communication, individual and group responses to stress; and discern how individuals cope with stress when health concerns are present.

• = Independent ▲ = Collaborative

C

- Establish rapport with families by providing accurate communication.
- Consider the use of family theory as a framework to help guide interventions (e.g., family stress theory, role theory, social exchange theory, family systems theory).
- Help family members recognize the need for help and teach them how to ask for it.
- Encourage expression of positive thoughts and emotions.
- Encourage family members to verbalize feelings. Spend time with them, sit down and make eye contact, and offer coffee and other nourishment.
- Mothers may require additional support in their role of caring for chronically ill children.
- Provide privacy during family visits. If possible, maintain flexible visiting hours to accommodate more frequent family visits. If possible, arrange staff assignments so the same staff members have contact with the family. Familiarize other staff members with the situation in the absence of the usual staff member.
- Determine whether the family is suffering from additional stressors (e.g., child care issues, financial problems, parental mental health issues).
- Examine antecedent factors within the family system (e.g., existing mental health issues, substance abuse, past traumas) that may be exacerbating the current situation.
- ▲ Refer the family with ill family members to appropriate resources for assistance as indicated (e.g., counseling, psychotherapy, financial assistance, or spiritual support).

Pediatric

- Assess the adolescent's perception of support from family and friends during crisis and illness. Also thoroughly assess adolescent's needs and concerns.
- Provide educational and psychosocial interventions such as coping skills training in treatment for families and their adolescents who have type 1 diabetes.
- Focus on the communication dynamics of families coping with chronic illness. Identify communication barriers and ways in which to enhance the communication process among parents, siblings, and other family members involved.

• = Independent   ▲ = Collaborative

C

- Encourage the use of family rituals such as connection, spirituality, love, recreation, and celebration, especially in single-parent families.
- Staff should involve the family in decision-making processes, especially during hospital discharge planning.
- Transitioning into parenthood is a major life event for individuals. Providing effective strategies and education to first-time parents can help them feel more prepared, confident, and supported during this transition.
- Teenage mothers may experience a variety of psychosocial complications during and after their pregnancy, including conflicts due to poor relational boundaries with their own mothers. This type of conflict may exacerbate maternal stress and negatively impact mother-infant interactions.

Geriatric

- Perform a holistic assessment of all needs of informal spousal caregivers.
- Help caregivers believe in themselves and their ability to handle the situation, taking life one day at a time, looking for positive aspects in each situation, and relying on their own individual expertise and experience. Encourage caregivers to establish their priorities and concentrate on caring for their own physical and emotional well-being.
- ▲ Refer caregivers of clients with Alzheimer's disease to a monthly psychoeducational support group (i.e., the Alzheimer's Association). Incorporate nonpharmacological support programs for caregivers.
- ▲ Consider the use of telephone support for caregivers of family members with illnesses such as cancer and dementia.
- Assist in finding transportation to enable family members to visit.

Multicultural

- Acknowledge racial/ethnic differences at the onset of care.
- Assess for the influence of cultural beliefs, norms, and values on the family's/community's perceptions of coping.
- Use culturally competent assessment procedures when working with families with different racial/ethnic backgrounds.

• = Independent   ▲ = Collaborative

- Provide culturally relevant interventions by understanding and utilizing treatment strategies that are acceptable and effective for a particular culture.
- Provide opportunities for families to discuss spirituality.
- Determine how the family's cultural context impacts their decisions in regard to managing and coping with a child's illness. Recognize and validate the cultural context.

Home Care

- The interventions described previously may be adapted for home care use.
- Assess the reason behind the breakdown of family coping.
- During the time of compromised coping, increase visits to ensure the safety of the client, support of the family, and assistance with coping strategies. Provide reassurance regarding expectations for prognosis as appropriate.
- ▲ Assess the needs of the caregiver in the home. Intervene to meet needs as appropriate, and explore all available resources that may be used to provide adequate home care (e.g., parish nursing as an effective adjunct, home health aide services to relieve the caregiver's fatigue). Encourage caregivers to attend to their own physical, mental, and spiritual health and give more specific information about the client's needs and ways to meet them.
- ▲ Refer the family to medical social services for evaluation and supportive counseling.
- ▲ Serve as an advocate, mentor, and role model for caregiving. Write down or contract for the care needed by the client.
- ▲ When a terminal illness is the precipitating factor for ineffective coping, offer hospice services and support groups as possible resources.
- Encourage the client and family to discuss changes in daily functioning and routines created by the client's illness. Validate discomfort resulting from changes.
- Support positive individual and family coping efforts.
- ▲ If compromised family coping interferes with the ability to support the client's treatment plan, refer for psychiatric home health care services for family counseling and implementation of a therapeutic regimen.

● = Independent   ▲ = Collaborative

C

Client/Family Teaching and Discharge Planning

- • Provide truthful information and support for the family and significant people regarding the client's specific illness or condition. Address grief issues that arise in the process, including anticipatory grief.
- ▲ Refer women with breast cancer and their family caregivers to support groups and other services that provide assistance with daily coping.
- • Promote individual and family relaxation and stress-reduction strategies.
- ▲ Provide a parent support and education group to provide opportunities for parents to access support, learn new parenting skills, and, ultimately, optimize their relationships with their children in families of children in residential care.

Disabled family Coping

NANDA-I Definition

Behavior of primary person (family member or significant other, or close friend) that disables his or her capacities and the client's capacities to effectively address tasks essential to either person's adaptation to the health challenge

Defining Characteristics

Abandonment; aggression; agitation; carrying on usual routines without regard for client's needs; client's development of dependence; depression; desertion; disregarding client's needs; distortion of reality regarding client's health problem; family behaviors that are detrimental to well-being; hostility; impaired individualization; impaired restructuring of a meaningful life for self; intolerance; neglectful care of client in regard to basic human needs; neglectful care of client in regard to illness treatment; neglectful relationships with other family members; prolonged over-concern for client; psychosomaticism; rejection; taking on illness signs of client

Related Factors (r/t)

Arbitrary handling of family's resistance to treatment; dissonant coping styles for dealing with adaptive tasks by the significant person and

● = Independent   ▲ = Collaborative

client; dissonant coping styles among significant people; highly ambivalent family relationships; significant person with chronically unexpressed feelings (e.g., guilt, anxiety, hostility, despair)

Client Outcomes

Family/Significant Person Will (Specify Time Frame):
• Identify normal family routines that will need to be adapted
• Participate positively in the client's care within the limits of his or her abilities
• Identify responses that are harmful
• Acknowledge and accept the need for assistance with circumstances
• Identify appropriate activities for affected family member

Nursing Interventions

• Families dealing with life-changing illnesses should be involved with the management process from the outset of treatment. Education and counseling should be provided early and repeatedly as learning and coping needs are reassessed. Caregivers should be invited to attend therapy sessions at an early stage.
▲ Health providers should be prepared to give specific information to families regarding the trajectory of a terminal illness.
• Nurses caring for clients with terminal cancer should recognize the need to treat family caregivers as "pseudo patients."
• Provide psychosocial intervention for parents dealing with a child who is suffering from a serious illness. Allow time for parents to express feelings. Recognize and validate parent's feelings of anxiety, depression, and stress.
• Assess social support of family members caring for survivors of traumatic brain injuries. Facilitate realistic expectations about caregiving.
• Assist families to identify physical and mental health effects of caregiving.
• Assist family members to find professional assistance for primary stressors such as financial issues and insurance coverage, or communicating with professionals.
• Handle dysfunctional family dynamics in an open, transparent, and professional way. Remain neutral when dealing with

family conflicts and avoid involvement in long-term prior conflicts.
- Respect and promote the spiritual needs of the client and family.

Pediatric

- Siblings of sick children should be considered at risk for emotional disturbances until a full assessment of the family and social support circumstances proves otherwise.
- Recognize predictors of anger in adolescents: anxiety, depression, exposure to violence, and trait anger.

Geriatric

- Assess family members who are caring for clients in long-term care facilities for compassion fatigue: symptoms include the inability to disengage from the suffering of the loved one, a growing feeling of hopelessness or despair, sadness or grief, and inattention to personal care or outside responsibilities. Encourage family members to attend to their own physical, emotional, and social needs. Develop relationships of trust with family caregivers, providing them with a sense of confidence in the level of care their loved ones will be receiving in their absence. Promote therapeutic relationships with family members who are assisting with care, allowing for sharing of concerns and emotions.

Multicultural

- Health care professionals working with African American adolescents who are coping with parental cancer should be sensitive to the potential for post-traumatic growth.

Home Care

- The interventions described previously may be adapted for home care use.
- Assess for strain in family caregivers.
- ▲ Provide psychosocial support to family members dealing with depressed or suicidal clients in the home setting.

• = Independent   ▲ = Collaborative

Client/Family Teaching and Discharge Planning

- Involve the client and family in the planning of care as often as possible; mutual goal setting is considered part of "client safety."
- Recognize that family decision-makers may need additional psychological support services.
- Educate family members regarding stress management techniques including massage and alternative therapies.

Readiness for enhanced family Coping

NANDA-I Definition

Effective management of adaptive tasks by family member involved with client's health challenge, who now exhibits desire and readiness for enhanced health and growth in regard to self and in relation to the client

Defining Characteristics

Chooses experiences that optimize wellness; family member attempts to describe growth impact of crisis; family member moves in directions of enriching lifestyle; family member moves in direction of health promotion; individual expresses interest in making contact with others who have experienced a similar situation

Client Outcomes

Client Will (Specify Time Frame):

- State a plan indicating strengths and areas for growth
- Perform tasks needed for change
- Evaluate changes and continually reevaluate plan for continued growth

Nursing Interventions

- Assess the structure, resources, and coping abilities of families.
- Acknowledge, assess, and support the spiritual needs and resources of families and clients.
- Establish rapport with families and empower their decision-making through effective and accurate communication.

● = Independent   ▲ = Collaborative

▲ Provide family members with educational and skill-building interventions to alleviate caregiving stress and to facilitate adherence to prescribed plans of care.

• Develop, provide, and encourage family members to use counseling services and interventions.

• Identify and refer to support programs that discuss experiences and challenges similar to those faced by the family (e.g., Alzheimer's Association).

▲ Incorporate the use of emerging technologies to increase the reach of interventions to support family coping.

• Refer to **Compromised family Coping** for additional interventions.

Pediatric

▲ Implement family-centered services for children and their caregivers.

• Identify the management styles of families and facilitate the use of more effective ways of coping with childhood illness.

• Provide educational and supportive interventions for families caring for children with illness and disability.

Geriatric

• Encourage family caregivers to participate in counseling and support groups.

▲ Provide educational interventions to family caregivers that focus on knowledge- and skill-building.

▲ Older adults should be provided with opportunities to engage their families and their communities.

Multicultural

• Acknowledge the importance of cultural influences in families and ensure that assessments and assessment tools account for such cultural differences.

▲ Understand and incorporate cultural differences into interventions to enhance the impact of nursing interventions.

• = Independent   ▲ = Collaborative

Decisional Conflict

NANDA-I Definition

Uncertainty about course of action to be taken when choice among competing actions involves risk, loss, or challenge to values and beliefs

Defining Characteristics

Delayed decision-making; physical signs of distress or tension (e.g., increased heart rate, increased muscle tension, restlessness); questioning moral principles while attempting a decision; questioning moral rules while attempting a decision; questioning moral values while attempting a decision; questioning personal beliefs while attempting a decision; questioning personal values while attempting a decision; self-focusing; vacillation among alternative choices; verbalizes feeling of distress while attempting a decision; verbalizes uncertainty about choices; verbalizes undesired consequences of alternative actions being considered

Related Factors (r/t)

Divergent sources of information; interference with decision-making; lack of experience with decision-making; lack of relevant information; moral obligations require performing action; moral obligations require not performing action; moral principles support courses of action; moral rules support mutually inconsistent courses of action; moral values support mutually inconsistent courses of action; multiple sources of information; perceived threat to value system; support system deficit; unclear personal beliefs; unclear personal values

Client Outcomes

Client Will (Specify Time Frame):
* State the advantages and disadvantages of choices
* Share fears and concerns regarding choices and responses of others
* Seek resources and information necessary for making an informed choice
* Make an informed choice

• = Independent ▲ = Collaborative

D

Nursing Interventions

- Observe for factors causing or contributing to conflict (e.g., value conflicts, fear of outcome, poor problem-solving skills).
- Provide emotional support.
- Give the client time and permission to express feelings associated with decision-making.
- ▲ Use decision aids or computer-based decision aid to assist clients in making decisions.
- ▲ Initiate health teaching and referrals when needed.
- Facilitate communication between the client and family members regarding the final decision; offer support to the person actually making the decision.
- Provide detailed information on benefits and risks using functional terms and probabilities tailored to clinical risk, plus steps for considering the issues and means for making a decision, including values clarification and decision aids, when clients are faced with difficult treatment choices.

Geriatric

- Carefully assess clients with dementia regarding ability to make decisions.
- ▲ Support previous wishes for clients with dementia.
- If end-of-life discussions are being avoided, nurses can facilitate discussions of health care choices among older adults and their family members.
- Discuss the purpose of a living will, medical power of attorney, and advance directives.
- Discuss choices or changes to be made (e.g., moving in with children, into a nursing home, or into an adult foster care home).

Multicultural

- Assess for the influence of cultural beliefs, norms, and values on the client's decision-making conflict.
- Provide support for client's decision-making.
- Identify who will be involved in the decision-making process.
- Use cross-cultural decision aids whenever possible to enhance an informed decision-making process.

● = Independent   ▲ = Collaborative

D

Home Care

- The interventions described previously may be adapted for home care use.
- ▲ Before providing any home care, assess the client plan for advance directives (living will and power of attorney). If a plan exists, place a copy in the client file. If no plan exists, offer information on advance directives according to agency policy. Refer for assistance in completing advance directives as necessary. Do not witness a living will.
- Assess the client and family for consensus (or lack thereof) regarding the issue in conflict.
- Refer to the care plan for **Anxiety** as indicated.

Client/Family Teaching and Discharge Planning

- ▲ Refer to family therapy as needed.
- Instruct the client and family members to provide advance directives in the following areas:
  - Person to contact in an emergency
  - Preference (if any) to die at home or in the hospital
  - Desire to sign a living will
  - Desire to donate an organ
  - Funeral arrangements (i.e., burial, cremation)
- Inform the family of treatment options; encourage and defend self-determination.
- Identify reasons for family decisions regarding care. Explore ways in which family decisions can be respected.
- Recognize and allow the client to discuss the selection of complementary therapies available, such as spiritual support, relaxation, imagery, exercise, lifestyle changes, diet (e.g., macrobiotic, vegetarian), and nutritional supplementation.
- ▲ Provide the Physician Orders for Life-Sustaining Treatment (POLST) form for clients and families faced with end-of-life choices across the health care continuum.

Readiness for enhanced Decision-Making

NANDA-I Definition

D A pattern of choosing courses of action that is sufficient for meeting short- and long-term health-related goals and can be strengthened

Defining Characteristics

Expresses desire to enhance decision-making; expresses desire to enhance congruency of decisions with goals; expresses desire to enhance congruency of decisions with personal values; expresses desire to enhance congruency of decisions with sociocultural goals; expresses desire to enhance congruency of decisions with sociocultural values; expresses desire to enhance risk benefit analysis of decisions; expresses desire to enhance understanding of choices for decision-making; expresses desire to enhance understanding of the meaning of choices; expresses desire to enhance use of reliable evidence for decisions

Client Outcomes

Client Will (Specify Time Frame):
- Review treatment options with providers
- Ask questions about the benefits and risks of treatment options
- Communicate decisions about treatment options to providers in relation to personal preferences, values and goals

Nursing Interventions

- Support and encourage clients and their representatives to engage in health care decisions.
- Respect personal preferences, values, needs, and rights.
- Determine the degree of participation desired by the client.
- Provide information that is appropriate, relevant, and timely.
- Determine the health literacy of clients and their representatives prior to helping with decision-making.
- Tailor information to the specific needs of individual clients, according to principles of health literacy.
- Motivate clients to be as independent as possible in decision-making.
- Identify the client's level of choice in decision-making.

• = Independent ▲ = Collaborative

- Focus on the positive aspects of decision-making, rather than decisional conflicts.
- Design educational interventions for decision support.
- Provide clients with the benefits of decisions at the same time as helping them to identify strategies to reduce the barriers for healthful decisions.
- Acknowledge the complexity of everyday self-care decisions related to self-management of chronic illnesses.

Geriatric

- The above interventions may be adapted for geriatric use. Facilitate collaborative decision-making.

Multicultural

- Use existing decision aids for particular types of decisions, or develop decision aids as indicated.

Home Care

- The above interventions may be adapted for home care use.
- Develop clinical practice guidelines that include shared decision-making.

Client/Family Teaching and Discharge Planning

- Before teaching clients ages 9 to 20, identify client preferences in involvement with decision-making.

Ineffective Denial

NANDA-I Definition

D

Conscious or unconscious attempt to disavow the knowledge or meaning of an event to reduce anxiety/fear, but leading to the detriment of health

Defining Characteristics

Delays seeking health care attention to the detriment of health; displaces fear of impact of the condition; displaces source of symptoms to other organs; displays inappropriate affect; does not admit fear of death; does not admit fear of invalidism; does not perceive personal relevance of danger; does not perceive personal relevance of symptoms; makes dismissive comments when speaking of distressing events; makes dismissive gestures when speaking of distressing events; minimizes symptoms; refuses health care attention to the detriment of health; unable to admit impact of disease on life pattern; uses self-treatment

Related Factors (r/t)

Anxiety; fear of death; fear of loss of autonomy; fear of separation; lack of competency in using effective coping mechanisms; lack of control of life situation; lack of emotional support from others; overwhelming stress; threat of inadequacy in dealing with strong emotions; threat of unpleasant reality

Client Outcomes

Client Will (Specify Time Frame):
- Seek out appropriate health care attention when needed
- Use home remedies only when appropriate
- Display appropriate affect and verbalize fears
- Actively engage in treatment program related to identified "substance" of abuse
- Remain substance-free
- Demonstrate alternate adaptive coping mechanism

Nursing Interventions

- Assess the client's and family's understanding of the illness, the treatments, and expected outcomes.
- Allow client time for adjustment to his/her situation.

• = Independent   ▲ = Collaborative

- Spend time with the client: listen and allow time for response.
- Aid the client in making choices regarding treatment and actively involve him/her in the decision-making process.
- Explain the necessity of adherence to the prescribed treatment plan to promote feelings of wellness.
- Allow the client to express and use denial as a coping mechanism if appropriate to treatment.
- Avoid confrontation and consider the client as an equal partner in health care.
- Support the client's spiritual coping measures.
- Develop a trusting, therapeutic relationship with the client/family.
▲ Assist the client in utilizing existing and additional sources of support.
- Refer to care plans **Defensive Coping** and **Dysfunctional Family Processes.**

Geriatric

- Allow the client to explain his/her concepts of health care needs, then use reality-focused techniques whenever possible to provide feedback.
- Encourage communication among family members.
- Recognize denial and be aware that grieving may prolong denial.

Multicultural

- Assess for the influence of cultural beliefs, norms, and values involved in the client's understanding of and ability to acknowledge health status.
- Discuss with the client those aspects of his or her health behavior/lifestyle that will remain unchanged by health status and those aspects of health behavior that will need to be modified to improve health status.
- Assess the role of fatalism in the client's ability to acknowledge health status.

• = Independent   ▲ = Collaborative

D

Home Care

- Previously mentioned interventions may be adapted for home care utilization.
- ▲ Observe family interaction and roles. Refer the client/family for follow-up if prolonged denial is a risk.
- Encourage communication between family members, particularly when dealing with the loss of a significant person.

Client/Family Teaching and Discharge Planning

- Instruct client and family to recognize the signs and symptoms of recurring illness and the appropriate responses to alteration in client's health status.
- Consider the client's belief in and use of complementary therapies in self-managing his/her disease.
- Teach family members that denial may continue throughout the adjustment to treatment and they should not be confrontational.
- ▲ Inform family of available community support resources.

Impaired Dentition

NANDA-I Definition

Disruption in tooth development/eruption patterns or structural integrity of individual teeth

Defining Characteristics

Abraded teeth, absence of teeth; asymmetrical facial expression; crown caries; erosion of enamel; excessive calculus; excessive plaque; halitosis, incomplete eruption for age (may be primary or permanent teeth); loose teeth; malocclusion; missing teeth; premature loss of primary teeth; root caries; tooth enamel discoloration; tooth fracture(s); tooth misalignment, toothache, worndown teeth

Related Factors (r/t)

Barriers to self-care; bruxism; chronic use of coffee; chronic use of tea; chronic use of red wine; chronic use of tobacco; chronic vomiting; deficient knowledge regarding dental health; dietary habits; economic barriers to professional care; excessive use of abrasive cleaning agents; excessive intake of fluorides; genetic predisposition; ineffective oral hygiene; lack of access to professional care; nutritional deficits; selected prescription medications; sensitivity to cold; sensitivity to heat

Client Outcomes

Client Will (Specify Time Frame):

• Have clean teeth, healthy pink gums
• Be free of halitosis
• Explain how to perform oral care
• Demonstrate ability to masticate foods without difficulty
• State free of pain in mouth

Nursing Interventions

▲ Inspect oral cavity/teeth at least once daily and note any discoloration, presence of debris, amount of plaque buildup, presence of lesions such as white lesions or patches, edema, or bleeding, and intactness of teeth. Refer to a dentist or periodontist as appropriate.

• If the client is free of bleeding disorders and is able to swallow, encourage the client to brush teeth with a soft toothbrush using fluoride-containing toothpaste at least two times per day. Do not use foam swabs or lemon glycerin swabs to clean the teeth.

• Encourage the client to floss the teeth at least once per day if free of a bleeding disorder, or if the client is unable, floss the teeth for the client.

• Determine the client's mental status and manual dexterity; if the client is unable to care for self, nursing personnel must provide dental hygiene. The nursing diagnosis **Bathing/hygiene Self-care deficit** is then applicable.

• If the client is unable to brush own teeth, follow this procedure:
1. Position the client sitting upright or on side.
2. Use a soft-bristle baby toothbrush.
3. Use fluoride toothpaste and tap water or saline as a solution.
4. Brush teeth in an up-and-down manner.
5. Suction as needed.

• = Independent   ▲ = Collaborative

D

- Monitor the client's nutritional and fluid status to determine if adequate. Recommend the client eat a balanced diet and limit between-meal snacks.
- Recommend the client stop or at least decrease intake of soft drinks.
- Instruct the client with halitosis to clean the tongue when performing oral hygiene. Brush tongue with a tongue scraper or toothbrush and follow with a mouth rinse.
- Determine the client's usual method of oral care. Whenever possible, build on the client's existing knowledge base and current practices to develop an individualized plan of care.
- Tell the client to direct the toothbrush at a 45-degree angle toward the tooth surfaces, not horizontally.
- Use an antimicrobial mouthwash as ordered or tap water or saline only for a mouth rinse. Avoid the use of hydrogen peroxide, or alcohol-based mouthwashes.
- ▲ Recommend client see a dentist at prescribed intervals, generally two times per year if teeth are in satisfactory condition.
- ▲ If there are any signs of bleeding when the teeth are brushed, refer the client to a dentist or, if obvious signs of inflamed gums, a periodontist. Bleeding along with halitosis is associated with gingivitis. If platelet numbers are decreased, or if the client is edentulous, use moistened Toothettes or a specially made very soft toothbrush for oral care.
- Recognize that good dental care/oral care can be effective in preventing hospital acquired (or extended care acquired) pneumonia.
- Provide scrupulous dental care to critically ill clients, including ventilated clients to prevent ventilator-associated pneumonia.
- If teeth are nonfunctional for chewing, modification of oral intake (e.g., edentulous diet, soft diet) may be necessary. The nursing diagnosis **Imbalanced Nutrition: less than body requirements** may apply.
- If the client is unable to swallow, keep suction nearby when providing oral care.
- See care plan for **Impaired Oral Mucous Membrane.**

● = Independent   ▲ = Collaborative

Pregnant Client

- Encourage the expectant mother to eat a healthy, balanced diet that is rich in calcium.
- Advise the pregnant mother not to smoke.
- Advise the expectant mother to practice good care of her teeth, to protect her child's teeth once born.

Infant Oral Hygiene

- Gently wipe baby's gums with a washcloth or sterile gauze at least once a day.
- Never allow the child to fall asleep with a bottle containing milk, formula, fruit juice, or sweetened liquids. If the child needs a comforter between regular feedings, at night, or during naps, fill a bottle with cool water or give the child a clean pacifier recommended by the dentist or physician. Never give child a pacifier dipped in any sweet liquid. Avoid filling child's bottle with liquids such as sugar water and soft drinks.
- ▲ When multiple teeth appear, brush with small toothbrush with small (pea-size) amount of fluoride toothpaste. Recommend that child either use a fluoride gel or fluoride varnish.
- Advise parents to begin dental visits at 1 year of age.

Older Children

- ▲ Encourage the family to talk with the dentist about dental sealants, which can help prevent cavities in permanent teeth.
- Recommend the child use dental floss to help prevent gum disease. The dentist will give guidelines on when to start using floss.
- Recommend to parents that they not permit the child to smoke or chew tobacco, and stress the importance of setting a good example by not using tobacco products themselves.
- Recommend the child drink fluoridated water when possible.
- Recommend the child use toothpaste containing fluoride.

Geriatric

- Provide dentists with accurate medication history to avoid drug interactions and client harm. If the client is taking anticoagulants, the INR should be reviewed before providing dental care.

• = Independent   ▲ = Collaborative

D

- Help clients brush own teeth, or provide dental care after breakfast and before bed every day.
- If the client has dementia or delirium, and exhibits care-resistant behavior such as fighting, biting, or refusing care, utilize the following method:
  1. Ensure client is in a quiet environment such as own bathroom, sitting or standing at the sink to prime memory for appropriate actions
  2. Approach the client at eye level within his/her range of vision
  3. Approach with a smile, and begin conversation with a touch of the hand and gradually move up
  4. Use mirror-mirror technique, standing behind the client, and brush and floss teeth
  5. Use respectful adult speech, not elderspeak—sing-song voice, calling "deary," "honey," etc.
  6. Promote self-care when client brushes own teeth if possible
  7. Utilize distractors when needed, singing, talking, reminiscing, or use of a teddy bear
- ▲ Ensure that dentures are removed and cleaned regularly, preferably after every meal and before bedtime. Soak dentures at night in cold water.
- ▲ Support other caregivers providing oral hygiene.

Multicultural

- Assess for the influence of cultural beliefs, norms, and values on the client's understanding of dental care.
- Assess for barriers to access to dental care, such as lack of insurance.

Home Care

- Assess client patterns for daily and professional dental care and related patterns (e.g., smoking, nail biting). Assess for environmental influences on dental status (e.g., fluoride).
- Assess client facilities and financial resources for providing dental care.
- Request dietary log from the client, adding column for type of food (i.e., soft, pureed, regular).

• = Independent   ▲ = Collaborative

• Observe a typical meal to assess first-hand the impact of impaired dentition on nutrition.
• Assist the client with accessing financial or other resources to support optimum dental and nutritional status.

D

Client/Family Teaching and Discharge Planning

• Teach how to inspect the oral cavity and monitor for problems with the teeth and gums.
• Teach how to implement a personal plan of dental hygiene, including appropriate brushing of teeth and tongue and use of dental floss. Utilize motivational interviewing to facilitate increased compliance in dental care.
• Advise clients to change their toothbrush every 3 to 4 months, because after that toothbrushes are less effective in removing plaque and are a source of bacterial contamination of the mouth and teeth.
• Teach the client the value of having an optimal fluoride concentration in drinking water, and to brush teeth twice daily with toothpaste containing fluoride.
• Teach clients of all ages the need to decrease intake of sugary foods and to brush teeth regularly.
• Inform individuals who are considering tongue piercing of the potential complications such as chipping and cracking of teeth and possible trauma to the gingiva. If piercing is done, teach the client how to care for the wound and prevent complications.

Risk for delayed Development

NANDA-I Definition

At risk for delay of 25% or more in one or more of the areas of social or self-regulatory behavior, or in cognitive, language, gross, or fine motor skills

Risk Factors

Prenatal

Economically disadvantaged; endocrine disorders; genetic disorders; illiteracy; inadequate nutrition; inadequate prenatal care; infections;

• = Independent   ▲ = Collaborative

lack of prenatal care; late prenatal care; maternal age <15 years; maternal age >35 years; substance abuse; unplanned pregnancy; unwanted pregnancy

D Individual

Adopted child; behavior disorders; brain damage (e.g., hemorrhage in postnatal period, shaken baby, abuse, accident); chronic illness; congenital disorders; failure to thrive; foster child; frequent otitis media; genetic disorders; hearing impairment; inadequate nutrition; lead poisoning; natural disasters; positive drug screen(s); prematurity; seizures; substance abuse; technology-dependent; treatment-related side effects (e.g., chemotherapy, radiation therapy, radiation therapy, pharmaceutical agents); vision impairment

Environmental

Economically disadvantaged; violence

Caregiver

Abuse; learning disabilities; mental illness; severe learning disability

Client Outcomes

Client/Parents/Primary Caregiver Will (Specify Time Frame):

- Infant/Child/Adolescent will achieve expected milestones in all areas of development (physical, cognitive, and psychosocial)
- Parent/Caregiver will verbalize understanding of potential impediments to normal development and demonstrate actions or environmental/lifestyle changes necessary to provide appropriate care in a safe, nurturing environment

Nursing Interventions

Preconception/Pregnancy

- Assess for alcohol/drug use during pregnancy. Expectant mothers should be instructed that no amount of alcohol consumption is safe during pregnancy.
- Advise expectant mothers to stop smoking and assist with methods of smoking cessation.

• = Independent   ▲ = Collaborative

- Recommend that women of childbearing age take 400 mcg of folic acid daily in order to reduce the risk of neural tube defects.

Neonate/Infant

- Encourage mother/baby interactions when caring for premature infants.
- ▲ Support early advanced developmental screening tests for male infants who are born prematurely or are medically fragile at birth.
- ▲ Be aware that socioeconomic factors are predictive of delayed infant development (physical and cognitive) and encourage continued screening along with follow-up care for these infants. Arrange appropriate social services referrals.
- ▲ Make arrangements for close follow-up monitoring of opioid-exposed infants.

Toddler/Preschooler/School-age

- Provide support and education to parents of toddlers with developmental disabilities (i.e., Down syndrome, cerebral palsy).
- Encourage parents of toddlers to obtain age-appropriate developmental screenings to detect early problems.
- ▲ Discuss advantages of early speech-language intervention with parents of toddlers having delayed development in communication.
- Educate parents on the importance of providing oral care for children with mild/moderate disabilities. Parents may need to assume the responsibility of brushing for the child.
- ▲ Encourage mothers with postpartum depression to seek assistance and support as appropriate to ensure normal development of their children.
- Teach new mothers the importance of breastfeeding.

Multicultural

- Recognize cultural risks associated with higher infant mortality.

• = Independent   ▲ = Collaborative

D

Diarrhea

NANDA-I Definition

Passage of loose, unformed stools

Defining Characteristics

Abdominal pain; at least three loose liquid stools per day; cramping; hyperactive bowel sounds; urgency

Related Factors (r/t)

Psychological

Anxiety; high stress levels

Situational

Adverse effects of pharmaceuticals; alcohol abuse; contaminants; travel; laxative abuse; radiation; toxins; tube feedings

Physiological

Infectious processes; inflammation; irritation; malabsorption; parasites

Client Outcomes

Client Will (Specify Time Frame):

• Defecate formed, soft stool every 1 to 3 days
• Maintain the perirectal area free of irritation
• State relief from cramping and less or no diarrhea
• Explain cause of diarrhea and rationale for treatment
• Maintain good skin turgor and weight at usual level
• Have negative stool cultures

Nursing Interventions

• Assess pattern of defecation, or have the client keep a diary that includes the following: time of day defecation occurs; usual stimulus for defecation; consistency, amount, and frequency of stool; type of, amount of, and time food consumed; fluid intake; history of bowel habits and laxative use; diet; exercise patterns; obstetrical/gynecological, medical, and surgical histories; medications; alterations in perianal sensations; and present bowel regimen.

• = Independent ▲ = Collaborative

- Recommend use of standardized tool both to consistently assess and then treat diarrhea.
- Inspect, auscultate, palpate, and percuss the abdomen in that order.
- ▲ Use an evidence-based bowel management protocol which includes obtaining a stool specimen, immediate cessation of any ordered laxative, use of soluble fiber supplement, and if continued diarrhea, use of loperamide. Consistently monitor and report bowel activity during this time.
- ▲ Identify cause of diarrhea if possible based on history (e.g., rotavirus or norovirus exposure; HIV infection; food poisoning; medication effect; radiation therapy; protein malnutrition; laxative abuse; stress). See Related Factors (r/t).
- ▲ Recognize that a workup for diarrhea will consist of laboratory work such as a complete blood count with differential and blood cultures if the client is febrile. Also obtain stool specimens as ordered, to either rule out or diagnose an infectious process (e.g., ova and parasites, *C. difficile* infection, bacterial cultures for food poisoning).
- ▲ If the client has watery diarrhea, a low-grade fever, abdominal cramps, and a history of antibiotic therapy, especially clindamycin, cephalosporins, and fluoroquinoline antibiotics, consider possibility of *C. difficile* infection.
- Review other factors such as increased age, extended use of enteral feedings, and gastrointestinal procedures and surgeries that increase the risk of diarrhea.
- Use standard precautions when caring for clients with diarrhea to prevent spread of infectious diarrhea; use gloves and handwashing.
- ▲ If the client has diarrhea associated with antibiotic therapy, consult with the primary care practitioner regarding the use of probiotics, such as yogurt with active cultures, to treat diarrhea, or probiotic dietary supplements; or preferably use probiotics to prevent diarrhea when first beginning antibiotic therapy.
- ▲ If a probiotic is ordered, administer it with food. Recommend that it be taken through the antibiotic course and 10 to 14 days after it has finished.

• = Independent   ▲ = Collaborative

D

▲ Recognize that *C. difficile* can commonly recur after treatment, and that reculturing of stool should be done before initiating retreatment.

• Ask the client to examine intake of high fructose corn syrup and fructose sweeteners in relation to onset of diarrhea symptoms. If diarrhea is associated with fructose ingestion, intake should be limited or eliminated.

▲ If the client has infectious diarrhea, consider avoiding use of medications that slow peristalsis.

• Assess for dehydration by observing skin turgor over sternum and inspecting for longitudinal furrows of the tongue. Watch for excessive thirst, fever, dizziness, lightheadedness, palpitations, excessive cramping, bloody stools, hypotension, and symptoms of shock.

▲ Refer to the care plans **Deficient Fluid Volume** and **Risk for Electrolyte Imbalance** if appropriate.

▲ If the client has chronic diarrhea causing fecal incontinence at intervals, consider suggesting use of dietary fiber from psyllium or gum arabic after consultation with primary practitioner.

▲ If diarrhea is chronic and there is evidence of malnutrition, consult with primary care practitioner for a dietary consult and possible use of a hydrolyzed formula (a clear liquid supplement containing increased protein and calories) such as Ensure Alive, Resource Breeze Fruit Beverage, or Citrotein to maintain nutrition while the gastrointestinal system heals.

• Encourage the client to eat small, frequent meals, eating foods that are easy to digest at first (e.g., bananas, crackers, pretzels, rice, potatoes, clear soups, applesauce), but switch to a regular diet as soon as tolerated. Also recommend avoiding milk products, foods high in fiber, and caffeine (dark sodas, tea, coffee, chocolate).

• Provide a readily available bathroom, commode, or bedpan.

• Thoroughly cleanse and dry the perianal and perineal skin daily and as needed (PRN) using a cleanser capable of stool removal. Refer to perirectal skin care in the care plan **Bowel Incontinence.**

• = Independent   ▲ = Collaborative

D

▲ If the client has enteral tube feedings and diarrhea, consider infusion rate, position of feeding tube, tonicity of formula, possible formula contamination, and excessive intake of hyper-osmolar medications, such as sorbitol commonly found in the liquid version of medications. Consider changing the formula to a lower osmolarity, lactose-free, or high-fiber feeding.

• Do not administer bolus enteral feedings into the small bowel.

▲ Dilute liquid medications before administration through the enteral tube and flush the enteral feeding tube with sufficient water before and after medication administration.

• Teach clients with cancer the types of diarrhea they may encounter, emphasizing not only chemotherapy and radiation induced diarrhea, but also *C. difficile,* along with associated signs and symptoms, and treatments.

▲ For chemotherapy induced diarrhea (CID) and radiation induced diarrhea (RID), review rationale for pharmacological interventions selected such as loperamide and octreotide, along with soluble fiber and probiotic supplements. Consult a registered dietitian to assist with recommendations to alleviate diarrhea, decrease dehydration, and maintain nutritional status.

Pediatric

▲ Assess for mild or moderate signs of dehydration with both acute and persistent diarrhea: Mild (increased thirst and dry mouth or tongue); Moderate (decreased urination, no wet diapers for 3+ hours, feeling weak or lightheaded, irritability or listlessness, few or no tears when crying). Refer to primary care practitioner for treatment.

▲ Recommend that the parents give the child oral rehydration fluids to drink in the amounts specified by the physician, especially during the first 4 to 6 hours to replace lost fluid. Once the child is rehydrated, an orally administered maintenance solution should be used along with food. Continue even if child vomits.

• Recommend the mother resume breastfeeding as soon as possible.

• = Independent   ▲ = Collaborative

- Recommend parents not give the child flat soda, fruit juices, gelatin dessert, or instant fruit drink.
- Recommend parents give children foods with complex carbohydrates, such as potatoes, rice, bread, cereal, yogurt, fruits, and vegetables. Avoid fatty foods, foods high in simple sugars, and milk products.
- ▲ Recommend rotavirus vaccine within the child's vaccination schedule.

Geriatric

- ▲ Evaluate medications the client is taking. Recognize that many medications can result in diarrhea, including digitalis, propranolol, angiotensin-converting enzyme (ACE) inhibitors, histamine-receptor antagonists, nonsteroidal antiinflammatory drugs (NSAIDs), anticholinergic agents, oral hypoglycemia agents, antibiotics, and others.
- ▲ Monitor the client closely to detect whether an impaction is causing diarrhea; remove impaction as ordered.
- ▲ Seek medical attention if diarrhea is severe or persists for more than 24 hours, or if the client has history of dehydration or electrolyte disturbances, such as lassitude, weakness, or prostration.
- Provide emotional support for clients who are having trouble controlling unpredictable episodes of diarrhea.

Home Care

- Previously mentioned interventions may be adapted for home care use.
- Assess the home for general sanitation and methods of food preparation. Reinforce principles of sanitation for food handling.
- Assess for methods of handling soiled laundry if the client is bed bound or has been incontinent. Instruct or reinforce Universal Precautions with family and blood-borne pathogen precautions with agency caregivers.
- When assessing medication history, include over-the-counter (OTC) drugs, both general and those currently being used to treat the diarrhea. Instruct clients not to mix OTC medications when self-treating.

● = Independent   ▲ = Collaborative

- Evaluate current medications for indication that specific interventions are warranted.
▲ Evaluate the need for a home health aide or homemaker service referral.
- Evaluate the need for durable medical equipment in the home.

Client/Family Teaching and Discharge Planning

- Encourage avoidance of coffee, spices, milk products, and foods that irritate or stimulate the gastrointestinal tract.
- Teach appropriate method of taking ordered antidiarrheal medications; explain side effects.
- Explain how to prevent the spread of infectious diarrhea (e.g., careful handwashing, appropriate handling and storage of food, and thoroughly cleaning the bathroom and kitchen).
- Help the client to determine stressors and set up an appropriate stress reduction plan, if stress is the cause of diarrhea.
- Teach signs and symptoms of dehydration and electrolyte imbalance.
- Teach perirectal skin care.
▲ Consider teaching clients about complementary therapies such as probiotics, after consultation with primary care practitioner.

Risk for Disuse Syndrome

NANDA-I Definition

At risk for a deterioration of body systems as the result of prescribed or unavoidable musculoskeletal inactivity

Risk Factors

Altered level of consciousness; mechanical immobilization; paralysis; prescribed immobilization; severe pain

NOTE: Complications from immobility can include pressure ulcer, constipation, stasis of pulmonary secretions, thrombosis, urinary tract infection and/or retention, decreased strength or endurance, orthostatic hypotension, decreased range of joint motion, disorientation, disturbed body image, and powerlessness.

● = Independent   ▲ = Collaborative

Client Outcomes

Client Will (Specify Time Frame):

- Maintain full range of motion in joints
- Maintain intact skin, good peripheral blood flow, and normal pulmonary function
- Maintain normal bowel and bladder function
- Express feelings about imposed immobility
- Explain methods to prevent complications of immobility

Nursing Interventions

- When client's condition is stable, screen for mobility skills in the following order: (1) bed mobility; (2) supported and unsupported sitting; (3) transition movements such as sit to stand, sitting down, and transfers; and (4) standing and walking activities. Use a tool such as the Assessment Criteria and Care Plan for Safe Patient Handling and Movement.
- Assess the level of assistance needed by the client and express in terms of amount of effort expended by the person assisting the client. The range is as follows: total assist, meaning client performs 0% to 25% of task and, if client requires the help of more than one caregiver, it is referred to as a dependent transfer; maximum assist, meaning client gives 25% of effort while caregiver performs majority of the work; moderate assist, meaning client gives 50% of effort; minimal assist, meaning client gives 75% of effort; contact guard assist, meaning no physical assist is given but caregiver is physically touching client for steadying, guiding, or in case of loss of balance; stand by assist, meaning caregiver's hands are up and ready in case needed; supervision, meaning supervision of task is needed even if at a distance; modified independent, meaning client needs assistive device or extra time to accomplish task; and independent, meaning client is able to complete task safely without instruction or assistance.
- ▲ Request a referral to a physical therapist as needed so that client's range of motion, muscle strength, balance, coordination, and endurance can be part of the initial evaluation.
- Incorporate bed exercises such as flexing and extending feet and quadriceps or use of Thera-Bands for upper extremities into nursing care to help maintain muscle strength and tone.

• = Independent   ▲ = Collaborative

D

▲ If not contraindicated by the client's condition, obtain a referral to physical therapy for use of tilt table to help determine
the cause of syncope.
• Perform range of motion exercises for all possible joints at
least twice daily; perform passive or active range of motion
exercises as appropriate.
• Use specialized boots to prevent pressure ulcers on the heels
and footdrop; remove boots twice daily to provide foot care.
• When positioning a client on the side, tilt client 30 degrees or
less while lying on side.
• Assess skin condition at least daily and more frequently if
needed. Utilize a risk assessment tool such the Braden Scale
or the Norton Scale to predict the risk of developing pressure
ulcers.
• Discuss with staff and management a "safe handling" policy
that may include a "no lift" policy.
• Turn clients at high risk for pressure/shear/friction frequently.
Turn clients **at least** every 2 to 4 hours on a pressure-reducing
mattress/every 2 hours on standard foam mattress.
• Provide the client with a pressure-relieving horizontal support
surface. For further interventions on skin care, refer to the care
plan for **Impaired Skin Integrity.**
• Help the client out of bed as soon as able.
• When getting the client up after bed rest, do so slowly and
watch for signs of postural (orthostatic) hypotension, tachycardia, nausea, diaphoresis, or syncope. Take the blood pressure lying, sitting, and standing, waiting 2 minutes between
each reading.
• Obtain assistive devices such as braces, crutches, or canes
to help the client reach and maintain as much mobility as
possible.
▲ Apply graduated compression stockings as ordered. Ensure
proper fit by measuring accurately. Remove the stockings at
least twice a day, in the morning with the bath and in the
evening to assess the condition of the extremity, then reapply.
Knee length is preferred rather than thigh length.
• Observe for signs of VTE, including pain, tenderness, and
swelling in the calf and thigh. Also observe for new onset of
breathlessness.

• = Independent   ▲ = Collaborative

D

- Have the client cough and deep breathe or use incentive spirometry every 2 hours while awake.
- Monitor respiratory functions, noting breath sounds and respiratory rate. Percuss for new onset of dullness in lungs.
- Note bowel function daily. Provide increased fluids, fiber, and natural laxatives such as prune juice as needed.
- Increase fluid intake to 2000 mL/day within the client's cardiac and renal reserve.
- Encourage intake of a balanced diet with adequate amounts of fiber and protein

Critical Care

▲ Recognize that the client who has been in an intensive care environment may develop a neuromuscular dysfunction acquired in the absence of causative factors other than the underlying critical illness and its treatment, resulting in extreme weakness. The client may need a workup to determine the cause before satisfactory ambulation can begin.
▲ Consider use of a continuous lateral rotation therapy bed.
▲ For the stable client in the intensive care unit, consider mobilizing the client in a four-phase method from dangling at the side of the bed to walking if there is sufficient knowledgeable staff available to protect the client from harm.

Geriatric

- Get the client out of bed as early possible and ambulate frequently after consultation with the physician.
- Use the Exercise Assessment and Screening for You (EASY), which was developed to identify benefits of exercise and to assist older adults to select safe and effective exercises. This tool decreases barriers to exercise.
▲ Refer the client to physical therapy for resistance strength exercise training.
- Monitor for signs of depression: flat affect, poor appetite, insomnia, many somatic complaints.
- Keep careful track of bowel function in the elderly; do not allow the client to become constipated.

Home Care

- Some of the previous interventions may be adapted for home care use.
- ▲ Begin discharge planning as soon as possible with case manager or social worker to assess need for home support systems and community or home health services.
- ▲ Become oriented to all programs of care for the client before discharge from institutional care.
- ▲ Confirm the immediate availability of all necessary assistive devices for home.
- Perform complete physical assessment and recent history at initial home visit.
- ▲ Refer to physical and occupational therapies for immediate evaluations of the client's potential for independence and functioning in the home setting and for follow-up care.
- Allow the client to have as much input and control of the plan of care as possible.
- Assess knowledge of all care with caregivers. Review as necessary.
- ▲ Support the family of the client in assumption of caregiver activities. Refer for home health aide services for assistance and respite as appropriate. Refer to medical social services as appropriate.
- ▲ Institute case management of frail elderly to support continued independent living, if possible in the home environment.

Client/Family Teaching and Discharge Planning

- Teach client/family how to perform range-of-motion exercises in bed if not contraindicated; this is referred to as a Home Exercise Program.
- Teach the family how to turn and position the client and provide all care necessary.

NOTE: Nursing diagnoses that are commonly relevant when the client is on bed rest include **Constipation, Risk for impaired Skin Integrity, Disturbed Sleep Pattern, Adult Failure to Thrive,** and **Powerlessness.**

● = Independent   ▲ = Collaborative

Deficient Diversional Activity

NANDA-I Definition

D

Decreased stimulation from (or interest or engagement in) recreational or leisure activities

Defining Characteristics

Client's statements regarding boredom (e.g., wish there was something to do, to read, etc.); usual hobbies cannot be undertaken in hospital

Related Factors (r/t)

Environmental lack of diversional activity

Client Outcomes

Client Will (Specify Time Frame):

- Engage in personally satisfying diversional activities

Nursing Interventions

- Observe for signs of deficient diversional activity: restlessness, unhappy facial expression, and statements of boredom and discontent.
- Observe ability to engage in activities that require good vision and use of hands.
- Discuss activities with clients that are interesting and feasible in the present environment.
- Encourage the client to share feelings about situation of inactivity.
- Encourage the client to participate in any available social or recreational opportunities in the health care environment.
- Encourage a mix of physical and mental activities if possible (e.g., crafts, crossword puzzles).
- Provide videos and/or DVDs of movies for recreation and distraction.
- Provide magazines of interest, books of interest.
- Provide books on CD and CD player, and electronic versions of books for listening or reading as available.
- Set up a puzzle in a community space, or provide individual puzzles as desired.

• = Independent   ▲ = Collaborative

- Provide access to a portable computer so that the client can access email and the Internet. Give client a list of interesting websites, including games and directions on how to perform Web searches if needed.
- Help client find a support group for the appropriate condition on the Internet if interested.
▲ Arrange animal-assisted therapy if desired, with a dog, cat, or bird for the client to interact with and care for, if possible.
- Encourage the client to schedule visitors so that they are not all present at once or at inconvenient times.
- If clients are able to write, help them keep journals or engage them in opportunities for creative writing in a group; if clients are unable to write, have them record thoughts on tape, or on videotape.
▲ Request recreational or art therapist to assist with activities.
▲ Refer to occupational therapy.
- Provide a change in scenery; get the client out of the room as possible.
- Help the client to experience nature through looking at a nature scene from a window, or walking through a garden if possible.
- Structure the environment as needed to promote optimal comfort and sensory diversity (e.g., have family bring in posters, banners, or a sound system; change lighting; change direction bed faces).
- Work with family to provide music that is enjoyable to the client.
- Structure the client's schedule around personal wishes for time of care, relaxation, and participation in fun activities.
- Spend time with the client when possible, giving the client full attention and being present in the moment, or arrange for a friendly visitor.

Pediatric

▲ Request an order for a child life specialist or, if not available, a play therapist for children.
- Promote a referral to a music therapist.
- Consider art therapy for children living with chronic illness who have activity restrictions.

● = Independent   ▲ = Collaborative

D

- Provide activities such as video projects and use of computer-based support groups for children, such as Starbright World, a computer network where teenagers interact virtually, sharing their experiences and escaping hospital routines (www.starbrightworld.org).
- Provide animal-assisted therapy for hospitalized children.
- Provide computer games and virtual reality experiences for children, which can be used as distraction techniques during venipuncture or other procedures.

Geriatric

- Assess the interests of older adults and the types of activities that they enjoy; encourage creative expression such as story-telling, drama, dance, painting, writing, or music.
- If the client is able, arrange for him or her to attend group senior citizen activities.
- Promote activity for older adults through the use of exergames (video games combined with exercise).
- Encourage involvement in dance.
- Encourage involvement in gardening.
- Encourage clients to use their ability to help others by volunteering.
- Provide an environment that promotes activity (e.g., one that has adequate lighting for crafts, large-print books, and adequate acoustics).
- Balance effortful activities with restful activities.
- Provide tai chi as an activity.
- Provide opportunities for storytelling.
- ▲ Use reminiscence therapy in conjunction with the expression of emotions. Refer to a reminiscence group if available. Arrange for intergenerational volunteering for individuals with mild to moderate dementia.
- Use the Eden Alternative for older adults; bring in appropriate plants for the elderly client to care for, animals such as birds, fish, dogs, and cats as appropriate for the client and children to visit.
- For clients who love gardening but who may have difficulty being outside, bring in seeds, soil, and pots for indoor

gardening experiences. Use seeds such as sunflower, pumpkin, and zinnia that grow rapidly.
- For clients with depressive symptoms, facilitate regular music listening.
- For clients in assisted-living facilities, provide leisure educational programs and pleasant dining experiences.
- For clients who are interested in writing, promote writing groups.
- Prescribe activities to engage passive dementia clients based on their extraversion and openness.
- Initiate opportunities for creative expression such as a TimeSlips storytelling group or Memories in the Making project to foster meaningful activities for clients with dementia.
- ▲ Provide recreational therapy exercises in the morning for clients with dementia in the extended care facility, and in geropsychiatric programs.

Home Care

- Many of the previously listed interventions may be administered in the home setting.
- Explore with the client previous interests; consider related activities that are within the client's capabilities.
- ▲ Assess the client for depression. Refer for mental health services as indicated.
- Assess the family's ability to respond to the client's psychosocial needs for stimulation. Assist as able.
- ▲ Refer to occupational therapy.
- Introduce (or continue) friendly volunteer visitors if the client is willing and able to have the company. If transportation is an issue or if the client does not want visitors in the home, consider alternatives (e.g., telephone contacts, computer messaging).
- For clients who are interested and capable, suggest involvement in a community gardening experience.
- If the client is dying, and is interested, assist in making a videotape, audiotape, or memory book for family members with treasured stories, memoirs, pictures, and video clips.

● = Independent   ▲ = Collaborative

E

Client/Family Teaching and Discharge Planning

- Work with the client and family on learning diversional activities in which the client is interested (e.g., knitting, hooking rugs, writing memoirs).
- If the client is in isolation, give the client complete information on why isolation is needed and how it should be accomplished, especially guidelines for visitors; provide diversional activities and encourage visitation.

Risk for Electrolyte Imbalance

NANDA-I Definition

At risk for change in serum electrolyte levels that may compromise health

Risk Factors

Diarrhea; endocrine dysfunction; fluid imbalance (e.g., dehydration, water intoxication); impaired regulatory mechanisms (e.g., diabetes insipidus, syndrome of inappropriate secretion of antidiuretic hormone); renal dysfunction; treatment-related side effects (e.g., medications, drains); vomiting

Client Outcomes

Client Will (Specify Time Frame):

- Maintain a normal sinus heart rhythm with a regular rate
- Have a decrease in edema
- Maintain an absence of muscle cramping
- Maintain normal serum potassium, sodium, calcium, and phosphorus
- Maintain normal serum pH

Nursing Interventions

- ▲ Monitor vital signs at least three times a day, or more frequently as needed. Notify provider of significant deviation from baseline.
- ▲ Monitor cardiac rate and rhythm. Report changes to provider.

• = Independent   ▲ = Collaborative

- Monitor intake and output and daily weights.
- Monitor for abdominal distention and discomfort.
- Monitor the client's respiratory status and muscle strength.
- Assess cardiac status and neurological alterations.
▲ Review laboratory data as ordered and report deviations to provider.
- Review the client's medical and surgical history for possible causes of altered electrolytes.
▲ Complete pain assessment. Assess and document the onset, intensity, character, location, duration, aggravating factors, and relieving factors. Notify the provider for any increase in pain or discomfort or if comfort measures are not effective.
▲ Monitor the effects of ordered medications such as diuretics and heart medications.
▲ Administer parenteral fluids as ordered and monitor their effects.

Geriatric

- Monitor electrolyte levels carefully, including sodium levels and potassium levels, with both increased and decreased levels possible.

Client/Family Teaching and Discharge Planning

- Teach client/family the signs of low potassium and the risk factors.
- Teach client/family signs of high potassium and the risk factors.
- Teach client/family the signs of low sodium and the risk factors.
- Teach client/family the signs of high sodium and the risk factors.
- Teach client/family the importance of hydration during exercise.
- Teach client/family the warning signs of dehydration.
- Teach client about any medications prescribed. Medication teaching includes the drug name, its purpose, administration instructions such as taking it with or without food, and any side effects to be aware of.
▲ Instruct the client to report any adverse medication side effects to his/her provider.

● = Independent   ▲ = Collaborative

Disturbed Energy Field

NANDA-I Definition

Disruption of the flow of energy surrounding a person's being results in disharmony of the body, mind, and/or spirit

Defining Characteristics

Perceptions of changes in patterns of energy flow around the body, such as movement (i.e., tingling, wave, spike, bulge) or lack of movement (i.e., congestion, density, hole, diminished flow); sounds (i.e., tone, words); temperature change (i.e., warmth, coolness); and/or visual changes (i.e., image, color)

Related Factors (r/t)

Slowing or blocking of energy flows secondary to:
   Maturational Factors:
      Pregnancy, age-related developmental difficulties or crisis
         (i.e., school, retirement)
   Pathophysiologic Factors:
      Illness, injury, degeneration
   Situational Factors:
      Anxiety, fear, grieving, pain
   Treatment-Related Factors:
      Chemotherapy, immobility, labor and delivery, peri- and
         postoperative experience

Client Outcomes

Client Will (Specify Time Frame):

- State sense of well-being
- State feelings of support
- State feeling of relaxation
- State decreased pain
- State decreased anxiety
- State increased ability to cope
- Demonstrate evidence of physical relaxation (e.g., decreased blood pressure, pulse, respiration rate, muscle tension)

• = Independent   ▲ = Collaborative

Nursing Interventions

- Consider using Therapeutic Touch (TT) and/or Healing Touch (HT) for clients with anxiety, tension, pain, or other conditions that indicate a disruption in the flow of energy.
- Consider HT treatments for clients with psychological depression.
- Administer TT and/or HT as described in the following discussion (may also include Reiki practice).
- Refer to care plans for **Anxiety, Acute Pain,** and **Chronic Pain.**

Guidelines for Therapeutic Touch and Healing Touch

- TT and HT may be practiced by anyone with the requisite preparation, desire, and commitment.
- Those who are not licensed health care professionals may practice TT and HT within their families, religious or spiritual community, and with friends.
- NOTE: Nurses who are not trained in TT or HT should consider spending quiet time with clients listening to their concerns.
- TT is conducted according to the standards for its practice.
- HT is conducted according to the code of ethics and standards of practice developed by Healing Touch International, Inc.
- Administer TT and HT according to the guidelines established by the prospective therapies and programs.

Pediatric

- Consider using TT or HT for pediatric clients with adjunct therapies to decrease stress, anxiety, and pain.
- Teach that when working with the very young, old, or ill, or in the head area, TT should be gentle and used only for short periods.

Geriatric

- Consider TT and HT for agitated clients with Alzheimer's disease.
- Consider TT for elderly with postsurgical pain.

● = Independent ▲ = Collaborative

E

Multicultural

- Assess for the influence of cultural beliefs, norms, and values on the client's sense of disharmony of mind and spirit.
- Assess for the presence of specific culture-bound syndromes that may manifest as disturbances in energy or spirit.
- Validate the client's feelings and concerns related to sense of disharmony or energy disturbance.

Home Care

- See Guidelines for TT and HT.
- Help the client and family accept TT and HT as healing interventions.
- Assist the family with providing an appropriate space in which TT and/or HT can be administered.
- ▲ Consider complementary therapies such as Therapeutic Touch for clients in community mental health programs.
- ▲ In the presence of a psychiatric disorder, refer for psychiatric home health care services for client reassurance and implementation of therapeutic regimen.

Client/Family Teaching and Discharge Planning

- Teach the TT and/or specific HT technique to clients and family members.
- Teach that when working with the very young, old, or ill, or in the head area, TT should be gentle and used only for short periods.
- Teach the client how to use guided imagery.
- Consider the use of progressive muscle relaxation, autogenic training, relaxation response, biofeedback, emotional freedom technique, guided imagery, diaphragmatic breathing, transcendental meditation, cognitive-behavioral therapy, mindfulness-based stress reduction, and emotional freedom technique.

Nurses/Staff

- The practice of Healing Touch, both in the giving and the receiving, can improve well-being.

• = Independent ▲ = Collaborative

Impaired Environmental Interpretation Syndrome

NANDA-I Definition

Consistent lack of orientation to person, place, time, or circumstances over more than 3 to 6 months, necessitating a protective environment

Defining Characteristics

Chronic confusional states; consistent disorientation; inability to concentrate; inability to follow simple directions; inability to reason; loss of occupation; loss of social functioning; slow in responding to questions

Related Factors (r/t)

Dementia; depression; Huntington's disease

Client Outcomes, Nursing Interventions, and Client/Family Teaching

Refer to care plan for **Chronic Confusion** or **Wandering** if appropriate.

Risk for dry Eye

NANDA-I Definition

At risk for eye discomfort or damage to the cornea and conjunctiva due to reduced quantity or quality of tears to moisten the eye

Risk Factors

Aging; autoimmune diseases (rheumatoid arthritis, diabetes mellitus, thyroid disease, gout, osteoporosis, etc.); contact lenses; environmental factors (air conditioning, excessive wind, sunlight exposure, air pollution, low humidity); female gender; history of allergy; hormones; lifestyle (e.g., smoking, caffeine use, prolonged reading); mechanical ventilation therapy; neurological lesions with sensory or motor reflex loss (lagophthalmos, lack of spontaneous blink reflex due to decreased consciousness and other medical conditions); ocular surface damage; place of living; treatment-related side effects (e.g., pharmaceutical agents such as angiotensin-converting enzyme inhibitors, antihistamines, diuretics, steroids, antidepressants, tranquilizers, analgesics, sedatives, neuromuscular blockage agents; surgical operations); vitamin A deficiency

• = Independent   ▲ = Collaborative

E

Client Outcomes

Client Will (Specify Time Frame):

- Experience comfort of the eyes without itching or burning of the eyes, and a feeling of dryness
- Demonstrate how to place drops in the eyes if drops are ordered
- State has clear vision

Nursing Interventions

- Watch for symptoms of dry eyes, which include blurring of vision, heaviness of eyelids, irritation and gritty sensation, light sensitivity, pain, decreased vision, redness of eyes, reflex tears, stinging and ocular discomfort.
- ▲ If symptoms are present, refer client to an ophthalmologist for diagnosis and treatment.
- ▲ Apply warm compresses over the closed eyes if ordered.
- Review medications that the client is taking for possible initiation of dry eye.
- ▲ Insert ordered eye drops.
- ▲ Watch for symptoms of blepharitis including crusting and irritation at the base of the lashes and adjacent redness of the eyelid which may accompany dry eye and refer for treatment as needed.

Geriatric

- Recognize that symptoms of dry eye are more common in geriatric clients and also can be very debilitating in advanced disease states.

Critical Care

- ▲ Provide protection for client's eyes during use of a ventilator or when unconscious by instilling ordered drops or ointment or using an ordered device to maintain eye moisture.

Client/Family Teaching and Discharge Planning

- Teach clients that the following activities such as watching television, computer use, and driving are associated with decreased blinking that can cause dry eye.

• = Independent   ▲ = Collaborative

- Teach clients methods to decrease problems with dry eye including the following:
  - Avoiding spending long periods of time in dry and windy or hot dry weather
  - Avoiding spending time in air-conditioned rooms or smoky environments
  - Protecting eyes from wind and dust
  - Drinking plenty of water to keep well hydrated
  - Avoiding sleeping in contacts
  - Getting plenty of sleep
- ▲ Teach client to consult with physician regarding use of omega-3 supplements to decrease dry eye.
- Teach client using eye drops how to self-administer eye drops, and to keep drops in the refrigerator.
- Warn clients with dry eyes that driving at night can be dangerous.

Adult Failure to Thrive

NANDA-I Definition

Progressive functional deterioration of a physical and cognitive nature. The individual's ability to live with multisystem diseases, cope with ensuing problems, and manage his or her care is remarkably diminished.

Defining Characteristics

Altered mood state; anorexia; apathy; cognitive decline: demonstrated difficulty responding to environmental stimuli; demonstrated difficulty in concentration; demonstrated difficulty in decision-making; demonstrated difficulty in judgment; demonstrated difficulty in memory; demonstrated difficulty in reasoning; decreased perception; consumption of minimal to no food at most meals (i.e., consumes <75% of normal requirements); decreased participation in activities of daily living; decreased social skills; expresses loss of interest in pleasurable outlets; frequent exacerbations of chronic health problems; inadequate nutritional intake; neglect of home environment; neglect of financial responsibilities; physical decline (e.g., fatigue, dehydration, incontinence of bowel and bladder); self-care deficit; social withdrawal; unintentional weight loss (e.g., 5% in 1 month, 10% in 6 months); verbalizes desire for death

• = Independent   ▲ = Collaborative

F

Related Factor (r/t)

Depression

Client Outcomes

Client Will (Specify Time Frame):

- Resume highest level of functioning possible
- Express feelings
- Participate in activities of daily living (ADLs)
- Participate in social interactions
- Consume adequate dietary intake for weight and height
- Maintain usual weight
- Maintain adequate fluid intake with no signs of dehydration
- Maintain clean personal and home environment

Nursing Interventions

Psychosocial

- Elderly clients who have failure to thrive (FTT) should be evaluated by review of their ADLs, cognitive function, and mood; a comprehensive history and physical examination; selected laboratory studies and screening for alcohol and substance abuse.
- Assess for depression with a geriatric depression scale. Be alert for depression in clients newly admitted to nursing homes.
- Screen for depression in persons with adult macular degeneration (AMD) and low vision or vision loss.
- ▲ Carefully assess for elder abuse and refer for treatment.
- Encourage the client to make decisions independently; offer choices.
- Instill hope; assist client to manage chronic conditions through education and social support.
- Provide music for clients with dementia, pain, acute confusion, and functional deficits.
- ▲ Consider the use of light therapy.
- ▲ Provide opportunities for visitation from animals.
- Encourage clients to reminisce and share and compile life histories.

● = Independent   ▲ = Collaborative

- Complete a spiritual assessment and support the client's spirituality; encourage clients to connect with their preferred faith community, and to pray if they wish.
- Evaluate the social support system and help the client to identify ways he might increase social support.
- Encourage older adult clients to take part in activities and social relationships according to their capacity and wishes.
- Help clients identify and practice activities that promote usefulness.
- Provide physical touch or massage for clients. Touch the client's hand or arm when speaking with him or her; offer hugs with permission.

Physiological

▲ Assess possible causes for adult FTT and treat or alleviate any underlying problems such as dysphagia, malnutrition, dehydration, depression, infection, diarrhea, renal failure, polypharmacy, sensory impairments, and illnesses caused by physical and cognitive changes.
- Assess for signs of fatigue and mental status changes that may indicate an infection is present.
- Monitor weight loss, food intake (leaving 25% or more of food uneaten at most meals), psychiatric/mood diagnoses, and decreased ability to participate in ADLs.
- Assess for signs of dehydration; the Dehydration Risk Appraisal Checklist is a potential tool for determining this risk in nursing home residents.
- Play soothing music during mealtimes to increase the amount of food eaten and promote decreased agitation.
- Decrease noise and increase lighting in the dining area.
- Serve "family-style" meals.
▲ Refer to a dietitian for individualized nutrition therapy; include the older adult in food choice decisions.
- Refer to care plan **Readiness for enhanced Nutrition** for additional interventions.
- Assess how often the frail older adult goes outdoors; encourage outside activities.
- Provide creative opportunities for interaction with the natural environment.

• = Independent   ▲ = Collaborative

F

- Assess grip strength periodically and monitor for a decline in strength.
- Assess and monitor physical function in terms of the client's ability to complete with tools such as the Katz Index or Lawton Scale.
- Assess frailty with a tool such as the Edmonton Frail Scale.
- Provide strength and resistance training.
- Promote participation in an exercise-based balance program.
- Implement dance therapy.
▲ Refer for possible pharmacological intervention.
- Refer to care plans for **Imbalanced Nutrition: less than body requirements, Hopelessness, Spiritual Distress, Readiness for enhanced Spiritual Well-Being, Social Isolation, Chronic Sorrow, Chronic low Self-Esteem.**

Multicultural

- Assess for the influence of cultural beliefs, norms, and values on the family's or caregiver's understanding of FTT.
- Actively listen and be sensitive to how communication is shared culturally; some cultures combine communication with eye contact, and some avoid eye contact.
▲ Refer culturally diverse clients to appropriate social, medical, mental health, and spiritual services.
- Refer to a dietitian who can suggest the least restrictive diet that considers ethnic and cultural preferences.
- Promote participation in a community-based exercise program that focuses on strength, endurance, and balance.

Home Care

- The above interventions may be adapted for home care use.
- If FTT is attributable to a dementing illness, refer to care plan for **Chronic Confusion.**
▲ Institute case management or coordinated care of frail elders in the community.

Client/Family Teaching and Discharge Planning

▲ Consider use of a nurse-managed telehealth system with clients who have been discharged early from the hospital to monitor symptoms, provide education, and make referrals if necessary.

• = Independent   ▲ = Collaborative

▲ Refer for medical evaluation when cognitive changes are noticed.
• Encourage family to provide and encourage social interaction with the client.
• Instruct the family to monitor the elder person's weight.
▲ Provide referral for evaluation of hearing and appropriate hearing aids.
▲ Refer for psychotherapy and possible medication if the etiology is depression.

Risk for Falls

NANDA-I Definition

Increased susceptibility to falling that may cause physical harm

Risk Factors (Intrinsic and Extrinsic)

Adults

Age 65 or older; history of falls; fear of falling; living alone; lower limb prosthesis; use of assistive devices (e.g., walker, cane); wheelchair use

Children

Less than 2 years of age; bed located near window; lack of automobile restraints; lack of gate on stairs; lack of window guard; lack of parental supervision; male gender when less than 1 year of age; unattended infant on elevated surface (e.g., bed/changing table)

Cognitive

Diminished mental status

Environment

Cluttered environment; dimly lit room; no antislip material in bath; no antislip material in shower; restraints; throw rugs; unfamiliar room; weather conditions (e.g., wet floors, ice)

Medications

Angiotensin-converting enzyme (ACE) inhibitors; alcohol use; antianxiety agents; antihypertensive agents; diuretics; hypnotics; narcotics/opiates; tranquilizers; tricyclic antidepressants

• = Independent ▲ = Collaborative

Physiological

Anemias; arthritis; diarrhea; decreased lower extremity strength; difficulty with gait; faintness when extending neck; foot problems; hearing difficulties; impaired balance; impaired physical mobility; incontinence; neoplasms (i.e., fatigue; limited mobility); neuropathy; orthostatic hypotension; postoperative conditions; postprandial blood sugar changes; presence of acute illness; proprioceptive deficits; sleeplessness; urgency; vascular disease; visual difficulties

Client Outcomes

Client Will (Specify Time Frame):

- Remain free of falls
- Change environment to minimize the incidence of falls
- Explain methods to prevent injury

Nursing Interventions

- **Safety guidelines.** Complete a fall-risk assessment for older adults in acute care using a valid and reliable tool such as the Hendrich II model. Recognize that risk factors for falling include recent history of falls, fear of falling, confusion, depression, altered elimination patterns, cardiovascular/respiratory disease impairing perfusion or oxygenation, postural hypotension, dizziness or vertigo, primary cancer diagnosis, and altered mobility.
- Screen all clients for balance and mobility skills (supine to sit, sitting supported and unsupported, sit to stand, standing, walking and turning around, transferring, stooping to floor and recovering, and sitting down). Use tools such as the Balance Scale by Tinetti or the Get Up and Go Scale.
- Recognize that when people attend to another task while walking, such as carrying a cup of water, clothing, or supplies, they are more likely to fall.
- Carefully assist a mostly immobile client up. Be sure to lock the bed and wheelchair and have sufficient personnel to protect the client from falls. When rising from a lying position, have the client change positions slowly, dangle legs, and stand next to the bed prior to walking to prevent orthostatic hypotension.
- Use a "high-risk fall" armband/bracelet and fall risk room sign to alert staff for increased vigilance and mobility assistance.

• = Independent   ▲ = Collaborative

▲ Evaluate the client's medications to determine whether medications increase the risk of falling; consult with physician regarding the client's need for medication if appropriate.

• Orient the client to environment. Place the call light within reach and show how to call for assistance; answer call light promptly.

• Use one quarter- to one half-length side rails only, and maintain bed in a low position. Ensure that wheels are locked on bed and commode. Keep dim light in room at night.

• Routinely assist the client with toileting on his or her own schedule. Always take the client to bathroom on awakening and before bedtime. Keep the path to the bathroom clear, label the bathroom, and leave the door open.

▲ Avoid use of restraints if at all possible. Obtain a physician's order if restraints are deemed necessary, and use the least restrictive device.

• In place of restraints, use the following:
  ■ Well-staffed and educated nursing personnel with frequent client contact with careful consideration during shift changes
  ■ Nursing units designed to care for clients with cognitive or functional impairments
  ■ Nonskid footwear, sneakers preferable
  ■ Adequate lighting, night-light in bathroom
  ■ Toilet frequently
  ■ Frequently assess need for invasive devices, tubes, IVs
  ■ Hide tubes with bandages to prevent pulling of tubes
  ■ Consider alternative IV placement site to prevent pulling out IV
  ■ Alarm systems with ankle, above-the-knee, or wrist sensors
  ■ Bed or wheelchair alarms
  ■ Wedge cushions on chairs to prevent slipping
  ■ Increased observation of the client
  ■ Locked doors to unit
  ■ Low or very low height beds
  ■ Border-defining pillow/mattress to remind the client to stay in bed

• If the client has an acute change in mental status (delirium), recognize that the cause is usually physiological and is a

F

• = Independent   ▲ = Collaborative

medical emergency. Consider possible causes for delirium. Consult with the physician or health care provider immediately. See interventions for **Acute Confusion.**

- If the client has chronic confusion due to dementia, implement individualized strategies to enhance communication. NOTE: See interventions for **Chronic Confusion.**

F

- Ask family to stay with the client to assist with ADLs and prevent the client from accidentally falling or pulling out tubes.
▲ If the client is unsteady on feet, have two nursing staff members alongside when walking the client. Consider referral to physical therapy for gait training and strengthening.
- Place a fall-prone client in a room that is near the nurses' station.
▲ Refer to physical therapy or other programs for exercise programs that target strength, balance, flexibility, or endurance.

Geriatric

- Assess fall risk using a falls risk assessment tool such as the Hendrich II Fall Risk Model, Stratify Tool, or Morse Falls Scale.
- Complete a post-fall assessment for older adults.
▲ If new onset of falling, assess for lab abnormalities, and signs and symptoms of infection and dehydration, and check blood pressure and pulse rate supine, sitting, and standing for hypotension and orthostatic hypotension. If the client has a borderline high blood pressure, the risk of falling due to administration of antihypertensives may outweigh the benefits of the antihypertensive medication. Discuss with the health care provider on a client-to-client basis.
- Complete a fear of falling assessment for older adults. This includes measuring fear of falling, or the level of concern about falling, and falls self-efficacy, the degree of confidence a person has in performing common activities of daily living without falling.
- Encourage the client to wear glasses and use walking aids when ambulating.
- If the client experiences dizziness because of orthostatic hypotension when getting up, teach methods to decrease dizziness,

such as rising slowly, remaining seated several minutes before standing, flexing feet upward several times while sitting, sitting down immediately if feeling dizzy, and trying to have someone present when standing.
▲ Refer to physical therapy for strength training, using free weights or machines, and suggest participation in exercise programs.
▲ Implement evidence-based interventions to prevent falls. These include:
  ■ Exercise for balance, gait and strength training, such as tai chi or physical therapy
  ■ Environmental adaptation to reduce fall risk factors in the home and in daily activities
  ■ Cataract surgery when indicated
  ■ Medication reduction with particular attention to medications that affect the brain such as sleeping medications, anti-anxiety medications, and antidepressants
  ■ Assessment and treatment of postural hypotension
  ■ Identification and appropriate treatment of foot problems
  ■ Vitamin D supplementation for those with vitamin D deficiency

Home Care

• Some of the above interventions may be adapted for home care use.
• Implement evidence-based fall prevention practices to older adults in community settings and home health care programs.
▲ If delirium is present, assess for cause of delirium and/or falls with the use of an interdisciplinary team. Consult with the physician immediately. Assess and monitor for acute changes in cognition and behavior.
• Assess home environment for threats to safety including clutter, slippery floors, scatter rugs, and other potential hazards. Additionally, assess external environment (e.g., uneven pavement, unleveled stairs/steps).
▲ Instruct the client and family or caregivers on how to correct identified hazards for those with visual impairment. Refer to physical and occupational therapy services for assistance if needed.

• = Independent   ▲ = Collaborative

▲ Use a multifactorial assessment along with interventions targeted to the identified risk factors. Key components of the interventions include evaluating need for all medications; balance, gait and strength training; use of strategies to deal with postural hypotension, if present; home safety evaluation with needed modifications; and any needed cardiovascular treatment.

• Encourage the client to eat a balanced diet, with particular inclusion of vitamin D and calcium.

• If the client lives alone or spends a lot of time alone, teach the client what to do if he or she falls and cannot get up, and suggest he or she have a personal emergency response system or a mobile phone that is available from the floor.

• Ensure appropriate nonglare lighting in the home. Ask the client to install indoor strip or "runway" type of lighting to baseboards to help clients vision. Install motion-sensitive lighting that turns on automatically when the client gets out of bed to go to the bathroom.

• Have the client wear supportive, low-heeled shoes with good traction when ambulating. Avoid use of slip-on footwear. Wear appropriate footwear in inclement weather.

• Provide a signaling device for clients who wander or are at risk for falls.

• Provide medical identification bracelet for clients at risk for injury from dementia, diabetes, seizures, or other medical disorders.

• Suggest a tai chi class designed for the elderly to selected clients who have sufficient balance to participate.

Client/Family Teaching and Discharge Planning

• **Safety guidelines.** Teach the client and the family about the fall reduction measures that are being used to prevent falls.

• Teach the client how to safely ambulate at home, including using safety measures such as hand rails in bathroom, and need to avoid carrying things or performing other tasks while walking.

• Teach the client the importance of maintaining a regular exercise program. If the client is afraid of falling while walking outside, suggest he or she walks the length of a local mall.

• = Independent   ▲ = Collaborative

Dysfunctional Family Processes

NANDA-I Definition

Psychosocial, spiritual, and physiological functions of the family unit are chronically disorganized, which leads to conflict, denial of problems, resistance to change, ineffective problem solving, and a series of self-perpetuating crises

Defining Characteristics

Behavioral

Agitation; blaming; broken promises; chaos; complicated grieving; conflict avoidance; contradictory communication; controlling communication; criticizing; deficient knowledge about substance abuse; denial of problems; dependency; difficulty having fun; difficulty with intimate relationships; difficulty with life cycle transitions; diminished physical contact; disturbances in academic performance in children; disturbances in concentration; enabling maintenance of substance use pattern (e.g., alcohol); escalating conflict; failure to accomplish developmental tasks; family special occasions are substance-use centered; harsh self-judgment; immaturity; impaired communication; inability to accept a wide range of feelings; inability to accept help; inability to adapt to change; inability to deal constructively with traumatic experiences; inability to express wide range of feelings; inability to meet the emotional needs of its members; inability to meet the security needs of its members; inability to meet the spiritual needs of its members; inability to receive help appropriately; inadequate understanding of substance abuse; inappropriate expression of anger; ineffective problem-solving skills; lack of reliability; lying; manipulation; nicotine addiction; orientation toward tension relief rather than achievement of goals; paradoxical communication; power struggles; rationalization; refusal to get help; seeking affirmation, seeking approval; self-blaming; social isolation; stress-related physical illnesses; substance abuse; verbal abuse of children; verbal abuse of parent; verbal abuse of spouse

Feelings

Abandonment; anger; anxiety; being different from other people; being unloved; chronic low self-esteem; confuses love and pity; confusion; depression; dissatisfaction; distress; embarrassment; emotional control by others; emotional isolation; failure; fear; frustration; guilt;

hopelessness; hostility; hurt; insecurity; lack of identity; lingering resentment; loneliness; loss; mistrust; moodiness; powerlessness; rejection; reports feeling misunderstood; repressed emotions; responsibility for substance abuser's behavior; suppressed rage; shame; tension; unhappiness; vulnerability; worthlessness.

Roles and Relationships

Altered role function; chronic family problems; closed communication systems; deterioration in family relationships; disrupted family rituals; disrupted family roles; disturbed family dynamics; economic problems; family denial; family does not demonstrate respect for autonomy of its members; family does not demonstrate respect for individuality of its members; inconsistent parenting; ineffective spouse communication; intimacy dysfunction; lack of cohesiveness; lack of skills necessary for relationships; low perception of parental support; marital problems; neglected obligations; pattern of rejection; reduced ability of family members to relate to each other for mutual growth and maturation; triangulating family relationships

Related Factors (r/t)

Abuse of alcohol; addictive personality; biochemical influences; family history of alcoholism; family history of resistance to treatment; genetic predisposition; inadequate coping skills; lack of problem-solving skills

Client Outcomes

Family/Client Will (Specify Time Frame):

- State one way that alcoholism has affected the health of the family
- Identify three healthy coping behaviors that family members can employ to facilitate a shift toward improved family functioning
- Identify one Al-Anon meeting from Al-Anon meeting schedule that family members express a desire to attend
- Attend different types of meetings (lead, big book, discussion, beginner's meeting) to find a good match and commit to attending that group regularly

Nursing Interventions

- Refer to care plans for **Ineffective Denial** and **Defensive Coping** for additional interventions.

● = Independent   ▲ = Collaborative

▲ Behavioral screening and intervention (BSI) should be integrated into all health care settings. Different terminology has evolved for screening, intervention, and referral for various behavioral issues. The five A's—ask, advise, assess, assist, and arrange—apply to tobacco use. SBIRT (screening, brief intervention, and referral to treatment) pertains to alcohol and drug use.

• Screen clients for at-risk drinking during routine primary care visits and before surgery using the Alcohol Use Disorders Identification Test (AUDIT).

• Stress early treatment and brief intervention to resolve the problem.

• Provide brief (5- to 10-minute) education and individual counsel as a routine part of primary care.

▲ Refer for family therapy.

▲ Refer for possible use of medications to control problem drinking.

Pediatric

• Use closed-ended questions when questioning adolescents about drinking behavior.

• Provide a brief motivational interviewing and cognitive-behavioral based alcohol intervention group program for young people at risk of developing a problem with alcohol.

• Encourage parent communication about alcohol use with adolescents.

▲ Consider the Community Reinforcement Approach (CRA) that encourages clients to become progressively involved in alternative nonsubstance-related pleasant social activities, and to work on enhancing the enjoyment they receive within the "community" of their family and job.

▲ Educate family members about available educational and support programs and encourage no/limited alcohol use in the home.

• Work at strengthening adolescents' relationships in and out of the home.

• Provide school-based prevention programs using peer leaders at an early age.

● = Independent   ▲ = Collaborative

- Provide a school-based drug-prevention program to junior high students.

Geriatric

- Include assessment of possible alcohol abuse when assessing elderly family members.
▲ Provide alcohol treatment programs for geriatric clients in primary care settings.

Multicultural

- Acknowledge racial/ethnic differences at the onset of care.
- Use a family-centered approach when working with Latino, Asian American, African American, and Native American clients.
- Some less-acculturated Latino families may be unwilling to discuss family issues with health care providers until they perceive a close personal relationship with the provider.
- Use family strengthening interventions such as behavioral parent training, family skills training, in-home family support, brief family therapy, and family education when working with culturally diverse families.
- Work with families in a way that incorporates cultural elements.

Home Care

NOTE: In the community setting, alcoholism as cause of dysfunctional family processes must be considered in two categories: (1) when the client suffers personally from the illness, and (2) when a significant other suffers from the illness, that is, the client is not the active alcoholic but may depend on the alcoholic for caregiving. The following considerations apply to both situations with appropriate adaptation for the circumstances.

- The previous interventions may be adapted for home care use.
- Work with family members to support a sense of valued fit on their part; include them in treatment planning and identify the importance of their roles in the client's care. At the same time, encourage their pursuit of positive outside activities that enhance their sense of belonging.

• = Independent   ▲ = Collaborative

- Educate client and family regarding the interactions of alcohol use with medications and the therapeutic regimen.
- Alcoholism is a family disease.
- ▲ Refer for psychiatric home health care services for client reassurance and implementation of therapeutic regimen.
- Provide telephone prompting for clients to start alcohol treatment.

Client/Family Teaching and Discharge Planning

- Suggest the client complete a confidential Internet self-screening test for identification of problems and suggestions for treatment if a problem with alcohol is suspected. Many tools are available.
- Provide education for family.
- Facilitate participation in mutual help groups.

Interrupted Family Processes

NANDA-I Definition

Change in family relationships and/or functioning

Defining Characteristics

Changes in assigned tasks; changes in availability for affective responsiveness; changes in availability for emotional support; changes in communication patterns; changes in effectiveness in completing assigned tasks; changes in expressions of conflict with community resources; changes in expressions of conflict within family; changes in expressions of isolation from community resources; changes in mutual support; changes in participation in decision-making; changes in participation in problem-solving; changes in satisfaction with family; changes in somatic complaints; communication pattern changes; intimacy changes; pattern changes; power alliance changes; ritual changes; stress-reduction behavior changes

Related Factors (r/t)

Developmental crises; developmental transition; interaction with community; modification in family finances; modification in family

• = Independent ▲ = Collaborative

social status; power shift of family members; shift in family roles; shift in health status of a family member; situation transition; situational crises

Client Outcomes

Family/Client Will (Specify Time Frame):

- Express feelings (family)
- Identify ways to cope effectively and use appropriate support systems (family)
- Treat impaired family member as normally as possible to avoid overdependence (family)
- Meet physical, psychosocial, and spiritual needs of members or seek appropriate assistance (family)
- Demonstrate knowledge of illness or injury, treatment modalities, and prognosis (family)
- Participate in the development of the plan of care to the best of ability (significant person)

Nursing Interventions

- Motivate family members to speak openly about illnesses.
- Acknowledge the range of emotions and feelings that may be experienced when the health status of a family member changes; counsel family members that it is normal to be angry and afraid.
- Encourage family members to list their personal strengths.
- Establish relationships among clients, their families, and health care professionals.
- Encourage family to visit the client; adjust visiting hours to accommodate family's schedule.
- Allow and encourage family members to assist in the client's treatment.
- Consider the use of different instruction methods in assisting inexperienced older adults through interactive training systems.
- Refer to the care plan **Readiness for enhanced Family Processes** for additional interventions.

Pediatric

- Carefully assess potential for reunifying children placed in foster care with their birth parents.
- Allow and encourage family to assist in the client's care.
- ▲ Refer children and mothers exposed to violence in the home to Theraplay: an attachment-based intervention that uses the four core elements of nurturing, engagement, structure, and challenge in interactions between mother and her child.

Geriatric

- Encourage family members to be involved in the care of relatives who are in residential care settings.
- Support group problem solving among family members and include the older member.
- ▲ Refer family for counseling with a psychotherapist who is knowledgeable about gerontology.
- Refer to care plan for **Readiness for enhanced Family Processes** for additional interventions.

Multicultural

- Refer to the care plan **Readiness for enhanced Family Processes** for additional interventions.

Home Care

- The nursing interventions described in the care plan for **Compromised family Coping** should be used in the home environment with adaptations as necessary.
- Encourage family members to find meaning in a serious illness.

Client/Family Teaching and Discharge Planning

- Refer to Client/Family Teaching and Discharge Planning in **Compromised family Coping** and **Readiness for enhanced family Coping** for suggestions that may be used with minor adaptations.

● = Independent   ▲ = Collaborative

Readiness for enhanced Family Processes

NANDA-I Definition

A pattern of family functioning that is sufficient to support the well-being of family members and can be strengthened

F

Defining Characteristics

Activities support the growth of family members; activities support the safety of family members; balance exists between autonomy and cohesiveness; boundaries of family members are maintained; communication is adequate; energy level of family supports activities of daily living; expresses willingness to enhance family dynamics; family adapts to change; family functioning meets needs of family members; family resilience is evident; family roles are appropriate for developmental stages; family roles are flexible for developmental stages; family tasks are accomplished; interdependent with community; relationships are generally positive; respect for family members is evident

Client Outcomes

Family/Client Will (Specify Time Frame):

- Identify ways to cope effectively and use appropriate support systems (family)
- Meet physical, psychosocial, and spiritual needs of members or seek appropriate assistance (family)
- Demonstrate knowledge of potential environmental, lifestyle, and genetic risks to health and use appropriate measures to decrease possibility of risk (family)
- Focus on wellness, disease prevention, and maintenance (family and individual)
- Seek balance among exercise, work, leisure, rest, and nutrition (family and individual)

Nursing Interventions

- Assess the family's stress level and coping abilities during the initial nursing assessment.
- Consider the use of family-centered theory as the conceptual foundation to help guide interventions.

• = Independent   ▲ = Collaborative

- Use family-centered care and role modeling for holistic care of families.
- Discuss with family members and identify the perceptions of the health care experience.
- Support family needs, strengths, and resourcefulness through family interviews.
- Spend time with family members; allow them to verbalize their feelings.
- Encourage family members to find meaning in a serious illness.
- Provide family-centered care to explore and use all available resources appropriate for the situation (e.g., counseling, social services, self-help groups, pastoral care).
- Consider focus groups to provide insight to family perceptions of illness and/or disease prevention.

Pediatric

- Provide a parenting class series based on individual and couple changes in meaning and identity, roles, and relationships and interaction during the transition to parenthood. Address mother and father roles, infant communication abilities, and patterns of the first 3 months of life in a mutually enjoyable, possibility focused manner.
- Encourage families with adolescents to have family meals.
- ▲ Consider the use of adventure therapy for adolescents with cancer.

Geriatric

- Carefully listen to residents and family members in the long-term care facility.
- Support caregivers' awareness of the positive effects of their contribution to the well-being of parents.
- Teach family members about the impact of developmental events (e.g., retirement, death, change in health status, and household composition).
- Encourage social networks; social integration; and social engagement with friends, children, and relatives of the elderly.

• = Independent   ▲ = Collaborative

Fatigue

F

Multicultural

- Assess for the influence of cultural beliefs, norms, and values on the family's perceptions of normal functioning.
- Identify and acknowledge the stresses unique to racial/ethnic families.
- Assess and support spiritual needs of families.
- With the client's consent, facilitate a group meeting for family members to discuss how the family is functioning.
- Facilitate modeling and role playing for the client and family regarding healthy ways to start a discussion about the client's prognosis.
- Encourage family mealtimes.

Home Care

- The previous nursing interventions should be used in the home environment with adaptations as necessary.
- ▲ Encourage virtual support groups to family caregivers.
- ▲ Encourage caregivers of elderly clients with chronic obstructive pulmonary disease (COPD) receiving long-term oxygen therapy (LTOT) to seek additional services such as social services, respite care, and additional home health visits.

Client/Family Teaching and Discharge Planning

- Refer to Client/Family Teaching and Discharge Planning in **Readiness for enhanced family Coping** for suggestions that may be used with minor adaptations.

NANDA-I Definition

An overwhelming, sustained sense of exhaustion and decreased capacity for physical and mental work at usual level

Defining Characteristics

Compromised concentration; compromised libido; decreased performance; disinterest in surroundings; drowsy; feelings of guilt for not keeping up with responsibilities; inability to maintain usual level of

• = Independent   ▲ = Collaborative

physical activity; inability to maintain usual routines; inability to restore energy even after sleep; increase in physical complaints; increase in rest requirements; introspection; lack of energy; lethargic; listless; perceived need for additional energy to accomplish routine tasks; tired; verbalization of an unremitting lack of energy; verbalization of an overwhelming lack of energy

Related Factors (r/t)

Psychological
Anxiety; boring lifestyle; depression

Physiological
Anemia; disease states (e.g., cancer, multiple sclerosis, respiratory diseases, coronary diseases); increased physical exertion; lack of endurance; malnutrition; poor physical condition; pregnancy; sleep deprivation

Environmental
Humidity; lights; noise; temperature

Situational
Negative life events; occupation

Client Outcomes

Client Will (Specify Time Frame):
- Identify potential causes of fatigue
- Identify potential factors that aggravate and relieve fatigue
- Describe ways to assess and track patterns of fatigue over set periods of time (e.g., a week, a month)
- Describe ways in which fatigue affects the ability to accomplish goals and activities of daily living
- Verbalize increased energy and improved well-being
- Explain energy conservation plan to offset fatigue
- Explain energy restoration plan to offset fatigue

Nursing Interventions

- Assess severity of fatigue on a scale of 0 to 10 (average fatigue, worst and best levels); assess frequency of fatigue (number of days per week and time of day), activities and symptoms associated with increased fatigue (e.g., pain), ability to perform

• = Independent   ▲ = Collaborative

F

ADLs and instrumental ADLs, interference with social and role function, times of increased energy, ability to concentrate, mood, and usual pattern of activity. Consider use of an instrument such as the Profile of Mood State Short Form Fatigue Subscale, the Multidimensional Assessment of Fatigue, the Lee Fatigue Scale, the Multidimensional Fatigue Inventory, the HIV-Related Fatigue Scale, the Brief Fatigue Inventory, or the Dutch Fatigue Scale to assess fatigue accurately.

- Evaluate adequacy of nutrition and sleep hygiene (napping throughout the day, inability to fall asleep or stay asleep). Encourage the client to get adequate rest, limit naps (particularly in the late afternoon or evening), use a routine sleep/wake schedule, avoid caffeine in the late afternoon or evening, and eat a well-balanced diet with at least eight glasses of water a day. Refer to **Imbalanced Nutrition: less than body requirements** or **Insomnia** if appropriate.

▲ Collaborate with the primary care provider to identify physiological and/or psychological causes of fatigue that could be treated, such as anemia, pain, electrolyte imbalance (e.g., altered potassium levels), hypothyroidism, depression, or medication effect.

▲ Work with the primary care provider to determine if the client has chronic fatigue syndrome, paying attention to risk factors in particular populations.

- Encourage the client to express feelings, attribution of cause and behaviors about fatigue, including potential causes of fatigue, and possible interventions to alleviate fatigue. Such interventions could include setting small, easily achieved short-term goals and developing energy management techniques; use active listening techniques and help identify sources of hope.

- Encourage the client to keep a journal of activities that contribute to symptoms of fatigue, patterns of symptoms across days/weeks/months and feelings, including how fatigue affects the client's normal daily activities and roles.

- Help the client identify sources of support and essential and nonessential tasks to determine which tasks can be delegated to whom. Give the client permission to limit social and role demands if needed (e.g., switch to part-time employment, hire cleaning service).

▲ Collaborate with the primary care provider regarding the appropriateness of referrals to physical therapy for carefully monitored aerobic exercise program and possible physical aids, such as a walker or cane.

• Encourage the client to try complementary and alternative therapy such as guided imagery, massage therapy, mindfulness, and acupressure.

▲ Refer the client to diagnosis-appropriate support groups such as National Chronic Fatigue Syndrome Association, Multiple Sclerosis Association, or cancer fatigue websites such as the Oncology Nurses Association (http://www.ons.org) or the National Comprehensive Cancer Network.

▲ For a cardiac client, recognize that fatigue is common after a myocardial infarction or chronic cardiac insufficiency. Refer to cardiac rehabilitation for carefully prescribed and monitored exercise program.

• If fatigue is associated with cancer or cancer-related treatment, assess for other symptoms that may enhance fatigue (e.g., pain, insomnia or depression).

▲ Collaborate with primary care provider to identify attentional fatigue, which may manifest itself as the inability to direct attention necessary to perform usual activities.

▲ Collaborate with primary care providers to identify potential pharmacological treatment for fatigue.

Geriatric

• Evaluate fatigue in elderly clients routinely, particularly in clients with limited physical function and lower levels of social support.

• Review comorbid conditions that may contribute to fatigue, such as congestive heart failure, arthritis, obesity, and cancer.

• Identify recent losses; monitor for depression as a possible contributing factor to fatigue.

▲ Review medications for side effects.

• = Independent   ▲ = Collaborative

F

Home Care

- The above interventions may be adapted for home care use.
- Assess the client's history and current patterns of fatigue as they relate to the home environment and environmental and behavioral triggers of increased fatigue.
- ▲ Refer to occupational and/or physical therapy if substantial intervention is needed to assist the client in adapting to home and daily patterns.
- For clients receiving chemotherapy, intervene to:
  - Relieve symptom distress (negative mood, nausea, difficulty sleeping)
  - Encourage as much physical activity as possible
  - Support a positive attitude for the future
  - Support adequate recovery time between treatments
- Teach the client and family the importance of and methods for setting priorities for activities, especially those with high energy demand (e.g., home or family events). Instruct in realistic expectations and behavioral pacing.
- Assess effect of fatigue on the client's relatedness; recognize that the client's fatigue affects the whole family. Initiate the following interventions:
  - Avoid dismissing reports of fatigue; validate the client's experience and foster hope for eventual treatment, if not resolution, of the fatigue.
  - Identify with the client ways in which he or she continues to be a valued part of his or her social environment.
  - Identify with the client ways in which he or she continues to participate in equitable exchange with others.
  - Encourage the client to maintain regular family routines (e.g., meals, sleep patterns) as much as possible.
  - Initiate cognitive restructuring to refute the client's guilt-producing and negative thought patterns.
  - Assess and intervene with family's and friends' contributions to guilt-inducing self-talk.
  - Work with the client to inoculate against the negative thinking of others.
  - Explore family life and demands to identify accommodations.

• = Independent   ▲ = Collaborative

F

- Support the client's efforts at limit setting on the demands of others.
- Assist the client to move toward a state of parallelism by working to identify and relieve sources of physical or emotional discomfort. Degree of involvement, limited by fatigue, need not be changed.
▲ Refer for family therapy in the event the client's fatigue interferes with normal family functioning.

Client/Family Teaching and Discharge Planning

- Help client to reframe cognitively; share information about fatigue and how to live with it, including need for positive self-talk.
- Teach strategies for energy conservation (e.g., sitting instead of standing during showering, storing items at waist level).
- Teach the client to carry a pocket calendar, make lists of required activities, and post reminders around the house.
- Teach the importance of following a healthy lifestyle with adequate nutrition, fluids, and rest; pain relief; insomnia correction; and appropriate exercise to decrease fatigue (i.e., energy restoration).
- See **Hopelessness** care plan if appropriate.

Fear

NANDA-I Definition

Response to perceived threat that is consciously recognized as a danger

Defining Characteristics

Report of alarm; apprehension; being scared; increased tension; decreased self-assurance; dread; excitement; jitteriness; panic; terror

Cognitive

Diminished productivity; learning ability; problem-solving ability; identifies object of fear; stimulus believed to be a threat

● = Independent   ▲ = Collaborative

Behaviors

Attack or avoidance behaviors; impulsiveness; increased alertness; narrowed focus on the source of fear

Physiological

Anorexia; diarrhea; dry mouth; dyspnea; fatigue; increased perspiration, pulse, respiratory rate, systolic blood pressure; muscle tightness; nausea; pallor; pupil dilation; vomiting

Related Factors (r/t)

Innate origin (e.g., sudden noise, height, pain, loss of physical support); innate releasers (neurotransmitters); language barrier; learned response (e.g., conditioning, modeling from or identification with others); phobic stimulus; sensory impairment; separation from support system in potentially stressful situation (e.g., hospitalization, hospital procedures); unfamiliarity with environmental experience(s)

Client Outcomes

Client Will (Specify Time Frame):

- Verbalize known fears
- State accurate information about the situation
- Identify, verbalize, and demonstrate those coping behaviors that reduce own fear
- Report and demonstrate reduced fear

Nursing Interventions

- Assess source of fear with the client.
- Assess for a history of anxiety.
- Have the client draw the object of his or her fear.
- Discuss the situation with the client and help distinguish between real and imagined threats to well-being.
- Encourage the client to explore underlying feelings that may be contributing to the fear.
- Stay with clients when they express fear; provide verbal and nonverbal (touch and hug with permission and if culturally acceptable) reassurances of safety if safety is within control.
- Explore coping skills previously used by the client to deal with fear; reinforce these skills and explore other outlets.

• = Independent   ▲ = Collaborative

- Provide backrubs and massage for clients to decrease anxiety.
- Use Therapeutic Touch (TT) and Healing Touch techniques.
▲ Refer for cognitive-behavioral therapy.
▲ Animal-assisted therapy can be incorporated into the care of clients in hospice situations.
- Encourage clients to express their fears in narrative form.
- Refer to care plans for **Anxiety** and **Death Anxiety**.

Pediatric

- Use drawing and artistic expression to assist children express fear.
- Explore coping skills previously used by the client to deal with fear.
- Teach parents to use cognitive-behavioral strategies such as positive coping statements ("I am a brave girl [boy]. I can take care of myself in the dark") and rewards of bravery tokens for appropriate behavior.
- Screen for depression in clients who report social or school fears.
- Teach relaxation techniques to children to induce calmness.

Geriatric

- Establish a trusting relationship so that all fears can be identified.
- Monitor for dementia and use appropriate interventions.
- Provide a protective and safe environment, use consistent caregivers, and maintain the accustomed environmental structure.
- Observe for untoward changes if antianxiety drugs are taken.
- Assess for fear of falls in hospitalized clients with hip fractures to determine risk of poor health outcomes.
- Encourage exercises to improve physical skills and levels of mobility to decrease fear of falling.
- Assist the client in identifying and reducing risk factors of falls, including environmental hazards in and out of the home, the importance of good nutrition and activity, proper footwear, and how to stand up after a fall.

• = Independent   ▲ = Collaborative

Multicultural

- Assess for the presence of culture-bound anxiety and fear states.
- Assess for the influence of cultural beliefs, norms, and values on the client's perspective of a stressful situation.
- Identify what triggers fear response.
- Identify how the client expresses fear.
- Validate the client's feelings regarding fear.
- Assess for fears of racism in culturally diverse clients.

Home Care

- The previous interventions may be adapted for home care use.
- Assess to differentiate the presence of fear versus anxiety.
- Refer to care plan for **Anxiety.**
- During initial assessment, determine whether current or previous episodes of fear relate to the home environment (e.g., perception of danger in the home or neighborhood or of relationships that have a history in the home).
- Identify with the client what steps may be taken to make the home a "safe" place to be.
- ▲ Encourage the client to seek or continue appropriate counseling to reduce fear associated with stress or resolve alterations in irrational thought processes.
- ▲ Encourage the client to have a trusted companion, family member, or caregiver present in the home for periods when fear is most prominent. Pending other medical diagnoses, a referral to homemaker or home health aide services may meet this need.
- ▲ Offer to sit quietly with a terminally ill client as needed by the client or family, or provide hospice volunteers to do the same.

Client/Family Teaching and Discharge Planning

- Teach the client the difference between warranted and excessive fear.
- Teach clients to use guided imagery when they are fearful; have them use all senses to visualize a place that is "comfortable and safe" for them.

- Teach use of appropriate community resources in emergency situations (e.g., hotlines, emergency departments, law enforcement, judicial systems).
- Encourage use of appropriate community resources in non-emergency situations (e.g., family, friends, neighbors, self-help and support groups, volunteer agencies, churches, recreation clubs and centers, seniors, youths, others with similar interests).
- If fear is associated with bioterrorism, provide accurate information and ensure that health care personnel have appropriate training and preparation.

Ineffective infant Feeding Pattern

NANDA-I Definition

Impaired ability of an infant to suck or coordinate the suck/swallow response resulting in inadequate oral nutrition for metabolic needs

Defining Characteristics

Inability to coordinate sucking, swallowing, and breathing; inability to initiate an effective suck; inability to sustain an effective suck

Related Factors (r/t)

Anatomical abnormality; neurological delay; neurological impairment; oral hypersensitivity; prematurity; prolonged nil by mouth (NPO) status

Client Outcomes

Infant Will (Specify Time Frame):

- Consume adequate calories that will result in appropriate weight gain and optimal growth and development
- Have opportunities for skin-to-skin (kangaroo care) experiences
- Have opportunities for "trophic" (i.e., small volume of breast milk/formula) enteral feedings prior to full oral feedings
- Progress to stable, neurobehavioral organization (i.e., motor, state, self-regulation, attention-interaction)

• = Independent   ▲ = Collaborative

- Demonstrate presence of mature oral reflexes that are necessary for safe feeding
- Progress to safe, self-regulated oral feedings
- Coordinate the suck-swallow-breathe sequence while nippling
- Display clear behavioral cues related to hunger and satiety
- Display approach/engagement cues, with minimal avoidance/disengagement cues
- Have opportunities to pace own feeding, taking breaks as needed
- Display evidence of being in the "quiet-alert" state while nippling
- Progress to and engage in mutually positive parent/caregiver–infant/child interactions during feedings

Parent/Family Will (Specify Time Frame):

- Recognize necessity of adequate calories for appropriate weight gain and optimal growth and development
- Learn to read and respond contingently to infant's behavioral cues (e.g., hunger, satiety, approach/engagement, stress/avoidance/disengagement)
- Learn strategies that promote organized infant behavior
- Learn appropriate positioning and handling techniques
- Learn effective ways to relieve stress behaviors during nippling
- Learn ways to help infant coordinate suck-swallow-breathe sequence (i.e., external pacing techniques)
- Engage in mutually positive interactions with infant during feeding
- Recognize ways to facilitate effective feedings: feed in quiet-alert state; keep length of feeding appropriate; burp; prepare/structure environment; recognize signs of sensory overload; encourage self-regulation; respect need for breaks and breathing pauses; avoid pulling and twisting nipple during pauses; allow infant to resume sucking when ready; provide oral support (cheek and/or jaw) as needed; use appropriate nipple hole size and flow rate

Nursing Interventions

- Refer to care plans for **Disorganized Infant behavior, Risk for disorganized Infant behavior,** and **Effective, Ineffective,** and **Interrupted Breastfeeding** and assess as needed.
- Interventions follow a sequential pattern of implementation that can be adapted as appropriate.

• = Independent ▲ = Collaborative

- Assess coordination of infant's suck, swallow, and gag reflex.
▲ Provide developmentally supportive neonatal intensive care for preterm infants.
- Provide opportunities for kangaroo (i.e., skin-to-skin) care.
▲ Before the infant is ready for oral feedings, implement gavage feedings (or other alternative) as ordered, using breast milk whenever possible.
- Provide a naturalistic environment for tube feedings (naso-orogastric, gavage, or other) that approximates a pleasurable oral feeding experience: hold in semi-upright/flexed position; offer nonnutritive sucking; pace feedings; allow for semi-demand feedings contingent with infant cues; offer rest breaks; burp, as appropriate.
- Consider trophic (i.e., small volume) feedings for high-risk hospitalized infants if appropriate.
- Allow parent(s) to feed the infant when possible.
- Position preterm infant in semi-upright position, with head in neutral alignment, chin slightly tucked, back straight, shoulders/arms forward, hands in midline, hips flexed 90 degrees.
- Feed infant in the quiet-alert state.
- Determine the appropriate shape, size, and hole of nipple to provide flow rate for preterm infants.
- Implement pacing for infants having difficulty coordinating breathing with sucking and swallowing.
- Provide infants with jaw and/or cheek support, as needed.
- Allow appropriate time for nipple feeding to ensure infant's safety, limiting to 15 to 20 minutes for bottle feeding.
- Monitor length of breastfeeding so that it does not exceed 30 minutes.
- Encourage transitioning from scheduled to semi-demand feedings, contingent with infant behavior cues.
▲ Refer to a multidisciplinary team (e.g., neonatal/pediatric nutritionist, physical or occupational therapist, speech pathologist, lactation specialist) as needed.

Home Care

- The above appropriate interventions may be adapted for home care use.

● = Independent   ▲ = Collaborative

▲ Infants with risk factors and clinical indicators of feeding problems present prior to hospital discharge should be referred to appropriate community early-intervention service providers (e.g., community health nurses), early learning programs (individualized per states), occupational therapy, (speech pathologists, feeding specialists) to facilitate adequate weight gain for optimal growth and development.

Client/Family Teaching and Discharge Planning

- Provide anticipatory guidance for infant's expected feeding course.
- Teach various effective feeding methods and strategies to parent(s).
- Teach parents how to read, interpret, and respond contingently to infant cues.
- Help parents identify support systems prior to hospital discharge.
- Provide anticipatory guidance for the infant's discharge.

Readiness for enhanced Fluid balance

NANDA-I Definition

A pattern of equilibrium between fluid volume and chemical composition of body fluids that is sufficient for meeting physical needs and can be strengthened

Defining Characteristics

Dehydration; expresses willingness to enhance fluid balance; good tissue turgor; intake adequate for daily needs; moist mucous membranes; no evidence of edema; no excessive thirst; specific gravity within normal limits; stable weight; straw-colored urine; urine output appropriate for intake

Client Outcomes

Client Will (Specify Time Frame):

- Maintain light yellow urine output
- Maintain elastic skin turgor, moist tongue, and mucous membranes
- Explain measure that can be taken to improve fluid intake

● = Independent ▲ = Collaborative

Nursing Interventions

- Discuss normal fluid requirements.
- Recommend the client choose mainly water to meet fluid needs, although fruit juices and milk are also useful for hydration. The intake of beverages containing caffeine or alcohol is no longer thought to cause dehydration.
- Recommend the client choose and prepare foods with less salt, aiming for a maximum of 1500 mg per day, less than a teaspoon. The CDC recommends that all salt-sensitive Americans, including everyone 40 years or older, should decrease daily sodium intake.
- Recommend the client avoid intake of soft drinks with sugar; instead, encourage the client to drink water.
- Recommend the client note the color of urine at intervals when voiding. Normal urine is straw-colored or amber.
- Recommend client monitor weight at intervals for alterations.

Geriatric

- Encourage the elderly client to develop a pattern of drinking water regularly.
- Ensure that when food intake is reduced or limited, it is compensated with an increase in water/fluid intake.
- Incorporate regular hydration into daily routines, such as providing an extra glass of fluid with medication or during social activities. Consider using a beverage cart to routinely offer beverages to clients in extended care facilities.

Risk for imbalanced Fluid Volume

NANDA-I Definition

At risk for a decrease, increase, or rapid shift from one to the other of intravascular, interstitial, and/or intracellular fluid that may compromise health. This refers to body fluid loss, gain, or both

Risk Factors

Abdominal surgery; ascites; burns; intestinal obstruction; pancreatitis; receiving apheresis; sepsis; traumatic injury (e.g., fractured hip)

• = Independent   ▲ = Collaborative

Client Outcomes

- Lung sounds clear, respiratory rate 12 to 20, and free of dyspnea
- Urine output greater than 0.5 mL/kg/hr
- Blood pressure, pulse rate, temperature, and oxygen saturation within expected range
- Laboratory values within expected range, i.e., normal serum sodium, hematocrit, and osmolarity
- Extremities and dependent areas free of edema
- Mental orientation appropriate based on previous condition

F

Nursing Interventions

Surgical Clients

- Monitor the fluid balance. If there are symptoms of hypovolemia, refer to the interventions in the care plan **Deficient Fluid Volume.** If there are symptoms of hypervolemia, refer to the interventions in the care plan **Excess Fluid Volume.**

Preoperative

- Collect a thorough history and perform a preoperative assessment to identify clients with increased risk for hemorrhage or hypovolemia, that is, clients with recent traumatic injury, abnormal bleeding or clotting times, complicated renal/liver disease, diabetes, cardiovascular disease, major organ transplant, history of aspirin and/or NSAID use, anticoagulant therapy, or history of hemophilia, von Willebrand's disease, or disseminated intravascular coagulation.
- Recognize that NPO at midnight may or may not be appropriate for each surgical client. Guidelines from the American Society of Anesthesiologists (ASA) in 2011 recommend the following: healthy clients having elective surgery should be allowed to have clear liquids up to 2 hours prior to.
- Determine length of time the client has been without normal intake, NPO, or experienced fluid loss, i.e., vomiting, diarrhea, bleeding, etc.
- Determine and document the client's mental status.

• = Independent   ▲ = Collaborative

F

- Recognize that there is conflicting evidence regarding liberal intraoperative fluid management versus restrictive fluid management.
- Recognize that an individualized fluid management plan would be the best treatment plan at this time until further research is conducted on intraoperative fluid.
- Recognize that research has shown no evidence to support that using colloids versus crystalloids in hypovolemia reduces risk of death, pulmonary edema, or length of stay.
- Recognize the effects of general anesthetics, inhalational agents, and of regional anesthesia on perfusion in the body, and decreasing the blood pressure.
- Monitor for signs of intraoperative hypovolemia: dry skin, dry mucous membranes, tachycardia, decreased urinary output, decreased central venous pressure, hypotension, increased pulse, and/or deep rapid respirations.
- Monitor for signs of intraoperative hypervolemia: dyspnea, coarse crackles, increased pulse and respirations, and decreased urinary output, all of which could progress to pulmonary edema.
- In the critically ill surgical client with a pulmonary artery catheter, pulmonary artery pressures should be monitored as they can be helpful to determine fluid balance and guide fluid and vasoactive IV drip administration.
- Monitor the client for hyponatremia, that is, headache, anorexia, nausea and vomiting, diarrhea, tachycardia, general malaise, muscle cramps, weakness, lethargy, change in mental status, disorientation, seizures, and death.
- Monitor clients undergoing laparoscopic or hysteroscopic procedures for the development of hyponatremia, hypervolemia, and pulmonary edema when an irrigation fluid is used.
- Monitor clients undergoing TURP (transurethral resection of the prostate) procedures for development of hyponatremia, and hypervolemia with symptoms of TURP syndrome: headache, visual changes, agitation, lethargy, vomiting, muscle twitching, bradycardia, diminished pupillary reflexes, hypertension, and respiratory distress.

• = Independent   ▲ = Collaborative

F

- Measure the irrigation fluid used during urological and gyne-cological procedures accurately for volume deficit, that is, amount of irrigation used minus amount of irrigation recovered via suction.
- Monitor intraoperative intake and output including blood loss, urine output, and third-space losses, to provide an estimate of fluid volume.
- Monitor the client for fluid extravasation in and around the surgical area.
- Assess the liposuction client for fluid and electrolyte imbalance, including fluid overload and hyponatremia.
- Observe the surgical client for hyperkalemia, that is, dysrhythmias, heart block, asystole, abdominal distention, and weakness.
- Maintain the client's core temperature at normal levels, using warming devices as needed.

Postoperative

- Recognize that restrictive fluid management is supported postoperatively.
- Observe the client for development of tissue edema.
- Recognize that IV fluid replacement should not be based on hourly urine output only—weight, blood pressure, heart rate, output from any drains, and hemoglobin results should also be utilized.

Geriatric

- Check skin turgor of elderly client on the forehead, sub-clavian area, or inner thigh; also look for the presence of longitudinal furrows on the tongue and dry mucous membranes.
- Note the color of urine and compare against a urine color chart to monitor adequate fluid intake; also note BUN/creatinine lab results. Monitor elderly clients for excess fluid volume during the treatment of deficient fluid volume: listen to lung sounds, watch for edema, and note vital signs.

Pediatric

- Assess the pediatric client's weight, length of NPO status, underlying illness, and the surgical procedure to be performed.
- Recognize that newborns require very little fluid replacement when undergoing major surgical procedures during the first few days of life.
- Monitor pediatric surgical clients closely for signs of fluid loss.
- Administer fluids preoperatively until NPO status must be initiated, so that fluid deficit is decreased.
- Perform an assessment for signs of dehydration in the pediatric client.

Deficient Fluid Volume

NANDA-I Definition

Decreased intravascular, interstitial, and/or intracellular fluid. This refers to dehydration, water loss alone without change in sodium level

Defining Characteristics

Change in mental state; decreased blood pressure, pulse pressure and pulse volume; decreased skin and tongue turgor; decreased urine output; decreased venous filling; dry mucous membranes; dry skin; elevated hematocrit; increased body temperature; increased pulse rate; increased urine concentration; sudden weight loss (except in third spacing); thirst; weakness

Related Factors (r/t)

Active fluid volume loss; failure of regulatory mechanisms

Client Outcomes

Client Will (Specify Time Frame):

- Maintain urine output of 0.5 mL/kg/hour
- Maintain normal blood pressure, pulse, and body temperature
- Maintain elastic skin turgor; moist tongue and mucous membranes; and orientation to person, place, and time
- Explain measures that can be taken to treat or prevent fluid volume loss
- Describe symptoms that indicate the need to consult with health care provider

• = Independent   ▲ = Collaborative

Nursing Interventions

F

- Watch for early signs of hypovolemia, including thirst, restlessness, headaches, and inability to concentrate. Thirst is often the first sign of dehydration.
- Recognize symptoms of cyanosis, cold clammy skin, weak thready pulse, confusion, and oliguria as late signs of hypovolemia.
- Monitor pulse, respiration, and blood pressure of clients with deficient fluid volume every 15 minutes to 1 hour for the unstable client, every 4 hours for the stable client.
- Check orthostatic blood pressures with the client lying, sitting, and standing. Note skin turgor over bony prominences such as the hand or shin.
- Monitor for the existence of factors causing deficient fluid volume (e.g., vomiting, diarrhea, difficulty maintaining oral intake, fever, uncontrolled type 2 diabetes, diuretic therapy).
- Observe for dry tongue and mucous membranes, and longitudinal tongue furrows.
- Recognize that checking capillary refill may not be helpful in identifying fluid volume deficit. Capillary refill can be normal in clients with sepsis, increased body temperature dilates peripheral blood vessels, and capillary return may be immediate.
- Weigh client daily and watch for sudden decreases, especially in the presence of decreasing urine output or active fluid loss.
- Monitor total fluid intake and output every 4 hours (or every hour for the unstable client). Recognize that urine output is not always an accurate indicator of fluid balance.
- Note the color of urine and specific gravity.
- Provide fresh water and oral fluids preferred by the client (distribute over 24 hours [e.g., 1200 mL on days, 800 mL on evenings, and 200 mL on nights]); provide prescribed diet; offer snacks (e.g., frequent drinks, fresh fruits, fruit juice); instruct significant other to assist the client with feedings as appropriate.
- ▲ Provide oral replacement therapy as ordered and tolerated with a hypotonic glucose-electrolyte solution when the client has acute diarrhea or nausea/vomiting. Provide small, frequent quantities of slightly chilled solutions.

• = Independent   ▲ = Collaborative

▲ Administer antidiarrheals and antiemetics as ordered and appropriate.
▲ Hydrate the client with ordered isotonic IV solutions if prescribed.
• Assist with ambulation if the client has postural hypotension.

Critically Ill

• Monitor central venous pressure, right atrial pressure, and pulmonary capillary wedge pressure for decreases.
• Monitor serum and urine osmolality, serum sodium, BUN/creatinine ratio, and hematocrit for elevations.
▲ Insert an indwelling urinary catheter if ordered and measure urine output hourly. Notify physician if urine output is less than 0.5 mL/kg/hr.
▲ When ordered, initiate a fluid challenge of crystalloids (0.9% normal saline or lactated Ringer's) for replacement of intravascular volume; monitor the client's response to prescribed fluid therapy and fluid challenge, especially noting central venous pressure and pulmonary capillary wedge pressure readings, vital signs, urine output, blood lactate concentrations, and lung sounds.
• Position the client flat with legs elevated when hypotensive, if not contraindicated.
▲ Monitor trends in serum lactic acid levels and base deficit obtained from blood gases as ordered.
▲ Consult physician/provider if signs and symptoms of deficient fluid volume persist or worsen.

Pediatric

• Monitor the child for signs of deficient fluid volume, including sunken eyes, decreased tears, dry mucous membranes, poor skin turgor, and decreased urine output.
▲ Reinforce the physician's recommendation for the parents to give the child oral rehydration fluids to drink in the amounts specified, especially during the first 4 to 6 hours to replace fluid losses. Consider using diluted oral rehydration fluids. Once the child is rehydrated, an orally administered maintenance solution should be used along with food.

• = Independent   ▲ = Collaborative

F

- Recommend that the mother resume breastfeeding as soon as possible.
- Recommend that parents not give the child decarbonated soda, fruit juices, gelatin dessert, or instant fruit drink mix. Instead give child the oral rehydration fluids ordered, and when tolerated, food.
- Once the child has been rehydrated, begin feeding regular food other than avoiding milk products.

Geriatric

- Monitor elderly clients for deficient fluid volume carefully, noting new onset of weakness, dizziness, and postural hypotension.
- Evaluate the risk for dehydration using the Dehydration Risk Appraisal Checklist.
- Check skin turgor of elderly client on the forehead, subclavian area, or inner thigh; also look for the presence of longitudinal furrows on the tongue and dry mucous membranes.
- Encourage fluid intake by offering fluids regularly to cognitively impaired clients.
- Incorporate regular hydration into daily routines (e.g., extra glass of fluid with medication or social activities). Because of their low water reserves, it may be prudent for the elderly to learn to drink regularly when not thirsty. Consider use of a beverage cart and a hydration assistant to routinely offer increased beverages to clients in extended care.
- If client is identified as having chronic dehydration, flag the food tray to indicate to caregivers he should finish 75% to 100% of his food and fluids.
- Recognize that lower blood pressures and a higher BUN/creatinine ratio can be significant signs of dehydration in the elderly.
- Note the color of urine and compare against a urine color chart to monitor adequate fluid intake.
- Monitor elderly clients for excess fluid volume during the treatment of deficient fluid volume: listen to lung sounds, watch for edema, and note vital signs.

● = Independent ▲ = Collaborative

Home Care

- Teach family members how to monitor output in the home (e.g., use of commode "hat" in the toilet, urinal, or bedpan, or use of catheter and closed drainage). Instruct them to monitor both intake and output. Use common terms such as "cups" or glasses of water a day when providing education.
- When weighing the client, use same scale each day. Be sure scale is on a flat, not cushioned, surface. Do not weigh the client with scale placed on any kind of rug.
- Teach family about complications of deficient fluid volume and when to call physician.
- If the client is receiving IV fluids, there must be a responsible caregiver in the home. Teach caregiver about administration of fluids, complications of IV administration (e.g., fluid volume overload, speed of medication reactions), and when to call for assistance. Assist caregiver with administration for as long as necessary to maintain client safety.
- Identify an emergency plan, including when to call 911.
- Support the family/client in a palliative care situation to decide if it is appropriate to intervene for deficient fluid volume or to allow the client to die without fluids.

Client/Family Teaching and Discharge Planning

- Instruct the client to avoid rapid position changes, especially from supine to sitting or standing.
- Teach the client and family about appropriate diet and fluid intake.
- Teach the client and family how to measure and record intake and output accurately.
- Teach the client and family about measures instituted to treat hypovolemia and to prevent or treat fluid volume loss.
- Instruct the client and family about signs of deficient fluid volume that indicate they should contact health care provider.

● = Independent   ▲ = Collaborative

Excess Fluid Volume

NANDA-I Definition

Increased isotonic fluid retention

Defining Characteristics

Adventitious breath sounds; altered electrolytes; anasarca, anxiety, azotemia, blood pressure changes; change in mental status; changes in respiratory pattern, decreased hematocrit, decreased hemoglobin, dyspnea, edema, increased central venous pressure; intake exceeds output, jugular vein distention, oliguria; orthopnea; pleural effusion; positive hepatojugular reflex; pulmonary artery pressures; increased pulmonary congestion; restlessness; specific gravity changes; S_3 heart sound; weight gain.

Related Factors (r/t)

Compromised regulatory mechanism; excess fluid intake; excess sodium intake

Client Outcomes

Client Will (Specify Time Frame):
- Remain free of edema, effusion, anasarca
- Maintain body weight appropriate for the client
- Maintain clear lung sounds; no evidence of dyspnea or orthopnea
- Remain free of jugular vein distention, positive hepatojugular reflex, and gallop heart rhythm
- Maintain normal central venous pressure, pulmonary capillary wedge pressure, cardiac output, and vital signs
- Maintain urine output of 0.5 mL/kg/hr or more with normal urine osmolality and specific gravity
- Explain actions that are needed to treat or prevent excess fluid volume including fluid and dietary restrictions, and medications
- Describe symptoms that indicate the need to consult with health care provider

• = Independent ▲ = Collaborative

Nursing Interventions

- Monitor location and extent of edema, use the 1+ to 4+ scale to quantify edema; also measure the legs using a millimeter tape in the same area at the same time each day. Note differences in measurement between extremities.
- Monitor daily weight for sudden increases; use same scale and type of clothing at same time each day, preferably before breakfast.
- Monitor intake and output; note trends reflecting decreasing urine output in relation to fluid intake.
- Monitor vital signs; note decreasing blood pressure, tachycardia, and tachypnea. Monitor for S_3 heart sounds. If signs of heart failure are present, see the care plan for **Decreased Cardiac output.**
- Listen to lung sounds for crackles, monitor respirations for effort, and determine the presence and severity of orthopnea.
- Monitor serum and urine osmolality, serum sodium, BUN/creatinine ratio, and hematocrit for abnormalities.
- With head of bed elevated 30 to 45 degrees, monitor jugular veins for distention in the upright position; assess for positive hepatojugular reflex.
- Monitor the client's behavior for restlessness, anxiety, or confusion; use safety precautions if symptoms are present.
- ▲ Monitor for the development of conditions that increase the client's risk for excess fluid volume, including heart failure, renal failure, and liver failure, all of which result in decreased glomerular filtration rate and fluid retention.
- ▲ Provide a restricted-sodium diet as appropriate if ordered.
- ▲ Monitor serum albumin level and provide protein intake as appropriate.
- ▲ Administer prescribed diuretics as appropriate; check blood pressure before administration to ensure it is adequate. If IV administration of a diuretic, note and record the blood pressure and urine output following the dose.
- Monitor for side effects of diuretic therapy: orthostatic hypotension (especially if the client is also receiving ACE inhibitors), hypovolemia, and electrolyte imbalances (hypokalemia and hyponatremia).

• = Independent   ▲ = Collaborative

▲ Implement fluid restriction as ordered, especially when serum sodium is low; include all routes of intake. Schedule limited intake of fluids around the clock, and include the type of fluids preferred by the client.

• Maintain the rate of all IV infusions, carefully utilizing an IV pump.

• Turn clients with dependent edema frequently (i.e., at least every 2 hours).

▲ Provide ordered care for edematous extremities including compression, elevation, and muscle exercises.

• Promote a positive body image and good self-esteem. Refer to the care plan for **Disturbed Body Image.**

▲ Consult with physician if signs and symptoms of excess fluid volume persist or worsen.

Critically Ill

▲ Insert an indwelling urinary catheter if ordered and measure urine output hourly. Notify physician if less than 0.5 mL/kg/hr.

▲ Monitor central venous pressure, mean arterial pressure, pulmonary capillary wedge pressure, and cardiac output/index; note and report trends indicating increasing or decreasing pressures over time.

▲ Monitor the effects of infusion of diuretic drips. Perform continuous renal replacement therapy (CRRT) as ordered if the client is critically ill, hemodynamically unstable, and excessive fluid must be removed.

Geriatric

• Recognize that the presence of fluid volume excess is particularly serious in the elderly.

• Monitor electrolyte levels carefully, including sodium levels and potassium levels, with both increased and decreased levels possible. Refer to the care plan for **Risk for Electrolyte imbalance.**

Home Care

• Assess client and family knowledge of disease process causing excess fluid volume.

• = Independent   ▲ = Collaborative

- ▲ Teach about disease process and complications of excess fluid volume, including when to contact the physician/provider.
- • Assess client and family knowledge and compliance with medical regimen, including medications, diet, rest, and exercise. Assist family with integrating restrictions into daily living.
- ▲ Teach and reinforce knowledge of medications. Instruct the client not to use over-the-counter (OTC) medications (e.g., diet medications) without first consulting the physician/provider.
- ▲ Instruct the client to make the primary physician/provider aware of medications ordered by other physicians.
- • Identify emergency plan for rapidly developing or critical levels of excess fluid volume when diuresing is not safe at home.
- ▲ Teach about signs and symptoms of both excess and deficient fluid volume such as darker urine and when to call physician.

Client/Family Teaching and Discharge Planning

- • Describe signs and symptoms of excess fluid volume and actions to take if they occur.
- ▲ Teach client on diuretics to weigh self daily in the morning, and notify the physician/provider if there is a 2.2 lb (1.0 kg) or more weight gain.
- ▲ Teach the importance of fluid and sodium restrictions. Help the client and family to devise a schedule for intake of fluids throughout entire day. Refer to dietitian concerning implementation of low-sodium diet.
- • Teach clients how to measure and document intake and output with common household measurements such as cups.
- ▲ Teach how to take diuretics correctly: take one dose in the morning and second dose (if taken) no later than 4 PM. Adjust potassium intake as appropriate for potassium-losing or potassium-sparing diuretics. Note the appearance of side effects such as weakness, muscle cramps, hypertension, palpitations, or irregular heartbeat.
- • For the client undergoing hemodialysis, teach client the required restrictions in dietary electrolytes, protein and fluid. Spend time with the client to detect any factors that may interfere with the client's compliance with the fluid restriction or restrictive diet.

• = Independent   ▲ = Collaborative

Risk for Deficient Fluid Volume

NANDA-I Definition

At risk for experiencing decreased intravascular, interstitial, and/or intracellular fluid. This refers to a risk for dehydration, water loss alone without change in sodium.

G

Risk Factors

Active fluid volume loss; deficient knowledge; deviations affecting absorption of fluids; deviations affecting access of fluids; deviations affecting intake of fluids; excessive losses through normal routes (e.g., diarrhea); extremes of age; extremes of weight; factors influencing fluid needs (e.g., hypermetabolic state); failure of regulatory mechanisms; loss of fluid through abnormal routes (e.g., indwelling tubes); pharmaceutical agents (e.g., diuretics)

Client Outcomes, Nursing Interventions, and Client/Family Teaching

Refer to care plan for **Deficient Fluid** Volume.

Impaired Gas Exchange

NANDA-I Definition

Excess or deficit in oxygenation and/or carbon dioxide elimination at the alveolar-capillary membrane

Defining Characteristics

Abnormal arterial blood gases; abnormal arterial pH; abnormal breathing (e.g., rate, rhythm, depth); abnormal skin color (e.g., pale, dusky); confusion; cyanosis; decreased carbon dioxide; diaphoresis; dyspnea; headache upon awakening; hypercapnia; hypoxemia; hypoxia; irritability; nasal flaring; restlessness, somnolence; tachycardia; visual disturbances

Related Factors (r/t)

Ventilation-perfusion imbalance; alveolar-capillary membrane changes

• = Independent   ▲ = Collaborative

Client Outcomes

Client Will (Specify Time Frame):

* Demonstrate improved ventilation and adequate oxygenation as evidenced by blood gas levels within normal parameters for that client
* Maintain clear lung fields and remain free of signs of respiratory distress
* Verbalize understanding of oxygen supplementation and other therapeutic interventions

G

Nursing Interventions

* Monitor respiratory rate, depth, and ease of respiration. Watch for use of accessory muscles and nasal flaring.
* Auscultate breath sounds every 1 to 2 hours. Listen for diminished breath sounds, crackles, and wheezes.
* Monitor the client's behavior and mental status for the onset of restlessness, agitation, confusion, and (in the late stages) extreme lethargy.
* ▲ Monitor oxygen saturation continuously using pulse oximetry. Correlate arterial oxygen saturation blood gas results with pulse oximetry.
* Observe for cyanosis of the skin; especially note color of the tongue and oral mucous membranes.
* Position the client in a semirecumbent position with the head of the bed at a 30- to 45-degree angle to decrease the aspiration of gastric, oral, and nasal secretions.
* If the client has unilateral lung disease, position with head of bed at 30 to 45 degrees with "good lung down" for about 1 hour at a time.
* ▲ If the client is acutely dyspneic, consider having the client lean forward over a bedside table, resting elbows on the table if tolerated.
* Help the client deep breathe and perform controlled coughing. Have the client inhale deeply, hold the breath for several seconds, and cough two or three times with the mouth open while tightening the upper abdominal muscles as tolerated. Controlled coughing uses the diaphragmatic muscles, which

makes the cough more forceful and effective. If the client has
excessive fluid in the respiratory system, refer to the care plan
Ineffective Airway clearance.

▲ Monitor the effects of sedation and analgesics on the client's
respiratory pattern; use judiciously.

• Schedule nursing care to provide rest and minimize fatigue.

▲ Administer humidified oxygen through an appropriate device
(e.g., nasal cannula or Venturi mask per the physician's/pro-
vider order); aim for an oxygen (O_2) saturation level of 90%
oxygen saturation or above. Watch for onset of hypoventilation as evidenced by increased somnolence.

• Assess nutritional status including serum albumin level and
body mass index (BMI).

• Assist the client to eat small meals frequently and use dietary
supplements as necessary.

• If the client is severely debilitated from chronic respiratory disease, consider the use of a wheeled walker to help in
ambulation.

▲ Watch for signs of psychological distress including anxiety,
agitation, depression, and insomnia. Refer for counseling as
needed.

▲ Refer the COPD client to a pulmonary rehabilitation
program.

Critical Care

▲ Assess and monitor oxygen indices such as the PF ratio
($FIO_2:pO_2$), venous oxygen saturation/oxygen consumption
(SVO_2 or $ScVO_2$).

▲ Turn the client every 2 hours. Monitor mixed venous oxygen
saturation closely after turning. If it drops below 10% or fails
to return to baseline promptly, turn the client back into the
supine position, check vital signs, and evaluate oxygen status.
If the client does not tolerate turning, consider use of a kinetic
bed that rotates the client from side to side in a turn of at
least 40 degrees.

▲ If the client has adult respiratory distress syndrome with difficulty maintaining oxygenation, consider positioning the client
prone with the upper thorax and pelvis supported, allowing

the abdomen to protrude. Monitor oxygen saturation and turn back to supine position if desaturation occurs. If the client becomes ventilator dependent, refer to the care plan **Impaired spontaneous Ventilation.**

Geriatric

▲ Use central nervous system (CNS) depressants carefully to avoid decreasing respiration rate.

• Recognize that the elderly have decreased pulmonary function with age, and that results in decreased gas exchange and pulmonary reserve function. Also, the elderly are more vulnerable to develop pneumonia because of decreased immune function.

Home Care

• Work with the client to determine what strategies are most helpful during times of dyspnea. Educate and empower the client to self-manage the disease associated with impaired gas exchange.

▲ Collaborate with physicians regarding long-term oxygen administration for chronic respiratory failure clients with severe resting hypoxemia. Administer long-term oxygen therapy greater than 15 hours daily for pO_2 less than 55 or SaO_2 at or below 88%.

• Assess the home environment for irritants that impair gas exchange. Help the client to adjust the home environment as necessary (e.g., install an air filter to decrease the level of dust).

▲ Refer the client to occupational therapy as necessary to assist the client in adaptation to the home and environment and in energy conservation.

• Assist the client with identifying and avoiding situations that exacerbate impairment of gas exchange (e.g., stress-related situations, exposure to pollution of any kind, proximity to noxious gas fumes such as chlorine bleach).

• Refer to GOLD guidelines for management of home care and indications of hospital admission criteria.

• Instruct the client to keep the home temperature above 68° F (20° C) and to avoid cold weather.

G

- Instruct the client to limit exposure to persons with respiratory infections.
- Instruct the family in the complications of the disease and the importance of maintaining the medical regimen, including when to call a physician.
▲ Refer the client for home health aide services as necessary for assistance with activities of daily living.
- When respiratory procedures are being implemented, explain equipment and procedures to family members, and provide needed emotional support.
- When electrically based equipment for respiratory support is being implemented, evaluate home environment for electrical safety, proper grounding, and so on. Ensure that notification is sent to the local utility company, the emergency medical team, and police and fire departments.
▲ Watch for family role changes and coping ability. Refer the client to medical social services as appropriate for assistance in adjusting to chronic illness.
- Support the family of the client with chronic illness.

Client/Family Teaching and Discharge Planning

- Teach the client how to perform pursed-lip breathing and inspiratory muscle training, and how to use the tripod position. Have the client watch the pulse oximeter to note improvement in oxygenation with these breathing techniques.
- Teach the client energy conservation techniques and the importance of alternating rest periods with activity. See nursing interventions for **Fatigue.**
▲ Teach the importance of not smoking. Refer to smoking cessation programs, and encourage clients who relapse to keep trying to quit. Ensure that client receives appropriate medications to support smoking cessation from the primary health care provider.
▲ Instruct the family regarding home oxygen therapy if ordered (e.g., delivery system, liter flow, safety precautions, number of tanks needed).
▲ Teach the client the need to receive a yearly influenza vaccine.
- Teach the client relaxation techniques to help reduce stress responses and panic attacks resulting from dyspnea.

• = Independent   ▲ = Collaborative

Risk for dysfunctional Gastrointestinal Motility

NANDA-I Definition

At risk for increased, decreased, ineffective, or lack of peristaltic activity within the gastrointestinal system

Risk Factors

G

Abdominal surgery; aging; anxiety; change in food; change in water; decreased gastrointestinal circulation; diabetes mellitus; food intolerance (e.g., gluten, lactose); gastroesophageal reflux disease (GERD); immobility; infection (e.g., bacterial, parasitic, viral): pharmaceutical agents (e.g., antibiotics, laxatives, narcotics/opiates, proton pump inhibitors); prematurity; sedentary lifestyle; stress; unsanitary food preparation

Client Outcomes, Nursing Interventions, and Client/ Family Teaching

Refer to care plan for **Dysfunctional Gastrointestinal Motility.**

Dysfunctional Gastrointestinal Motility

NANDA-I Definition

Increased, decreased, ineffective, or lack of peristaltic activity within the gastrointestinal system

Defining Characteristics

Absence of flatus; abdominal cramping; abdominal distention; abdominal pain; accelerated gastric emptying; bile-colored gastric residual; change in bowel sounds (e.g., absent, hypoactive, hyperactive); diarrhea; dry stool; difficulty passing stool; hard stool; increased gastric residual; nausea; regurgitation; vomiting

Related Factors (r/t)

Aging; anxiety; enteral feedings; food intolerance (e.g., gluten, lactose); immobility; ingestion of contaminates (e.g., food, water); malnutrition; pharmaceutical agents (e.g., narcotics/opiates, laxatives, antibiotics, anesthesia); prematurity; sedentary lifestyle; surgery

• = Independent   ▲ = Collaborative

G

Client Outcomes

Client Will (Specify Time Frame):
- Be free of abdominal distention and pain
- Have normal bowel sounds
- Pass gas rectally at intervals
- Defecate formed, soft stool every day to every third day
- State has an appetite
- Be able to eat food without nausea and vomiting

Nursing Interventions

- Monitor for abdominal distention, and presence of abdominal pain.
- Auscultate for bowel sounds noting characteristics and frequency, also palpate, and percuss the abdomen.
- Review history noting any anorexia, dyspepsia, nausea/vomiting, abnormal characteristics of bowel movements, including frequency, consistency, and the presence of gas. Other symptoms may include relation of symptoms to meals, especially if aggravated by food, early satiety, postprandial fullness/bloating, and weight loss (more with severe gastroparesis).
- Have client keep a diary of time food and fluid was consumed as it compares to pattern of defecation, including, but not limited to, consistency, amount, and frequency of.
- Monitor for fluid deficits by checking skin turgor, and moisture of tongue. Refer to care plan **Deficient Fluid Volume** if relevant.
- ▲ Monitor for nutritional deficits by keeping close track of food intake. Review laboratory studies that affirm nutritional deficits, such as decreased albumin and serum protein levels, liver profile, glucose, and an electrolyte panel. Refer to care plan **Imbalanced Nutrition: less than body requirements** or **Risk for Electrolyte Imbalance** as appropriate.

Slowed Gastrointestinal Motility

- Monitor the client for signs and symptoms of decreased gastric motility, which may include delayed emptying, nausea

---

• = Independent   ▲ = Collaborative

after meals, vomiting, heartburn, diarrhea, feeling full quickly while eating, abdominal bloating and/or pain, anorexia, and reflux.

▲ Monitor daily laboratory studies, ensuring ordered glucose levels are done and evaluated.

▲ If client has nausea and vomiting, provide an antiemetic and intravenous fluids as ordered. Refer to the care plans for **Nausea.**

▲ Evaluate medications the client is taking.

• Obtain a thorough gastrointestinal history if the client has diabetes, as they are at high risk for gastroparesis and gastric reflux.

▲ Review laboratory and other diagnostic tools, including complete blood count (CBC), amylase, thyroid-stimulating hormone level, glucose with other metabolic studies, upper endoscopy, and gastric-emptying scintigraphy.

▲ Obtain nutritional consult, considering diets lower or higher in liquids or solids, especially fats, depending on gastric motility

▲ Recommend eating small meals and soft (well cooked) foods as they may relieve symptoms of slower motility.

▲ If client is unable to eat or retain food, consult with the registered dietitian and physician, considering further nutritional support in the form of enteral or parenteral feedings for the client with gastroparesis.

▲ If client is receiving gastric enteral nutrition (EN), evaluate gastric residual volume (GRV) per hospital protocol. See the care plan **Risk for Aspiration.**

▲ Administer prokinetic medications as ordered.

▲ For the client with nausea and vomiting associated with gastroparesis, review use of tricyclics, in addition to the traditional antiemetics and other prokinetic drugs.

▲ Recognize that acupuncture may be an option for both slowed and increased gastric motility.

Postoperative Ileus

• Observe for complications of delayed intestinal motility. Symptoms include abdominal pain and distention, nausea, cramping, anorexia, and sometimes bloating. Other signs include tympany to percussion, with absence of flatus, bowel sounds or bowel.

▲ Recommend chewing gum for the routine postoperative patient who is experiencing an ileus, is not at risk for aspiration, and has normal dentition.

• Determine if the client is a smoker.

• Help the client out of bed to walk at least two times per day.

▲ If postoperative ileus is associated with opioid pain medication, request an order for a peripherally acting opioid antagonist.

▲ Note serum electrolyte levels, especially potassium and magnesium.

Increased Gastrointestinal Motility

▲ Observe for complications of gastric surgeries such as dumping syndrome.

• Watch for nausea, vomiting, bloating, cramping, diarrhea, dizziness, and fatigue.

• Monitor for low blood sugar, weakness, sweating, and dizziness 1 to 3 hours after eating as this is when late rapid gastric emptying may occur.

▲ Order a nutritional consult to discuss diet changes. Encourage several small meals per day that are low in carbohydrates, and higher in fiber supplements and fat. Space fluids around meal times, not with them.

▲ Give intravenous fluids as ordered for the client complaining of diarrhea with weakness and dizziness.

▲ Review the client's medication profile, including current medication list, noting those that may increase gastric motility.

• Offer bathroom, commode, or bedpan assistance, depending on frequency, amount of diarrhea, and condition of client.

• Refer to the care plans for the nursing diagnoses of **Deficient Fluid Volume, Nausea, and Diarrhea** as relevant.

Pediatric

• Assess infants and children with suspected delayed gastric for fullness and vomiting.

• = Independent ▲ = Collaborative

- Continue to encourage the mother of a baby diagnosed with delayed gastric emptying to breastfeed, reinforcing the benefits of breastfeeding.
▲ If the infant is already on a bottle, encourage parents to discuss with the pediatrician a switch to a hypoallergenic formula.
▲ Observe for nutritional and fluid deficits with assessment of skin turgor, mucous membranes, fontanels, furrows of the tongue, electrolyte panel, fluid status, and cardiopulmonary function.
▲ Recommend gentle massage for preterm infants as appropriate.

Geriatric

- Closely monitor diet and medication use/side effects as they affect the gastrointestinal system. Watch for constipation.
▲ Watch for symptoms of dysphagia, gastroesophageal reflux disease, dyspepsia, irritable bowel syndrome, maldigestion, and reduced absorption of nutrients.
▲ If client takes metoclopramide for gastroesophageal reflux disease or slowed gastric motility, assess indication and side effects. Recognize that metoclopramide can cause drug-induced Parkinson's disease in the elderly, in addition to other neurotoxic side effects

Client/Family Teaching and Discharge Planning

- Teach the client and caregivers about their medications, reinforcing the side effects as they relate to gastrointestinal function.
▲ Recommend possible exercise programs if appropriate.
- Teach client and caregivers to report signs and symptoms that may indicate further complications including increased abdominal girth, projectile vomiting, and unrelieved acute cramping pain (bowel obstruction).
▲ Recommend signs and symptoms of dehydration with client and caregivers.

Risk for ineffective Gastrointestinal Perfusion

NANDA-I Definition

At risk for decrease in gastrointestinal circulation

Risk Factors

Abdominal aortic aneurysm; abdominal compartment syndrome; abnormal partial thromboplastin time; abnormal prothrombin time; acute gastrointestinal bleed; acute gastrointestinal hemorrhage; age ≥60 years; anemia; coagulopathy (e.g., sickle cell anemia); diabetes mellitus; disseminated intravascular coagulation; female gender; gastric paresis (e.g., diabetes mellitus); gastroesophageal varices; gastrointestinal disease (e.g., duodenal or gastric ulcer, ischemic colitis, ischemic pancreatitis); hemodynamic instability; liver dysfunction; myocardial infarction; poor left ventricular performance; renal failure; stroke; trauma; smoking; treatment-related side effects (e.g., cardiopulmonary bypass, medication, anesthesia, gastric surgery); vascular disease (e.g., peripheral vascular disease, aortoiliac occlusive disease)

Client Outcomes

Client Will (Specify Time Frame):

- Maintain blood pressure within normal limits
- Remain free from abdominal distention
- Tolerate feedings without nausea, vomiting, or abdominal discomfort
- Pass stools of normal color, consistency, frequency, and amount
- Describe prescribed diet regimen
- Describe prescribed medication regimen including medication actions and possible side effects
- Verbalize understanding of treatment regimen including monitoring for signs and symptoms that may indicate problems with gastrointestinal tissue perfusion, the importance of diet and exercise to gastrointestinal health

Nursing Interventions

▲ Complete pain assessment. Assess and document the onset, intensity, character, location, duration, aggravating factors, and relieving factors. Determine whether the pain is exacerbated by eating. Notify the provider for any increase in pain or discomfort or if comfort measures are not effective.

● = Independent   ▲ = Collaborative

G

- Monitor vital signs frequently as needed watching for hypotension and tachycardia.
- Encourage the client to eat small, frequent meals rather than three larger meals. Encourage the client to rest after eating to maximize blood flow to the stomach and improve digestion.
- Perform a physical abdominal examination including inspection, auscultation, percussion, and palpation. Complete the assessment in the described order.
- Monitor frequency, consistency, color, and amount of stools.
- Assess for abdominal distention. Measure abdominal girth and compare to client's accustomed waist or belt size.
▲ Monitor for gastrointestinal side effects from medication administrations, particularly NSAIDs. Discuss the possibility of prescribing a gastroprotective agent such as a proton pump inhibitor with the provider for clients requiring long-term administration of NSAIDs.
- Review the client's medical and surgical history. Certain conditions place clients at higher risk for ineffective tissue perfusion (e.g., diabetes mellitus, abdominal surgery, cardiothoracic surgery, trauma, mechanical ventilation). In addition to medical or surgical conditions, lifestyle choices such as smoking or cocaine and amphetamine use affect tissue perfusion.
- Recognize that any client who has been in a shock state is vulnerable to decreased gastrointestinal perfusion, and watch for symptoms as just identified.
- Encourage the client to ambulate or perform activity as tolerated, but vigorous activity or heavy lifting should be avoided for several hours after meals.
▲ Monitor intake and output to evaluate fluid and electrolyte balance, and review laboratory data as ordered.
▲ Prepare client for diagnostic or surgical procedures. Diagnostic studies may include abdominal x-ray to rapidly rule out intestinal obstruction, CT, angiography, and abdominal ultrasound. Surgical procedures include exploratory laparotomy, thrombectomy, surgical revascularization, and/or stent placement.
- Recognize that ineffective gastrointestinal perfusion may be an emergency situation necessitating immediate care to save bowel function or life of the client.

Pediatric

- Monitor vital signs frequently. Notify physician if significant deviation from baseline.
- Monitor oxygen saturation and provide oxygen therapy as ordered. Take steps to prevent hypovolemia and hypotensive episodes. Avoid periods of physiological stress, which can lead to hypoxemia. Minimize environmental stressors.
- Monitor tolerance of enteral feedings.
- Monitor patients at risk for abdominal compartment syndrome for signs of increased abdominal pressure.

Geriatric

▲ Recognize that decreased gastrointestinal perfusion, either acute or chronic, is much more common in the elderly.

▲ Be aware that gastrointestinal bleeding that is difficult to control in the elderly may be associated with decreased gastrointestinal perfusion.

Client/Family Teaching and Discharge Planning

- Provide client teaching related to risk factors for ineffective gastrointestinal tissue perfusion, signs and symptoms, lifestyle changes that can improve gastrointestinal functioning. Start with the client's base level of understanding and use that as a foundation for further education.
- Teach client about any medications prescribed. Medication teaching includes the drug name, its purpose, administration instructions such as taking it with or without food, and any side effects to be aware of. Instruct the client to report any adverse side effects to his/her provider.

Risk for unstable blood Glucose level

NANDA-I Definition

Risk for variation of blood glucose/sugar levels from the normal range

● = Independent   ▲ = Collaborative

Risk Factors

Deficient knowledge of diabetes management (e.g., action plan); developmental level; dietary intake; inadequate blood glucose monitoring; lack of acceptance of diagnosis; lack of adherence to diabetes management (e.g., action plan); lack of diabetes management (e.g., action plan); medication management; mental health status; physical activity level; physical health status; pregnancy; rapid growth periods; stress; weight gain; weight loss

Client Outcomes

Client Will (Specify Time Frame):

- Maintain A_{1C} less than 7% (normal level 4% to 6%)
- Maintain less stringent A_{1C} goals than 7% in clients with a history of severe hypoglycemia, advanced diabetes complications, or limited life expectancy
- Maintain outpatient preprandial blood glucose between 70 and 130 mg/dL; consult primary care provider for client-specific goals
- Maintain outpatient postprandial glucose below 180 mg/dL
- In gestational diabetes, maintain preprandial blood glucose ≤ 95 mg/dL, 1-hour pc level at or below 140 mg/dL, and 2-hour pc level at or below 120 mg/dL
- In a pregnant mother with preexisting type 1 or 2 diabetes, maintain premeal, bedtime, and overnight blood glucose 60-99 mg/dL, peak postprandial glucose 100-129 mg/dL, and A_{1C} <6%
- In critically ill hospitalized clients, maintain blood glucose between 140 and 180 mg/dL
- In noncritically ill hospitalized clients, maintain premeal blood glucose values below 140 mg/dL and random blood glucose values below 180 mg/dL. Higher levels may be acceptable in terminally ill patients.
- Demonstrate how to accurately test blood glucose
- Identify self-care actions to take to maintain target glucose levels
- Identify self-care actions to take if blood glucose level is too low or too high
- Demonstrate correct administration of prescribed medications

● = Independent   ▲ = Collaborative

Nursing Interventions

▲ Check blood glucose three or more times daily.

▲ Evaluate blood glucose levels in hospitalized clients
before administering oral hypoglycemic agents or insulin.
Adjust timing of medication appropriately with meal
times.

▲ Monitor blood glucose every 30 minutes to 2 hours for clients
on continuous insulin drips.

▲ Consider continuous glucose monitoring (CGM) in
clients with type 1 diabetes on intensive insulin
regimens.

▲ Evaluate A_{1C} level for glucose control over previous 2 to 3
months.

• Consider monitoring 1 to 2 hours post meal in individuals
who have premeal glucose values within target but have A_{1C}
values above target.

• Discuss with provider relaxing goals for clients who have
comorbid conditions, shortened life expectancy, frequent
hypoglycemia, or hypoglycemia unawareness.

• Monitor for signs and symptoms of hypoglycemia, such as
shakiness, dizziness, sweating, hunger, headache, pallor, behavior changes, confusion, or seizures.

▲ Be alert for hypoglycemia in clients receiving 0.6 unit/kg
insulin or more daily, and in clients receiving NPH
insulin.

▲ If client is experiencing signs and symptoms of hypoglycemia, test glucose and if result is below 70 mg/dL, administer
15 to 20 g glucose (½ cup fruit juice or regular [not diet]
soda, 1 cup milk, 1 small piece of fruit, or 3 to 4 glucose
tablets). Repeat test in 15 minutes and repeat treatment if
indicated. Once SMBG glucose returns to normal, the individual should consume a meal or snack to prevent recurrence
of hypoglycemia.

▲ Administer intramuscular/subcutaneous glucagon according
to agency protocol if client is hypoglycemic and is unable to
take oral carbohydrate. For severe hypoglycemia, an IV infusion of 10% dextrose or 25% to 50% IV bolus dextrose may
be used.

• = Independent   ▲ = Collaborative

- Monitor for signs and symptoms of hyperglycemia, such as increased thirst or urination, or high blood or urine glucose levels.
▲ Ensure an acutely ill client is receiving adequate fluids and carbohydrates. Adjustment in oral hypoglycemic or insulin therapy may be required.
▲ Test urine or blood for ketones in ketosis-prone clients during acute illness, trauma, surgery or stress.
▲ Prime IV tubing with 20 mL of diluted IU insulin solution before initiating insulin drip.
▲ Evaluate client's medication regimen for medications that can alter blood glucose.
▲ Refer client to dietitian for carbohydrate counting instruction.
▲ Refer overweight clients to dietitian for weight loss counseling.
- For interventions regarding foot care, refer to the care plan **Ineffective peripheral Tissue Perfusion.**

Geriatric

- Watch for age-related cognitive changes that can impair self-management of diabetes.
- Monitor for vision and dexterity impairments that may affect the older client's ability to accurately measure insulin doses.
- Encourage self-monitoring of blood glucose for residents of extended care facilities who are capable of doing so.
- Assist client to set up pill boxes or a reminder system for taking medications.
- Teach older clients the importance of verifying symptoms with a glucometer reading.

Pediatric

- Be aware that young children (younger than 6 or 7 years) may not be aware of symptoms of hypoglycemia.
▲ Teach adolescents older than 12 years to monitor blood glucose frequently as ordered.
- Teach self-efficacy measures to adolescents with type 1 diabetes who are involved in family conflict.

Home Care

▲ Teach family how to use an emergency glucagon kit (if prescribed).

Multicultural

- Provide culturally appropriate diabetes health education.
- Involve Hispanic community workers *(promotoras)* when working with Hispanic clients with diabetes.
- Encourage involvement of African American clients' family and friends in diabetes education activities.

Client/Family Teaching and Discharge Planning

- Provide "survival skills" education for hospitalized clients, including information about (1) diabetes and its treatment, (2) medication administration, (3) nutrition therapy, (4) self-monitoring of blood glucose, (5) symptoms and treatment of hypoglycemia, (6) basic foot care, and (7) follow-up appointments for in-depth training.
- Evaluate clients' monitoring technique initially at regular intervals.
- ▲ Refer client to a diabetes treatment and teaching program (DTTP) for training in flexible intensive insulin therapy and dietary freedom.
- ▲ Refer client for Blood Glucose Awareness Training (BGAT) or web-based training available at http://www.BGAThome.com for instruction in detection, anticipation, avoidance, and treatment of extremes in blood glucose levels.
- Teach client to maintain a blood glucose diary.
- Provide group-based training programs for instruction.
- Teach client the importance of at least 150 minutes/week of moderate-intensity aerobic physical activity (50% to 70% of maximum heart rate).
- Discuss recommending resistance training with client's provider.
- Teach client with type 1 diabetes to avoid vigorous activity if ketones are present in urine or blood.

● = Independent ▲ = Collaborative

- Teach clients who are treated with insulin or insulin-stimulating oral agents to eat added carbohydrates prior to exercise if glucose levels are below 100 mg/dL.
- Teach client and family members regarding sick day management, including importance of early contact with provider, continuing insulin or medication unless instructed otherwise, frequent monitoring, and oral intake.

G

Grieving

NANDA-I Definition

A normal, complex process that includes emotional, physical, spiritual, social, and intellectual responses and behaviors by which individuals, families, and communities incorporate an actual, anticipated, or perceived loss into their daily lives

Defining Characteristics

Alteration in activity level; alterations in dream patterns; alterations in immune function; alterations in neuroendocrine function; alteration in sleep patterns; anger; blame; detachment; despair; disorganization; experiencing relief; maintaining connection to the deceased; making meaning of the loss; pain; panic behavior; personal growth; psychological distress; suffering

Related Factors (r/t)

Anticipatory loss of significant object (e.g., possession, job, status, home, parts and processes of body); anticipatory loss of a significant other; death of a significant other; loss of significant object (e.g., possession, job, status, home, parts and processes of body)

Client/Family Outcomes

Client/Family Will (Specify Time Frame):

- Discuss meaning of the loss to his/her life and the functioning of the family
- Identify ways to support family members and articulate methods of support he or she requires from family and friends
- Accept assistance in meeting the needs of the family from friends/extended family

● = Independent ▲ = Collaborative

Nursing Interventions

Anticipatory Grieving Interventions

- Grieving of the client, and family/relatives of a critically ill and dying client for the losses experienced during the deteriorating illness, and the future that will be filled with loss.
- Develop a trusting relationship both with the client and with the family by using presence and therapeutic communication techniques.
- Keep the family apprised of the client's ongoing condition as much as possible. Consult with the family for decision-making as appropriate.
- Keep the family informed on clients' needs for physical care and support in symptom control, and inform them about health care options at the end of life including palliative care, hospice care, and home care.
- Encourage the family to touch the client as desired; when near death encourage holding the hand, or foot, or wherever can reach and is acceptable to the client and family member.
- Ask family members if receiving sufficient sleep. If a family member desires to be in the room for sleep, provide a reclining chair or portable bed if possible, and bedding to keep the family member comfortable. If needed, find housing for family member from out of town with support of case manager, or social worker.
- Ask family member when last ate if appropriate. Touch family members as appropriate.
- Listen to the family member's story.
- Encourage family members to show their caring feelings and talk to the client. Recognize and respect different feelings and wishes from both the family members and client.
- If necessary, refer a family member for counseling or minister/priest to help him cope with the existential questions and current overwhelming reality.
- Recognize that one family member may be in a state of caregiver role strain from a long caregiving situation. See the care plan **Caregiver Role Strain** if appropriate.
- Promote the family roles as appropriate.

● = Independent   ▲ = Collaborative

- Promote mutual goal setting where decisions are made together that affect the family.

Grieving Interventions When Death of a Loved One Occurs

- Utilize the following activities when interacting with the bereaved person:
  - Be present and attentive, use active empathetic listening.
  - Validate the client's feelings of grief, and feeling hurt, stressful, anxious, out of control, and further symptoms of grieving.
  - Provide time and space for the person to tell his story of loss.
  - Offer condolences: "I am sorry that you lost your husband."
  - Explain that the feelings will oscillate, as the person does grief work, from coping to accept the loss, to coping to build a new life without the loved one.
  - Intentionally schedule meetings with the family member(s) to provide support during grieving.
  - Refer to mental health providers as needed.
- Help the client utilize a method to give voice to his unique story of loss. Methods to do this include: Keeping a personal journal to record feelings and insights/Retelling of the loss narrative to a caring person/Music therapy techniques with a trained therapist, or listening to music that has significance to the relationship/Use of the "Virtual Dream," a dreamlike short story written by the grieving person to tell the narrative of the loss.
- Discuss coping methods with the grieving person. Common coping techniques used include exercise, telling the story of grief to a caring person, journaling, pets, and developing a legacy for the deceased.
- Encourage the family to create a quiet and comfortable healing environment, and follow comforting grief rituals such as prayer, interacting with nature, or lighting votive candles.
- ▲ Refer the family members for spiritual counseling if desired.

• = Independent   ▲ = Collaborative

- Help the family determine the best way and place to find social support. Encourage family members to continue to use supports as needed for years.
- Identify available community resources, including bereavement groups at local hospitals and hospice centers. Volunteers who provide bereavement support can also be effective.
- Watch for signs of complicated grieving. These include the absence of support in a person's social network, the presence of a concurrent life crisis, a highly ambivalent marital relationship that preceded the spouse's death, traumatic circumstances surrounding the death such as suicide, homicide or traffic accident, bereavement with young children, limited economic resources, high self-reproach, high pining, and persistent anger associated with grieving.

Pediatric/Parent

- Treat the child with respect, give him or her opportunity to talk about concerns, and answer questions honestly.
- Listen to the child's expression of grief.
- Help parents recognize that the grieving child does not have to be "fixed"; instead they need support going through an experience of grieving just as adults.
- Consider the use of art for children in hospice care who are dying or dealing with the death of a parent, sibling, or other family member.
▲ Refer grieving children and parents to a program to help facilitate grieving if desired, especially if the death was traumatic.
- Help the adolescent determine sources of support and how to use them effectively.
- Encourage grieving parents to take good care of their own health.
▲ Encourage grieving parents to seek mental health services as needed.
- Recognize that men and women often grieve differently, and explain this to parents if it becomes an issue.

- Recognize that mothers who have a miscarriage grieve and experience sorrow because of loss of the child.

Geriatric

- Monitor an older adult who has been treated for bereavement-related depression for relapse or recurrence.
- Provide support for the family when the loss is associated with dementia of the family member.
- Pay careful attention to the older adult's self-care.
- Determine the social supports of older adults.

Multicultural

- See Nursing Interventions in care plans for **Complicated Grieving** and **Chronic Sorrow.**

Home Care

- The interventions previously described may be adapted for home care use.
- Assessment of ADLs and IADLs is essential as part of comprehensive care after a home care client has suffered the loss of a loved one.
- Actively listen as the client grieves for his or her own death or for real or perceived loss. Normalize the client's expressions of grief for self. Demonstrate a caring and hopeful approach.
- ▲ Refer the client to medical social services as necessary for losses not related to death.
- ▲ Refer the bereaved to hospice bereavement programs, or an Internet self-help group.

Complicated Grieving

NANDA-I Definition

A disorder that occurs after the death of a significant other in which the experience of distress accompanying bereavement fails to follow normative (or cultural) expectations and manifests in functional impairment

● = Independent   ▲ = Collaborative

G

Defining Characteristics

Decreased functioning in life roles; decreased sense of well-being; depression; experiencing somatic symptoms of the deceased; fatigue; grief avoidance; longing for the deceased; low levels of intimacy; persistent emotional distress; preoccupation with thoughts of the deceased; rumination; searching for the deceased; self-blame; separation distress; traumatic distress; verbalizes anxiety; verbalizes distressful feelings about the deceased; verbalizes feeling dazed; verbalizes feeling empty; verbalizes feeling in shock; verbalizes feeling stunned; verbalizes feelings of anger; verbalizes feelings of detachment from others; verbalizes feelings of disbelief; verbalizes feelings of mistrust; verbalizes lack of acceptance of the death; verbalizes persistent painful memories; verbalizes self-blame; yearning

Related Factors (r/t)

Death of a significant other; emotional instability; lack of social support; sudden death of a significant other, dementia caregiving, loss of a child

Client Outcomes

Client Will (Specify Time Frame):

- Express appropriate feelings of guilt, fear, anger, or sadness
- Identify somatic distress associated with grief (e.g., anxiety, changes in appetite, insomnia, nightmares, loss of libido, decreased energy, altered activity levels)
- Seek support in dealing with grief-associated issues
- Identify personal strengths and effective coping strategies
- Function at a normal developmental level and begin to successfully and increasingly perform activities of daily living

Nursing Interventions

- Watch for signs of complicated grieving that include symptoms that persist at least 6 months after the death and are experienced at least daily or to a disabling degree. Symptoms include feeling emotionally numb, stunned, shocked, and that life is meaningless; dysfunctional thoughts and maladaptive behaviors; experiencing mistrust and estrangement from others; anger and bitterness over the loss; identity confusion; avoidance of the reality of the loss, or excessive proximity seeking to try to feel closer to the deceased, sometimes focused on wishes to die or suicidal statements and behavior; or difficulty moving on with life. Symptoms must be associated with functional impairment.

▲ Determine the client's state of grieving. Use a tool such as the Prolonged Grief Disorder Scale, the Grief Support in Health Care Scale, the Hogan Grief Reaction Checklist, and the Beck Depression Inventory.

▲ Determine whether the client is experiencing depression, suicidal tendencies, or other emotional disorders. Refer the client for counseling or therapy as appropriate.

• Educate the client and his or her support systems that grief resolution is not a sequential process and that the positive outcome of grief resolution is the integration of the deceased into the ongoing life of the griever.

▲ Assess caregivers, particularly younger caregivers, for pessimistic thinking and additional stressful life events and refer for appropriate support.

• See the Nursing Interventions in the care plans for **Grieving** and **Chronic Sorrow.**

Pediatric/Parent

▲ Refer grieving children and parents to a program to help facilitate grieving if desired, especially if the death was traumatic.

• Encourage grieving parents to take good care of their own health.

▲ Encourage grieving parents to seek mental health services as needed.

• Help the adolescent determine sources of support and how to use them effectively. If client is an adolescent exposed to a peer's suicide, watch for symptoms of traumatic grief as well as PTSD, which include numbness, preoccupation with the deceased, functional impairment, and poor adjustment to the loss.

See the pediatric and parent interventions in the care plans for **Grieving** and **Chronic Sorrow.**

• = Independent   ▲ = Collaborative

Geriatric

- Pay careful attention to the older adult's self-care.
- Those who have lived with elders with dementia and experienced significant feelings of loss before the loved one's death may be at risk for more intense feelings of grief after the death of the client with dementia.
- ▲ Elderly people experience complicated grieving with physical and mental health problems especially when the deceased is a child or spouse.

Multicultural

- Assess for the influence of cultural beliefs, norms, and values on the client's grief and mourning practices.
- Encourage discussion of the grief process.
- Identify whether the client had been notified of the health status of the deceased and was able to be present during illness and death.

Home Care

- Consider providing support via the Internet.

Risk for complicated Grieving

NANDA-I Definition

At risk for a disorder that occurs after the death of a significant other, in which the experience of distress accompanying bereavement fails to follow normative expectations and manifests in functional impairment

Risk Factors

Death of a significant other, lack of social support, emotional instability

Client Outcomes, Nursing Interventions, and Client/Family Teaching and Discharge Planning

Refer to care plan for **Complicated** Grieving.

● = Independent   ▲ = Collaborative

Risk for disproportionate Growth

NANDA-I Definition

At risk for growth above the 97th percentile or below the 3rd percentile for age, crossing two percentile channels

Risk Factors

Caregiver

Abuse; learning difficulties (mental handicap); mental illness; or severe learning disability

Environmental

Deprivation; economically disadvantaged; lead poisoning; natural disasters; teratogen; violence

Individual

Anorexia; caregiver's maladaptive feeding behaviors; chronic illness; individual maladaptive feeding behaviors; infection; insatiable appetite; malnutrition; prematurity; substance abuse

Prenatal

Congenital disorders; genetic disorders; maternal infection; maternal nutrition; multiple gestation; substance abuse; teratogen exposure

Client Outcomes

Client/Parents/Primary Caregiver Will (Specify Time Frame):

- State information related to possible teratogenic agents
- Identify components of healthy nutrition that will promote growth
- Maintain or improve weight to be within a healthy range for age and sex

Nursing Interventions

Preconception/Pregnancy

- Counsel women who smoke to quit smoking prior to conception if possible and to avoid smoking and secondhand smoke while pregnant.

● = Independent   ▲ = Collaborative

- Assess alcohol consumption of pregnant women and advise those that drink alcohol to discontinue all use of alcohol through the pregnancy.
- Assess and limit exposure to all drugs (prescription, "recreational," and over the counter) and give the mother information on known teratogenic agents.
- All women of childbearing age who are capable of becoming pregnant should take 400 mcg of folic acid daily.
▲ Promote a team approach toward preconception and pregnancy glucose control for women with diabetes.
▲ Advise women with mental health disorders to seek appropriate counseling prior to pregnancy.

Pediatric

- Consider regular breast milk and protein-fortified breast milk for low-birth-weight infants in the neonatal intensive care unit.
- Provide tube feedings per physician's orders when appropriate for clients with neuromuscular impairment.
- Provide for adequate nutrition and nutritional monitoring in clients with medical disorders requiring chronic medication and those with developmental delay.
- Adequate intake of vitamin D is set at 400 IU/day by the National Academy of Sciences. Because adequate sunlight exposure is difficult to determine, a supplement of 400 IU/day is recommended for the following groups to prevent rickets and vitamin D deficiency in healthy infants and children:
  - All breastfed infants unless they are weaned to at least 500 mL/day of vitamin D–fortified formula or milk
  - All non-breastfed infants who are ingesting less than 500 mL/day of vitamin D–fortified formula or milk
  - Children and adolescents who do not receive regular sunlight exposure, do not ingest at least 500 mL/day of vitamin D–fortified milk, or do not take a daily multivitamin supplement containing at least 400 IU of vitamin D
- Provide adequate nutrition to clients with active intestinal inflammation.

* Encourage limiting "screen time" (television, video games, Internet, smart phones, and tablets) to less than 2 hours/day for children.

Multicultural

* Assess the influence of cultural beliefs, norms, values, and expectations on parents' perceptions of normal growth and development.
* Focus nutritional education on promoting good nutrition and physically active lifestyles for healthy child development as opposed to only for prevention or reduction of overweight.
* Assess for the influence of acculturation.
* Assess whether the parents are concerned about the amount of food eaten.
* Assess the influence of family support on patterns of nutritional intake.
* Negotiate with clients regarding which aspects of healthy nutrition can be modified while still honoring cultural beliefs.
* Encourage parental efforts at increasing physical activity and decreasing dietary fat for their children.

Home Care

* The interventions previously described may be adapted for home care use.
* Assess parental perception of their child's weight.
* Assess family meal planning and family participation in meal-time activities such as eating together at a scheduled time.

Client/Family Teaching and Discharge Planning

* Educate families and children about providing healthy meals and healthy eating to improve learning ability.

Delayed Growth and Development

NANDA-I Definition

Deviations from age-group norms

● = Independent ▲ = Collaborative

Defining Characteristics

Altered physical growth; decreased response time; delay in performing skills typical of age group; difficulty in performing skills typical of age group; flat affect; inability to perform self-care activities appropriate for age; inability to perform self-control activities appropriate for age; listlessness

Related Factors (r/t)

G

Effects of physical disability; environmental deficiencies; inadequate caretaking; inconsistent responsiveness; indifference; multiple caretakers; prescribed dependence; separation from significant others; stimulation deficiencies

Client Outcomes

Client/Parents/Primary Caregiver Will (Specify Time Frame):

- Describe realistic, age-appropriate patterns of growth and development
- Promote activities and interactions that support age-related developmental tasks
- Display consistent, sustained achievement of age-appropriate behaviors (social, interpersonal, and/or cognitive) and/or motor skills
- Achieve realistic developmental and/or growth milestones based on existing abilities, extent of disability, and functional age
- Attain steady gains in growth patterns

Nursing Interventions

Pregnancy/Pediatric

- Counsel women who smoke to quit smoking prior to conception if possible and to avoid smoking and secondhand smoke while pregnant.
- To determine risk for or actual deviations in normal development, consider the use of a screening tool.
- Regularly compare height and weight measurements for the child or adolescent with established age-appropriate norms and previous measurements.

• = Independent   ▲ = Collaborative

- Provide opportunities for mother-infant skin-to-skin contact (kangaroo care) for preterm infants.
- Provide normal sleep-wake times for clients to promote growth and development.
▲ Engage the child in appropriate play activities. Refer the child to a child life therapist or recreational therapist (if available) for supplemental strategies.

Multicultural

- Assess the influence of cultural beliefs, norms, and values on the client's perceptions of child development.
- Assess and identify for possible environmental conditions, which may be a contributing factor to altered growth and development.
- Acknowledge racial and ethnic differences at the onset of care.
- Provide information on the effects of environmental risk exposure on growth and development.

Home Care

- The interventions previously described may be adapted for home care use.
- Assess whether exposure to violence or parental stress is contributing to developmental problems.
▲ Refer premature neonates for follow-up home care and assessment of functional performance.
▲ If possible, refer the family to a program of animal-assisted therapy.

Client/Family Teaching and Discharge Planning

- Encourage parents to take infants and children for routine health visits to the family physician or pediatrician.
- Encourage parents of children with language delays to approach their physician during regular visits regarding the delay.
- Provide parents and/or caregivers realistic expectations for attainment of growth and development milestones. Clarify expectations and correct misconceptions.
- Instruct the client regarding appropriate baby equipment and the importance of buying new equipment rather than used.

• = Independent   ▲ = Collaborative

- Elicit the involvement of parents and caregivers in social support groups and parenting classes.
- Assess whether parents may benefit from Internet/electronic support groups.
- See care plans **Risk for disproportionate Growth/Risk for delayed Development.**

H

Deficient community Health

NANDA-I Definition

Presence of one or more health problems or factors that deter wellness or increase the risk of health problems experienced by an aggregate

Defining Characteristics

Incidence of risks relating to hospitalization experienced by aggregates or populations; incidence of risks relating to physiological states experienced by aggregates or populations; incidence of risks relating to psychological states experienced by aggregates or populations; incidence of health problems experienced by aggregates or populations; no program available to enhance wellness for an aggregate or population; no program available to prevent one or more health problems for an aggregate or population; no program available to reduce one or more health problems for an aggregate or population; no program available to eliminate one or more health problems for an aggregate or population

Related Factors

Lack of access to public health care providers; lack of community experts; limited resources; program has inadequate budget; program has inadequate community support; program has inadequate consumer satisfaction; program has inadequate evaluation plan; program has inadequate outcome data; program partly addresses health problem

Client Outcomes

Community/Adolescents/Minority Clients Will (Specify Time Frame):
- Provide programs for healthy behaviors
- Demonstrate goal setting

• = Independent ▲ = Collaborative

- Describe and comply with healthy behaviors
- Describe and demonstrate compliance with HBV education and testing

Nursing Interventions

Refer to care plans: **Readiness for enhanced Community Coping, Ineffective Community Coping, Ineffective Health Maintenance, Impaired Home Maintenance, Risk for Other-directed Violence**

- Encourage healthy nutrition and exercise among community members using the resources available to the community.
- Facilitate goal setting in the community for behavior change related to diet and exercise for overweight and obese adults.

Pediatric

▲ Consider a community-based program for young people that encourages health-related behavior changes, increasing fruit and vegetable intake and engaging in activity.

▲ Support religious affiliation and positive school climates for adolescents, particularly for lesbian, gay, and bisexual youths in the community.

Geriatric

▲ Assess homeless elderly veterans in the community for suicidal behavior and make appropriate referrals.

▲ Provide community-dwelling older women with psychoeducation about aging skills and behaviors and cognitive function that includes group discussion.

Multicultural

- Provide information about the pervasiveness and deadly consequence of HBV for Asians in the United States.

Home Care and Client/Family Teaching and Discharge Planning

- The above interventions may be adapted for home care and client/family teaching.
- Provide support for establishment of a community garden.

• = Independent   ▲ = Collaborative

Risk-prone Health Behavior

NANDA-I Definition

Impaired ability to modify lifestyle/behaviors in a manner that improves health status

Defining Characteristics

Demonstrates nonacceptance of health status change; failure to achieve optimal sense of control; failure to take action that prevents health problems; minimizes health status change

Related Factors (r/t)

Excessive alcohol; inadequate comprehension; inadequate social support; low self-efficacy; low socioeconomic status; multiple stressors; negative attitude toward health care; smoking

Client Outcomes

Client Will (Specify Time Frame):

- State acceptance of change in health status
- Request assistance in altering behaviors to adapt to change
- State personal goals for dealing with change in health status and means to prevent further health problems
- State experience of a period of grief that is proportional to the actual or perceived effect of the loss
- Report and/or demonstrate behavior changes mutually agreed upon with nurse as evidence of positive adaptation

Nursing Interventions

- Assess the client's definitions of health and wellness and major barriers to health and wellness.
- Use motivational interviewing to help the client identify and change unhealthy behaviors.
- Allow the client adequate time to express feelings about the change in health status.
- Use open-ended questions to allow the client free expression (e.g., "Tell me about your last hospitalization" or "How does this time compare?").

• = Independent   ▲ = Collaborative

- Help the client work through the stages of grief that occur as part of a psychological adaptation to illness.
- Encourage visitation and communication with family/close relatives of clients including during episodes of critical illness.
- Discuss the client's current goals. If appropriate, have the client list goals so that they can be referred to and steps can be taken to accomplish them. Support hope that the goals will be accomplished.
- ▲ Encourage participation in appropriate wellness programs associated with health changes.
- Provide assistance with activities as needed.
- Give the client positive feedback for accomplishments, no matter how small. Support the client and family and promote their strengths and coping skills.
- Manipulate the environment to decrease stress; allow the client to display personal items that have meaning.
- Maintain consistency and continuity in daily schedule. When possible, provide the same caregiver.
- Promote use of positive spiritual influences.
- ▲ Refer to community resources. Provide general and contact information for ease of use.

Pediatric

- Encourage visitation of children when family members are in intensive care.
- ▲ Refer parents of critically ill children to an intervention program such as COPE, a theory-based intervention program.
- Use visualization and distraction during chest physiotherapy for children with cystic fibrosis.

Geriatric

- ▲ Assess for signs of depression resulting from illness-associated changes and make appropriate referrals.
- Use open-ended questions in screening for depression in the elderly.
- Support activities that promote usefulness of older adults.
- ▲ Encourage social support.

• = Independent   ▲ = Collaborative

- Monitor the client for agitation associated with health problems. Support family caring for elders with agitation.

Multicultural

- Assess for the influence of cultural beliefs, norms, and values on the client's ability to modify health behavior.
- Assess the role of fatalism on the client's ability to modify health behavior.
- Encourage spirituality as a source of support for coping.
- Negotiate with the client regarding the aspects of health behavior that will need to be modified.

Home Care

- The above interventions may be adapted for home care use.
- Take the client's perspective into consideration, and use a holistic approach in assessing and responding to client planning for the future.
- Assist the client to adapt to his/her diagnosis and to live with the disease.
- ▲ Refer the client to a counselor or therapist for follow-up care. Initiate community referrals as needed (e.g., grief counseling, self-help groups).
- Refer to care plan for **Powerlessness.**

Client/Family Teaching and Discharge Planning

- Assess family/caregivers for coping and teaching/learning styles.
- Foster communication between the client/family and medical staff.
- Educate and prepare families regarding the appearance of the client and the environment before initial exposure.
- Help the client to enjoy a sense of "wellness." Provide support for progress and support enjoyment of the physical, emotional, spiritual, and social aspects of life.
- Teach a client and his or her family relaxation techniques (controlled breathing, guided imagery) and help them practice.
- Allow the client to proceed at own pace in learning; provide time for return demonstrations (e.g., self-injection of insulin).

● = Independent   ▲ = Collaborative

- If long-term deficits are expected, inform the family as soon as possible.
- Provide clients with information on how to access and evaluate available health information via the Internet.

Ineffective Health Maintenance

NANDA-I Definition

Inability to identify, manage, and/or seek out help to maintain health

Defining Characteristics

Demonstrated lack of adaptive behaviors to environmental changes; demonstrated lack of knowledge about basic health practices; history of lack of health-seeking behavior; inability to take responsibility for meeting basic health practices; impairment of personal support systems; lack of expressed interest in improving health behaviors

Related Factors (r/t)

Cognitive impairment; complicated grieving; deficient communication skills; diminished fine motor skills; diminished gross motor skills; inability to make appropriate judgments; ineffective family coping; ineffective individual coping; insufficient resources (e.g., equipment, finances); lack of fine motor skills; lack of gross motor skills; perceptual impairment; spiritual distress; unachieved developmental tasks

Client Outcomes

Client Will (Specify Time Frame):

- Discuss fear of or blocks to implementing health regimen
- Follow mutually agreed on health care maintenance plan
- Meet goals for health care maintenance

Nursing Interventions

- Assess the client's feelings, values, and reasons for not following the prescribed plan of care. See Related Factors.
- Assess for family patterns, economic issues, and cultural patterns that influence compliance with a given medical regimen.

- Help the client to choose a healthy lifestyle and to have appropriate diagnostic screening tests.
- Assist the client in reducing stress.
- Help the client determine how to manage complex medication schedules (e.g., HIV/AIDS regimens or polypharmacy).
- Identify complementary healing modalities, such as herbal remedies, acupuncture, healing touch, yoga, or cultural shamans that the client uses in addition to or instead of the prescribed allopathic regimen.
- ▲ Refer the client to appropriate services as needed.
- Identify support groups related to the disease process.
- Use technology such as text messaging to remind clients of scheduled appointments.

Geriatric

- Assess the client's perception of health.
- Assist client to identify both life- and health-related goals.
- Provide information that supports informed decision-making.
- Discuss with the client and support person realistic goal-setting for changes in health maintenance.
- Educate the client about the symptoms of life-threatening illness, such as myocardial infarction (MI), and the need for timeliness in seeking care.

Multicultural

- Assess influence of cultural beliefs, norms, and values on the client's ability to modify health behavior.
- Assess the effect of fatalism on the client's ability to modify health behavior.
- Assess for use of and reasons for not using health services.
- Clarify culturally related health beliefs and practices.
- Provide culturally targeted education and health care services.

Home Care

- The interventions described previously may be adapted for home care use.
- ▲ Provide nurse-led case management.

• = Independent   ▲ = Collaborative

- Include a health-promotion focus for the client with disabilities, with the goals of reducing secondary conditions (e.g., obesity, hypertension, pressure sores), maintaining functional independence, providing opportunities for leisure and enjoyment, and enhancing overall quality of life.
- Encourage a regular routine for health-related behaviors.
- Provide support and individual training for caregivers before the client is discharged from the hospital.
- Assist client to develop confidence in ability to manage the health condition.
- Consider a written contract with the client to follow the agreed-upon health care regimen. Written agreements reinforce the verbal agreement and serve as a reference.
- Using self-care management precepts, instruct the client about possible situations to which he or she may need to respond; include the use of role playing. Instruct in generating hypotheses from available evidence rather than solely from experience.

Client/Family Teaching and Discharge Planning

- Provide the family with website addresses where information can be obtained from the Internet. (Most libraries have Internet access with printing capabilities.)
▲ Develop collaborative multidisciplinary partnerships.
- Tailor both the information provided and the method of delivery of information to the specific client and/or family.
- Obtain or design educational material that is appropriate for the client; use pictures if possible.
- Teach the client about the symptoms associated with discontinuation of medications, such as a selective serotonin reuptake inhibitor (SSRI).
- Explain nonthreatening aspects before introducing more anxiety-producing information regarding possible side effects of the disease or medical regimen.
- Treat tobacco use as a chronic problem. Tailor the smoking cessation program to the individual. Consider mixed groups of current and past smokers.

• = Independent   ▲ = Collaborative

Impaired Home Maintenance

NANDA-I Definition

Inability to independently maintain a safe, growth-promoting immediate environment

Defining Characteristics

Objective

Disorderly surroundings; inappropriate household temperature; insufficient clothes; insufficient linen; lack of clothes; lack of linen; lack of necessary equipment; offensive odors; overtaxed family members; presence of vermin; repeated unhygienic disorders; repeated unhygienic infections; unavailable cooking equipment; unclean surroundings

Subjective

Household members report difficulty in maintaining their home in a comfortable fashion; household members report financial crises; household members report outstanding debts; household members request assistance with home maintenance

Related Factors (r/t)

Deficient knowledge; disease; illness; impaired functioning; inadequate support systems; injury; insufficient family organization; insufficient family planning; insufficient finances; lack of role modeling; unfamiliarity with neighborhood resources

Client Outcomes

Client Will (Specify Time Frame):

- Maintain a healthy home environment
- Use community resources to assist with home care needs

Nursing Interventions

- Assess the concerns of family members, especially the primary caregiver, about long-term home care.
- ▲ Consider a predischarge home assessment referral to determine the need for accessibility and safety-related environmental changes.

• = Independent   ▲ = Collaborative

- Use an assessment tool to identify environmental safety hazards in the home.
- Establish a plan of care with the client and family based on the client's needs and the caregiver's capabilities.
- Assist family members to develop realistic expectations of themselves in the performance of their caregiving roles.
- Set up a system of relief for the main caregiver in the home, and plan for sharing of household duties.
▲ Initiate referral to community agencies as needed, including housekeeping services, Meals on Wheels (MOW), wheelchair-compatible transportation services, and oxygen therapy services.
▲ Obtain adaptive equipment and telemedical equipment, as appropriate, to help family members continue to maintain the home environment.
- Ask the family to identify support people.

Geriatric

- All of the previously mentioned interventions are applicable for the geriatric population.
- Explore community resources to assist with home maintenance (e.g., senior centers, Department of Aging, hospital case managers, the Internet, or church parish nurse).
- Support "aging in place" by providing assistive technology devices: home modification, daily living aids, mobility aids, seating and positioning devices, and sensory aids.
- Focus on the interaction between the older client and the technology, assisting the client to be an active participant in choices and uses.
- See the care plans for **Risk for Injury** and **Risk for Falls.**

Multicultural

- Acknowledge the stresses unique to racial/ethnic communities.

Home Care

- The previously mentioned interventions incorporate these resources.
▲ Refer clients with mental illness and medical conditions to in-home behavioral health case management.

● = Independent   ▲ = Collaborative

▲ Consider referral for new home safety technologies as they become available.

• See care plans **Contamination** and **Risk for Contamination.**

Client/Family Teaching and Discharge Planning

• Teach the caregiver the need to set aside some personal time every day to meet his or her own needs.

• Identify support groups within the community to assist families in the caregiver role.

• Provide counseling and support for clients and for caregivers of clients.

• Focus teaching on environmental hazards identified in the nursing assessment. Areas may include, but are not limited to:

■ **Home Safety.** Identify the need for and use of common safety devices in the home.

■ **Biological and Chemical Contaminants.** Assess for and reduce the presence of allergens, contaminants, and pollutants in the home.

■ **Food Safety.** Instruct client to avoid microbial food-borne illness by regularly washing hands, food contact surfaces, and fruits and vegetables.

■ **Environmental Stressors.** Assist clients and families with decision-making regarding potential conflicts in home maintenance priorities, given financial constraints.

• Teach clients to assess their homes for potential environmental health hazards in the home, including risks related to structure, moisture/mold, fire, pets, electrical, ventilation, pests, and lifestyle.

• See care plans **Contamination, Risk for Contamination, Risk for Falls, Risk for Infection,** and **Risk for Injury.**

Readiness for enhanced Hope

NANDA-I Definition

A pattern of expectations and desires for mobilizing energy on one's own behalf that is sufficient for well-being and can be strengthened

• = Independent ▲ = Collaborative

Defining Characteristics

Expresses desire to enhance ability to set achievable goals; expresses desire to enhance belief in possibilities; expresses desire to enhance congruency of expectations with desires; expresses desire to enhance hope; expresses desire to enhance interconnectedness with others; expresses desire to enhance problem solving to meet goals; expresses desire to enhance sense of meaning to life; expresses desire to enhance spirituality

Client Outcomes

Client Will (Specify Time Frame):

H

- Describe values, expectations, and meanings
- Set achievable goals that are consistent with values
- Design strategies to achieve goals
- Express belief in possibilities

Nursing Interventions

- Develop an open and caring and empathetic relationship that enables the client to discuss hope.
- Screen the client for hope using a valid and reliable instrument as indicated.
- Focus on the positive aspects of hope, rather than the prevention of hopelessness.
- Provide emotional support and encourage hope.
- Help the person to identify his or her desires and expectations.
- Use a family-oriented approach when discussing hope.
- Review internal and external resources to enhance hope.
- Identify spiritual beliefs and practices.
- Assist the person to consider possible adaptations to changes.

Home Care

- The above interventions may be adapted for home care use.

Client/Family Teaching and Discharge Planning

- Assess client and family hope prior to teaching.
- Incorporate client and family goal setting with teaching content.
- Provide information to the client and family regarding all aspects of the client's health condition.

• = Independent   ▲ = Collaborative

Hopelessness

NANDA-I Definition

Subjective state in which an individual sees limited or no alternatives or personal choices available and is unable to mobilize energy on own behalf

Defining Characteristics

Closing eyes; decreased affect; decreased appetite; decreased response to stimuli; decreased verbalization; lack of initiative; lack of involvement in care; passivity; shrugging in response to speaker; sleep pattern disturbance; turning away from speaker; verbal cues (e.g., despondent content, "I can't," sighing)

Related Factors (r/t)

Abandonment; deteriorating physiological condition; long-term stress; lost belief in spiritual power; lost belief in transcendent values; prolonged activity restriction; social isolation

Client Outcomes

Client Will (Specify Time Frame):
- Verbalize feelings, participate in care
- Make positive statements (e.g., "I can" or "I will try")
- Set goals
- Make eye contact, focus on speaker
- Maintain appropriate appetite for age and physical health
- Sleep appropriate length of time for age and physical health
- Express concern for another
- Initiate activity

Nursing Interventions

▲ Monitor and document the potential for suicide. (Refer the client for appropriate treatment if a potential for suicide is identified.) Refer to the care plan **Risk for Suicide** for specific interventions.
▲ Monitor potential for depression. (Refer the client for appropriate treatment if depression is identified.)

• = Independent   ▲ = Collaborative

- Monitor family caregivers for symptoms of hopelessness.
- Determine appropriate approaches based on the underlying condition or situation that is contributing to feelings of hopelessness.
- Assess for pain and respond with appropriate measures for pain relief.
- Facilitate access to resources to support spiritual well-being.
- Assist the client in looking at alternatives and setting goals that are important to him or her.
- Discussion of hope may be helpful in increasing hope.
- Provide accurate information.
- Encourage decision-making and problem solving.
- Spend one-on-one time with the client. Use empathy; try to understand what the client is saying and communicate this understanding to the client to create a nonjudgmental trusting environment to develop therapeutic relationships with the client.
- Teach alternative coping strategies such as physical activity.
- Review the client's strengths and resources with the client.
- Involve family and significant others in the plan of care.
- For additional interventions, see the care plans for **Readiness for enhanced Hope, Spiritual Distress, Readiness for enhanced Spiritual Well-Being,** and **Disturbed Sleep Pattern.**

Geriatric

- Previous interventions may be adapted for geriatric clients.
- ▲ If depression is suspected; confer with the primary physician regarding referral for mental health services.
- Take threats of self-harm or suicide seriously.
- Use reminiscence and life-review therapies to identify past coping skills.
- Encourage visits from children.
- Consider videoconferencing for elders in nursing homes with relatives as alternative to "live visits."
- Position the client by a window, take the client outside, or encourage such activities as gardening (if ability allows).

• = Independent   ▲ = Collaborative

- Provide esthetic forms of expression, such as dance, music, literature, and pictures.
- Consider "biblio and telephone therapy" (BBT).

Multicultural

- Assess for the influence of cultural beliefs, norms, and values on the client's feelings of hopelessness.
- Assess the effect of fatalism on the client's expression of hopelessness.
- ▲ Assess for depression and refer to appropriate services.
- Encourage spirituality as a source of support for hopelessness.

Home Care

- Previously mentioned interventions may be adapted for home care use.
- ▲ Assess for isolation within the family unit. Encourage the client to participate in family activities. If the client cannot participate, encourage him or her to be in the same area and watch family activities. Refer for telephone support.
- Reminisce with the client about his or her life.
- Identify areas in which the client can have control.
- If illness precipitated the hopelessness, discuss knowledge of and previous experience with the disease.
- ▲ Provide plant or pet therapy if possible.

Client/Family Teaching and Discharge Planning

- Provide information regarding the client's condition, treatment plan, and progress.
- Teach family caregivers skills to provide care in the home.
- Provide positive reinforcement, praise, and acknowledgment of the challenges of caregiving to family members.
- ▲ Refer the client to self-help groups, such as "I Can Cope" and "Make Today Count."
- ▲ When depression is identified by primary care physician in adolescents consider an Internet-based behavior change intervention

● = Independent   ▲ = Collaborative

Risk for compromised Human Dignity

NANDA-I Definition

At risk for perceived loss of respect and honor

Honoring an individual's dignity is imperative and consists of the following elements:

- Physical comfort (bathing, positioning, pain and symptom relief, touch, and a peaceful environment). Encompasses aspects of privacy, respect, and autonomy. Also includes staff expertise, effectiveness, and safety of care
- Psychosocial comfort (listening, sharing fears, giving permission, presence, not dying alone, family support and presence). Includes elements of client participation and choice. Clients feel at ease, safe, and protected; neither intimidated nor threatened
- Spiritual comfort (sharing love and caring words, being remembered, validating their lives, praying with and for, reading scripture and Bible, clergy and referral to other providers [i.e., hospice])

Risk Factors

Cultural incongruity; disclosure of confidential information; exposure of the body; inadequate participation in decision-making; loss of control of body functions; perceived dehumanizing treatment; perceived humiliation; perceived intrusion by clinicians; perceived invasion of privacy; stigmatizing label; use of undefined medical terms

Client Outcomes

Client/Caregiver Will (Specify Time Frame):

- Perceive that dignity is maintained throughout hospitalization/encounter
- Consistently call client by name of choice
- Maintain client's privacy

Nursing Interventions

- Be authentically present when with the client, try to limit extraneous thoughts of self or others, and concentrate on the well-being of the client.
- Accept the client as is, with unconditional positive regard.

● = Independent   ▲ = Collaborative

H

- Use loving, appropriate touch based on the client's culture. When first meeting the client, shake hands with younger clients; touch the arm or shoulder of older clients.
- Determine the client's perspective about his/her health. Example questions include: "Tell me about your health." "What is it like to be in your situation?" "Tell me how you perceive yourself in this situation." "What meaning are you giving to this situation?" "Tell me about your health priorities." "Tell me about the harmony you wish to reach."
- Create a loving, healing environment for the client to help meet physical, psychological, and spiritual needs as possible.
- Determine the client's preferences for when and how nursing care is needed and follow the client's guidelines if at all possible.
  - Knowing what they are doing
  - Know when it's necessary to call the medical provider
  - Treat me as an individual
  - Give my treatments and medications on time
  - Check my condition very closely
  - Give my pain medication on time
  - Know how to handle equipment
  - Keep my family informed of my progress
  - Don't give up on me when I am difficult to get along with
- Include the client in all decision-making; if the client does not choose to be part of the decision, or is no longer capable of making a decision, use the named surrogate decision maker.
- Encourage the client to share his or her feelings, both positive and negative as appropriate and as the client is willing.
- Ask the client what he/she would like to be called and use that name consistently.
- Maintain privacy at all times.
- Avoid authoritative care when the nurse knows what should be done, and the client is powerless.
- Actively listen to what the client is saying both verbally and nonverbally.
- Encourage the client to share thoughts about spirituality as desires.
- Utilize interventions to instill increased hope; see the care plan **Readiness for enhanced Hope.**

• = Independent   ▲ = Collaborative

- For further interventions on spirituality, see the care plan for **Readiness for enhanced Spiritual Well-Being.**

Geriatric

- Always ask the client how he or she would like to be addressed. Avoid calling elderly clients "sweetie," "honey," "Gramps," or other terms that can be demeaning unless this is acceptable in the client's culture, or requested by the client.
- Treat the elderly client with the utmost respect, even if delirium or dementia is present with confusion.
- Avoid use of restraints. Consider all aspects of restraint use including IVs, Foleys, and chemicals.

Multicultural

- Assess for the influence of cultural beliefs, norms, and values on the client's way of communicating, and follow the client's lead in communicating in matters of eye contact, amount of personal space, voice tones, and amount of touching. If in doubt, ask the client.

Home Care

- Most of the interventions described previously may be adapted for home care use.
- Recognize that the client with the caregiver has complete autonomy in the home.

Client/Family Teaching and Discharge Planning

- Teach family and caregivers the need for the dignity of the client to be maintained at all times.

Hyperthermia

NANDA-I Definition

Body temperature elevated above normal range

Elevated body temperature can be either fever (pyrexia) or hyperthermia. Fever is a regulated rise in the core body temperature to 1° to 2° C higher than the client's normal body temperature as

• = Independent   ▲ = Collaborative

an innate immune response to a perceived threat and is regulated by the hypothalamus. Hyperthermia is an unregulated rise in body temperature that occurs when a client either gains heat through an increase in the body's heat production or has developed an inability to effectively dissipate heat. Hyperthermia is *not* adaptive and should be treated as a medical emergency.

Defining Characteristics

Flushed skin; increase in body temperature above normal range; tachycardia; tachypnea; warm to touch; seizures in children

Related Factors (r/t)

Anesthesia; decreased perspiration; dehydration; exposure to hot environment; inappropriate clothing; increased metabolic rate; medications; trauma; neurological disorder/injury; strenuous physical activity in hot climates

Client Outcomes

Client Will (Specify Time Frame):

- Maintain core body temperature within adaptive levels (less than 104° F, 40° C)
- Remain free of complications of malignant hyperthermia (MH)
- Remain free of complication of neuroleptic malignant syndrome (NMS)
- Remain free of dehydration
- Verbalize signs and symptoms of heat stroke and actions to prevent heat stroke
- Verbalize personal risks for malignant hyperthermia and neuroleptic malignant syndrome to be reported during health history reviews to all health care professionals including pharmacists

Nursing Interventions

Temperature Measurement

- Recognize that hyperthermia is a rise in body temperature above 40° C [104° F] that is not regulated by the hypothalamus resulting in an uncontrolled increase in body temperature exceeding the body's ability to lose heat, and is a medical emergency

● = Independent   ▲ = Collaborative

- Measure and record a client's temperature using two modes of temperature monitoring every hour and more frequently as clinically indicated. Continuous temperature monitoring using an indwelling method of temperature measurement is usually indicated to monitor effectiveness of interventions in lowering the body temperature.
- Use the same site and method (device) for temperature measurement for a given client so that temperature trends are assessed accurately; record site of temperature measurement.
▲ Work with the physician to help determine the cause of the temperature increase, hyperthermia, which will often help direct appropriate treatment.

Refer to care plan for **Ineffective Thermoregulation** for interventions managing fever (pyrexia).

Heat Stroke

- Recognize that heat stroke may be separated into two categories: classic and exertional.
- Watch for risk factors for classic heat stroke, which include:
  - Medications especially diuretic agents, anticholinergic agents, antiparkinson medications
  - Alcoholism
  - Mental illness
- Risk factors of exertional heat stroke include:
  - Preexisting illness
  - Drug use (e.g., alcohol, amphetamines, ecstasy)
  - Wearing protective clothing (uniforms and athletic gear) that limits heat dissipation
- Recognize signs and symptoms of hyperthermia which include: core body temperature greater than 40° C (104° F), tachycardia, tachypnea, dizziness, weakness, vomiting, headache, confusion, delirium, seizures, coma, acute kidney injury (rhabdomyolysis), hot dry skin (classic heat stroke).
- Recognize that antipyretic agents are of no use in treatment of hyperthermia.
▲ Assess fluid loss and facilitate oral intake or administer intravenous fluids as ordered to accomplish fluid replacement and support the cardiovascular system. Refer to the care plan for **Deficient Fluid Volume.**

- Use external cooling measures carefully: loosen or remove excessive clothing, give a tepid water bath, provide cool liquids if the client is alert enough to swallow, fan the client's face.
- Recognize that cooling with ice packs, cooled intravenous solution, a hypothermia blanket may be required to lower the body temperature. When using a cooling blanket, choose a circulating water cooling device if available and set the temperature regulator to 0.5° to 1° C (1° to 2° F) below the client's current temperature to prevent shivering.
- ▲ Continually assess the client's neurological and other organ function, especially kidney function, for signs of injury from hyperthermia.

Malignant Hyperthermia

- ▲ If the client has just received general anesthesia, especially halothane, sevoflurane, isoflurane, or succinylcholine, recognize that the hyperthermia may be caused by malignant hyperthermia and requires immediate treatment to prevent death.
- Recognize that signs and symptoms of malignant hyperthermia typically occur suddenly after exposure to the anesthetic agent and include rapid rise in core body temperature, muscle rigidity, arrhythmias, tachycardia, tachypnea, hypercarbia, rhabdomyolysis, and acute kidney injury, and elevated serum calcium and potassium, progressing to disseminated intravascular coagulation and cardiac arrest.
- ▲ If the client has malignant hyperthermia, begin treatment as ordered, including cessation of the anesthetic agent and intravenous administration of dantrolene sodium, stat, along with antiarrhythmics, and continued support of the cardiovascular system.
- Provide client and family education when malignant hyperthermia occurs, as it is an inherited muscle disorder.

Neuroleptic Malignant Syndrome

- ▲ Recognize that neuroleptic malignant syndrome is a rare condition associated with clients who are taking typical and atypical antipsychotic agents.

- Watch for signs and symptoms that can range from mild to severe and include a sudden change in mental status, rapid rise in body temperature, muscle rigidity, tachycardia, tachypnea, elevated or labile blood pressure, diaphoresis, rhabdomyolysis, and acute kidney injury.
▲ Begin treatment when diagnosed, including cessation of the neuroleptic or dopamine antagonist agent; ordered administration of dantrolene, bromocriptine, levodopa, amantadine, or nifedipine; and continued support of the cardiovascular and renal systems.
- A client health history that reports extrapyramidal reaction to any medication should be further explored for risk of neuroleptic malignant syndrome, as this syndrome can occur at any time during a client's treatment with typical and atypical antipsychotic agent.
- Recognize that clients receiving rapid dose escalation of antipsychotic agents (e.g., haloperidol) intramuscularly for acute treatment of delirium may be at increased risk of developing neuroleptic malignant syndrome.

Pediatric

- Assess risk factors of malignant hyperthermia as this has an increased prevalence in the pediatric population.
▲ Administer dantrolene and oxygen as ordered if malignant hyperthermia is present.

Geriatric

- Help the client seek medical attention immediately if elevated core temperature is present. To diagnose the hyperthermia, assess for possible precipitating factors, including changes in medication, environmental changes, and recent medical interventions or infectious exposures.
- In hot weather, encourage the client to wear lightweight cotton clothing.
- Provide education on the importance of drinking eight glasses of fluid per day (within their cardiac and renal reserves) regardless of whether they are thirsty. Assess for the need for and presence of fans or air conditioning, and also appropriate clothing.

• = Independent　　　　▲ = Collaborative

▲ In hot weather, monitor the elderly client for signs of heat stroke: rising temperature, orthostatic blood pressure drop, weakness, restlessness, mental status changes, faintness, thirst, nausea, and vomiting. If signs are present, move the client to a cool place, have the client lie down, give sips of water, check orthostatic blood pressure, spray with lukewarm water, cool with a fan, and seek medical assistance immediately.

• During warm weather, help the client obtain a fan or an air conditioner to increase evaporation, as needed. Help the elderly client locate a cool environment to which the client can go for safety in hot weather.

• Take the temperature of the elderly client in hot weather.

Home Care

• Some of the interventions described previously may be adapted for home care use.

• Determine whether the client or family has a functioning thermometer, and know how to use it. Please refer to the interventions above on taking a temperature.

• Help the client and caregivers prevent and monitor for heat stroke/hyperthermia during times of high outdoor temperatures.

• To prevent heat-related injury in athletes, laborers, and military personnel, instruct them to acclimate gradually to the higher temperatures, increase fluid intake, wear vapor-permeable clothing, and take frequent rests.

• In the event of temperature elevation above the adaptive range, institute measures to decrease temperature (e.g., get the client out of the sun and into a cool place, remove excess clothing, have the client drink fluids, spray the client with lukewarm water, and fan with cool air). Initiate emergency transport.

Client/Family Teaching and Discharge Planning

▲ Instruct to increase fluids to prevent heat-induced hyperthermia and dehydration in the presence of fever.

• Teach the client to stay in a cooler environment during periods of excessive outdoor heat or humidity. If the client does go out, instruct him or her to avoid vigorous physical activity; wear lightweight, loose-fitting clothing; and wear a hat to minimize sun exposure.

• = Independent   ▲ = Collaborative

Hypothermia

NANDA-I Definition

Body temperature below normal range

Defining Characteristics

Body temperature below normal range; cool skin; cyanotic nail beds; hypertension; pallor; piloerection; shivering; slow capillary refill; tachycardia

Related Factors (r/t)

Aging; consumption of alcohol; damage to hypothalamus; decreased ability to shiver; decreased metabolic rate; evaporation from skin in cool environment; exposure to cool environment; illness; inactivity; inadequate clothing; malnutrition; medications; trauma; drowning; medically induced targeted temperature hypothermia

Client Outcomes

Client Will (Specify Time Frame):

- Maintain body temperature within normal range
- Identify risk factors of hypothermia
- State measures to prevent hypothermia
- Identify symptoms of hypothermia and actions to take when hypothermia is present
- If hypothermia is medically induced client/family will state goals for hypothermia treatment

Nursing Interventions

Temperature Measurement

- Recognize hypothermia as a drop in core body temperature below 35° C [95° F].
- Take the temperature at least hourly; if more than mild hypothermia is present (temperature lower than 35° C [95° F]), use a continuous temperature-monitoring device, preferably two of them, one in the rectum, the other in the esophagus.

• = Independent   ▲ = Collaborative

- Measure and record the client's temperature hourly and with changes in client condition (e.g., chills, change in metal status) using a core or near core temperature measurement method. Avoid peripheral temperature measurement sites. If client is critically ill, use an indwelling method of temperature measurement.
- Use the same site and method (device) for temperature measurement for a given client so that temperature trends are assessed accurately and record site of temperature measurement.
- Bladder temperature may be used as an indwelling urinary catheter and is often inserted in the management of hypothermia to monitor diuresis.
- See the care plan for **Ineffective Thermoregulation** as appropriate.

Accidental Hypothermia

- Recognize that there are three types of accidental hypothermia (environmental causes):
  - Acute hypothermia, also called immersion hypothermia, often from sudden exposure to cold through immersion in cold water or snow
  - Exhaustion hypothermia, caused by exposure to cold in association with lack of food and exhaustion
  - Chronic hypothermia that occurs over days or weeks and primarily affects the elderly
- Remove the client from the cause of the hypothermic episode (e.g., cold environment, cold or wet clothing) and bring into a warm environment. Cover the client with warm blankets and apply a covering to the head and neck to conserve body heat.
- Watch the client for signs of hypothermia: shivering, slurred speech, confusion, clumsy movements, fatigue, dehydration.
- ▲ Administer oxygen as ordered.
- Monitor the client's vital signs every hour and as appropriate. Note changes associated with hypothermia, such as initially increased pulse rate, respiratory rate, and blood pressure as well as diuresis with mild hypothermia, and then decreased pulse rate, respiratory rate, and blood pressure as well as oliguria with moderate to severe hypothermia.

● = Independent   ▲ = Collaborative

▲ Attach electrodes and a cardiac monitor. Watch for dysrhythmias.

▲ Monitor for signs of coagulopathy (e.g., oozing of blood from any open areas or from intravascular catheter sites or mucous membranes). Also note results of clotting studies as available.

• For mild hypothermia (core temperature of 32.2° to 35° C [90° to 95° F]), rewarm client passively:
  ■ Set room temperature to 21° to 24° C (70° to 75° F)
  ■ Keep the client dry; remove any damp or wet clothing
  ■ Layer clothing and blankets and cover the client's head; use insulated metallic blankets
  ■ Offer warm fluids; avoid alcohol or caffeine

▲ For moderate hypothermia (core temperature 28° to 32.1° C [82.4° to 90° F]), use active external rewarming methods. The rewarming rate should not exceed 0.5° to 1° C (1.8° F) per hour. Methods include the following:
  ■ Forced-air warming blankets
  ■ Circulate water through external heat exchange pads
  ■ Radiant heat sources

▲ For severe hypothermia (core temperature below 28° C [82.4° F]), use active core-rewarming techniques as ordered:
  ■ Recognize that extracorporeal blood rewarming methods, such as coronary artery bypass, are most effective
  ■ Use of an intravascular countercurrent in-line heat exchange to deliver warmed fluid or blood
  ■ Use of heated and humidified oxygen through the ventilator as ordered
  ■ Administering heated intravenous (IV) fluids at prescribed temperature
  ■ Heated irrigation of the gastrointestinal tract (nasogastric lavage) or bladder irrigations as ordered.

• Rewarm clients slowly, generally at a rate of 0.5° to 1° C every hour.

• Check blood pressure frequently when rewarming; watch for hypotension.

▲ Administer IV fluids, using a rapid infuser IV fluid warmer as ordered.

• Determine the factors leading to the hypothermic episode; see Related Factors.

H

• = Independent   ▲ = Collaborative

▲ Request a social service referral to help the client obtain the heat, shelter, and food needed to maintain body temperature.

▲ Encourage proper nutrition and hydration.

Targeted Temperature Hypothermia

- Recognize that targeted temperature management, also called therapeutic hypothermia, is the active lowering of the client's body temperature, in a controlled manner, to preserve neurological function after an acute myocardial injury or cardiac arrest.

- Recognize that controlled cooling of clients should be considered for all unconscious survivors of out-of-hospital ventricular tachycardia arrest as well as clients experiencing in-hospital arrests. The optimal targeted temperature for therapy is between 32° and 34° C for up to 48 hours.

- Monitor core or near core temperatures continuously using two methods of temperature monitoring.

- Recognize that cooling may be achieved noninvasively, using fluid-filled cooling devices that are placed next to the client's skin, or invasively, infusing iced solution.

- Obtain vital signs hourly (or via continuous monitoring) to include continuous electrocardiogram monitoring. Observe for signs of hypotension, bradycardia, and arrhythmias. Mechanical ventilation is required to protect the client's airway and breathing during treatment.

▲ Observe for shivering and administer sedation agents or paralytic agents as prescribed.

- Closely inspect the skin prior to and throughout the cooling intervention to prevent skin breakdown associated with the treatment. Implement frequent turning and other pressure reduction interventions as indicated.

▲ Monitor and treat serum electrolytes (e.g., potassium, magnesium, calcium, and phosphorus) and serum glucose closely during targeted hypothermia and during rewarming of the client. Electrolytes will fluctuate as the client is rewarmed.

▲ Observe for signs and symptoms of coagulopathy during targeted hypothermia treatment. Hemoconcentration may be noticed as fluids shift during treatment.

• = Independent   ▲ = Collaborative

- Rewarming should occur in a controlled manner with a rise in body temperature of 0.5° to 1° C per hour and targeted goal of normothermia, 37° C.
▲ Neurological and cognitive function should be assessed during targeted temperature treatment and after rewarming.

Pediatric

- Recognize that pediatric clients have a decreased ability to adapt to temperature extremes. Take the following actions to maintain body temperature in the infant/child:
  - Keep the head covered.
  - Use blankets to keep the client warm.
  - Keep the client covered during procedures, transport, and diagnostic testing.
  - Keep the room temperature at 22.2° C (72 °F).
▲ For the preterm or low-birth-weight newborn, use specially designed bags, skin-to-skin care, transwarmer mattresses, and radiant warmers to keep the infant warm.

Geriatric

- Normal aging often includes changes in touch-related sensations, making it harder to differentiate cool and cold.
- Recognize that the elderly can develop indoor hypothermia from air conditioning or ice baths.
- Assess neurological signs frequently, watching for confusion and decreased level of consciousness.
- Recognize that the elderly often wear socks and sweaters to protect themselves from feeling cold, even in warmer weather.

Home Care

Hypothermia is not a symptom that appears in the normal course of home care. When it occurs, it is a clinical emergency, and the client/family should access emergency medical services immediately.
- Some of the interventions described earlier may be adapted for home care use.
- Before a medical crisis occurs, confirm that the client or family has a thermometer and can read it. Instruct as needed. Verify that the thermometer registers accurately.

• = Independent ▲ = Collaborative

- Instruct the client or family to take the temperature when the client displays cyanosis, pallor, or shivering.
▲ Monitor temperature every hour, as noted previously. If the temperature of the client begins dropping below the normal range, apply layers of clothing or blankets, or adjust environmental heat to the comfort level. Do not overheat. Contact a physician.
▲ If temperature continues to drop, activate the emergency system and notify a physician.
▲ If the client is in hospice care or is terminally ill, follow advance directives, client wishes, and the physician's orders. Keep the client free of pain.

Client/Family Teaching and Discharge Planning

- Teach the client and family signs of hypothermia and the method of taking the temperature (age-appropriate).
- Teach the client methods to prevent hypothermia: wearing adequate clothing, including a hat and mittens; heating the environment to a minimum of 20° C (68° F); and ingesting adequate food and fluid.
▲ Teach the client and family about medications such as sedatives, opioids, and anxiolytics that predispose the client to hypothermia (as appropriate).

Disturbed personal Identity

NANDA-I Definition

Inability to maintain an integrated and complete perception of self

Defining Characteristics

Contradictory personal traits; delusional description of self; disturbed body image; gender confusion; ineffective coping; ineffective relationships; ineffective role performance; reports feelings of emptiness; reports feelings of strangeness; reports fluctuating feeling about self; unable to distinguish between inner and outer stimuli; uncertainty about cultural values (e.g., beliefs, religion, moral questions); uncertainty about goals; uncertainty about ideological values

● = Independent   ▲ = Collaborative

Related Factors (r/t)

Chronic low self-esteem; cult indoctrination; cultural discontinuity; discrimination; dysfunctional family processes; ingestion of toxic chemicals; inhalation of toxic chemicals; manic states; multiple personality disorder; organic brain syndromes; perceived prejudice; psychiatric disorders (e.g., psychosis, depression, dissociative disorder); situational crisis; situational low self-esteem; social role change; stages of development; stages of growth; use of psychoactive agents

Client Outcomes

Client Will (Specify Time Frame):

* Demonstrate new purposes for life
* Show interests in surroundings
* Perform self-care and self-control activities appropriate for age
* Acknowledge personal strengths
* Engage in interpersonal relationships

Nursing Interventions

* Assess and support family strengths of commitment, appreciation, and affection toward each other, positive communication, time together, a sense of spiritual well-being, and the ability to cope with stress and crisis.
* ▲ Assess for suicidal ideation and make appropriate referral for clients with schizophrenia and bipolar disorder.
* ▲ Assess women with mood disorders for reproductive and metabolic disorders and make appropriate referrals for treatment.
* ▲ Assess and make appropriate referrals for clients with obesity and depression.
* ▲ Assess lymphocyte counts and make appropriate referrals for clients with bulimia nervosa (BN), who may present with psychopathological variables associated with psychological instability (depression, hostility, impulsivity, self-defeating personality traits, and borderline personality symptoms).
* Use empathetic communication and encourage the client and family to verbalize fears, express emotions, and set goals. Be present for clients physically or by telephone.

● = Independent   ▲ = Collaborative

- Empower the client to set realistic goals and to engage in problem solving.
- Encourage expression of positive thoughts and emotions.
- Encourage the client to use spiritual coping mechanisms such as faith and prayer.
- Help the clients with serious and chronic conditions such as depression, cancer diagnosis, and chemotherapy treatment to maintain social support networks or assist in building new ones.
▲ Refer women facing diagnostic and curative breast cancer surgery for psychosocial support.
▲ Refer for cognitive-behavioral therapy (CBT).
▲ Refer clients with borderline personality disorder (BPD) and dual-diagnosed BPD and substance-dependent female clients for dialectical behavior therapy (DBT) and psychoanalytical-orientated day-hospital therapy.
- Refer to the care plans for **Readiness for enhanced Communication** and **Readiness for enhanced Spiritual Well-Being**.

Pediatric

- Encourage exercise for children and adolescents to promote positive self-esteem, to enhance coping, and to prevent behavioral and psychological problems.
▲ Evaluate and refer children and adolescents for eating disorder prevention programs to include medical care, nutritional intervention, and mental health treatment and care coordination.
- Provide gifted children with low self-esteem with appropriate support.
- Suggest that parents with children diagnosed with cancer use computer-mediated support groups to exchange messages with other parents.

Geriatric

- Consider the use of telephone support for caregivers of family members with dementia.
- Encourage clients to discuss "life history."

● = Independent   ▲ = Collaborative

▲ Refer the older client to self-help support groups, such as the Red Hat Society for older women.
▲ Refer the client with Alzheimer's disease who is terminally ill to hospice.

Multicultural

• Assess an individual's sociocultural background in teaching self-management and self-regulation as a means of supporting hope and coping with a diagnosis of type 2 diabetes.
• Encourage spirituality as a source of support for coping.
• Refer to care plan for **Ineffective Coping**.

Home Care

• The interventions described previously may be adapted for home care use.
• Provide an Internet-based health coach to encourage self-management for clients with chronic conditions such as depression, impaired mobility, and chronic pain.
▲ Refer the client to mutual health support groups.
▲ Refer the client to a behavioral program that teaches coping skills via "Lifeskills" workshop and/or video.
▲ Refer prostate cancer clients and their spouses to family programs that include family-based interventions of communication, hope, coping, uncertainty, and symptom management.
▲ Refer combat veterans and service members directly involved in combat, as well as those providing support to combatants, including nurses, for mental health services.

Client/Family Teaching and Discharge Planning

▲ Teach the client about available community resources (e.g., therapists, ministers, counselors, self-help groups, family-education groups).
▲ Teach coping skills to family caregivers of cancer clients.
▲ Teach caregivers the COPE intervention (creativity, optimism, planning, expert information) to assist with symptom management.

• = Independent   ▲ = Collaborative

Risk for disturbed personal Identity

NANDA-I Definition

Risk for the inability to maintain an integrated and complete perception of self

Risk Factors

Chronic low self-esteem; cult indoctrination; cultural discontinuity; discrimination; dysfunctional family processes; ingestion of toxic chemicals; inhalation of toxic chemicals; manic states; multiple personality disorder; organic brain syndromes; perceived prejudice; psychiatric disorders (e.g., psychoses, depression, dissociative disorder); situational crises; situational low self-esteem; social role change; stages of development; stages of growth; use of psychoactive pharmaceutical agents

Client Outcomes, Nursing Interventions, and Client/Family Teaching and Discharge Planning

Refer to care plan **Disturbed personal Identity.**

Readiness for enhanced Immunization Status

NANDA-I Definition

A pattern of conforming to local, national, and/or international standards of immunization to prevent infectious disease(s) that is sufficient to protect a person, family, or community and can be strengthened

Defining Characteristics

Expresses desire to enhance behavior to prevent infectious disease; expresses desire to enhance identification of possible problems associated with immunizations; expresses desire to enhance identification of providers of immunizations; expresses desire to enhance immunization status; expresses desire to enhance knowledge of immunization standards; expresses desire to enhance record keeping of immunizations

Client Outcomes

Client/Caregiver Will (Specify Time Frame):

- Review appropriate recommended immunization schedule with provider annually and/or at well check-ups

• = Independent   ▲ = Collaborative

- Ask questions about the benefits and risks of immunizations prior to scheduled immunization
- Ask questions regarding the risks of choosing not to be immunized prior to scheduled immunization
- Accurately respond to provider's questions related to pertinent information regarding individual health status as it relates to contraindications for individual vaccines during office visits when immunizations are scheduled
- Inform provider of the health status of close contacts and household members during office visits when immunizations are scheduled and during peak infectious disease seasons
- Provide evidence of an understanding of the risks and benefits of individual immunization decisions during annual physical exam and/or well check-ups
- Provide evidence of an understanding of the benefits of community immunization during peak infectious disease seasons
- Communicate decisions about immunization decisions to provider in relation to personal preferences, values, and goals annually
- Communicate/provide documentation to health care provider ongoing personal record of immunizations annually
- Reinforce the client's responsibility to maintain an accurate record of immunization annually

Nursing Interventions

Psychosocial

- Assess barriers to immunization:
  - Anxiety related to injection/parenteral pharmacological therapy
  - Anxiety related to immunization side effects
  - Knowledge of risk associated with disease
  - Cost of health care
- Assess client-provider relationship.
- Assess client/caregiver level of participation in decision-making process.
- Assess sources of information client has previously turned to.
- Assist client/caregiver to find appropriate educational resources.

• = Independent   ▲ = Collaborative

- Assess cultural or religious beliefs that may relate to either the decision-making process or specific immunizations such as for sexually transmitted diseases.

Physiological

- Perform comprehensive interview to elicit information regarding the client's susceptibility to adverse reactions to specific vaccines according to the manufacturer guidelines.
- Identify clients for whom a specific vaccine is contraindicated.
▲ Report potential or actual adverse effects.
- Inform client/caregiver of the vaccine-specific risks to both women of childbearing age and the fetus.
- Discuss pregnancy planning with appropriate clients considering immunization.
- Identify high-risk individuals for specific vaccine-preventable diseases.
- Identify high-risk groups for specific vaccine-preventable disease.
- Identify high-risk populations for specific vaccine-preventable disease.
- Assess client's recent travel history and future travel plans.
- Identify vulnerable populations and marginalized populations.
- Tailor educational programs specific to these marginalized and vulnerable populations.
- Adopt recommendations made by national and international professional groups advocating the use of Immunization Central Registries and standing orders.
- Support access to health care that enables clients to access well-preventive care on a walk-in basis during times that are consistent with client schedules.

Multicultural

- Assess cultural beliefs and practices that may have an impact on the educational and decision-making process specific to immunization as well as vaccine-specific illness.
- Actively listen and be sensitive to how communication is shared culturally.
- Employ culturally sensitive educational strategies to maximize the individual, family, or community response.

• = Independent   ▲ = Collaborative

Home Care

- The foregoing interventions may be adapted for home care use.
- Develop clinical practice guidelines that include shared decision-making.
- Implement home care strategies that will enhance decision-making and ability to maintain current immunization status.
- Implement mechanisms to contact the client/caregiver at appropriate intervals with reminder literature or phone contact.

Client/Family Teaching and Discharge Planning

- Before teaching, evaluate the client preference for involvement with the decision-making process.
- Use community-based and school-based interventions to teach school-age children and thereby provide vicarious education to the family.
- Develop curricula and media that enhance immunization education.
- Employ media and curricula in office waiting rooms.
- Develop and distribute client log books that provide record-keeping and foster ownership of the responsibility of current immunization status.

Ineffective Impulse Control

NANDA-I Definition

A pattern of performing rapid, unplanned reactions to internal or external stimuli without regard for the negative consequences of these reactions to the impulsive individual or to others

Defining Characteristics

Acting without forethought; asking personal questions of others despite their discomfort; inability to save money or regulate finances; inhibition; irritability; pathological gambling; sensation seeking; sexual promiscuity; sharing personal details inappropriately; temper outbursts; too familiar with strangers; violence

● = Independent   ▲ = Collaborative

Related Factors

Anger; chronic low self-esteem; co-dependency; compunction; delusion; denial; disorder of cognition; disorder of development; disorder of mood; disorder of personality; disturbed body image; economically disadvantaged; environment that might cause frustration; environment that might cause irritation; fatigue; hopelessness; ineffective coping; insomnia; organic brain disorders; smoker; social isolation; stress vulnerability; substance abuse; suicidal feeling; unpleasant physical symptoms

Client Outcomes

Client will (Specify Time Frame):

* Be free from harm
* Cooperate with behavioral modification plan
* Verbalize adaptive ways to cope with stress by means other than impulsive behaviors
* Delay gratification and use adaptive coping strategies in response to stress
* Verbalize understanding that behavior is unacceptable
* Accept responsibility for own behavior

Nursing Interventions

▲ Refer to mental health treatment for cognitive-behavioral therapy (CBT).
* Implement motivational interviewing for clients with impulse control disorders.
* Teach client mindfulness meditation techniques. Mindfulness meditation includes observing experiences in the present moment, describing those experiences without judgments or evaluations, and participating fully in one's current context.
* Refer to self-help groups such as Gambler's Anonymous or Overeaters Anonymous as needed.
* Remove positive reinforcements associated with excessive behavior.
* Assist the client to recognize patterns and cues of impulsive behavior.

• = Independent   ▲ = Collaborative

- Teach clients to utilize urge surfing techniques when impulses are triggered. A core skill associated with urge surfing is the ability to observe within oneself the rise and fall of urges and to "surf" or stay with these urges without acting on them.
- Implement cue elimination procedures as a stimulus control technique.

Pediatric

- Implement in-situ training to address impulsive behavior followed by role-play, differential reinforcement, corrective feedback and rehearsal in young children and adolescents.
- Refer to mental health treatment for CBT.

Geriatric

- Maintain increased surveillance of the client whenever use of dopamine agonists has been initiated. Implement fall risk screening and precautions for geriatric clients with inattention and impulse control symptoms.
- Monitor caregivers for evidence of caregiver burden.

Client/Family Teaching and Discharge Planning

- Provide families with information about addiction or marriage counseling.
- Families should be encouraged to employ practical measures to manage behavior such as limiting access to credit cards and restricting Internet access gambling and casino websites.

Functional urinary Incontinence

NANDA-I Definition

Inability of usually continent person to reach toilet in time to avoid unintentional loss of urine

Defining Characteristics

Able to completely empty bladder; amount of time required to reach toilet exceeds length of time between sensing the urge to void and

• = Independent   ▲ = Collaborative

uncontrolled voiding; loss of urine before reaching toilet; may be incontinent only in the early morning; senses need to void.

Related Factors (r/t)

Cognitive disorders (delirium, dementia, severe, or profound retardation); neuromuscular limitations impairing mobility or dexterity; environmental barriers to toileting

Client Outcomes

Client Will (Specify Time Frame):

- Eliminate or reduce incontinent episodes
- Eliminate or overcome environmental barriers to toileting
- Use adaptive equipment to reduce or eliminate incontinence related to impaired mobility or dexterity
- Use portable urinary collection devices or urine containment devices when access to the toilet is not feasible

Nursing Interventions

- Take a history and perform a physical assessment focusing on bothersome lower urinary tract symptoms, cognitive status, functional status (particularly physical mobility and dexterity), frequency and severity of leakage episodes, alleviating and aggravating factors, and reversible or modifiable causes of urinary incontinence.
- ▲ Consult with the client and family, the client's physician/ provider, and other health care professionals concerning treatment of incontinence in the elderly client undergoing detailed geriatric evaluation.
- Teach the client, the client's care providers, or the family to complete a bladder diary; each 24-hour period is subdivided into 1- to 2-hour periods and includes number of urinations occurring in the toilet, actual episodes of incontinence and amount of urine leaked, reasons for episode of incontinence, type and amount of liquid intake, number of bowel movements, and incontinence pads or other products used.
- ▲ Consult with the physician/provider about discontinuing antimuscarinic medications in clients receiving cholinesterase reuptake inhibitors for Alzheimer's-type dementia.

• = Independent   ▲ = Collaborative

- Assess the client in an acute care or rehabilitation facility for risk factors for functional incontinence.
- Assess the client for coexisting or premorbid urinary incontinence.
- Assess clients, regardless of frailty or age, residing in a long-term care facility for UI.
- Assess the home, acute care, or long-term care environment for accessibility to toileting facilities, paying particular attention to the following:
  - Distance of the toilet from the bed, chair, and living quarters
  - Characteristics of the bed, including presence of side rails and distance of the bed from the floor
  - Characteristics of the pathway to the toilet, including barriers such as stairs, loose rugs on the floor, and inadequate lighting
  - Characteristics of the bathroom, including patterns of use, lighting, height of the toilet from the floor, presence of handrails to assist transfers to the toilet, and breadth of the door and its accessibility for a wheelchair, walker, or other assistive device
- Assess the client for mobility, including the ability to rise from chair and bed, transfer to the toilet, and ambulate, and the need for physical assistive devices such as a cane, walker, or wheelchair.
- ▲ Assess the client for dexterity, including the ability to manipulate buttons, hooks, snaps, loop and pile closures, and zippers as needed to remove clothing. Consult a physical or occupational therapist to promote optimal toilet access as indicated.
- Assess the functional and cognitive status using a tool such as the Mini Mental Status Examination for the elderly client with functional incontinence.
- Remove environmental barriers to toileting in the acute care, long-term care, or home setting. Assist the client in removing loose rugs from the floor and improving lighting in hallways and bathrooms.
- Provide an appropriate, safe urinary receptacle such as a three-in-one commode, female or male hand-held urinal, no-spill

● = Independent   ▲ = Collaborative

urinal, or containment device when toileting access is limited by immobility or environmental barriers.

▲ Help the client with limited mobility to obtain evaluation by a physical therapist and to obtain assistive devices as indicated; assist the client in selecting shoes with a nonskid sole to maximize traction when arising from a chair and transferring to the toilet.

• Assist the client in altering the wardrobe to maximize toileting access. Select loose-fitting clothing with stretch waistbands rather than buttoned or zippered waist; minimize buttons, snaps, and multilayered clothing; and substitute a loop-and-pile closure or other easily loosened systems such as Velcro for buttons, hooks, and zippers in existing clothing.

• Begin a prompted voiding program or patterned urge response toileting program for the elderly client in the home or a long-term care facility who has functional incontinence and dementia:

  ■ Determine the frequency of current urination using an alarm system or check-and-change device.

  ■ Record urinary elimination and incontinent patterns in a bladder log to use as a baseline for assessment and evaluation of treatment efficacy.

  ■ Begin a prompted toileting program based on the results of this program; toileting frequency may vary from every 1.5 to 2 hours to every 4 hours.

  ■ Praise the client when toileting occurs with prompting.

  ■ Refrain from any socialization when incontinent episodes occur; change the client and make her or him comfortable.

Geriatric

• Institute aggressive continence management programs for the cognitively intact, community-dwelling client in consultation with the client and family.

• Monitor the elderly client in a long-term care facility, acute care facility, or home for dehydration.

Home Care

• The interventions described previously may be adapted for home care use.

• = Independent   ▲ = Collaborative

- Assess current strategies used to reduce urinary incontinence, including limitation of fluid intake, restriction of bladder irritants, prompted or scheduled toileting, and use of containment devices.
- Encourage a mindset and program of self-care management.
- For a memory-impaired older adult client, implement an individualized, scheduled toileting program (on a schedule developed in consultation with the caregiver, approximately every 2 hours, with toileting reminders provided and existing patterns incorporated, such as toileting before or after meals).
- Teach the family the general principles of bladder health, including avoidance of bladder irritants, adequate fluid intake, and a routine schedule of toileting. (Refer to the care plan for **Impaired Urinary Elimination.**)
- Teach prompted voiding to the family and client for the client with mild to moderate dementia (refer to previous description).
- Inspect the perineal and perianal skin for evidence of incontinence-associated dermatitis, including inflammation, vesicles in skin exposed to urinary leakage, and especially skin folds or denudation of the skin, particularly when incontinence is managed by absorptive pads or containment briefs.
- Begin a preventive skin care regimen for all clients with urinary and/or fecal incontinence and treat clients with incontinence-associated dermatitis or related skin damage.
- Advise the client about the advantages of using disposable or reusable insert pads, pad-pant systems, or replacement briefs specifically designed for urinary incontinence (or double urinary and fecal incontinence) as indicated.
- Assist the family with arranging care in a way that allows the client to participate in family or favorite activities without embarrassment. Elicit discussion of the client's concerns about the social or emotional burden of incontinence.
- ▲ Refer to occupational therapy for help in obtaining assistive devices and adapting the home for optimal toilet accessibility.
- ▲ Consider the use of an indwelling catheter for continuous drainage in the client who is both homebound and bed-bound

and is receiving palliative or end-of-life care (requires a physician's/provider order).

▲ When an indwelling urinary catheter is in place, follow prescribed maintenance protocols for managing the catheter, taping and replacing the catheter, drainage bag, and care of perineal skin and urethral meatus. Teach infection control measures adapted to the home care setting.

• Assist the client in adapting to the catheter. Encourage discussion of the client's response to the catheter.

Client/Family Teaching and Discharge Planning

• Work with the client, family, and their extended support systems to assist with needed changes in the environment and wardrobe, and other alterations required to maximize toileting access.

• Work with the client and family to establish a reasonable and manageable prompted voiding program using environmental and verbal cues to remind caregivers of voiding intervals, such as television programs, meals, and bedtime.

• Teach the family to use an alarm system for toileting or to carry out a check-and-change program and to maintain an accurate log of voiding and incontinence episodes.

Overflow urinary Incontinence

NANDA-I Definition

Involuntary loss of urine associated with overdistention of the bladder

Defining Characteristics

Bladder distention; high post-void residual volume; nocturia; observed involuntary leakage of small volumes of urine; reports involuntary leakage of small volumes of urine

Related Factors (r/t)

Bladder outlet obstruction; detrusor external sphincter dyssynergia; poor detrusor contraction strength; fecal impaction; severe pelvic prolapse; side effects of medications with anticholinergic actions; side

• = Independent   ▲ = Collaborative

effects of calcium channel blockers; side effects of medication with alpha-adrenergic agonistic effects; urethral obstruction

Client Outcomes, Nursing Interventions, and Client/Family Teaching and Discharge Planning

Refer to care plan for **Urinary Retention.**

Reflex urinary Incontinence

NANDA-I Definition

Involuntary loss of urine at somewhat predictable intervals when a specific bladder volume is reached.

Involuntary loss of urine caused by a defect in the spinal cord between the nerve roots at or below the first cervical segment and those above the second sacral segment. Urine elimination occurs at unpredictable intervals; micturition may be elicited by tactile stimuli, including stroking of inner thigh or perineum.

Defining Characteristics

Inability to voluntarily inhibit voiding; inability to voluntarily initiate voiding; incomplete emptying with lesion above pontine micturition center; incomplete emptying with lesion above sacral micturition center; no sensation of bladder fullness; no sensation or urge to void; no sensation of voiding; predictable pattern of voiding; sensation of urgency without voluntary inhibition of bladder contraction; sensations associated with full bladder (e.g., sweating, restlessness, abdominal discomfort)

NOTE: Reflex urinary incontinence may be associated with sweating and acute elevation in blood pressure and pulse rate in clients with spinal cord injury. Refer to the care plan for **Autonomic Dysreflexia.**

Related Factors (r/t)

Neurological impairment above level of pontine micturition center; neurological impairment above level of sacral micturition center; tissue damage (e.g., due to radiation cystitis, inflammatory bladder conditions, radical pelvic surgery)

Client Outcomes

Client Will (Specify Time Frame):

- Follow prescribed schedule for bladder emptying
- Have intact perineal skin

• = Independent   ▲ = Collaborative

- Remain clear of symptomatic urinary tract infection
- Demonstrate how to apply containment device or insert intermittent catheter or be able to provide caregiver with instructions for performing these procedures

Nursing Interventions

- Ask the client to complete a bladder diary/log to determine the pattern of urine elimination, any incontinence episodes, and current bladder management program. An electronic voiding diary may be kept whenever feasible.
- ▲ Consult with the physician concerning current bladder function and the potential of the bladder to produce hydronephrosis, vesicoureteral reflux, febrile urinary tract infection, or compromised renal function.
- ▲ Consult with the physician and physical therapist concerning the neuromuscular ability to perform bladder management.
- Inspect the perineal and perigenital skin for signs of incontinence-associated dermatitis and pressure ulcers.
- ▲ In consultation with the rehabilitation team, counsel the client and family concerning the merits and potential risks associated with each possible bladder management program, including spontaneous voiding, intermittent self-catheterization, reflex voiding with condom catheter containment, and indwelling suprapubic catheterization.

Intermittent Self-Catheterization

- Begin intermittent catheterization as ordered using sterile technique; the client may be taught to use clean technique in the home situation.
- Schedule the frequency of intermittent catheterization based on the frequency/volume records of previous catheterizations, functional bladder capacity, and the impact of catheterization on the quality of the client's life.
- Teach the client managed by intermittent or indwelling catheter to recognize signs of symptomatic urinary tract infection and to seek care promptly when these signs occur. The signs of symptomatic infection are the following:
  - ■ Discomfort over the bladder or during urination

● = Independent   ▲ = Collaborative

- Acute onset of urinary incontinence
- Fever
- Markedly increased spasticity of muscles below the level of the spinal lesion
- Malaise, lethargy
- Hematuria
- Autonomic dysreflexia (hyperreflexia) symptoms

▲ Recognize that intermittent catheterization is typically associated with asymptomatic bacteriuria, and the indwelling catheter is routinely associated with asymptomatic colonization.

▲ Teach intermittent catheterization as the client approaches discharge as directed. Instruct the client and at least one family member in the performance of catheterization. Teach the client with quadriplegia how to instruct others to perform this procedure.

▲ Teach the client managed by intermittent catheterization to self-administer antispasmodic (parasympatholytic) medications as ordered and to recognize and manage potential side effects as needed.

Condom Catheter

- For a male client with reflex incontinence who does not have urinary retention and cannot manage the condition effectively with spontaneous voiding, does not choose to perform intermittent catheterization, or cannot perform catheterization, teach the client and his family to obtain, select, and apply an external collective device and urinary drainage system. Assist the client and family to choose a product that adheres to the glans penis or penile shaft without allowing seepage of urine onto surrounding skin or clothing; that avoids provoking hypersensitivity reactions on the skin; and that includes a urinary drainage reservoir that is easily concealed under the clothing and does not cause irritation to the skin of the thigh.
- Teach the client whose incontinence is managed by a condom catheter to routinely inspect the skin with each catheter change for evidence of lesions caused by pressure from the containment device or by exposure to urine, to cleanse the penis thoroughly, and to reapply a new device daily or every other day.

Geriatric

- If difficulties are encountered in client teaching, refer the elderly client to a nurse who specializes in care of the aging client with urinary incontinence.

Home Care

- The interventions described previously may be adapted for home care use.
- Teach the client what the complications of reflex incontinence are and when to report changes to a physician or primary nurse.
- If the client is taught intermittent self-catheterization, arrange for contingency care in the event that the client is unable to perform self-catheterization.
- Assess and instruct the client and family in care of the catheter and supplies in the home.
- Encourage a mindset and program of self-care management.
- Assist the family with arranging care in a way that allows the client to participate in family or favorite activities without embarrassment. Elicit discussion of the client's concerns about the social or emotional burden of incontinence.

Client/Family Teaching and Discharge Planning

- Teach the client to ensure good hydration. Total daily fluid intake should be approximately 2.7 liters per day for women, and 3.7 liters per day for men.
- Teach the client with a spinal injury the signs of autonomic dysreflexia, its relationship to bladder fullness, and management of the condition. Refer to the care plan for **Autonomic Dysreflexia.**
- Teach the client and several significant others the techniques of intermittent catheterization, indwelling catheter care and removal, or condom catheter management as appropriate.
- Teach the client and family techniques to clean catheters used for intermittent catheterization (if clean technique is ordered, including washing with soap and water and allowing to air dry), and using microwave cleaning techniques.

● = Independent   ▲ = Collaborative

Stress urinary Incontinence

NANDA-I Definition

Sudden leakage of urine with activities that increase intraabdominal pressure

Defining Characteristics

Observed urine loss with physical exertion (sign of stress incontinence); reported loss of urine associated with physical exertion or activity (symptom of stress incontinence); urine loss associated with increased abdominal pressure (urodynamic stress urinary incontinence)

Related Factors (r/t)

Urethral hypermobility/pelvic organ prolapse (genetic factors/familial predisposition, multiple vaginal deliveries, delivery of infant large for gestational age, forceps-assisted or breech delivery, obesity, changes in estrogen levels at climacteric, extensive abdominopelvic, or pelvic surgery); urethral sphincter mechanism incompetence (multiple urethral suspensions in women, radical prostatectomy in men, uncommon complication of transurethral prostatectomy or cryosurgery of prostate, spinal lesion affecting sacral segments 2 to 4 or cauda equina, pelvic fracture)

NOTE: Defining Characteristics and Related Factors adapted from the work of NANDA-I.

Client Outcomes

Client Will (Specify Time Frame):

- Report fewer stress incontinence episodes and/or a decrease in the severity of urine loss
- Experience reduction in frequency of urinary incontinence episodes as recorded on voiding diary (bladder log)
- Identify containment devices that assist in management of stress incontinence

Nursing Interventions

- Take a focused history addressing risk factors for stress incontinence: pregnancy, parity, large babies, forceps or breech deliveries, obesity, chronic cough, physical activity, previous urinary

● = Independent   ▲ = Collaborative

tract or gynecological surgery, medications such as diuretics, lithium, adrenergic blockers, and diabetes and smoking.

- Ask about onset and duration of urinary leakage and related lower urinary tract symptoms, including voiding frequency (day/night), urgency, severity (small, moderate, large amounts) of urinary leakage, and factors provoking urine loss (diuretics, bladder irritants, alcohol), focusing on the differential diagnosis of stress, urge or mixed stress and urge urinary symptoms. Consider using a symptom questionnaire that elicits relevant lower urinary tract symptoms and provides differentiation between stress and urge incontinence symptoms.

- To assess for mixed urinary incontinence (a combination of stress and urge incontinence), ask the following questions: (1) Can you delay urination for a 2-hour movie or car ride? (2) How often do you arise at night to urinate? (3) When you have the urge to urinate, can you reach the toilet without leaking?

- Assess the severity of incontinence as well as impact on the individual's lifestyle; inquire about incontinence pad use and change in daily, social, or recreational activities, as well as emotional impact.

- Inspect the perineal skin for evidence of incontinence-associated dermatitis, including inflammation, vesicles in skin exposed to urinary leakage, and especially skin folds or denudation of the skin, particularly when incontinence is managed by absorptive pads or containment briefs.

- Attempt to reproduce the sign of stress urinary incontinence by asking the client to perform the Valsalva maneuver or to cough while observing the urethral meatus for urine loss.

▲ Perform a focused physical assessment, including bladder palpation after voiding to check for retention, inspection of the perineal skin, vaginal examination to determine hypoestrogenic changes in the mucosa (may contribute to urge incontinence), and reproduction of stress urinary incontinence with the cough test. Also, constipation should be assessed.

- Determine the client's current use of containment devices; evaluate the devices for their ability to adequately contain urine loss, protect clothing, and control odor. Assist the client

● = Independent ▲ = Collaborative

in identifying containment devices specifically designed to contain urinary leakage.

- Teach the client to complete a bladder diary by recording voiding frequency, the frequency and degree of urinary incontinence episodes, their association with urgency (a sudden and strong desire to urinate that is difficult to defer), fluid intake, and pad usage over a 3- to 7-day period. An electronic voiding diary may be kept whenever feasible.

▲ With the client and in close consultation with the physician, review treatment options, including behavioral management; drug therapy; use of a pessary, vaginal device, or urethral insert; and surgery. Outline their potential benefits, efficacy, and side effects.

- Begin a pelvic floor muscle training program.
- Teach the client undergoing pelvic floor muscle training to identify, contract, and relax the pelvic floor muscles without contracting distal muscle groups (e.g., abdominal muscles or gluteus muscles) using verbal feedback based on vaginal or anal palpation, biofeedback, or electrical stimulation, utilizing the assistance of an incontinence specialist or physician as necessary.
- Incorporate principles of exercise physiology into a pelvic muscle training program using the following strategies:
  - Begin a graded exercise program, usually starting with 5 to 10 repetitions and advancing gradually to no more than 35 to 50 repetitions every day or every other day based on baseline and ongoing evaluation of maximal strength and endurance.
  - Continue exercise sessions over a period of 3 to 6 months.
  - Integrate muscle training into activities of daily living.
  - Assess progress every 2 weeks during the first month and every 4 to 6 weeks thereafter.
- Teach the principles of bladder training to women with stress urinary incontinence:
  - Assist the client in completing a bladder diary over a period of a minimum of 3 days or up to 7 days.
  - Review the results with the client, determining typical voiding frequency and establishing goals for voiding frequency.

• = Independent   ▲ = Collaborative

- Using baseline voiding frequency, as determined by the diary, teach the client to urinate by the clock when awake, typically every 30 to 120 minutes.
- Encourage adherence to the program with timing devices, as well as verbal encouragement and support, and address individual reasons for schedule interruption.
- Gradually increase the time between urinations to the negotiated goal. Time intervals between voiding are typically increased in increments of 15 to 30 minutes for clients with a baseline frequency of less than every 60 minutes and increments of 25 to 30 minutes for clients with a baseline frequency of more than every 60 minutes.

- Teach the client to self-administer duloxetine and imipramine as ordered, and to monitor for adverse side effects.
- Teach the client to self-administer topical (vaginal) estrogens as directed, and to monitor for adverse side effects.
▲ Refer the female client with stress urinary incontinence and pelvic organ prolapse who wishes to employ a pessary to manage stress incontinence to a nurse specialist or gynecologist with expertise in the placement and maintenance of these devices.
- Discuss potentially reversible or controllable risk factors, such as weight loss, with the client with stress incontinence and assist the client to formulate a strategy to eliminate these conditions.
- Provide information about support resources such as the National Association for Continence, The Simon Foundation for Continence, or the Total Control Program.
▲ Refer the client with persistent stress incontinence to a continence service, physician, or nurse who specializes in the management of this condition.

Geriatric

- Evaluate the elderly client's functional and cognitive status to determine the effect of functional limitations on the frequency and severity of urine loss and on plans for management.

Home Care

- The interventions described previously may be adapted for home care use.

- Elicit discussion of the client's concerns about the social or emotional burden of stress incontinence.
- Encourage a mindset and program of self-care management; assist the client to develop an action plan for continence.
- Implement a bladder-training program as outlined previously.
▲ Consider the use of an indwelling catheter for continuous drainage in the client with severe stress urinary incontinence who is homebound, bed-bound, and receiving palliative or end-of-life care (requires a physician's order).
▲ When an indwelling catheter is in place, follow the prescribed maintenance protocols for managing the catheter, drainage bag, and perineal skin and urethral meatus. Teach infection control measures adapted to the home care setting.
- Assist the client in adapting to the catheter. Encourage discussion of the client's response to the catheter.

Client/Family Teaching and Discharge Planning

- Teach the client to perform pelvic muscle exercise using an audiotape or videotape if indicated.
- Teach the client the importance of avoiding dehydration and instruct the client to consume fluid at the rate of 30 mL/kg of body weight daily (0.5 ounce/pound/day).
- Teach the client the importance of avoiding constipation by a combination of adequate fluid intake, adequate intake of dietary fiber, and exercise.
▲ Teach the client to apply and remove support devices such as a urethral insert.
- Teach the client to select and utilize incontinence supplies.

Urge urinary Incontinence

NANDA-I Definition

Involuntary passage of urine occurring soon after a strong sense of urgency to void

Urge incontinence is defined within the context of overactive bladder syndrome. The overactive bladder is characterized by bothersome urgency (a sudden and strong desire to urinate that is not easily deferred). Overactive bladder is typically associated with frequent daytime voiding and nocturia, and approximately 37% will experience urge urinary incontinence.

Defining Characteristics

Diurnal urinary frequency (voiding more than once every 2 hours while awake); nocturia (awakening three or more times per night to urinate); voiding more than eight times within a 24-hour period as recorded on a voiding diary (bladder log); bothersome urgency (a sudden and strong desire to urinate that is not easily deferred); symptom of urge incontinence (urine loss associated with desire to urinate); enuresis (involuntary passage of urine while asleep)

Related Factors (r/t)

Neurological disorders (brain disorders, including cerebrovascular accident, brain tumor, normal pressure hydrocephalus, traumatic brain injury); inflammation of bladder (calculi; tumor, including transitional cell carcinoma and carcinoma in situ; inflammatory lesions of the bladder; urinary tract infection); bladder outlet obstruction (see **Urinary retention**); stress urinary incontinence (mixed urinary incontinence; these conditions often coexist but relationship between them remains unclear); idiopathic causes (associated factors include depression, sleep apnea, and obesity).

Note: Defining Characteristics and Related Factors adapted from the work of NANDA-I.

Client Outcomes

Client Will (Specify Time Frame):
- Report relief from urge urinary incontinence or a decrease in the frequency of incontinent episodes
- Identify containment devices that assist in the management of urge urinary incontinence

Nursing Interventions

- Take a focused history addressing onset, diurnal frequency (voiding more than once every 2 hours while awake), nocturia, severity of symptoms, alleviating and aggravating factors, medical history, and current management.

• = Independent   ▲ = Collaborative

- Inquire about urgency, daytime frequency, nocturia, involuntary leakage, leakage accompanied by or preceded by urgency, and whether the amount of urine loss is a moderate or large volume.
▲ In close consultation with a physician or advanced practice nurse, consider administering a symptom questionnaire that elicits relevant lower urinary tract symptoms and differentiates stress and urge incontinence symptoms.
- Assess the severity of incontinence as well as the impact on the individual's lifestyle; inquire about incontinence pad use and change in daily, social, or recreational activities, as well as emotional impact.
▲ Perform a focused physical assessment, including bladder palpation after voiding to check for retention; bladder scanning for postvoid residual; inspection of the perineal skin; vaginal examination to determine hypoestrogenic changes in the mucosa (may contribute to urge incontinence); pelvic examination to determine the presence, location, and severity of vaginal wall prolapse; and reproduction of stress urinary incontinence with the cough test. Anal tone and constipation should be assessed.
- Inspect the perineal and perianal skin for evidence of incontinence-associated dermatitis, including inflammation, vesicles in skin exposed to urinary leakage, and especially skin folds or denudation of the skin, particularly when incontinence is managed by absorptive pads or containment briefs.
- Teach the client to complete a bladder diary by recording voiding frequency, the frequency and degree of urinary incontinence episodes and their association with urgency (a sudden and strong desire to urinate that is difficult to defer) or other circumstances surrounding the episode, fluid intake, and pad usage over a 3- to 7-day period. An electronic bladder diary may be kept whenever feasible. In addition to these parameters, the client may be asked to record voided volume and fluid intake.
▲ Review all medications the client is receiving, paying particular attention to sedatives, opioid analgesics, diuretics, antidepressants, psychotropic drugs, and cholinergics. Consult

the physician or nurse practitioner about altering or eliminating these medications if they are suspected of affecting incontinence.

- Assess the client for urinary retention (see the care plan for **Urinary retention**).
- Assess the client for functional limitations (environmental barriers, limited mobility or dexterity, impaired cognitive function; refer to the care plan for **Functional urinary Incontinence**).

▲ Consult the physician concerning diabetic management or pharmacotherapy for urinary tract infection when indicated.

▲ Assess for signs and symptoms of atrophic vaginal changes in the perimenopausal or postmenopausal woman, including vaginal dryness, tenderness to touch, mucosal dryness, friability, and discomfort with gentle palpation. Specifically query the woman with atrophic vaginitis concerning associated lower urinary tract symptoms (usually voiding frequency, urgency, and dysuria). Refer the woman with atrophic vaginal changes and bothersome lower urinary tract symptoms to a gynecologist, urologist, or women's health nurse practitioner for further evaluation and management. Teach the principles of bladder training to women with urge urinary incontinence.

■ Assist the client in completing a voiding diary over a period of a minimum of 3 days or up to 7 days.

■ Review the results with the client, determining typical voiding frequency and establishing goals for voiding frequency based on the longest time interval between voids that is comfortable for the client.

■ Using baseline voiding frequency, as determined by the diary, teach the client to void first thing in the morning, every time the predetermined voiding interval passes, and before going to bed at night.

■ Encourage adherence to the program with timing devices and verbal encouragement and support, and address individual reasons for schedule interruption.

■ Teach distraction and urge suppression techniques (see later discussion) to control urgency while the client postpones urination.

• = Independent   ▲ = Collaborative

- Gradually increase the time between urinations to the negotiated goal. Time intervals between voiding are typically increased in increments of 15 to 30 minutes for clients with a baseline frequency of less than every 60 minutes and increments of 25 to 30 minutes for clients with a baseline frequency of more than every 60 minutes. The voiding interval should be increased by 15 to 30 minutes each week (based on the client's tolerance) until a voiding interval of 3 to 4 hours is achieved. Utilize a bladder diary to monitor progress.

▲ With the assistance of an incontinence specialist or physician, teach the client undergoing pelvic floor muscle training to identify, contract, and relax the pelvic floor muscles without contracting distal muscle groups (e.g., abdominal muscles and gluteal muscles). Instruct the client that the pelvic floor muscles are the same ones used to hold gas in the rectum. To locate them, instruct the client to slow down or stop the urine stream when almost finished voiding. Teach them that when they contract the pelvic floor muscles, the client will not see or feel any movement on the outside of the body. Teach the client that these muscles may not be very strong; begin with contracting them 10 times, holding each contraction for 3 seconds and resting for 3 seconds. Gradually work up to holding the contraction for 6 to 10 seconds, then resting for 6 to 10 seconds. Exercise in sets of 10 at first, doing at least 30 to 50 a day. If the client seems to have difficulty isolating these muscles, request a physical therapist or incontinence specialist to use vaginal or anal palpation, biofeedback, or electrical stimulation to assist with feedback.

• Review with the client the types of beverages consumed, focusing on the intake of caffeine, which is associated with a transient effect on lower urinary tract symptoms. Advise all clients to reduce or eliminate intake of caffeinated beverages or over-the-counter medications of dietary aids containing caffeine. Identify and counsel the client to eliminate other bladder irritants that may exacerbate incontinence, such as smoking, carbonated beverages, citrus, sugar substitutes, and tomato products.

• = Independent   ▲ = Collaborative

- Review with the client the volume of fluids consumed; fluids may be reduced to alleviate urinary frequency, especially in the evening after 6 PM or 3 to 4 hours before bedtime to reduce nocturia.
- Teach the client methods to avoid constipation such as increasing dietary fiber, moderately increasing fluid intake, exercising, and establishing a routine defecation schedule.
- Instruct in techniques of urge suppression. When a strong or precipitous urge to urinate is perceived, teach the client to avoid running to the toilet. Instead, she or he should pause, sit down, relax the entire body, and perform repeated, rapid pelvic muscle contractions until the urge is relieved. Teach the client to utilize distraction: count backwards from 100 by sevens, recite a poem, write a letter, balance a checkbook, do handwork such as knitting, take five deep breaths, focusing on breathing. Relief is followed by micturition within 5 to 15 minutes, using nonhurried movements when locating a toilet and voiding.
- Teach the client to use urge suppression strategies on waking during the night. If the urge subsides, the client should be encouraged to go back to sleep. If after a minute or two it does not, clients should be instructed to get up to void to avoid sleep interruption. Teach the client to interrupt or slow the urinary stream during voiding once a day.
▲ Teach the client to self-administer antimuscarinic (anticholinergic) drugs as directed. Teach dosage and administration of the medication and the importance of combining pharmacotherapy with scheduled voiding, adequate fluid intake, restriction of bladder irritants, and urge suppression techniques.
- Assist the client in selecting, obtaining, and applying a containment device for urine loss as indicated.
- Provide the client with information about incontinence support groups such as the National Association for Continence and the Simon Foundation for Continence. A helpful website titled Total Control (http://www.totalcontrolprogram.com/Pelvic+Health/Bladder+Health) can be accessed to give support and information to women with incontinence.

● = Independent   ▲ = Collaborative

Geriatric

- Assess the functional and cognitive status of the elderly client with urge incontinence; utilize interventions to improve mobility.
- Plan care in long-term or acute care facilities based on knowledge of the elderly client's established voiding patterns, paying particular attention to patterns of nocturia.
- Carefully monitor the elderly client for potential adverse effects of antispasmodic medications, including a severely dry mouth interfering with the use of dentures, eating, or speaking, or confusion, nightmares, constipation, mydriasis, or heat intolerance.

Home Care

- The interventions described previously may be adapted for home care use.
- Teach the importance of avoiding dehydration or excessive fluid consumption and the paradoxical relationship between dehydration and symptoms of urgency.
- Teach the family and client to identify and correct environmental barriers to toileting within the home.
- Encourage the client to develop an action plan for of self-care management of incontinence. Implement a bladder-training program as appropriate, including self monitoring activities (reducing caffeine intake, adjusting amount and timing of fluid intake, decreasing long voiding intervals while awake, making dietary changes to promote bowel regularity), bladder training, and pelvic muscle exercise.
- Help the client and family to identify and correct environmental barriers to toileting within the home.

Client/Family Teaching and Discharge Planning

- Teach the client and family to recognize foods and beverages that are likely to irritate the bladder.
- Teach the family and client to recognize and manage side effects of antispasmodic medications used to treat urge incontinence.
- Help the client and family to recognize and manage side effect of anticholinergic medications used to manage irritative lower urinary tract symptoms.

• = Independent   ▲ = Collaborative

Risk for urge urinary Incontinence

NANDA-I Definition

At risk for involuntary passage of urine occurring soon after a sudden, strong sensation of urgency to void

Risk Factors

Atrophic urethritis, atrophic vaginitis, effects of alcohol; effects of caffeine; effects of pharmaceutical agents, detrusor hyperactivity with impaired bladder contractility, fecal impaction, impaired bladder contractility, ineffective toileting habits, involuntary sphincter relaxation, small bladder capacity

Bowel Incontinence

NANDA-I Definition

Change in normal bowel elimination habits characterized by involuntary passage of stool

Defining Characteristics

Constant dribbling of soft stool, fecal odor; inability to delay defecation; fecal staining of bedding; fecal staining of clothing; inability to recognize urge to defecate; inattention to urge to defecate; recognizes rectal fullness but reports inability to expel formed stool; red perianal skin; self-report of inability to recognize rectal fullness; urgency

Related Factors (r/t)

Abnormally high abdominal pressure; abnormally high intestinal pressure; chronic diarrhea; colorectal lesions; dietary habits; environmental factors (e.g., inaccessible bathroom); general decline in muscle tone; immobility; impaired cognition; impaired reservoir capacity; incomplete emptying of bowel; laxative abuse; loss of rectal sphincter control; lower motor nerve damage; medications; rectal sphincter abnormality; impaction; stress; toileting self-care deficit; upper motor nerve damage

Client Outcomes

Client Will (Specify Time Frame):

- Have regular, complete evacuation of fecal contents from the rectal vault (pattern may vary from every day to every 3 days)

• = Independent   ▲ = Collaborative

- Have regulation of stool consistency (soft, formed stools)
- Reduce or eliminate frequency of incontinent episodes
- Exhibit intact skin in the perianal/perineal area
- Demonstrate the ability to isolate, contract, and relax pelvic muscles (when incontinence related to sphincter incompetence or high-tone pelvic floor dysfunction)
- Increase pelvic muscle strength (when incontinence related to sphincter incompetence)
- Identify triggers that precipitate change in bowel continence

Nursing Interventions

- In a private setting, directly question client about the presence of fecal incontinence. If the client reports altered bowel elimination patterns, problems with bowel control, or "uncontrollable diarrhea," complete a focused nursing history including previous and present bowel elimination routines, dietary history, frequency and volume of uncontrolled stool loss, and aggravating and alleviating factors.
- Recognize that risk factors for fecal incontinence include older individuals, female sex, impaired mobility, cognitive impairment, and structural or functional impairment of bowel function.
- Recognize that additional risk factors for bowel incontinence in hospitalized clients include antibiotic therapy, medications, nasogastric feeding, immobility, inability to communicate elimination needs, acute disease processes and procedures (e.g., cancer, abdominal surgery), sedation, and mechanical ventilation.
- ▲ Conduct a health history assessment that includes a review of current bowel patterns/habits to include constipation and use of laxatives; pelvic floor injury with childbirth; acute trauma to organs, muscles, or nerves involved in defecation; gastrointestinal inflammatory disorders; functional disability; and medications.
- ▲ Closely inspect the perineal skin and skin folds for evidence of skin breakdown in clients with incontinence.
- ▲ In close consultation with a physician or advanced practice nurse, consider routine use of a validated tool that focuses on bowel elimination patterns.

• = Independent   ▲ = Collaborative

▲ Complete a focused physical assessment, including inspection of perineal skin, pelvic muscle strength assessment, digital examination of the rectum for presence of impaction and anal sphincter strength, and evaluation of functional status (mobility, dexterity, visual acuity).

- Complete an assessment of cognitive function; explore for a history of dementia, delirium, or acute confusion.
- Document patterns of stool elimination and incontinent episodes through a bowel record, including frequency of bowel movements, stool consistency, frequency and severity of incontinent episodes, precipitating factors, and dietary and fluid intake.
- Assess stool consistency and its influence on risk for stool loss.
- Identify conditions contributing to or causing fecal incontinence.
- Improve access to toileting:
  - Identify usual toileting patterns and plan opportunities for toileting accordingly.
  - Provide assistance with toileting for clients with limited access or impaired functional status (mobility, dexterity, access).
  - Institute a prompted toileting program for persons with impaired cognitive status.
  - Provide adequate privacy for toileting.
  - Respond promptly to requests for assistance with toileting.
- Review the client's nutritional history and evaluate methods to normalize stool consistency with dietary adjustments (e.g., avoiding high fat content foods) and use of fiber.
- Encourage the client to keep a nutrition log to track foods that irritate the bowel.
- For hospitalized clients receiving tube feeding–associated fecal incontinence, involve the nutrition specialist to evaluate the formula composition, osmolality, and fiber content.
- For the client with intermittent episodes of fecal incontinence related to acute changes in stool consistency, begin a bowel reeducation program consisting of:
  - Cleansing the bowel of impacted stool if indicated
  - Normalizing stool consistency by adequate intake of fluids (30 mL/kg of body weight/day) and dietary or supplemental fiber

- Establishing a regular routine of fecal elimination based on established patterns of bowel elimination (patterns established prior to onset of incontinence)

▲ Implement a scheduled stimulation defecation program for persons with neurological conditions causing fecal incontinence:
  - Cleanse the bowel of impacted fecal material before beginning the program.
  - Implement strategies to normalize stool consistency, including adequate intake of fluid and fiber and avoidance of foods associated with diarrhea.
  - Determine a regular schedule for bowel elimination (typically every day or every other day) based on prior patterns of bowel elimination.
  - Provide a stimulus before assisting the client to a position on the toilet; digital stimulation, a stimulating suppository, "mini-enema," or pulsed evacuation enema may be used for stimulation.

▲ Begin a reeducation or pelvic floor muscle exercise program for the person with sphincter incompetence or high-tone pelvic floor muscle dysfunction of the pelvic muscles, or refer persons with fecal incontinence related to sphincter dysfunction to a nurse specialist or other therapist with clinical expertise in these techniques of care.

▲ Consider a pelvic muscle training program or radiofrequency stimulation program in clients with urgency to defecate and fecal incontinence related to recurrent diarrhea or fecal incontinence associated with myogenic disorders affecting the pelvic floor muscles.

- Institute a structured skin care regimen that incorporates three essential steps: cleanse, moisturize, and protect:
  - Select a cleanser with a pH range comparable to that of normal skin (usually labeled "pH balanced").
  - Moisturize with an emollient to replace lipids removed with cleansing, and protect with a skin. Products containing petrolatum, dimethicone, or zinc oxide base or a no-sting skin barrier should be used.

- Routine incontinence care should include daily perineal skin cleansing and following each episode of incontinence.
- When feasible, select a product that combines two or all three of these processes into a single step. Ensure that products are available at the bedside when caring for a client with total incontinence in an inpatient facility.

▲ Use of absorptive pads or adult containment briefs that are applied next the client's skin increases the risk of incontinence-associated dermatitis. Absorbent underpads that wick moisture away from skin may be used with immobile clients.

▲ Consult the physician or advanced practice nurse if a fungal infection is suspected. An antifungal cream or powder beneath a protective ointment may be indicated

• Assist the client to select and apply a containment device for occasional episodes of fecal incontinence. A fecal containment device will prevent soiling of clothing and reduce odors in the client with uncontrolled stool loss.

• In the client with frequent episodes of fecal incontinence and limited mobility, monitor the sacrum and perineal area for pressure ulcerations.

• With acutely ill clients, anticipate and evaluate the cause of acute diarrhea. Anticipate diarrhea associated with treatment or specific interventions (e.g., medications, initiation of tube feedings).

▲ Consult a physician or advanced practice nurse about insertion of a bowel management system in the critically ill client when conservative measures have failed and fecal incontinence is excessive and/or produces perianal skin injury or incontinence-associated dermatitis.

• Evaluate all elderly clients for established or acute fecal incontinence when the elderly client enters the acute or long-term care facility and intervene as indicated.

• Determine the client's cognitive level using a screening tool such as the Mini-Mental State Exam (MMSE), the CAM, or Mini-Cog.

■ Teach nursing colleagues, nonprofessional care providers, family, and client the importance of providing toileting opportunities and adequate privacy for the client in an acute or long-term care facility.

Home Care

• The preceding interventions may be adapted for home care use.

• Assess and teach a bowel management program to support continence. Address timing, diet, fluids, and actions taken independently to deal with bowel incontinence.

• Instruct caregiver to provide clothing that is nonrestrictive, can be manipulated easily for toileting, and can be changed with ease.

• Evaluate self-care strategies of community-dwelling elders; strengthen adaptive behaviors, and councel elders about altering strategies that compromise general health.

• Assist the family in arranging care in a way that allows the client to participate in family or favorite activities without embarrassment.

▲ If the client is limited to bed (or bed and chair), provide a commode or bedpan that can be easily accessed. Involve occupational and physical therapy services as indicated to promote safe transfers.

▲ If the client is frequently incontinent, refer for home health aide services to assist with hygiene and skin care.

▲ Refer the family to support services to assist with in-home management of fecal incontinence as indicated.

NOTE: Refer to nursing diagnoses **Diarrhea** and **Constipation** for detailed management of these related conditions.

Disorganized Infant behavior

NANDA-I Definition

Disintegrated physiological and neurobehavioral responses of infant to the environment

● = Independent   ▲ = Collaborative

Defining Characteristics

Attention-Interaction System
Abnormal response to sensory stimuli (e.g., difficult to soothe, unable to sustain alert status)

Motor System
Altered primitive reflexes; changes to motor tone; finger splaying; fisting; hands to face; hyperextension of extremities; jitteriness; startles; tremors; twitches; uncoordinated movement

Physiological
Arrhythmias; bradycardia; oxygen desaturation; feeding intolerances; skin color changes; tachycardia; time-out signals (e.g., gaze, grasp, hiccough, cough, sneeze, sigh, slack jaw, open mouth, tongue thrust)

Regulatory System
Inability to inhibit startle; irritability

State-Organization System
Active-awake (fussy, worried gaze); diffuse sleep; irritable crying; quiet-awake (staring, gaze aversion); state-oscillation

Caregiver
Cue misreading; deficient knowledge regarding behavioral cues; environmental stimulation contribution

Environmental
Lack of containment within environment; physical environment inappropriateness; sensory deprivation; sensory inappropriateness; sensory overstimulation

Individual
Illness; immature neurological system; low postconceptual age; prematurity

Postnatal
Feeding intolerance; invasive procedures; malnutrition; motor problems; oral problems; pain

• = Independent   ▲ = Collaborative

Prenatal
Congenital disorders; genetic disorders; teratogenic exposure

Client Outcomes

Client Will (Specify Time Frame):
Infant/Child
- Display physiological/autonomic stability: cardiopulmonary, digestive functioning
- Display signs of organized motor system
- Display signs of organized state system: ability to achieve and maintain a state, and transition smoothly between states
- Demonstrate progress toward effective self-regulation
- Demonstrate progress toward or ability to maintain calm attention
- Demonstrate progress or ability to engage in positive interactions
- Demonstrate ability to respond to sensory information in an adaptive way

Parent/Significant Other
- Recognize infant/child behaviors as complex communication system that express specific needs and wants (e.g., hunger, pain, stress desire to engage or disengage)
- Educate parents/caregivers to recognize infant's four avenues of communication: autonomic/physiological, motor, state, attention/interaction
- Recognize how infants respond to environmental sensory input through stress/avoidance and approach/engagement behaviors
- Recognize and support infant's self-regulatory, coping behaviors used to regain or maintain homeostasis
- Teach parents to "tune in" to their own interactive style and how that affects their infant's behavior
- Teach parents ways to adapt their interactive style in response to infant's style of communication
- Identify appropriate positioning and handling techniques that will enhance normal motor development
- Promote infant/child's attention capabilities that support visual and auditory development
- Engage in pleasurable parent-infant interactions that encourage bonding and attachment

- Structure and modify the environment in response to infant/child's behavior and personal needs
- Identify available community resources that provide early intervention services, emotional support, community health nursing, and parenting classes

Nursing Interventions

- Recognize the five neuro-behavior systems through which infants communicate organization and/or disorganization/stress (i.e., physiological/autonomic, motor, states, attention/interactional, self-regulatory).
- Recognize behavior used to communicate stress/avoidance and approach/engagement.
- Individualized developmental care for low-birth-weight, preterm infants has been shown to positively influence neurodevelopmental outcomes.
- Provide optimal physical (inanimate) environment, social (animate) environment including caregiver-infant interactions for premature and medically fragile infants.
- Provide infants with adequate pain management during stressful and painful procedures.
- Identify appropriate body positions that optimize body alignment (neck, trunk, semiflexed, and midline orientation of extremities, with spine in straight alignment).
- Identify and use best positions that encourage longer periods of sleep.
- Provide care that encourages infant state organization—ability to achieve and maintain quiet-sleep and quiet-awake states, and transition smoothly between sleep and awake states.
- Provide infants opportunities for nonnutritive sucking.
- Encourage parents to identify and support infant's attention capabilities.
- Provide parents opportunities to experience physical closeness through loving touch, massage, cuddling, skin-to-skin (kangaroo care), and rocking that enhances parent-infant attachment.
- Encourage parents to be active collaborators in their infant's care.

● = Independent   ▲ = Collaborative

- Provide infants with positive sensory experiences (i.e., visual, auditory, tactile, vestibular, proprioceptive) to enhance development of sensory pathways.
▲ Provide information or refer to community-based follow-up programs for preterm/at-risk infants and their families.

Multicultural

- Assess for the influence of cultural beliefs, norms, and values on the family's perceptions of infant/child behavior.

Client/Family Teaching and Discharge Planning

- Ask parents what they need to help them care for their premature infant.
- Educate parents on the positive effects of pacifier use after NICU discharge, including breastfed infants
- Provide information on techniques to promote sleep for infants.
- Nurture parents so that they in turn can nurture their infant/child.
- Have knowledge of community early intervention services and follow-up programs for preterm and at-risk infants and families.

Home Care

- The preceding interventions may be adapted for home care use.
- Educate families in ways of preparing the home environment.
- Prepare families for realistic challenges of caring for preterm and at-risk infants prior to discharge.
- Encourage families to teach friends/visitors to recognize and respond to infant's unique behavioral cues.
- Provide families information about community resources, developmental follow-up services, and parent-to-parent support programs. Primary care physician (PCP) follow-up should include all infants born prematurely for early identification of adverse neurological development.

• = Independent   ▲ = Collaborative

Readiness for enhanced organized Infant behavior

NANDA-I Definition

A pattern of modulation of the physiological and behavioral systems of functioning (i.e., autonomic, motor, state-organization, self-regulatory, and attentional-interactional systems) in an infant that is sufficient for well-being and can be strengthened

Defining Characteristics

Definite sleep-wake states; response to stimuli (e.g., visual, auditory); stable physiological measures; use of some self-regulatory behaviors

Risk for disorganized Infant behavior

NANDA-I Definition

Risk for alteration in integrating and modulation of the physiological and behavioral systems of functioning (i.e., autonomic, motor, state, organizational, self-regulatory, and attentional-interactional systems)

Risk Factors

Environmental overstimulation; invasive procedures; lack of containment within environment; motor problems; oral problems; pain; painful procedures; prematurity

Risk for Infection

NANDA-I Definition

At increased risk for being invaded by pathogenic organisms

Risk Factors

Chronic disease (diabetes mellitus, obesity); deficient knowledge to avoid exposure to pathogens; inadequate primary defenses (altered peristalsis, broken skin) (e.g., intravenous catheter placement, invasive procedures), change in pH of secretions, decrease in ciliary action, premature rupture of amniotic membranes, prolonged rupture of amniotic membranes, smoking, stasis of body fluids, traumatized tissue (e.g., trauma, tissue destruction); inadequate secondary defenses: decreased hemoglobin, immunosuppression (e.g., inadequate acquired immunity,

• = Independent   ▲ = Collaborative

pharmaceutical agents including immunosuppressants, steroids, monoclonal antibodies, immunomodulators), leukopenia, suppressed inflammatory response); inadequate vaccination; increased environmental exposure to pathogens, outbreaks; invasive procedures; malnutrition

Client Outcomes

Client Will (Specify Time Frame):

* Remain free from symptoms of infection
* State symptoms of infection
* Demonstrate appropriate care of infection-prone site
* Maintain white blood cell count and differential within normal limits
* Demonstrate appropriate hygienic measures such as handwashing, oral care, and perineal care

Nursing Interventions

* Consider targeted surveillance for methicillin-resistant *Staphylococcus aureus* (MRSA) (screen clients at risk for MRSA on admission).
* ▲ Observe and report signs of infection such as redness, warmth, discharge, and increased body temperature.
* ▲ Assess temperature of neutropenic clients; report a single temperature of greater than 100.5° F.
* Oral or tympanic thermometers may be used to assess temperature in adults and infants.
* ▲ Note and report laboratory values (e.g., white blood cell count and differential, serum protein, serum albumin, and cultures).
* Assess skin for color, moisture, texture, and turgor (elasticity). Keep accurate, ongoing documentation of changes.
* Carefully wash and pat dry skin, including skinfold areas. Use hydration and moisturization on all at-risk surfaces.
* Refer to care plan for **Risk for impaired Skin Integrity.**
* Monitor client's vitamin D level.
* Refer to care plan **Readiness for enhanced Nutrition** for additional interventions.
* Use strategies to prevent health care–acquired pneumonia: assess lung sounds, and sputum color and characteristics; use sterile water rather than tap water for mouth care of

immunosuppressed clients; use sterile technique when suctioning; suction secretions above tracheal tube before suctioning; drain accumulated condensation in ventilator tubing into a fluid trap or other collection device before repositioning the client; assess patency and placement of nasogastric tubes; elevate the client's head to 30 degrees or higher to prevent gastric reflux of organisms in the lung.

- Encourage fluid intake.
- Use appropriate "hand hygiene" (i.e., handwashing or use of alcohol-based hand rubs).
- When using an alcohol-based hand rub, apply ample amount of product to palm of one hand and rub hands together, covering all surfaces of hands and fingers, until hands are dry. Note that the volume needed to reduce the number of bacteria on hands varies by product.
- Follow standard precautions and wear gloves during any contact with blood, mucous membranes, nonintact skin, or any body substance except sweat. Use goggles and gowns when appropriate. Standard precautions apply to all clients. You must assume all clients are carrying blood-borne pathogens.
- Follow transmission-based precautions for airborne-, droplet-, and contact-transmitted microorganisms:
  ▲ **Airborne:** Isolate the client in a room with monitored negative air pressure, with the room door closed and the client remaining in the room. Always wear appropriate respiratory protection when you enter the room. Limit the movement and transport of the client from the room to essential purposes only. Have the client wear a surgical mask during transport.
  ▲ **Droplet:** Keep the client in a private room, if possible. If not possible, maintain a spatial separation of 3 feet from other beds or visitors. The door may remain open. Wear a surgical mask when you must come within 3 feet of the client. Some hospitals may choose to implement a mask requirement for droplet precautions for anyone entering the room. Limit transport to essential purposes and have the client wear a mask if possible.

• = Independent   ▲ = Collaborative

▲ **Contact:** Place the client in a private room if possible or with someone (cohorting) who has an active infection from the same microorganism. Wear clean, nonsterile gloves when entering the room. When providing care, change gloves after contact with any infective material such as wound drainage. Remove the gloves and clean your hands before leaving the room and take care not to touch any potentially infectious items or surfaces on the way out. Wear a gown if you anticipate your clothing may have substantial contact with the client or other potentially infectious items. Remove the gown before leaving the room. Limit transport of the client to essential purposes and take care that the client does not contact other environmental surfaces along the way. Dedicate the use of noncritical client care equipment to a single client. If use of common equipment is unavoidable, adequately clean and disinfect equipment before use with other clients.

- Use alternatives to indwelling catheters whenever possible (external catheters, incontinence pads, bladder control techniques). Sterile technique must be used when inserting urinary catheters.
- If a urinary catheter is necessary, follow catheter management practices: All indwelling catheters should be connected to a sterile, closed drainage system (i.e., not broken), except for good clinical reasons. Cleanse the perineum and meatus twice daily using soap and water.
- Use evidence-based practices and educate personnel in care of peripheral catheters: use aseptic technique for insertion and care, label insertion sites and all tubing with date and time of insertion, inspect every 8 hours for signs of infection, record, and report.
- Use sterile technique wherever there is a loss of skin integrity.
- Ensure the client's appropriate hygienic care with handwashing; bathing; oral care; and hair, nail, and perineal care performed by either the nurse or the client.
- Recommend responsible use of antibiotics; use antibiotics sparingly.
- Carefully screen and treat women with infertility who may have female genital tuberculosis.

• = Independent   ▲ = Collaborative

NOTE: Many of the preceding interventions are appropriate for the pediatric client.
- Follow meticulous hand hygiene when working with premature infants.
- Cluster nursing procedures to decrease number of contacts with infants, allowing time for appropriate hand hygiene.
- Avoid the prophylactic use of topical cream in premature infants.
- Encourage early enteral feeding with human milk.
- Monitor recurrent antibiotic use in children. Instruct parents on appropriate indicators for medical visits and the risks associated with overuse of antibiotics.

Geriatric

- Suspect pneumonia when the client has symptoms of lethargy or confusion. Assess response to treatment, especially antibiotic therapy.
- Most clients develop HCAP by either aspirating contaminated substances or inhaling airborne particles. Refer to care plan for **Risk for Aspiration.**
- Carefully screen elderly women with incontinence for urinary tract infections
- ▲ Observe and report if the client has a low-grade temperature or new onset of confusion. Use an electronic axillary thermometer.
- ▲ Recommend that the geriatric client receive an annual influenza immunization and one-time pneumococcal vaccine.
- Recognize that chronically ill geriatric clients have an increased susceptibility to infection; practice meticulous care of all invasive sites.

Home Care

- Some of the above interventions may be adapted for home care use.
- Assess and treat wounds in the home.
- Review standards for surveillance of infections in home care.
- Maintain strong infection-prevention policies.

▲ Monitor for the occurrence of infectious exacerbation of chronic obstructive pulmonary disease (COPD); refer to physician for treatment.

▲ Refer for nutritional evaluation; implement dietary changes to support recovery and address antibiotic side effects.

Client/Family Teaching and Discharge Planning

• Teach the client risk factors contributing to surgical wound infection (e.g., diabetes and higher body mass index).

• Teach the client and family the importance of hand hygiene in preventing postoperative infections.

• Encourage high-risk persons, including health care workers, to get vaccinated.

• Influenza: Teach symptoms of influenza and importance of vaccination for influenza.

• Teach the client and family how to take a temperature. Encourage the family to take the client's temperature between 4 PM and 10 PM at least once daily.

Risk for Injury

NANDA-I Definition

At risk for injury as a result of environmental conditions interacting with the individual's adaptive and defensive resources

NOTE: This nursing diagnosis overlaps with other diagnoses such as **Risk for Falls, Risk for Trauma, Risk for Poisoning, Risk for Suffocation, Risk for Aspiration,** and if the client is at risk of bleeding, **Ineffective Protection.** Refer to care plans for these diagnoses if appropriate.

Risk Factors

External

Biological (e.g., immunization level of community, microorganism); chemical (e.g., poisons, pollutants, drugs, pharmaceutical agents, alcohol, nicotine, preservatives, cosmetics, dyes); human (e.g., nosocomial agents; staffing patterns; cognitive, affective, psychomotor factors); mode of transport; nutritional (e.g., vitamins, food types); physical

• = Independent   ▲ = Collaborative

(e.g., design, structure, and arrangement of community, building, and/
or equipment)

Internal

Abnormal blood profile (e.g., leukocytosis/leukopenia, altered clotting
factors, thrombocytopenia, sickle cell, thalassemia, decreased hemoglobin); biochemical dysfunction; developmental age (physiological,
psychosocial); effector dysfunction; immune/autoimmune dysfunction; integrative dysfunction; malnutrition; physical (e.g., broken skin,
altered mobility); psychological (affective orientation); sensory dysfunction; tissue hypoxia

Client Outcomes

Client Will (Specify Time Frame):

- Remain free of injuries
- Explain methods to prevent injuries
- Demonstrate behaviors that decrease the risk for injury.

Nursing Interventions

- Prevent iatrogenic harm to the hospitalized client by following the National Patient Safety goals:

Accuracy of Client Identification

- Use at least two methods (e.g., client's name and medical
  record number or birth date) to identify the client before
  administering medications, blood products, treatments, or
  procedures.
- Prior to beginning any invasive or surgical procedure, have
  a final verification to confirm the correct client, the correct procedure, and the correct site for the procedure using
  active communication techniques.
- Label containers used for blood and other specimens in the
  presence of the client.

Effectiveness of Communication Among Care Staff

- When taking verbal or telephone orders, the orders should
  be written down and then read back for verification to the
  individual giving the order.

● = Independent   ▲ = Collaborative

- Standardize use of abbreviations, acronyms, symbols, and dose designations that are used in the institution.
- Ensure critical test results and values are recorded and reported in a timely manner.
- Utilize a standardized approach of "handing off" communications, including opportunities to ask and answer questions.
- Use only approved abbreviations.

Medication Safety

- Standardize and limit the number of drug concentrations utilized by the institution (e.g., concentrations of medications such as morphine in patient-controlled analgesia [PCA] pumps).
- Label all medications and medication containers (e.g., syringes, medication cups, or other solutions on or off the surgical field).
- Identify all of the client's current medications upon admission to a health care facility, and ensure that all health care staff have access to the information.
- Ensure that accurate medicine information is sent with the client throughout his/her care.
- Reconcile all medication at discharge, and provide list to the client.
- Improve the effectiveness of alarm systems in the clinical area.
- Standardize a list of medications that look alike or sound alike. This list needs to be updated yearly.
- Identify and take extra care with clients who are on blood-thinning medications.

Infection Control

- Reduce the risk of infections by following Centers for Disease Control and Prevention (CDC) hand hygiene guidelines.
- Clients who obtain injuries or die from infectious disease must be documented.
- Utilize proven guidelines to prevent infections that are difficult to treat.

• = Independent   ▲ = Collaborative

- Utilize proven guidelines to prevent infection of the blood from central lines.
- Utilize safe practices to treat the surgical site of the client.

Fall Prevention

- Evaluate all clients for fall risk and take appropriate actions to prevent falls.

Client Involvement in Care

- Educate the client and family on how to recognize and report concerns about safety issues.

Identify Clients with Safety Risks

- Identify which clients are at risk for harming themselves.

Identify Clients Who Are Susceptible to Changes in Health Status

- Educate staff on how to recognize changes in client condition, how to respond quickly, and how to alert specially trained staff to intervene if needed.
- Prevent errors in surgery.
- Standardize steps to educate staff so documents for surgery are ready prior to surgery.
- Educate staff to mark the body part scheduled for surgery and engage the client in this process as well.
- See care plan for **Risk for Falls.**
- ▲ Avoid use of restraints if at all possible. Restraint-free is now the standard of care for hospitals and long-term care facilities. Obtain a physician's order if restraints are necessary.
- In place of restraints, use the following:
  - Well-staffed and educated nursing personnel with frequent client contact
  - Continuity of care with familiar staff
  - Nursing units designed to care for clients with cognitive or functional impairments
  - Avoiding use of IVs or tubes that are susceptible to being removed
  - Alarm systems with ankle, above-the-knee, or wrist sensors

- Bed or wheelchair alarms
- Increased observation of the client
- Providing exercise to diffuse and deflect client behavior
- Low or very-low height beds
- Border-defining pillow/mattress to remind the client to stay in bed
- Mobility exercise to strength muscles and steady gait
- Floor mats and transfer poles for client safety

- For an agitated client, consider providing individualized music of the client's choice.
- Review drug profile for potential side effects that may increase risk of injury.
- Use one quarter- to one half-length side rails only, and maintain bed in a low position. Ensure that wheels are locked on bed and commode. Keep dim light in room at night.
- If the client has a new onset of confusion (delirium), refer to the care plan for **Acute Confusion.** If the client has chronic confusion, see the care plan for **Chronic Confusion.**
- Ask family to stay with the client to prevent the client from accidentally falling or pulling out tubes.
- Remove all possible hazards in environment such as razors, medications, and matches.
- Place an injury-prone client in a room that is near the nurse's station.
- Help clients sit in a stable chair with armrests. Avoid use of wheelchairs and geri-chairs except for transportation as needed.
▲ Refer to physical therapy for strengthening exercises and gait training to increase mobility.
▲ For the agitated psychotic client, use nonphysical forms of behavior management, such as verbal intervention or show of force. If medication is required, use oral medications if at all possible.

Pediatric

- Teach parents the need for close supervision of all young children playing near water.
- If child has epilepsy, recommend showers instead of tub baths, and no unsupervised swimming is ever allowed.

● = Independent   ▲ = Collaborative

- Assess the client's socioeconomic status.
- Never leave young children unsupervised around cooking areas.
- Teach parents and children the need to maintain safety for the exercising child, including wearing helmets when biking.
- Encourage parents to insist on using breakaway bases for baseball.
- Provide parents of children with traumatic brain injury with written instruction, emergency phone numbers and ensure that instructions are understood before child is discharged from health care setting. Instruct them to observe for the following symptoms: nausea, mild headache, dizziness, irritability, lethargy, poor concentration, loss of appetite, and insomnia
- Teach both parents and children the need for gun safety.

Geriatric

- Encourage the client to wear glasses and hearing aids and to use walking aids when ambulating.
- If the client experiences dizziness because of orthostatic hypotension when getting up, teach methods to decrease dizziness, such as rising slowly, remaining seated several minutes before standing, flexing feet upward several times while sitting, sitting down immediately if feeling dizzy, and trying to have someone present when standing.
- Discourage driving at night.
- Acknowledge racial/ethnic differences at the onset of care.
- Assess for the influence of cultural beliefs, norms, and values on the client's perceptions of risk for injury.
- Assess whether exposure to community violence is contributing to risk for injury.
- Use culturally relevant injury prevention programs whenever possible.
- Validate the client's feelings and concerns related to environmental risks.

Home Care and Client/Family Teaching and Discharge Planning

- See **Risk for Trauma** for more Nursing Interventions.

• = Independent   ▲ = Collaborative

Insomnia

NANDA-I Definition

A disruption in amount and quality of sleep that impairs functioning

Defining Characteristics

Observed changes in affect, observed lack of energy, increased work/school absenteeism, reports changes in mood, reports decreased health status, reports decreased quality of life, reports difficulty concentrating, reports difficulty falling asleep, reports difficulty staying asleep, reports dissatisfaction with sleep (current), reports increased accidents, reports lack of energy, reports nonrestorative sleep, reports sleep disturbances that produce next-day consequences, reports waking up too early

Related Factors (r/t)

Activity pattern (e.g., timing, amount), anxiety, depression, environmental factors (e.g., ambient noise, daylight/darkness exposure, ambient temperature/humidity, unfamiliar setting), fear, frequent daytime naps, gender-related hormonal shifts, grief, inadequate sleep hygiene (current), intake of stimulants, intake of alcohol, impairment of normal sleep pattern (e.g., travel, shift work), interrupted sleep, pharmaceutical agents, parental responsibilities, physical discomfort (e.g., pain, shortness of breath, cough, gastroesophageal reflux, nausea, incontinence/urgency), stress (e.g., ruminative pre-sleep pattern)

Client Outcomes

Client Will (Specify Time Frame):

- Verbalize plan to implement sleep-promoting routines
- Fall asleep with less difficulty a minimum of four nights out of seven
- Wake up less frequently during night a minimum of four nights out of seven
- Sleep a minimum of 6 hours most nights and more if needed to meet next stated outcome
- Awaken refreshed and not be fatigued during day most of the time

• = Independent   ▲ = Collaborative

Nursing Interventions

- Obtain a sleep history including time needed to initiate sleep, duration of awakenings after the first sleep onset, total night-time sleep amounts, and satisfaction with sleep amounts. Also explore bedtime routines, use of medications and stimulants, and use of complementary/alternative therapies for stress management and relaxation before bedtime.
- From the history, assess the degree and chronic nature of insomnia.
- Avoid negative associations with ability to sleep.
- If feasible, have client arise from bed to participate in calming activities whenever anxious about failure to fall asleep.
- Avoid a focus on the clock and subsequent worry about sleep time lost to sleeplessness.
- Focus on positive aspects of life.
- ▲ Assist clients with chronic insomnia to select nights for sleeping pill use if complete discontinuance of sleeping pills is not feasible.
- ▲ For clients with chronic insomnia, refer to a nurse practitioner or other professional trained in cognitive-behavioral therapies.
- ▲ Assess pain medication use and, when feasible, recommend pain medications that promote rather than interfere with sleep. (See **Acute Pain** and **Chronic Pain** care plans.)
- ▲ Assess level of anxiety. If chronic insomnia is accompanied by anxiety, use relaxation techniques. (See further Nursing Interventions for **Anxiety.**)
- ▲ Assess for signs of depression: depressed mood state, statements of hopelessness, poor appetite. Refer for counseling as appropriate.
- ▲ Assess for signs of sleep apnea and restless leg syndrome; if present, refer to an accredited sleep clinic for evaluation.
- ▲ Assess for signs of substance overuse/abuse including prescription, OTC, and illicit drugs, as well as alcohol, caffeine, and theophylline use. Suggest lifestyle change and refer for addiction counseling as appropriate.
- Supplement other interventions with teaching about sleep and sleep promotion. (See further Nursing Interventions for **Readiness for enhanced Sleep.**)

● = Independent   ▲ = Collaborative

Geriatric

- Assessment of medications used for pain and other symptoms in the elderly is important because pain medications may be interfering with the client's ability to initiate and maintain sleep.
- Most interventions discussed previously may be used with geriatric clients. Passive body heating via full-immersion or foot baths should be used with great caution in the elderly because of multiple safety issues that are more prevalent with the elderly, including burns, dehydration, and potential for slips/falls in bath area.
- In addition see the Geriatric section of Nursing Interventions for **Readiness for enhanced Sleep.**

Home Care

- Assessments and interventions discussed previously may be adapted for use in home care.
- In addition, see the Home Care section of Nursing Interventions for **Readiness for enhanced Sleep.**

Client/Family Teaching and Discharge Plannning

- Teach family about normal sleep and promote adoption of behaviors that enhance it. See Nursing Interventions for **Readiness for enhanced Sleep.**
- Teach family about sleep deprivation and how to avoid it. See Nursing Interventions for **Sleep Deprivation.**
- Advise family of importance of not disrupting sleep of others unnecessarily. See Nursing Interventions for **Sleep Disruption.**
- Advise family of importance of minimizing noise and light in the sleep environment. See Nursing Interventions for **Disturbed Sleep Pattern.**
- Help family differentiate insomnia from externally caused sleep disruption and resultant sleep deprivation: Family members may have direct control over interruptions in sleep and thus may help limit sleep deprivation directly.

• = Independent   ▲ = Collaborative

Decreased Intracranial Adaptive Capacity

NANDA-I Definition

Intracranial fluid dynamic mechanisms that normally compensate for increases in intracranial volumes are compromised, resulting in repeated disproportionate increases in intracranial pressure (ICP) in response to a variety of noxious and nonnoxious stimuli

Defining Characteristics

Baseline ICP greater than 10 mm Hg; disproportionate increases in ICP following a single environmental or nursing maneuver stimulus; repeated increases in ICP of greater than 10 mm Hg for more than 5 minutes following any of a variety of external stimuli; volume-pressure response test variation (volume-pressure ratio of 2, pressure-volume index of less than 10); wide-amplitude ICP waveform

Related Factors (r/t)

Brain injuries: decreased cerebral perfusion less than or equal to 50 to 60 mm Hg; sustained increase in ICP greater than 10 to 15 mm Hg; systemic hypotension with intracranial hypertension

Client Outcomes

Client Will (Specify Time Frame):

- Experience fewer than five episodes of disproportionate increases in intracranial pressure (DIICP) in 24 hours
- Have neurological status changes that are not triggered by episodes of DIICP
- Have cerebral perfusion pressure (CPP) remaining greater than 60 to 70 mm Hg in adults

Nursing Interventions

▲ To assess ICP and CPP effectively:
- Maintain and display ICP and CPP continuously as ICP data guide therapy and predict outcome.
- Maintain ICP less than 20 mm Hg and CPP greater than 60 mm Hg.

• = Independent   ▲ = Collaborative

- Monitor neurological status frequently (hourly in acute situations) using the Glasgow Coma Scale (GCS), noting changes in eye opening, motor response to painful stimuli, and awareness of self, time, and place.
- Monitor pupillary size and reaction to light during all neurological assessments.
- Monitor brain temperature.
- Monitor brain tissue oxygen ($PbtO_2$).

▲ To prevent harmful increases in ICP:
  - Elevate head of bed 30 to 45 degrees with head in midline position.
  - Administer sedation per collaborative protocol.
  - Administer pain medication per collaborative protocol.
  - Maintain glycemic control per collaborative protocol.
  - Maintain normothermia.
  - Maintain optimal oxygenation and ventilation, applying positive end expiratory pressure (PEEP) as needed and avoiding hyperventilation.
  - Premedicate clients with adequate sedation and limit endotracheal suction passes to two in order to limit ICP increases.

▲ To prevent harmful decreases in CPP:
  - See care plan for **Risk for ineffective Cerebral tissue perfusion.**

▲ To treat sustained intracranial hypertension (ICP greater than 20 mm Hg):
  - Remove or loosen rigid cervical collars.
  - Administer a bolus dose of mannitol and/or hypertonic saline per collaborative protocol.
  - Drain CSF from an intraventricular catheter system per collaborative protocol.
  - Administer barbiturates per collaborative protocol, and monitor blood pressure closely during medication administration.
  - Induce moderate hypothermia (32° to 35° C) per collaborative protocol.

▲ To treat decreased CPP (sustained CPP < 60 mm Hg):

> ■ Administer norepinephrine to raise MAP per collaborative protocol.
> ■ Administer hypertonic saline per collaborative protocol.

Neonatal Jaundice

NANDA-I Definition

The yellow-orange tint of the neonate's skin and mucous membranes that occurs after 24 hours of life as a result of unconjugated bilirubin in the circulation

Defining Characteristics

Abnormal blood profile (e.g., hemolysis; total serum bilirubin greater than 2 mg/dL; total serum bilirubin in the high-risk range on age in hour-specific nomogram); abnormal skin bruising; yellow mucous membranes; yellow-orange skin; yellow sclera

Related Factors (r/t)

Abnormal weight loss (greater than 7% to 8% in breastfeeding newborn; 15% in term infant); feeding pattern not well established; infant experiences difficulty making transition to extrauterine life; neonate age 1 to 7 days; stool (meconium) passage delayed

Client Outcomes

Client (Infant) Will (Specify Time Frame):
* Establish effective feeding pattern (breast or bottle)
* Receive bilirubin assessment and screening within the first week of life to identify potentially harmful levels of serum bilirubin
* Receive appropriate therapy to enhance indirect bilirubin excretion
* Receive nursing assessments to determine risk for severity of jaundice
* Maintain hydration: moist buccal membranes, 4 to 6 wet diapers in 24 hour period, weight loss no greater than 8% of birth weight
* Evacuate stool within 48 hours of birth, and pass 3 or 4 stools per 24 hours by day 4 of life

• = Independent   ▲ = Collaborative

Client (Parent[s]) Will (Specify Time Frame):

- Receive information on neonatal jaundice prior to discharge from birth hospital
- Verbalize understanding of physical signs of jaundice prior to discharge
- Verbalize signs requiring immediate health practitioner notification: sleepy infant who does not awaken easily for feedings, fewer than 4 to 6 wet diapers in 24-hour period by day 4, fewer than 3 to 4 stools in 24 hours by day 4, breastfeeds fewer than 8 times per day
- Demonstrate ability to operate home phototherapy unit if prescribed

Nursing Interventions

- Evaluate maternal and delivery history for risk factors for neonatal jaundice (RhD, ABO, G6PD deficiency, direct Coombs).
- Perform neonatal gestational age assessment once the newborn has had an initial period of interaction with mother and father.
- Encourage breastfeeding within the first hour of the neonate's life.
- Encourage skin-to-skin mother-newborn contact shortly after delivery.
- Assess infant's skin color at birth and every 8 hours thereafter until birth hospital discharge for the appearance of jaundice.
- Encourage and assist mother with frequent breastfeeding (at least 8 to 12 times per day in the first week of life).
- Assist parents with bottle-feeding neonate.
- Avoid feeding supplements such as water, dextrose water, or any other milk substitutes in breastfeeding neonate.
- Assess neonate's stooling pattern in first 48 hours of life.
- ▲ Collect and evaluate laboratory blood specimens as prescribed or per unit protocol.
- ▲ Monitor transcutaneous bilirubin level in jaundiced neonate per unit protocol or at least once every 8 hours.

● = Independent ▲ = Collaborative

- Perform hour-specific total serum bilirubin risk assessment before newborn's birth center discharge and document the results.
- Monitor newborn for signs of inadequate breast milk or formula intake: dry oral mucous membranes, fewer than 4 to 6 wet diapers per 24 hours, no stool in 24 hours, body weight loss greater than 7% to 8% in breastfeeding infant.
- Assess late preterm infant (born between 34 weeks and 36⅔ weeks' gestation) for ability to breastfeed successfully and adequate intake of breast milk.
- Assist mother with breastfeeding and assess latch-on.
- Encourage alternate methods for providing expressed breast milk if maternal health status is compromised (use of expressed breast milk) and assist mother with collection of breast milk via use of breast pump or hand expression.
- Encourage father's participation in newborn care by changing diapers, helping position newborn for breastfeeding, and holding newborn while mother rests. Weigh newborn daily.
▲ When phototherapy is ordered, place seminude infant (diaper only) under prescribed amount of phototherapy lights.
- Protect infant's eyes from phototherapy light source with eye shields. Remove eye shields periodically when infant is removed from light source for feeding and parent-infant interaction.
- Monitor infant's hydration status, fluid intake, skin status, and body temperature while undergoing phototherapy.
▲ Collect and evaluate laboratory blood specimens (total serum bilirubin) while infant is undergoing phototherapy.
- Encourage continuation of breastfeeding and brief infant care activities such as changing diapers while infant is being treated with phototherapy; phototherapy may be interrupted for breastfeeding.
- Provide emotional support for parent(s) of infant undergoing phototherapy.

Multicultural

- Assess infants of Chinese ethnicity for early rising bilirubin levels, especially when breastfeeding.

• = Independent   ▲ = Collaborative

- Encourage early and exclusive breastfeeding among Chinese and other Asian newborns.
- Assess Chinese and other Asian newborns suspected of being jaundiced with a serum bilirubin level or transcutaneous monitor.

Client/Family Teaching and Discharge Planning

- Teach the breastfeeding mother and support persons about the appearance of jaundice (yellow or orange color of skin) after birth center discharge, and provide health care resource telephone number for parents to call for concerns related to newborn's care.
- Teach parents regarding the signs of inadequate milk intake: fewer than 3 to 4 stools by day 4, fewer than 4 to 6 wet diapers in 24 hours, and dry oral mucous membranes; additional danger signs include a sleepy baby that does not awaken for breastfeeding or appears lethargic (decreased activity level from usual newborn pattern).
- Teach parents to avoid placing infant in sunlight at home to treat jaundice.
▲ Teach the parent(s) about the importance of medical follow-up in the first several days of life for the evaluation of jaundice.
- Teach parents about the use of phototherapy (hospital or home, as prescribed), the proper use of the phototherapy equipment, feedings, and assessment of hydration, body temperature, skin status, and urine and stool output.

Quality and Safety in Nursing

- **Patient Safety:** Minimizes risk of harm to patient
- Knowledge: Nurses continually assess newborns for risk factors associated with the development of jaundice
- Skills: Nurses use transcutaneous and serum bilirubin measurements to determine the newborn's bilirubin risk according to the hour-specific nomogram
- Attitudes: Nurses appreciate their role as one of promoting safety for the newborn at risk for developing jaundice
- Knowledge: Nurses implement patient-focused strategies to promote serum bilirubin reduction; these include but are

not limited to placing the newborn to mother's breast in first hours of life and encouraging frequent (every 2 hours) breastfeeding
- Skills: Nurses identify individual clinical risk factors in the neonate that place him/her at risk for jaundice
- Attitudes: Nurses value their role as a health care team member to promote the safe care of the newborn at discharge from the birth center and beyond
- Knowledge: Nurses understand use of phototherapy to reduce levels of indirect bilirubin
- Skills: Nurses use phototherapy lights appropriately
- Skills: Nurses assess infant for untoward effects of phototherapy
- Attitudes: Nurses appreciate the role of phototherapy as a treatment
- Attitudes: Nurses value their role in the promotion of safety with the use of phototherapy
- Quality and Safety Education for Nurses: *http://www.qsen.org/ksas_graduate.php#safety* and *http://www.qsen.org/about_qsen.php*

Risk for neonatal Jaundice

NANDA-I Definition

At risk for the yellow-orange tint of the neonate's skin and mucous membranes that occurs after 24 hours of life as a result of unconjugated bilirubin in the circulation

Risk Factors

- Abnormal weight loss (greater than 7% to 8% in breastfeeding newborn; 15% in term infant)
- Feeding pattern not well established
- Infant experiences difficulty making transition to extrauterine life
- Neonate age 1 to 7 days
- Prematurity
- Stool (meconium) passage delayed

● = Independent   ▲ = Collaborative

Nursing Interventions

- Evaluate maternal and delivery history for risk factors for neonatal jaundice (RhD, ABO, G6PD deficiency, direct Coombs).
- Perform neonatal gestational age assessment once the newborn has had an initial period of interaction with mother and father.
- Encourage breastfeeding within the first hour of the neonate's life.
- Encourage skin-to-skin mother-newborn contact shortly after delivery.
- Assess infant's skin color at birth and every 8 hours thereafter until birth hospital discharge for the appearance of jaundice.
- Encourage and assist mother with frequent breastfeeding (at least 8 to 12 times per day in the first week of life).
- Assist parents with bottle feeding neonate.
- Avoid feeding supplements such as water, dextrose water, or any other milk substitutes in breastfeeding neonate.
- Assess neonate's stooling pattern in first 48 hours of life.
- Identify clinical risk factors that place the infant at greater risk of developing neonatal jaundice: exclusive breastfeeding, preterm birth (less than 37 weeks' gestation), previous sibling with jaundice, East Asian ethnicity, and significant bruising.
- ▲ Collect and evaluate laboratory blood specimens as determined by presence of clinical risk factors or as prescribed.
- ▲ Monitor transcutaneous bilirubin level in jaundiced neonate per unit protocol or at least once every 8 hours. The transcutaneous bilirubin levels are a screening tool and not used as a diagnostic measure.
- ▲ Perform hour-specific total serum bilirubin risk assessment prior to newborn's birth center discharge and document the results.
- Monitor newborn for signs of inadequate breast milk or formula intake: dry oral mucous membranes, fewer than 4 to 6 wet diapers per 24 hours, no stool in 24 hours, body weight loss greater than 7% to 8% in breastfeeding infant.
- Assist mother with breastfeeding and assess latch-on.
- Encourage alternate methods for providing expressed breast milk if maternal health status is compromised (use of expressed breast milk) and assist mother with collection of breast milk via use of breast pump or hand expression.

• = Independent   ▲ = Collaborative

- Encourage father's participation in newborn care by changing diapers, helping position newborn for breastfeeding, and holding newborn while mother rests.
- Weigh late preterm infant and the term newborn daily who is at high risk for inadequate caloric intake daily for the first week of life.

Multicultural

▲ Assess infants of Chinese ethnicity for early rising bilirubin levels, especially when breastfeeding.
- Encourage early and exclusive breastfeeding among Chinese and other Asian newborns.
▲ Assess Chinese and other Asian newborns suspected of being jaundiced with a serum bilirubin level or transcutaneous monitor.

Client/Family Teaching and Discharge Planning

- Teach the breastfeeding mother and support persons about the appearance of jaundice (yellow or orange color of skin) after birth center discharge, and provide health care resource telephone number for parents to call for concerns related to newborn's care.
- Teach parents regarding the signs of inadequate milk intake: fewer than 3 to 4 stools by day 4, fewer than 4 to 6 wet diapers in 24 hours, and dry oral mucous membranes; additional danger signs include a sleepy baby who does not awaken for breastfeeding, or appears lethargic (decreased activity level from usual newborn pattern).
- Teach parents to avoid placing infant in sunlight at home to treat jaundice.
▲ Teach the parent(s) about the importance of medical follow-up in the first several days of life for the evaluation of jaundice, especially in the late preterm infant.

Quality and Safety in Nursing

- **Client Safety:** Minimizes risk of harm to client
- Knowledge: Nurses continually assess newborns for risk factors associated with the development of jaundice

- Skills: Nurses use transcutaneous and serum bilirubin measurements to determine the newborn's bilirubin risk according to the hour-specific nomogram
- Attitudes: Nurses appreciate their role as one of promoting safety for the newborn at risk for developing jaundice
- Knowledge: Nurses implement client-focused strategies to promote serum bilirubin reduction; these include but are not limited to placing the newborn to mother's breast in first hours of life and encouraging frequent (every 2 hours) breastfeeding
- Skills: Nurses identify individual clinical risk factors in the neonate that place him/her at risk for jaundice
- Attitudes: Nurses value their role as a health care team member to promote the safe care of the newborn at discharge from the birth center and beyond
- Quality and Safety Education for Nurses: *http://www.qsen.org/ksas_graduate.php#safety* and *http://www.qsen.org/about_qsen.php*

Deficient Knowledge

NANDA-I Definition

Absence or deficiency of cognitive information related to a specific topic

Defining Characteristics

Exaggerated behaviors; inaccurate follow-through of instruction; inaccurate performance of test; inappropriate behaviors (e.g., hysterical, hostile, agitated, apathetic); reports the problem

Related Factors (r/t)

Cognitive limitation; information misinterpretation; lack of exposure; lack of interest in learning; lack of recall; unfamiliarity with information resources

Client Outcomes

Client Will (Specify Time Frame):
- Explain disease state, recognize need for medications, and understand treatments

● = Independent   ▲ = Collaborative

- Describe the rationale for therapy/treatment options
- Incorporate knowledge of health regimen into lifestyle
- State confidence in one's ability to manage health situation and remain in control of life
- Demonstrate how to perform health-related procedure(s) satisfactorily
- Identify resources that can be used for more information or support after discharge

Nursing Interventions

- Consider the client's ability and readiness to learn (e.g., mental acuity, ability to see or hear, existing pain, emotional readiness, motivation, and previous knowledge) when teaching clients.
- Assess personal context and meaning of illness (e.g., perceived change in lifestyle, financial concerns, cultural patterns, and lack of acceptance by peers or coworkers).
- Offer anticipatory educational interventions that support self-regulation and self-management.
- Monitor how clients process information over time.
- Use individualized approaches that focus on client priorities and preferences.
- Engage client as a partner in the educational decision process.
- Assess the client's literacy skill when using written information.
- Provide visual aids to enhance learning.
- Consider coordinated, multifaceted methods of disbursing information over multiple sessions.
- Use teaching methods that reinforce learning and allow adequate time for mastery of content.
- Help the client locate appropriate follow-up resources for continuing information and support.
- Use computer- and web-based methods as appropriate.
- Use outreach and community educational intervention as appropriate.

Pediatric

- Use family-centered approaches when teaching children and adolescents.

● = Independent   ▲ = Collaborative

- Use communication strategies to enhance learning that are uniquely tailored for children and/or adolescents.
- Use educational strategies that are appropriate to the developmental needs of the child or adolescent.
- Consider using recreational playthings for younger children such as puppets in combination with structured sessions as a therapeutic education intervention for young children.
- Provide anticipatory guidance as necessary for procedures and about the course of illness for both parents and preschool children.
- Educational strategies that are participatory are recommended for adolescents.
- Consider the benefits of computer and web learning as a teaching methodology.

Geriatric

- Involve older clients in setting their own goals and participating in the decision-making process.
- Ensure that the client uses necessary reading aids (e.g., eyeglasses, magnifying lenses, large-print text) or hearing aids if necessary.
- Consider using self-paced learning and methods of reinforcing learning.
- Repeat and reinforce information during several brief sessions.
- Discuss healthy lifestyle changes that promote safety, health promotion, and health maintenance for older clients.
- Offer opportunities for practice of psychomotor skills.
- ▲ Refer elderly clients for postdischarge follow-up as they transition from hospital to home in regard to their treatment and medication regimens.
- Consider using technology, including interactive computer programs and other creative interventions, to disperse health education to older adults.
- Consider the use of creative interventions, such as art, poetry, and writing, to help an older adult learn.

Multicultural

- Acknowledge racial/ethnic differences at the onset of care.
- Consider involving bilingual members of a community who are considered outside the traditional health care

K

• = Independent   ▲ = Collaborative

system who may assist in the teaching of community health issues.
- Assess the extent of understanding of language and cultural practices when teaching clients who may not understand English.
- Assess for the influence of cultural beliefs, norms, and values on the client's knowledge base.
- Assess for cultural/ethnic self-care practices.
- Use teaching methods that are culturally sensitive and support client customs, values, and lifestyle.
- Be aware of the potential influence of medical interpreters in information sharing and decision-making and of the possible difficulties for clients when using medical interpreters.

Home Care

- All of the previously mentioned interventions are applicable to the home setting.
- Assess the client/family learning needs, information needs, and current level of knowledge.
- Encourage family and peer support.
- Encourage caregivers to practice skills prior to discharge.
- Consider the emerging field of telehealth and assistive technology as a method for supporting ongoing education for symptom, treatment, and self-care management.

Readiness for enhanced Knowledge

NANDA-I Definition

A pattern of cognitive information related to a specific topic, or its acquisition, that is sufficient for meeting health-related goals and can be strengthened

Defining Characteristics

Behaviors congruent with expressed knowledge; describes previous experiences pertaining to the topic; explains knowledge of the topic; expresses an interest in learning

● = Independent ▲ = Collaborative

Client Outcomes

Client Will (Specify Time Frame):
* Meet personal health-related goals
* Explain how to incorporate new health regimen into lifestyle
* List sources to obtain information

Nursing Interventions

▲ Include clients as members of the health care team in mutual goal setting when providing education.
* Support client priorities, preferences, and choice.
* Seek teachable moments to encourage health promotion.
* Use motivational strategies to promote client participation and sustain learning.
* Use a consultative, interactive teaching approach.
* Consider using lifestyle and health promotion programs delivered in workplace or community sites outside traditional health care environments.
* Use interactive and web-based technologies as appropriate to individualize health education interventions.
* Facilitate individualized proactive planning with clients before visits to their health care provider.
* Provide appropriate health care information and screening for clients with physical disabilities.
* Encourage peer group support as appropriate to enhance learning.
* Use a combination of teaching methods.
* Refer to care plan for **Deficient Knowledge.**

Pediatric
* Involve children and especially adolescents in designing health promotion programs and teaching methods.
▲ Consider settings outside traditional health care centers and interdisciplinary approaches for engaging children and adolescents in preventive health care.
* Provide a developmentally appropriate environment when addressing health education needs of adolescents.
* Refer to **Deficient Knowledge** care plan.

Geriatric and Multicultural
* Refer to **Deficient Knowledge** care plan.

• = Independent   ▲ = Collaborative

Latex Allergy Response

NANDA-I Definition

A hypersensitive reaction to natural latex rubber products

Defining Characteristics

Life-Threatening Reactions Occurring Less Than 1 Hour after Exposure to Latex

Protein

Bronchospasm; cardiac arrest; contact urticaria progressing to generalized symptoms; dyspnea; edema of the lips; edema of the throat; edema of the tongue; edema of the uvula; hypotension; respiratory arrest; syncope; tightness in chest; wheezing

Orofacial Characteristics

Edema of eyelids; edema of sclera; erythema of the eyes; facial erythema; facial itching; itching of the eyes; oral itching; nasal congestion; nasal erythema; nasal itching; rhinorrhea; tearing of the eyes

Gastrointestinal/Characteristics

Abdominal pain; nausea

Generalized Characteristics

Flushing; generalized discomfort; generalized edema; increasing complaint of total body warmth; restlessness

Type IV Reactions Occurring More Than 1 Hour After Exposure to Latex Protein

Discomfort reaction to additives such as thiurams and carbamates; eczema; irritation; redness

Related Factors (r/t)

Hypersensitivity to natural latex rubber protein

Client Outcomes

Client Will (Specify Time Frame):
- Identify presence of natural rubber latex (NRL) allergy
- List history of risk factors
- Identify type of reaction

     • = Independent   ▲ = Collaborative

- State reasons not to use or to have anyone use latex products
- Experience a latex-safe environment for all health care procedures
- Avoid areas where there is powder from NRL gloves
- State the importance of wearing a medical alert bracelet and wear one
- State the importance of carrying an emergency kit with a supply of nonlatex gloves, antihistamines, and an autoinjectable epinephrine syringe (EpiPen), and carry one

Nursing Interventions

- Identify clients at risk: those persons who are most likely to exhibit a sensitivity to NRL that may result in varying degrees of reactivity. Consider the following client groups:
  - Persons with neural tube defects including spina bifida, myelomeningocele/meningocele.
  - Children who have experienced three or more surgeries, particularly as a neonate, and adults who have undergone multiple surgeries.
  - Atopic individuals (persons with a tendency to have multiple allergic conditions) including allergies to food products. Particular allergies to fruits and vegetables including bananas, avocado, celery, fig, chestnut, papaya, potato, tomato, melon, and passion fruit are significant.
  - Persons who possess a known or suspected NRL allergy by having exhibited an allergic or anaphylactic reaction, positive skin testing, or positive IgE antibodies against latex.
  - Persons who have had an ongoing occupational exposure to NRL, including health care workers, rubber industry workers, bakers, laboratory personnel, food handlers, hairdressers, janitors, policemen, and firefighters.
- Take a thorough history of the client at risk.
- Question the client about associated symptoms of itching, swelling, and redness after contact with rubber products such as rubber gloves, balloons, and barrier contraceptives, or swelling of the tongue and lips after dental examinations.
- Consider the use of a provocation test (cutaneous, sublingual, mucous, conjunctival) for latex allergy diagnosis confirmation.
- Consider a blood test to measure serum IgE levels.

L

• = Independent   ▲ = Collaborative

- All latex-sensitive clients are treated as if they have NRL allergy.
- Clients with spina bifida and others with a positive history of NRL sensitivity or NRL allergy should have all medical/surgical/dental procedures performed in a latex-controlled environment.
- In select high-risk atopic individuals, a specific immunotherapy regimen should be discussed with their health care provider.
▲ The most effective approach to preventing NRL anaphylaxis is complete latex avoidance.
▲ Materials and items that contain NRL must be identified and latex-free alternatives must be found.
▲ In health care settings, general use of latex gloves having negligible allergen content, powder-free latex gloves, and nonlatex gloves and medical articles should be considered in an effort to minimize exposure to latex allergen.
▲ If latex gloves are chosen for protection from blood or body fluids, a reduced-protein, powder-free glove should be selected.
- See Box II-1 for examples of products that may contain NRL and safe alternatives that are available.

Home Care

- Assess the home environment for presence of NRL products (e.g., balloons, condoms, gloves, and products of related allergies, such as bananas, avocados, and poinsettia plants).
- At onset of care, assess client history and current status of NRL allergy response.
▲ Seek medical care as necessary.
- Do not use NRL products in caregiving.
- Assist the client in identifying and obtaining alternatives to NRL products.

Client/Family Teaching and Discharge Planning

- Provide written information about NRL allergy and sensitivity.
▲ Instruct the client to inform health care professionals if he or she has an NRL allergy, particularly if the client is scheduled for surgery.

• = Independent   ▲ = Collaborative

- Teach the client what products contain NRL and to avoid direct contact with all latex products and foods that trigger allergic reactions.
- See Box II-2 for examples of products found in the community that may contain NRL and safe alternatives that are available.
- Teach the client to avoid areas where powdered latex gloves are used, as well as where latex balloons are inflated or deflated.
- Instruct the client with NRL allergy to wear a medical identification bracelet and/or carry a medical identification card.
- Instruct the client to carry an emergency kit with a supply of nonlatex gloves, antihistamines, and an autoinjectable epinephrine syringe (EpiPen).

BOX II-1	Products that May Contain Latex and Latex-Free Alternatives Used in Health Care Settings

Frequently Contain Latex	Latex-Free Alternative
Ace wraps	Teds, pneumatic boots
Airways	Hudson airways, oxygen masks
Ambu (bag-valve) masks (black or blue reusable)	Clear, disposable Ambu bags
Band-Aids	Sterile dressing with plastic tape or Tegaderm
Blood pressure cuffs	Dura-Cuf Critikon Vital Answers or use over gown or stockinette
Catheter, indwelling	Silocone Foley (Kendall, Argyle, Baxter)
Catheter, straight	Plastic (Mentor, Bard)
	Double, triple lumen (Bard, Rusch)
Chux	Disposable underpads
Disposable gloves, latex, nonsterile	SensiCare gloves
Dressings—moleskin, Micropore, Coban (3M)	Tegaderm (3M), Steri-Strips
Electrode pads	3M, Baxter electrocardiogram pads
	Dantec surface electrocardiogram pads
Endotracheal tubes	Mallinckrodt, Sheridan, Portex tube stylets
	Laryngeal mask airway
Gloves, sterile and exam, surgical and medical	Vinyl, neoprene gloves (Neolon, Tachylon, Tru-Touch, Elastryn)
Heplock-PRN adapter	Use stopcock to inject medications

Continued

● = Independent   ▲ = Collaborative

BOX II-I	Products that May Contain Latex and Latex-Free Alternatives Used in Health Care Settings—cont'd

Frequently Contain Latex	Latex-Free Alternative
IV solutions and tubing systems	Baxter, Abbott, Walrus tubing Walrus anesthesia sets are latex-free Abbott IV fluid
Medication syringes	Becton Dickinson angiocaths and syringes Concord Portex, Bard syringes
Medication vial	Remove latex stopper
Oral and nasal airways	Hudson airways, oxygen masks
OR caps with elastic (bouffant)	Caps with ties
Oxygen tubing	Nasal, face mask
Stethoscope tubing	Do not let tubing touch client, cover with web roll
Suction tubing	Mallinckrodt, Yankauer, Davol suction catheters
Tape—cloth, adhesive, paper	Plastic, silk, 3M Microfoam Blenderm, Durapore
Tourniquets	Latex-free tourniquet (blue)

Data from American Association of Nurse Anesthetists: *AANA latex protocol,* Park Ridge, IL, 1998, Author, pp 1–9; National Institute for Occupational Safety and Health: *Preventing allergic reactions to natural rubber latex in the workplace,* Cincinnati, July 1998, Author; Hepner DL, Castells MC: Latex allergy: an update, *Anesth Analg* 96(4):1219–1229, 2003.

BOX II-2	Latex Products and Safe Alternatives Outside of the Health Care Setting

Containing Latex	Latex-Free Alternative
Balloons	Mylar balloons
Balls, Koosh ball	Vinyl, Thornton sport ball
Belt for clothing	Leather or cloth belts
Beach shoes	Cotton socks
Bungee cords	Rope or twine
Cleaning/kitchen gloves	Vinyl gloves
Condoms	Polyurethane Avanti for males Polyurethane Reality for females
Crib mattress pads	Heavy cotton pads
Elastic bands	Paper clips, staples, twine
Elastic on legs, waist of clothing, disposable diapers, rubber pants	Velcro closures Cloth diapers

• = Independent   ▲ = Collaborative

BOX II-2	Latex Products and Safe Alternatives Outside of the Health Care Setting—cont'd
Containing Latex	**Latex-Free Alternative**
Halloween rubber masks	Plastic mask or water-based paints
Pacifiers	Plastic pacifier "The First Years"
	Silicone—Pur, Gerber, Soft-Flex
Racquet handles	Leather handles
Raincoats/slickers	Nylon or synthetic waterproof coats
Swim fins	Clear plastic fins
Telephone cords	Clear cords

Data from American Association of Nurse Anesthetists: *AANA latex protocol,* Park Ridge, IL, 1998, Author, pp 1–9; National Institute for Occupational Safety and Health: *Preventing allergic reactions to natural rubber latex in the workplace,* Cincinnati, July 1998, Author; Hepner DL, Castells MC: Latex allergy: an update, *Anesth Analg* 96(4):1219–1229, 2003.

L

Risk for Latex Allergy Response

NANDA-I Definition

Risk of hypersensitivity to natural latex rubber products

Risk Factors

Allergies to avocados; allergies to bananas; allergies to chestnuts; allergies to kiwis; allergies to poinsettia plants; allergies to tropical fruits; history of allergies; history of asthma; history of reaction to latex; multiple surgical procedures, especially from infancy; professions with daily exposure to latex.

Client Outcomes

Client Will (Specify Time Frame):

* State risk factors for natural rubber latex (NRL) allergy
* Request latex-free environment
* Demonstrate knowledge of plan to treat NRL allergic reaction

Nursing Interventions

* Clients at high risk need to be identified, such as those with frequent bladder catheterizations, occupational exposure to latex, past history of atopy (hay fever, asthma, dermatitis,

• = Independent   ▲ = Collaborative

or food allergy to fruits such as bananas, avocados, papaya, chestnut, or kiwi); those with a history of anaphylaxis of uncertain etiology, especially if associated with surgery; health care workers; and females exposed to barrier contraceptives and routine examinations during gynecological and obstetric procedures.

- Clients with spina bifida are a high-risk group for NRL allergy and should remain latex free from the first day of life.
- Children who require regular medical treatments at home (catheterization, home ventilation, etc.) should be assessed for NRL allergy.
- Assess for NRL allergy in clients who are exposed to "hidden" latex.
- See care plan for **Latex Allergy Response.**

Home Care

▲ Ensure that the client has a medical plan if a response develops. Prompt treatment decreases potential severity of response.
- See care plan for **Latex Allergy Response.** Note client history and environmental assessment.

Client/Family Teaching and Discharge Planning

▲ A client who has had symptoms of NRL allergy or who suspects he or she is allergic to latex needs to give this information to health care providers.
▲ Provide written information about latex allergy and sensitivity.
- Health care workers should avoid the use of latex gloves and seek alternatives such as gloves made from nitrile.
- Health care institutions should develop prevention programs for the use of latex-free gloves and the absence of powdered gloves; they should also establish latex-safe areas in their facilities.

L

• = Independent   ▲ = Collaborative

Risk for impaired Liver Function

NANDA-I Definition

At risk for a decrease in liver function that may compromise health

Risk Factors

Hepatotoxic medications (e.g., acetaminophen, statins); HIV co-infection; substance abuse (e.g., alcohol, cocaine); viral infection (e.g., hepatitis A, B, C, E, Epstein-Barr)

Client Outcomes

Client Will (Specify Time Frame):

- State the upper limit of the amount of acetaminophen can safely take per day
- Have normal liver enzymes, serum and urinary bilirubin levels, white blood cell count (WBC), red blood cell count (RBC)
- Be free of unexplained weight loss, jaundice, pruritus, bruising, petechiae, gastrointestinal bleeding, hemorrhage
- Be free of abdominal tenderness/pain, increased abdominal girth, and have normal-colored stool and urine
- Be able to eat frequent small meals per day without nausea and/or vomiting
- If alcohol abuse is factor, state relationship between abuse and worsening gastrointestinal and liver disease

Nursing Interventions

▲ Watch for signs of liver dysfunction including fatigue, nausea, jaundice of the eyes or skin, pruritus, gastrointestinal bleeding, coagulopathy, infections, increasing abdominal girth, fluid overload, shortness of breath, mental status changes, light-colored stools, dark urine, and increased serum and urinary bilirubin levels.

▲ Evaluate liver function tests.

▲ Discuss with the client/family preparations for other diagnostic studies, such as ultrasounds, CT, and MRI exams.

▲ Evaluate coagulation studies such as international normalized ratio (INR), prothrombin time (PT), and partial thromboplastin time (PTT), especially with bleeding of the mouth or gums.

- Monitor for signs of hemorrhage, especially in the upper GI tract, as it is the most frequent site.
- Obtain a list of all medications, including over-the-counter NSAIDs, acetaminophen, and herbal remedies. Review risk of drug-induced liver disease. The list includes some antibiotics, anticonvulsants, antidepressants, antiinflammatory drugs, antiplatelets, antihypertensives, calcium channel blockers, cyclosporine, lipid-lowering drugs, chemotherapy drugs, oral hypoglycemics, tranquilizers, and more. If taking either OTC medications or herbals, discuss signs and symptoms of toxic hepatitis.
- ▲ In clients receiving drugs associated with liver injury, review risk factors in order to prevent potentially severe drug reactions.
- ▲ Determine the total amount of acetaminophen the client is taking per day. The amount of acetaminophen ingested should not exceed 3.25 g per day, or even lower in the client with chronic alcohol intake.
- ▲ Evaluate the serum acetaminophen-protein adducts in the client with possible liver failure from excessive intake of acetaminophen.
- ▲ If the client is on statin medications, ensure that liver enzyme testing is done at intervals.
- ▲ If the client is an alcoholic, refer to a cessation program.
- ▲ Provide frequent smaller meals for easier digestion. Provide diet with optimal carbohydrates, proteins, and fats. Consult with a registered dietitian to discuss best nutritional support.
- ▲ Recognize that severe malnutrition may result in acute liver failure, which is reversible with improved nutrition.
- ▲ Review medical history with the client, recognizing that obesity and type 2 diabetes, along with hypertriglyceridemia and polycystic ovarian syndrome are major risk factors in the development of liver disease, specifically nonalcoholic fatty liver disease.
- Encourage vaccinations for hepatitis A and B for all ages.

● = Independent   ▲ = Collaborative

- Measure abdominal girth if individual presents with abdominal distention and pain.
- Assess for tenderness and/or pain level in the right upper quadrant.
- Use standard precautions for handling of blood and body fluids. Review sterile techniques when giving intravenous solution and/or medications.
▲ Observe for signs and symptoms of mental status changes such as confusion from encephalopathy. Assess ammonia level if mental changes occur.

Pediatric/Parents

▲ Prescreen pregnant women for hepatitis B surface antigens. If found, recommend nursing case management during pregnancy.
▲ Recommend implementation of postexposure prophylaxis, including the HBV vaccine birth dose within 12 hours postpartum, for an infant born to a hepatitis B surface antigen-positive woman. This consists of a birth dose of hepatitis B immune globulin (HBIG) and the HBV vaccine on an accelerated schedule. Recommend that this child also undergo serology testing to confirm a protective immune response 3 to 9 months after completing the three-dose vaccine series.
- Encourage vaccinations for hepatitis A and B for all ages.
▲ Recognize that children can develop fatty liver disease, which can result in liver failure. Most children are asymptomatic, but others complain of malaise, fatigue, or vague recurrent abdominal pain.
▲ During a well-baby visit, assess for signs of potential liver problems. Observe for prolonged jaundice, pale stools, and urine that is anything other than colorless. Consult with physician to order a split bilirubin as needed.

Home Care

- Encourage rest, optimal nutrition (high carbohydrates, sufficient protein, essential vitamins and minerals) during initial inflammatory processes of the liver.

● = Independent   ▲ = Collaborative

Client/Family Teaching and Discharge Planning

- Teach the client and family to examine all medications the client is taking, looking for acetaminophen as an ingredient, and reinforce the 3.25-g upper limit of intake of acetaminophen to protect liver function.
- For the caregiver or client with hepatitis A, B, or C, teach the need for careful handwashing, use of gloves, and other precautions to prevent spread of any of these diseases.
- Teach avoidance of high-risk behaviors that cause hepatitis and ways to avoid those behaviors.
- Educate clients and their caregivers about treatment options and interventions for hepatitis. Recommend other informational support: risk factors, side effects of the different treatment options, and dietary advice.
- Recommend psychological support if possible during education sessions.
- For those clients with mental health problems, collaborate with outreach programs to teach signs/symptoms of hepatitis, risk factors, and factors that increase transmission.

L

Risk for Loneliness

NANDA-I Definition

At risk for experiencing discomfort associated with a desire or need for more contact with others

Risk Factors

Affectional deprivation; cathectic deprivation; physical isolation; social isolation

Client Outcomes

Client Will (Specify Time Frame):

- Maintain one or more meaningful relationships (growth-enhancing versus codependent or abusive in nature)
- Sustain relationships that allow self-disclosure and demonstrate a balance between emotional dependence and independence

     • = Independent   ▲ = Collaborative

- Participate in personally meaningful activities and interactions, that are ongoing, positive, and relevant socially
- Demonstrate positive use of time alone when socialization is not possible

Nursing Interventions

- Assess the client's perception of loneliness. (Is the person alone by choice, or are there other factors that contribute to the feelings of loneliness? Is the client in one of the at-risk populations for loneliness?)
- Use active listening skills. Establish a therapeutic relationship and spend quality time with the client.
- Assess the client's ability and/or inability to meet his/her physical, psychosocial, spiritual, and financial needs; assess how unmet needs challenge the client's ability to socially integrate. NOTE: See care plan for **Disturbed Body Image** if loneliness is associated with chronic illness and/or afflictions (MS, skin disturbance, mental illness etc.).
- ▲ Assess the isolated, bereaved client for risk of suicide and make appropriate referrals as necessary.
- ▲ Assess the client who is alone for substance abuse and make appropriate referrals.
- Evaluate the client's desire for social interaction in relation to actual social interaction.
- Assist the client with identifying loneliness as a feeling and also aid in further identifying the causes related to this feeling.
- Explore ways to increase the client's support system and participation in groups and organizations.
- Encourage the client to be involved in meaningful social relationships and provide support of one's personal attributes.
- Encourage the client to develop closeness in at least one relationship.

Adolescents

- Assess the client's social support system.
- Evaluate the family stability of younger and middle adolescent clients; advocate and encourage healthy, growth-producing relationships with both family and other support systems.

● = Independent   ▲ = Collaborative

- Evaluate peer relationships.
- Encourage social support for clients with disabilities such as mental illness, visual impairment, or deafness and make appropriate referrals when necessary.
- For older adolescents, encourage close relationships with peers and involvement with groups and organizations.

Geriatric

- Assess the client's adaptive sensory functions or any other health deviations that may limit or decrease his or her ability to interact with others.
- Assess older caregivers of persons with chronic conditions such as Alzheimer's or other dementias, Parkinson's etc. for depression related to loneliness.
- Identify support systems in elderly populations.
- When relocation is necessary for older adults, evaluate relocation stress as a contributing factor to loneliness.
- Identify risk factors for loneliness in older persons confined to extended care facilities (ECFs).
- Encourage support by friends and family when the decision to stop driving must be made.
- Provide activities that are pleasurable to the client.
- Refer to the care plan for **Social Isolation** for additional interventions.

Multicultural

- Refer to the care plan for **Social Isolation**.

Home Care

- ▲ The preceding interventions may be adapted for home care use.
- ▲ Assess for depression with the lonely elderly client and make appropriate referrals.
- If the client has unexplained somatic complaints, evaluate these complaints to ensure that physical needs are being met, and assess for a possible relationship between somatic complaints and loneliness.
- Identify alternatives to being alone (e.g., telephone contact, Internet).
- Refer to the care plan for **Social Isolation**.

● = Independent   ▲ = Collaborative

Client/Family Teaching and Discharge Planning

- Identify the type of loneliness that the client is experiencing—emotional and/or social.
- Encourage family members' involvement, if possible, in helping to alleviate client's loneliness.
- Include the family, if possible, in all client-teaching activities, and give them accurate information.
- Provide appropriate education for clients and their support persons about disease transmission and treatment if applicable.
- Refer to the care plan for **Social Isolation** for additional interventions.

M

Risk for disturbed Maternal/Fetal Dyad

NANDA-I Definition

At risk for disruption of the symbiotic maternal/fetal dyad as a result of comorbid or pregnancy-related conditions

Risk Factors

Complications of pregnancy (e.g., premature rupture of membranes, placenta previa or abruption, late prenatal care, multiple gestation, malnutrition); compromised O_2 transport (e.g., anemia, cardiac disease, asthma, hypertension, seizures, premature labor, hemorrhage); impaired glucose metabolism (e.g., diabetes, steroid use); physical abuse; substance abuse (e.g., tobacco, alcohol, drugs); treatment-related side effects (e.g., medications, surgery, chemotherapy)

Client Outcomes

Client Will (Specify Time Frame):
- Cope with discomforts of high-risk pregnancy until delivery of baby
- Adhere to prescribed regimens to maintain homeostasis during pregnancy

● = Independent   ▲ = Collaborative

Nursing Interventions

- Standardize internal and external transport forms using SBAR format (situation, background, assessment, recommendation) to provide safe and efficient transport of a high-risk pregnant client.
- ▲ Arrange for psychotherapeutic support when woman expresses intense fear related to high-risk pregnancy and fetal outcomes.
- Screen all antepartum clients for depression using a tool that evaluates the biopsychosocial-spiritual dimensions in a culturally sensitive way.
- Offer flexible visiting hours; private space for families; and nursing support for management of family stressors, including music and recreation therapy, when a woman is hospitalized with a high-risk pregnancy.
- Focus on the abilities of a woman with disabilities by encouraging her to identify her support system, resources, and needs for modification of her environment.
- Recognize patterns of physical abuse in all pregnant and postpartum women, regardless of age, race, and socioeconomic status.
- Perform accurate blood pressure readings at each client's clinic encounter.
- Provide educational materials and support for personal autonomy about genetic counseling and testing options prior to pregnancy, that is, preimplantation genetic testing, or during pregnancy, that is, fetal nuchal translucency ultrasound, quadruple screen, cystic fibrosis.
- Identify adherence barriers and assist with meal selections to maintain optimal and safe pregnancy weight gain (25 to 35 pounds; 15 to 25 if overweight).
- Use an analogy to explain the pathophysiology of gestational diabetes to teach a pregnant woman about management and treatment.
- Utilize the 5As (tobacco cessation interventions) to treat tobacco use and dependence in pregnant women.
- When questioning at-risk clients regarding recreational drug use, ask if they have used substances such as marijuana or

cocaine within the last month, instead of questioning if have used within the last few days.

▲ Refer clients who self-report drug abuse or have positive toxicology screens to a comprehensive addiction program designed for the pregnant woman.

• Encourage pregnant women to utilize electronic resources, such as Text4Baby or whattoexpect.com, to track pregnancy progress and provide education and motivation to make healthy lifestyle choices (abstinence from poor nutrition, smoking, alcohol, etc.).

Impaired Memory

M

NANDA-I Definition

Inability to remember or recall bits of information or behavioral skills; impaired memory may be attributed to pathophysiological or situational causes that are either temporary or permanent

Defining Characteristics

Experience of forgetting; forgets to perform a behavior at a scheduled time; inability to determine if a behavior was performed; inability to learn new information; inability to learn new skills; inability to perform a previously learned skill; inability to recall events; inability to recall factual information; inability to retain new information; inability to retain new skills

Related Factors (r/t)

Anemia; decreased cardiac output; excessive environmental disturbances; fluid and electrolyte imbalance; hypoxia; neurological disturbances

Client Outcomes

Client Will (Specify Time Frame):

• Demonstrate use of techniques to help with memory loss
• State has improved memory for everyday concerns

• = Independent   ▲ = Collaborative

Nursing Interventions

- Assess overall cognitive function and memory. The emphasis of the assessment is everyday memory, the day-to-day operations of memory in real-world ordinary situations. Use an assessment tool such as the Mini-Mental State Examination (MMSE).
- Determine whether onset of memory loss is gradual or sudden. If memory loss is sudden, refer the client to a physician or neuropsychologist for evaluation.
- Determine amount and pattern of alcohol intake.
- Note the client's current medications and intake of any mind-altering substances such as benzodiazepines, ecstasy, marijuana, cocaine, or glucocorticoids.
- Note the client's current level of stress. Ask if there has been a recent traumatic event.
- If stress was associated with memory loss, refer to a stress reduction clinic. If not available, suggest that the client meditate, receive massages, and participate in moderate physical activity, all of which may promote stress reduction and reduce anxiety and depression.
- Encourage the client to develop an aerobic exercise program.
- Determine the client's sleep patterns. If insufficient, refer to care plan for **Disturbed Sleep Pattern.**
- Determine the client's blood sugar levels. If they are elevated, refer to physician for treatment and encourage healthy diet and exercise.
- If signs of depression such as weight loss, insomnia, or sad affect are evident, refer the client for psychotherapy.
- ▲ Perform a nutritional assessment. If nutritional status is marginal, confer with a dietitian and primary care practitioner to evaluate whether the client needs supplementation with foods or vitamins. Teach the client the need to eat a healthy diet with adequate intake of whole grains, fruits, and vegetables to decrease cerebrovascular infarcts.
- Question the client about cholesterol level. If it is high, refer to physician or dietitian for help in lowering. Encourage the client to eat a healthy diet, avoiding saturated fats and trans fatty acids.

• = Independent   ▲ = Collaborative

- Suggest clients use cues, including alarm watches, electronic organizers, calendars, lists, or pocket computers, to trigger certain actions at designated times.
- Encourage the client to participate in a multicomponent cognitive rehabilitation program that recommends stress and relaxation training, physical activity, external memory devices, such as a calendar for appointments and reminder lists.
- Help the client set up a medication box that reminds the client to take medication at needed times; assist the client with refilling the box at intervals if necessary.
- If safety is an issue with certain activities (e.g., the client forgets to turn off stove after use or forgets emergency telephone numbers), suggest alternatives such as using a microwave or whistling teakettle for heating water and programming emergency numbers in telephone so that they are readily available.
- Refer the client to a memory clinic (if available), a neuropsychologist, or an occupational therapist.
- For clients with memory impairments associated with dementia, see care plan for **Chronic Confusion.**

Geriatric

- Assess for signs of depression.
- Evaluate all medications that the client is taking to determine whether they are causing the memory loss, particularly drugs used to treat an overactive bladder.
- Evaluate all herbal and/or nutraceutical products that the individual might be using to improve memory function.
- Recommend that elderly clients maintain a positive attitude and active involvement with the world around them and that they maintain good nutrition.
- Encourage the elderly to believe in themselves and to work to improve their memory.
- Refer the client to a memory class that focuses on helping older adults learn memory strategies
- Help family label items such as the bathroom or sock drawer to increase recall.

Multicultural

- Assess for the influence of cultural beliefs, norms, and values on the family or caregiver's understanding of impaired memory.
- When assessing memory in Mexican Americans, the MMSE has been tested.
- Inform the client's family or caregiver of meaning of and reasons for common behavior observed in the client with impaired memory, which can vary depending on race and ethnicity.
- Attempt to validate family members' feelings regarding the impact of the client's behavior on family lifestyle.

Home Care

- The preceding interventions may be adapted for home care use.
- Assess the client's need for outside assistance with recall of treatment, medications, and willingness/ability of family to provide needed support.
- Identify a checking-in support system (e.g., Lifeline or significant others).
- Keep furniture placement and household patterns consistent.

Client/Family Teaching and Discharge Planning

- When teaching the client, determine what the client knows about memory techniques and then build on that knowledge.
- When teaching a skill to the client, set up a series of practice attempts that will enhance motivation. Begin with simple tasks so that the client can be positively reinforced and progress to more difficult concepts.
- Teach clients to use memory techniques such as concentrating and attending, repeating information, making mental associations, and placing items in strategic places so that they will not be forgotten.

Impaired bed Mobility

NANDA-I Definition

Limitation of independent movement from one bed position to another

Defining Characteristics

Impaired ability to move from supine to sitting; to move from sitting to supine; to move from supine to prone; to move from prone to supine; to move from supine to long sitting; to move from long sitting to supine; to "scoot" or reposition self in bed; to turn from side to side

Related Factors (r/t)

Cognitive impairment; deconditioning; deficient knowledge; environmental constraints (i.e., bed size, bed type, treatment equipment, restraints); insufficient muscle strength; musculoskeletal impairment; neuromuscular impairment; obesity; pain; sedating medications. NOTE: Specify level of independence using a standardized functional scale

Client Outcomes

Client Will (Specify Time Frame):

* Demonstrate optimal independence in positioning, exercising, and performing functional activities in bed
* Demonstrate ability to direct others on how to do bed positioning, exercising, and functional activities

Nursing Interventions

* Critically think/set priorities to use the most therapeutic bed positions based on client's history, risk profile, preventive needs; realize positioning for one condition may negatively affect another.
* Assess client's risk for aspiration; if present, elevate HOB to 30 degrees and elevate HOB to 90 degrees during oral intake.
* Raise head of bed (HOB) to 30 degrees for clients with acute increased intracranial pressure (ICP) and brain injury. Refer to care plan for **Decreased Intracranial Adaptive Capacity.**

• = Independent   ▲ = Collaborative

- ▲ Consult physician for HOB elevation of clients with acute stroke and monitor their response. Refer to care plan for **Decreased Intracranial Adaptive Capacity.**
- Raise HOB as close to 45 degrees as possible for critically ill, ventilated clients to prevent pneumonia (this height may place clients at higher risk for pressure ulcers).
- Assist client to sit as upright as possible during meals/ingestion of pills if dysphagic. Refer to care plan for **Impaired Swallowing.**
- Periodically sit client as upright as tolerated in bed and dangle client, if vital signs/oxygen saturation levels remain stable.
- Maintain HOB at lowest elevation that is medically possible to prevent shear-related injury; check sacrum often.
- Trial prone positioning for clients with acute respiratory distress syndrome (ARDS), acute lung injury (ALI), and amputation and monitor their tolerance/response.
- Assess client's risk for falls using a valid tool, establish individualized fall prevention strategies, and perform postfall assessment to further refine fall prevention interventions.
- Lock bed brakes, use low-rise beds at lowest position with floor mats next to them, avoid use of side rails, and apply personal exit alarms on confused clients.
- ▲ Avoid use of bedrails and restraints unless ordered by physician.
- Place call light, bedside table, and telephone within reach of clients.
- Use a formalized screening tool to identify persons at high risk for thromboembolism (DVT).
- ▲ Implement thromboembolism prophylaxis/treatment as ordered (e.g., anticoagulants, antiembolic stockings, elastic leg wraps, sequential compression devices, feet/ankle exercises, and hydration). Refer to care plan for **Ineffective peripheral Tissue Perfusion.**
- Use a formal tool to assess for risk of pressure ulcers.
- Implement the following interventions to prevent pressure ulcers and complications of immobility:
  - ■ Position sitting clients with special attention to the individual's anatomy, postural alignment, distribution of weight,

M

and support of feet; heel protection devices should completely offload (float) the heel.

- Turn (logroll) clients at high risk for pressure/shear/friction frequently and regularly.
- Use statis/dynamic bed surfaces and assess for "bottoming out" under susceptible bony areas (body sinks into mattress, thus the recommended 1 inch between mattress/bones is absent). Refer to care plan for **Risk for impaired Skin Integrity.**
- Use heel protection devices that completely float or offload heels.
- Implement a 2-hour on/off schedule for heel protector boots or high-top tennis shoes with socks underneath on clients with paralyzed feet, and check condition of heels when removed.
- Strictly maintain leg abduction in persons with a surgical hip pinning or replacement by placing an abductor splint/pillow between legs.
- Use devices such as trapeze, friction-reducing slide sheets, mechanical lateral transfer aids, and ceiling-mounted or floor lifts to move (rather than drag) dependent/obese persons in bed.
- Apply elbow pads to comatose/restrained clients and to those who use elbows to prop/scoot up in bed; apply nocturnal elbow splint as ordered if ulnar nerve palsy exists or if painful elbow with paresthesia in ulnar side of fourth/fifth fingers develops.

- Explain importance of exhaling versus holding one's breath (Valsalva maneuver) and straining during bed activities.
- Reassess pain level, especially before movement/exercising, and accept clients' pain rating and level they think is appropriate for comfort, then administer analgesics based on pain rating. Refer to **Acute Pain** or **Chronic Pain.**
- Use special beds/equipment to move bariatric (very obese) clients, such as mattress overlay, sliding/roller board, trapeze, stirrup, and pulley attached to overhead traction system (holds one leg up during pericare).
- Place bariatric clients in free-standing or ceiling-mounted lifts with padded slings while changing bed linen.

- Place bariatric beds along a corner wall.
- Identify/modify hospital beds with large gaps between bed rail/mattress that create an entrapment hazard. Ensure that mattresses fit the bed; instill gap fillers/rail inserts, then monitor effectiveness.

Exercise

- Test strength in bilateral grips, arms at elbow flexion and extension, bilateral arm abduction and adduction, bilateral leg or thigh raise (one at a time in bed or chair), and quadriceps and hamstring strength to extend and flex at knee to assess baseline and interval strength gains.
- Perform passive range of motion (ROM) of three repetitions, at least twice a day, to immobile joints.
- Perform ROM slowly/rhythmically. Do not range beyond point of pain. Range only to point of resistance in those with loss of sensation/mentation.
- Range/move a hemiplegic arm with the shoulder slightly externally rotated (hand up).
- ▲ Emphasize client's practice of exercises taught by therapists (muscle setting, strengthening, contraction against resistance, and weight lifting).

Bed Positioning

- Incorporate the following measures to promote normal tone and prevent complications in clients with neurological impairment:
  - Use a flat head pillow when clients are supine. Use a small pillow behind the head and/or between shoulder blades if neck extension occurs.
  - Abduct the shoulders of persons with high paraplegia or quadriplegia horizontally to 90 degrees briefly two or three times a day while supine.
  - Position a hemiplegic shoulder fairly close to the client's body.
- ▲ Elevate paralyzed forearm(s) on a pillow when supine and apply Isotoner gloves; elevate edematous legs on a pillow and apply elastic wraps and compression garments as ordered.

- Tilt hemiplegics onto both unaffected/affected sides with the affected shoulder slightly forward (move/lift the affected shoulder, *not* the forearm/hand).
- ▲ Apply resting wrist and hand splints. Strictly adhere to on/off orders. Routinely check underlying skin for signs of pressure/poor circulation.
- ▲ Range weak/paralyzed ankle joints before applying foot splints, boots, or high-top tennis shoes on rotation schedule recommended by the physical therapist; routinely assess underlying skin for signs of pressure.
- ▲ Recognize that components of normal bed mobility include rolling, bridging, scooting, long sitting, and sitting upright. Activity starts with the client supine, flat in bed, and promotes normal movements that are bilateral, segmental, well timed, and involve set positions such as weight bearing and trunk centering. Refer to physical therapist (PT) for individualized instructions/strategies.

Geriatric

- Assess caregivers' strength, health history, and cognitive status to predict ability/risk for assisting bed-bound clients at home. Explore alternatives if risk is too high. Refer to care plan for **Caregiver Role Strain.**
- Assess the client's stamina and energy level during bed activities/exercises; if limited, spread out activities and allow rest breaks.

Home Care

- ▲ Utilize nurse case managers, care coordinators, or social workers to assess support systems and identify need for durable medical equipment, assistive technology, and home health services.
- Encourage use of the client's bed unless contraindicated. Raise HOB with commercial blocks or grooved-out pieces of wood under legs; set bed against walls in a corner.
- Suggest home modifications and rearranging rooms/furniture to meet sleeping/toileting/living needs on one level.

● = Independent   ▲ = Collaborative

- Stress psychological/physical benefits of clients being as self-sufficient as possible with bed mobility/care even though it may be time-consuming.
- Offer emotional support and help client identify usual coping responses to help with adjustment and loss issues.
- Discuss support systems available for caregivers to help them cope. Please refer to care plan for **Caregiver Role Strain.**
▲ In the presence of medical disorders, institute case management for the frail elderly to support continued independent living.
- Refer to the Home Care interventions of the care plan for **Impaired physical Mobility.**

Client/Family Teaching and Discharge Planning

- Use various sensory modalities to teach client/caregivers correct ROM, exercises, positioning, self-care activities, and use of devices. Readiness and learning styles vary but may be enhanced with visual/auditory/tactile/cognitive stimulus as follows:
  ■ Provide visual information such as demonstrations, sketches, instructional videos, written directions/schedules, notes.
  ■ Provide auditory information such as verbal instructions, recorded audiotapes, timers, reading aloud written directions, and self-talk during activities.
  ■ Use tactile stimulation such as motor task practice/repetition, return demonstrations, note taking, manual guidance, or staff's-hand-on-client's-hand technique.
- Schedule time with family/caregivers for education and practice; for nursing as well as physical therapy and occupational therapy. Suggest family come prepared with questions and wear comfortable, safe clothing/shoes.
- Implement safe approaches for caregivers/home care staff and reinforce adequate number of people and handling equipment (friction pads, slide boards, lifts, etc.) during bed mobility, exercise, toileting, and bathing.
- Coordinate bariatric equipment for home use before discharge, including a weight-rated bed, a wheelchair or mobility device (scooter) and lift device; doorways may need to be widened, floors reinforced, and ramps may need to be added for safety.

• = Independent   ▲ = Collaborative

Impaired physical Mobility

NANDA-I Definition

A limitation in independent, purposeful physical movement of the body or of one or more extremities

Defining Characteristics

Decreased reaction time; difficulty turning; engages in substitutions for movement (e.g., increased attention to other's activity, controlling behavior, focus on pre-illness disability/activity); exertional dyspnea; gait changes; jerky movements; limited ability to perform gross motor skills; limited ability to perform fine motor skills; limited range of motion; movement-induced tremor; postural instability; slowed movement; uncoordinated movements

Related Factors (r/t)

M

Activity intolerance; altered cellular metabolism; anxiety; body mass index above 75th age-appropriate percentile; cognitive impairment; contractures; cultural beliefs regarding age-appropriate activity; deconditioning; decreased endurance; depressive mood state; decreased muscle control; decreased muscle mass; decreased muscle strength; deficient knowledge regarding value of physical activity; developmental delay; discomfort; disuse; joint stiffness; lack of environmental supports (e.g., physical or social); limited cardiovascular endurance; loss of integrity of bone structures; malnutrition; medications; musculoskeletal impairment; neuromuscular impairment; pain; prescribed movement restrictions; reluctance to initiate movement; sedentary lifestyle; sensoriperceptual impairments

Suggested functional level classifications include the following:
0—Completely independent
1—Requires use of equipment or device
2—Requires help from another person for assistance, supervision, or teaching
3—Requires help from another person and equipment device
4—Dependent (does not participate in activity)

Client Outcomes

Client Will (Specify Time Frame):
- Meet mutually defined goals of increased ambulation and exercise that include individual choice, preference and enjoyment in the exercise prescription.

● = Independent   ▲ = Collaborative

- Verbalize feeling of increased strength and ability to move.
- Verbalize less fear of falling and pain with physical activity.
- Demonstrate use of adaptive equipment (e.g., wheelchairs, walkers, gait belts, weighted walking vests) to increase mobility.
- Increase exercise to 20 minutes per day for those who were previously sedentary (less than 150 minutes per week). NOTE: Light to moderate intensity exercise may be beneficial in deconditioned persons. In very deconditioned individuals exercise bouts of less than 10 minutes are beneficial.
- Increase pedometer step counts by 1000 steps per day every 2 weeks to reach a daily step count of at least 7000 steps per day, with a daily goal for most healthy adults of 10,000 steps per day (approximately 5 miles).
- Perform resistance exercises that involve all major muscle groups (legs, hips, back, chest, abdomen, shoulders, and arms) performed 2 or 3 days per week.
- Perform flexibility exercise (stretching) for each of the major muscle-tendon groups 2 days per week for 10 to 60 seconds to improve joint range of motion; greatest gains occur with daily exercise.
- Engage in neuromotor exercise 20 to 30 minutes per day including motor skills (e.g., balance, agility, coordination, and gait), proprioceptive exercise training, and multifaceted activities (e.g., tai chi and yoga) to improve and maintain physical function and reduce falls in those at risk for falling (older persons).
- Engage in purposeful moderate-intensity cardiorespiratory (aerobic) exercise for 30 to 60 minutes per day on at least 5 days per week for a total of 2 hours and 30 minutes (150 minutes) per week.

Nursing Interventions

NOTE: Adults with disabilities should follow the adult guidelines; however, if not possible these persons should be as physically active as their abilities allow and avoid inactivity. Use "start low and go slow" approach for intensity and duration of physical activity if client highly deconditioned, functionally limited, or has chronic conditions affecting performance of physical tasks. When progressing client's activities, use an individualized and tailored approach based on client's tolerance and preferences.

• = Independent   ▲ = Collaborative

- Screen for mobility skills in the following order: (1) bed mobility; (2) supported and unsupported sitting; (3) transition movements such as sit to stand, sitting down, and transfers; and (4) standing and walking activities. Use a tool such as the Assessment Criteria and Care Plan for Safe Patient Handling and Movement.
- Screen for additional measures of physical function to assess strength of muscle groups, including unassisted leg stand, use of a balance platform, elbow flexion and knee extension strength, grip strength, timed chair stands, and the 6-minute walk.
- Assess the client for cause of impaired mobility. Determine whether cause is physical, psychological, or motivational. Refer to care plans for **Risk for Falls, Acute** or **Chronic Pain, Ineffective Coping,** or **Hopelessness.**
- Use Self-Efficacy for Exercise Scale and the Outcome Expectation for Exercise Scale to determine client's self-efficacy and outcome expectations toward exercise.
- Monitor and record the client's ability to tolerate activity and use all four extremities; note pulse rate, blood pressure, dyspnea, and skin color before and after activity. Refer to the care plan for **Activity Intolerance.**
- ▲ Before activity, observe for and, if possible, treat pain with massage, heat pack to affected area, or medication. Ensure that the client is not oversedated.
- ▲ Consult with physical therapist for further evaluation, strength training, gait training, and development of a mobility plan.
- Obtain any assistive devices needed for activity, such as gait belt, weighted vest, walker, cane, crutches, or wheelchair, before the activity begins.
- If the client is immobile, perform passive ROM exercises at least twice a day unless contraindicated; repeat each maneuver three times.
- ▲ If the client is immobile, consult with physician for a safety evaluation before beginning an exercise program; if program is approved, begin with the following exercises:
  - Active ROM exercises using both upper and lower extremities (e.g., flexing and extending at ankles, knees, hips)

M

• = Independent   ▲ = Collaborative

- Chin-ups and pull-ups using a trapeze in bed (may be contraindicated in clients with cardiac conditions)
- Strengthening exercises such as gluteal or quadriceps sitting exercises
- If client is immobile, consider use of vertical transfer techniques such as a transfer chair or gait belt pending weight-bearing status and client cooperation.
- Help the client achieve mobility and start walking as soon as possible if not contraindicated.
- Use a gait-walking belt when ambulating the client.
▲ Apply any ordered brace before mobilizing the client.
- Initiate a "No Lift" policy where appropriate assistive devices are used for manual lifting.
- Increase independence in ADLs, encouraging self-efficacy and discouraging helplessness as the client gets stronger.
▲ If the client has osteoarthritis or rheumatoid arthritis, ask for a referral to a physical therapist to begin an exercise program that includes aerobic exercise, resistance exercise, and flexibility exercise (stretching).
▲ If client has had a cerebrovascular accident (CVA) with hemiparesis, consider use of constraint-induced movement therapy (CIMT), where the functional extremity is purposely constrained and the client is forced to use the involved extremity.
- If the client has had a CVA, recognize that balance and *mobility* are likely impaired, and engage client in fall prevention strategies and protect from falling.
- If the client does not feed or groom self, sit side-by-side with the client, put your hand over the client's hand, support the client's elbow with your other hand, and help the client feed self; use the same technique to help the client comb hair.

Geriatric

- Assess ability to move using valid and reliable criterion-referenced standards for fitness testing (e.g., Senior Fitness Test) designed for older adults that can predict the level of capacity associated with maintaining physical independence into later years of life (e.g., get up and go test).

- Help the mostly immobile client achieve mobility as soon as possible, depending on physical condition.
- For a client who is mostly immobile, minimize cardiovascular deconditioning by positioning the client in the upright position several times daily.
▲ Refer the client to physical therapy for resistance exercise training as able, involving all major muscle groups (e.g., abdominal crunch, leg press, leg extension, leg curl, and calf press).
- Use the Function-Focused Care (FFC) rehabilitative philosophy of care with older adults in residential nursing facilities to prevent avoidable functional decline. The primary goals of FFC are to alter how direct care workers (DCWs) provide care to residents to maintain and improve time spent in physical activity and improve or maintain function.
- If client is scheduled for an elective surgery that will result in admission into the intensive care unit (ICU) and immobility, or recovery from a joint replacement, for example, initiate a prehabilitation program that includes a warm-up, aerobic activity, strength, flexibility, neuromotor, and functional task work.
▲ Evaluate the client for signs of depression (flat affect, insomnia, anorexia, frequent somatic complaints), anxiety or cognitive impairment (use Mini-Mental State Exam [MMSE]). Refer for treatment and counseling as needed.
- Watch for orthostatic hypotension when mobilizing elderly clients. Have the client dangle at the side of the bed with legs hanging over the edge of the bed, flex and extend feet several times after sitting up, then stand up slowly with someone holding the client. If client becomes lightheaded or dizzy, return him to bed immediately.
- Do not routinely assist with transfers or bathing activities unless necessary.
- Use gestures and nonverbal cues when helping clients move if they are anxious or have difficulty understanding and following verbal instructions.
- Recognize that wheelchairs are not a good mobility device and often serve as a mobility restraint.

M

• = Independent   ▲ = Collaborative

- Ensure that chairs fit clients. Chair seat should be 3 inches above the height of the knee. Provide a raised toilet seat if needed.
- If the client is mainly immobile, provide opportunities for socialization and sensory stimulation (e.g., television and visits). Refer to the care plan for **Deficient Diversional Activity.**
- Recognize that immobility and a lack of social support and sensory input may result in confusion or depression in the elderly. Refer to nursing interventions for **Acute Confusion** or **Hopelessness** as appropriate.

Home Care

- The preceding interventions may be adapted for home care use.
- ▲ Begin discharge planning as soon as possible with a personal health navigator (e.g., nurse care coordinator or case manager) to assess need for home support systems, assistive devices, and community or home health services.
- ▲ Assess home environment for factors that create barriers to physical mobility. Refer to occupational therapy services if needed to assist the client in restructuring home environment and daily living patterns.
- ▲ Refer to home health aide services to support the client and family through changing levels of mobility. Reinforce need to promote independence in mobility as tolerated.
- ▲ Refer to physical therapy for gait training, strengthening, and balance training. Physical therapists can provide direct interventions as well as assess need for assistive devices (e.g., cane, walker).
- Discuss with client and caregiver the possibility of a service dog to support the more immobile client.
- Assess skin condition at every visit. Establish a skin care program that enhances circulation and maximizes position changes.
- Once the client is able to walk independently, suggest the client enter an exercise program, or walk with a friend.
- Provide support to the client and family/caregivers during long-term impaired mobility. Refer to the care plan for **Caregiver Role Strain.**

• = Independent   ▲ = Collaborative

▲ Institute a personal health navigator (e.g., nurse care coordinator or case manager) and transitional care management of frail older adults to support continued independent living.

Client/Family Teaching and Discharge Planning

- Consider using motivational interviewing techniques when working with both children and adult clients to increase their activity.
- Teach the client progressive mobilization (e.g., dangle legs, get out of bed slowly when transferring from the bed to the chair).
- Teach the client relaxation techniques such as deep breathing and stretching to use during activity.
- Teach the client to use assistive devices such as a cane, a walker, gait belt, weighted vest, or crutches or wheelchair to increase mobility.
- Teach family members and caregivers to work with clients actively during self-care activities using a restorative care philosophy for eating, bathing, grooming, dressing, and transferring to restore the client to maximum function and independence.
- Work with the client using self-efficacy interventions using single or multiple methods. Teach client and family members to assess fear of falling and develop strategies to mitigate its effect on mobility progression.
- Work with the client using theory-based interventions (e.g., social cognitive theoretical components such as self-efficacy; transtheoretical model).

M

Impaired wheelchair Mobility

NANDA-I Definition

Limitation of independent operation of wheelchair within environment

Defining Characteristics

Impaired ability to operate: manual or powered wheelchair on curbs; manual or powered wheelchair on even surface; manual or power

• = Independent   ▲ = Collaborative

wheelchair on an uneven surface; manual or powered wheelchair on an incline; manual or powered wheelchair on a decline

Related Factors (r/t)

Cognitive impairment; deconditioning; deficient knowledge; depressed mood; environmental constraints (e.g., stairs, inclines, uneven surfaces, unsafe obstacles, distances, lack of assistive devices or person, wheelchair type); impaired vision; insufficient muscle strength; limited endurance; musculoskeletal impairment (e.g., contractures); neuromuscular impairment; obesity; pain

Client Outcomes

Client Will (Specify Time Frame):

* Demonstrate independence in operating and moving a wheelchair or other device with wheels
* Demonstrate the ability to direct others in operating and moving a wheelchair or other device
* Demonstrate therapeutic positioning, pressure relief, and safety principles while operating and moving wheelchair or other device equipped with wheels

Nursing Interventions

* Assist client to put on and take off equipment (e.g., braces, orthoses, abdominal binders) in bed.
* Inspect skin where orthoses, braces, and other equipment rested, once they are removed.
▲ Obtain referrals for physical and occupational therapy, or wheelchair seating clinic.
* Recognize that use of support surfaces (on chairs and beds) redistributes pressure and should be used an adjunct to reduce the risk of developing pressure ulcers in addition to repositioning the client on a regular schedule.
* Intervene to maintain continence or use absorbent diapers to help prevent skin breakdown due to wet, macerated skin. Some wheelchair cushions have moisture-wicking characteristics
* Maintain nutrition and hydration, which help to maintain skin integrity.

● = Independent ▲ = Collaborative

▲ Obtain physical therapist (PT), occupational therapist (OT), or wheelchair clinic referral for cushion reevaluation if signs of pressure emerge.

• Emphasize importance of weight shifts every 15 minutes with safety belts in place (leaning forward/laterally) for about 2 minutes for clients with paralysis with ability to move the trunk of their body.

• Ensure that client and family know how and when to relieve weight bearing and the importance of pressure relief program and demonstrate compliance with it.

• Utilize a passive standing position of wheelchair to relieve weight bearing, or, if applicable, manually stand client or use a sit-to-stand lift with sling for a few minutes.

• Routinely assess client's sitting posture and frequently reposition him/her into alignment.

• Sit dysphagic clients as upright as possible in individualized wheelchair versus geri-chair when eating.

• Implement use of friction-coated projection hand rims and leather gloves for clients to propel manual wheelchairs.

• Manually guide or explain how to push forward on both wheel rims to move ahead, push the right rim to turn left and vice versa, and pull backward on both wheel rims to back up.

• Recommend that clients back wheelchairs into an elevator. If entering face first, instruct them to turn chair around to face the elevator doors.

• Reinforce principle of descending a curb backward ("popping a wheelie") if balance, trunk control, strength, and timing are adequate.

• Ascend curbs in a forward position by popping a wheelie or having aide tilt chair back, place front wheels over curb, and roll chair up. If surface is muddy or sandy, ascend backwards.

• During assisted wheelies, helper must hold wheelchair until all four wheels are back on the ground and client has control of wheelchair.

▲ Follow therapist's recommendations for how clients should propel manual wheelchairs to prevent upper extremity pain and joint degeneration.

M

• = Independent   ▲ = Collaborative

▲ Inform clients that ultra-lightweight, pushrim-activated, power-assisted, or electric wheelchairs may be more therapeutic than manual ones.

• Help clients transition from a manual to a powered wheelchair/scooter if progressive disability occurs.

▲ Reduce floor clutter and establish safety rules for drivers of electric/power mobility devices; make referrals to PT or OT for driver reevaluations if accidents occur or client's health deteriorates.

• Request and receive client's permission before moving unoccupied wheelchair in room or out to hallway.

• Reinforce compensatory strategies for unilateral neglect and agnosia (visual scanning, self-talk, self-questioning as to what could be wrong) as clients propel wheelchair through doorways and around obstacles. Refer to care plan for **Unilateral Neglect.**

• Offer support to help clients cope with issues related to physical disability.

• Provide information on support group and Internet resource options.

• Provide information about advocacy, accessibility, assistive technology, and issues under the Americans with Disabilities Act.

▲ Make social service or wheelchair clinic referral to educate clients on financial coverage/regulations of third-party payers and Health Care Financing Association for wheelchairs.

• Suggest that clients test-drive wheelchairs and try out cushions/postural supports before purchasing them.

Geriatric

• Avoid using restraints on fidgeting clients who slide down in a wheelchair; rather, assess for deformities, spinal curvatures, abnormal tone, discomfort, and limited joint range.

• Ensure proper seat depth/leg positioning and use custom footrests (not elevated leg rests) to prevent elders from sliding down in wheelchairs.

▲ Assess for side effects of medications and potential need for dosage readjustments to increase wheelchair tolerance.

• = Independent   ▲ = Collaborative

- Allow client to propel wheelchair independently at his or her own speed.

Home Care

- Assess home environment for barriers and a support system for emergency and contingency care (e.g., Lifeline).
- Recommend the following changes to the home to accommodate the use of a wheelchair:
  - Arrange traffic patterns so they are wide enough to maneuver a wheelchair.
  - Recognize that a 5-foot turning space is necessary to maneuver wheelchairs; doorways need to be 32 to 36 inches wide; and entrance ramps/paths should slope 1 inch per foot.
  - Replace door hardware with fold-back hinges, remove doorway encasements (if too narrow), remove/replace thresholds (if too high), hang wall-mounted sinks/handrails, grade floors in showers for roll-in chairs, use nonskid/nonslip floor coverings (e.g., nonwaxed wood, linoleum, or Berber carpet).
  - Rearrange room functions, furniture, and storage so that toileting, sleeping, bathing, and preparing/eating meals can safely take place on one level of the home.
- ▲ Request PT/OT referrals to evaluate wheelchair skills and safety, to suggest home modifications and ways to propel wheelchairs on irregular surfaces and get back into a chair after a fall.
- Suggest community resources for servicing and tuning up wheelchairs and/or locating parts so clients can service their own chairs; an annual tune-up is recommended.

Client/Family Teaching and Discharge Planning

- ▲ Assess pain levels of long-term wheelchair users and make referrals to therapists or wheelchair clinics for modifications as needed.
- Instruct and have client return demonstrate re-inflation of pneumatic tires; encourage client to monitor tire pressure every 2 to 3 weeks.

M

• = Independent   ▲ = Collaborative

- Instruct family/clients to remove large wheelchair parts (leg rests, armrests) when lifting wheelchair into car for transport; when reassembling it, check that all parts are fastened securely and temperature is tepid.
- Teach the importance of using seatbelts or chair tie-downs when riding in motor vehicles in a wheelchair. If unavailable, clients in wheelchairs should be transported in large heavy vehicles only.
- For further information, refer to care plan for **Impaired Transfer Ability.**

M

Moral Distress

NANDA-I Definition

Response to the inability to carry out one's chosen ethical/moral decision/action

Defining Characteristics

Expresses anguish (e.g., powerlessness, guilt, frustration, anxiety, self-doubt, fear) over difficulty acting on one's moral choice

Related Factors (r/t)

Conflict among decision makers; conflicting information guiding ethical decision-making; conflicting information guiding moral decision-making; cultural conflicts; end-of-life decisions; loss of autonomy; physical distance of decision maker; time constraints for decision-making; treatment decisions

Client Outcomes

Client Will (Specify Time Frame):

- Be able to act in accordance with values, goals, and beliefs
- Regain confidence in the ability to make decisions and/or act in accord with values, goals, and beliefs
- Express satisfaction with the ability to make decisions consistent with values, goals, and beliefs
- Have choices respected

● = Independent   ▲ = Collaborative

Nursing Interventions

- Ask about the nature of the problem and determine that moral distress is present. Expert opinion recommends this as the first step in the 4As to Rise Above Moral Distress model.
- Affirm the distress, commitment, "to take care of yourself" and your obligations. Validate feelings and perceptions with others.
- Prepare to take Action, implement strategies to "initiate the changes you desire." Anticipate and manage setbacks.
- Assess sources and severity of distress.
- Give voice/recognition to moral distress and express concerns about constraints to supportive individuals.
- Engage in problem solving.
- Engage in interdisciplinary problem-solving forums including family meeting and/or interdisciplinary rounds.
- Implement multidisciplinary interventions/strategies to address moral distress.
- Identify/use a support system.
- Initiate an ethics consult or ethics committee review.

Pediatric

- Consider the developmental age of children when evaluating decisions and conflict.

Multicultural

- Acknowledge and understand that cultural differences may influence a client's moral choices.

Geriatric and Home Care

- Previous interventions may be adapted for geriatric or home care use.

Nausea

NANDA-I Definition

A subjective, unpleasant, wavelike sensation in the back of the throat, epigastrium, or the abdomen that may lead to the urge or need to vomit

• = Independent   ▲ = Collaborative

Defining Characteristics

Aversion to food; gagging sensation; increased salivation; increased swallowing; report of nausea; sour taste in mouth

Related Factors (r/t)

Biophysical

Biochemical disorders (e.g., uremia, diabetic ketoacidosis, pregnancy); esophageal disease; gastric distention; gastric irritation; increased intracranial pressure; intraabdominal tumors; labyrinthitis; liver capsule stretch; localized tumors (e.g., acoustic neuroma, primary or secondary brain tumors, bone metastases at base of skull); meningitis; Ménière's disease; motion sickness; pain; pancreatic disease; splenetic capsule stretch; toxins (e.g., tumor-produced peptides, abnormal metabolites due to cancer)

Situational

Anxiety; fear; noxious odors; noxious taste; pain; psychological factors; unpleasant visual stimulation

Treatment-Related

Gastric distention; gastric irritation: pharmaceuticals

Client Outcomes

Client Will (Specify Time Frame):

* State relief of nausea
* Explain methods clients can use to decrease nausea and vomiting (N&V)

Nursing Interventions

▲ Determine cause or risk for N&V (e.g., medication effects, infectious causes, disorders of the gut and peritoneum, central nervous system causes [including anxiety], endocrine and metabolic causes [including pregnancy], postoperative-related status).

▲ Evaluate and document the client's history of N&V, with attention to onset, duration, timing, volume of emesis, frequency of pattern, setting, associated factors, aggravating factors, and past medical and social histories.

● = Independent   ▲ = Collaborative

- Document each episode of nausea and/or vomiting separately, as well as effectiveness of interventions.
- Identify and eliminate contributing causative factors. This may include eliminating unpleasant odors or medications that may be contributing to nausea.
▲ Implement appropriate dietary measures such as NPO status as appropriate; small, frequent meals; and low-fat meals. It may be helpful to avoid foods that are spicy, fatty, or highly salty. Reverting to previous practices when ill in the past and consuming "comfort foods" may also be helpful at this time.
▲ Recognize and implement interventions and monitor complications associated with N&V. This may include administration of intravenous fluids and electrolytes.
▲ Administer appropriate antiemetics, according to emetic cause, by most effective route, considering the side effects of the medication, with attention to and coverage for the timeframes that the nausea is anticipated.
- Consider nonpharmacologic interventions such as acupressure, acupuncture, music therapy, distraction, and slow, deliberate movements.
- Provide oral care after the client vomits.

Nausea in Pregnancy

- There are no studies of dietary or other lifestyle interventions with any evidence to support traditional advice and interventions. It is often recommended that the woman eat dry crackers or dry toast in bed before arising and then get up slowly. Additional advice includes eating small frequent meals, drinking small amounts of fluids often, avoid foods with offensive odors, and avoiding preparing food or shopping when nauseated.
▲ Discuss with the primary care practitioner the possibility of using the P6 acupressure point stimulation to help relieve nausea.
▲ Recognize that ginger ingestion may help nausea. Ginger is available in a number of forms including tea, biscuits, and capsules.

N

• = Independent   ▲ = Collaborative

▲ Recognize that there are currently no FDA-approved drugs for the treatment of morning sickness, N&V of pregnancy, or hyperemesis gravidarum. There are, however, several pharmacologic treatments outlined by the American College of Obstetrics and Gynecology (ACOG).

Nausea Following Surgery

▲ Evaluate for risk factors for postoperative nausea and vomiting (PONV). Strong evidence suggests that client-related risk factors such as female gender, history of PONV, history of motion sickness, nonsmoking behavior, and environmental risk factors such as postoperative opioid use, emetogenic surgery (type and duration), and volatile anesthetics may increase the risk for PONV. Prolonged NPO status, more than 6 hours, has been associated with postop nausea.

▲ Medicate the client prophylactically for nausea as ordered, throughout the period of risk.

▲ Alleviate postoperative pain using ordered analgesic agents (refer to care plan for **Acute Pain**).

• Consider the use of nonpharmacological techniques, such as P6 acupoint stimulation, as an adjunct for controlling PONV, which has been shown to be effective.

• Use of therapeutic suggestions and ginger may not work as effectively in postdischarge nausea and vomiting (PDNV).

• Include client education on the management of PONV for all outpatients and discuss key assessment criteria.

Nausea Following Chemotherapy

• Perform risk assessment prior to chemotherapy administration. Risk factors include female gender, younger age, history of low alcohol consumption, history of morning sickness during pregnancy, anxiety, previous history of chemotherapy, client expectancy of nausea, and emetic potential of the regimen.

▲ Consult with physician regarding antiemetic strategy, either prophylactic or when N&V occurs.

• Consider teaching your client to learn how to use acupressure for nausea, applying pressure bilaterally at P6 points using fingers or bands to decrease the amount and severity of nausea.

• = Independent   ▲ = Collaborative

▲ Consider the use of ginger root *(Zingiber officinale)* to relieve nausea.
- Consider massage for symptom relief of nausea.
- Consider the use of yoga for CINV.

Geriatric

There are no specific guidelines that address the prophylaxis of CINV in the elderly. Risk still needs to be assessed, although many elderly clients are often treated with less emetic chemotherapy. Chemotherapy, however, can cause increased toxicity due to age-related decreases in organ function, comorbidities, and drug-drug interactions secondary to polypharmacy. Additionally, adherence may be an issue, due to cognitive decline, impaired senses, and economic issues.

Pediatric

- Interventions for CINV should be implemented prior to and after chemotherapy.
- Relatively few studies exist examining the antiemetic medications used for CINV in children. It appears that 5-HT$_3$ antagonists combined with dexamethasone are better than older agents.

Home Care

- Previously mentioned interventions may be adapted for home care use.
▲ In hospice care clients, assess for causes of nausea, such as constipation, bowel obstruction, adverse effects of medications, and onset of increased intracranial pressure. Refer the client to a primary care practitioner if needed.
- Assist the client and family with identifying and avoiding irritants in the home that exacerbate nausea (e.g., strong odors from food, plants, perfume, and room deodorizers). All medications except antiemetics should be given after meals to minimize the risk of nausea.

Client/Family Teaching and Discharge Planning

- Teach the client techniques to use before and after chemotherapy, including antiemetics/medication management schedules and relaxation techniques, guided imagery, hypnosis, and music therapy.

• = Independent   ▲ = Collaborative

Noncompliance

NANDA-I Definition

Behavior of person and/or caregiver that fails to coincide with a health-promoting or therapeutic plan agreed on by the person (and/or family and/or community) and health care professional. In the presence of an agreed-on, health-promoting, or therapeutic plan, person's or caregiver's behavior is fully or partially nonadherent and may lead to clinically ineffective or partially ineffective outcomes

Defining Characteristics

Behavior indicative of failure to adhere; evidence of development of complications; evidence of exacerbation of symptoms; failure to keep appointments; failure to progress; objective tests (e.g., physiological measures, detection of physiological markers)

Related Factors (r/t)

Health System

Access to care, communication skills of the provider, convenience of care, credibility of provider, difficulty In client-provider relationship, individual health coverage, provider continuity, provider regular follow-up, provider reimbursement, satisfaction with care, teaching skills of the provider

Health Care Plan

Complexity, cost, duration, financial flexibility of plan, intensity

Individual Factors

Cultural influences, developmental abilities, health beliefs; deficient knowledge relevant to the regimen behavior; individual's value system, motivational forces, personal abilities, significant others, skill relevant to the regimen behavior, spiritual values

Network

Involvement of members in health plan; perceived beliefs of significant others; social value regarding plan

NOTE: The nursing diagnosis **Noncompliance** is judgmental and places blame on the client. The authors recommend use of the diagnosis **Ineffective Self-Health Management** in place of the diagnosis **Noncompliance.** The diagnosis **Ineffective Self-Health**

• = Independent ▲ = Collaborative

Management has interventions that are developed by both the health care providers and the client. It is a more respectful and efficacious nursing diagnosis than **Noncompliance.**

Readiness for enhanced Nutrition

NANDA-I Definition

A pattern of nutrient intake that is sufficient for meeting metabolic needs and can be strengthened

Defining Characteristics

Attitude toward drinking is congruent with health goals; attitude toward eating is congruent with health goals; consumes adequate fluid; consumes adequate food; eats regularly; expresses knowledge of healthy fluid choices; expresses knowledge of healthy food choices; expresses willingness to enhance nutrition; follows an appropriate standard for intake (e.g., the American Diabetic Association guidelines); safe preparation for fluids; safe preparation for food; safe storage for food and fluids

Client Outcomes

Client Will (Specify Time Frame):
- Explain how to eat according to the U.S. Dietary Guidelines
- Design dietary modifications to meet individual long-term goal of health, using principles of variety, balance, and moderation
- Maintain weight within normal range for height and age

Nursing Interventions
- Ask the client to keep a 1- to 3-day food diary where everything eaten or drunk is recorded. Analyze the quality, quantity, and pattern of food intake.
- Advise the client to measure food periodically. Help the client learn usual portion sizes.
- Help the client determine his or her body mass index (BMI). Use a chart or a website such as http://www.cdc.gov/healthyweight/assessing/bmi/index.html.
- Recommend the client follow the U.S. Dietary Guidelines to determine foods to eat, which can be found at http://www.cnpp.usda.gov/Publications/DietaryGuidelines/2010/PolicyDoc/ExecSumm.pdf.

• = Independent   ▲ = Collaborative

- Recommend the client use Super Tracker (http://www. choosemyplate.gov/food-groups) to determine the number of calories to eat and gain more information on how to eat in a healthy fashion. To lose weight, the client must eat fewer calories.
- Recommend the client eat a healthy breakfast every morning.
- Recommend the client avoid eating in fast food restaurants.
- Demonstrate the use of food labels to make healthful choices. Alert the client/family to focus on serving size, total fat, and simple carbohydrate.

Carbohydrates/Sugars

- Encourage the client to **decrease** intake of sugars, including intake of soft drinks, desserts, and candy. Limit sugar intake to 6.5 teaspoons of added sugars for women and 9.5 teaspoons of added sugar for men daily.
- Share with client the names of sugars include glucose, dextrose, corn syrup, maple syrup, brown sugar, molasses, evaporated cane juice, sucrose, honey, orange juice concentrate, grape juice concentrate, apple juice concentrate, brown rice syrup, high-fructose corn syrup, agave, and fructose.
- Limit intake of fruit juice to 1 cup per day.
- Recommend the client eat whole grains whenever possible, and explain how to find whole grains using the food label.
- Evaluate the client's usual intake of fiber. Recommended intake is 25 g per day for women and 38 g per day for men. Increase intake of whole grains, beans, fruits, and vegetables to obtain needed fiber. Wheat bran is an excellent source of fiber, but cannot be tolerated by all people; beans are the second-best source of fiber.
- Recommend the client eat five to nine fruits and vegetables per day, with a minimum of two servings of fruit and three servings of vegetables. Encourage client to eat a rainbow of fruits and vegetables because bright colors are associated with increased nutrients.

Fats

- Recommend the client limit intake of saturated fats and avoid trans fatty acids completely; instead increase intake of vegetable oils such as polyunsaturated and monounsaturated oils.

- Recommend client use low-fat choices when selecting and cooking meat, and also when selecting dairy products.
- Recommend that the client eat cold-water fish such as salmon, tuna, or mackerel at least two times per week to ensure adequate intake of omega-3 fatty acids. If unwilling to eat fish, suggest sources such as flaxseed, soy, or walnuts. NOTE: Fish oil capsules should be taken cautiously; some brands can be contaminated with mercury or pesticides. Intake of excessive omega-3 fatty acids can result in bleeding.

Protein

- Recommend the client decrease intake of red meat and processed meats, instead eat more poultry, fish, soy, and dairy sources of protein.
- Recommend the client eat meatless meals at intervals and try alternative sources of protein, including nuts, especially almonds (one handful), and nut butters.
- Recommend the client eat beans and soy as an alternative to animal proteins at intervals. Introduce the client to soy products such as flavored soy milk and tofu.

Fluid and Electrolytes

- Recommend the client choose and prepare foods with less salt, aiming for a maximum of 2300 mg per day.
- If the client drinks alcohol, encourage him or her to drink in moderation—no more than one drink per day for women and two drinks per day for men.
- Recommend client increase intake of water, to at least 2000 mL or 2 quarts per day. A guideline is 1 to 1.5 mL of fluid for each calorie needed, so an average intake would be between 2000 and 3000 mL/day, or at least 8 cups of fluid.

Supplements

- Recommend that clients utilize dietary supplements such as vitamins and minerals only after consulting with their primary care practitioner.

N

Pediatric

* Recommend that families eat together for at least one meal per day.
* Recommend involving the family in planning meals and food preparation. Children can learn about nutrition as they help plan and make meals.
* Suggest that parents work at being good role models of healthy eating.
* Recommend that the family try new foods, either a new food or recipe every week.
* Suggest the parents keep healthy snacks on hand. Store the snacks in a purse, the car, a desk drawer.
* Plan ahead before eating out.

Geriatric

* Utilize a nutritional screening tool designed for the elderly such as the Mini Nutrition Assessment (MNA), the Malnutrition Universal Screening Tool (MUST), or the Nutrition Risk Screening (NRS).
* Assess changes in lifestyle and eating patterns. Geriatric clients need to decrease portion size as they get older because they are not burning as many calories.
* Assess fluid intake. Recommend routine drinks of water regardless of thirst. Monitor elderly clients for deficient fluid volume carefully, noting new onset of weakness, dizziness, and postural hypotension.
* Observe for socioeconomic factors that influence food choices (e.g., funds, cooking facilities).

Multicultural

* Assess for the influence of cultural beliefs, norms, and values on the client's nutritional knowledge.
* Discuss with the client those aspects of his or her diet that will remain unchanged.

Client/Family Teaching and Discharge Planning

* The majority of the preceding interventions involve teaching.
* Work with the family members regarding information on how to improve nutritional status.

• = Independent ▲ = Collaborative

Imbalanced Nutrition: less than body requirements

NANDA-I Definition

Intake of nutrients insufficient to meet metabolic needs

Defining Characteristics

Abdominal cramping; abdominal pain; aversion to eating; body weight 20% or more under ideal; capillary fragility; diarrhea; excessive loss of hair; hyperactive bowel sounds; lack of food; lack of information; lack of interest in food; loss of weight with adequate food intake; misconceptions; misinformation; pale mucous membranes; perceived inability to ingest food; poor muscle tone; reported altered taste sensation; reported food intake less than RDA (recommended daily allowance); satiety immediately after ingesting food; sore buccal cavity; steatorrhea; weakness of muscles required for swallowing or mastication

Related Factors (r/t)

Biological factors; economic factors; inability to absorb nutrients; inability to digest food; inability to ingest food; psychological factors

Client Outcomes

Client Will (Specify Time Frame):

- Progressively gain weight toward desired goal
- Weigh within normal range for height and age
- Recognize factors contributing to underweight
- Identify nutritional requirements
- Consume adequate nourishment
- Be free of signs of malnutrition

Nursing Interventions

▲ Use a nutritional screening tool to determine possibility of malnutrition on admission into any health care facility. Watch for recent weight loss of over 10 lb, 10% under healthy weight, not eating for more than 3 days, ½ normal eating for greater than 5 days, and body mass index (BMI) of less than 20, or other reasons why the client may be malnourished, and refer to a dietitian for a complete nutritional assessment.

● = Independent   ▲ = Collaborative

- Recognize that clients with acute disease or injury-related malnutrition, wounds, recent surgery, trauma, and a fever are using more calories and need increased calories to maintain their nutritional status.
- Recognize that clients with chronic disease-related malnutrition (cancer, rheumatoid arthritis, sarcopenic obesity, organ failure) may need calories to maintain nutritional status.
- Monitor for signs of malnutrition, including brittle hair that is easily plucked, bruises, dry skin, pale skin and conjunctiva, muscle wasting, marked decrease in body fat, smooth red tongue, cheilosis, and a "flaky paint" rash over lower extremities.
- Recognize that severe protein-calorie malnutrition can result in septicemia from impairment of the immune system, and organ failure including heart failure, liver failure, and respiratory dysfunction, especially in the critically ill client.
- ▲ Note laboratory test results as available: serum albumin, prealbumin, serum total protein, serum ferritin, transferrin, hemoglobin, hematocrit, and electrolytes.
- Weigh the client daily in acute care, weekly to monthly in extended care at the same time (usually before breakfast), with same amount of clothing.
- ▲ Monitor food intake; record percentages of served food that is eaten (25%, 50%, 75%, 100%). Keep a 3-day food diary to determine actual intake; consult with dietitian for actual calorie count if needed.
- Observe the client's relationship to food. Attempt to separate physical from psychological causes for eating difficulty.
- Evaluate the intake of the client using the United States Department of Agriculture's My Tracker online software, available at https://www.choosemyplate.gov/SuperTracker/default.aspx.
- If the client is a vegetarian, evaluate vitamin B_{12} and iron intake.
- Observe the client's ability to eat (time involved, motor skills, visual acuity, and ability to swallow various textures). If the client needs to be fed, allocate **at least 35 minutes** to feeding.

    NOTE: If the client is unable to feed self, refer to Nursing Interventions for **Feeding Self-Care deficit.** If the client has difficulty swallowing, refer to Nursing Interventions for **Impaired Swallowing.** If the client is receiving tube feedings, refer to the Nursing Interventions for **Risk for Aspiration.**

• If the client has a minimally functioning gastrointestinal tract and is on clear fluids, consult with dietitian regarding use of a clear liquid product that contains increased amounts of protein and calories such as Ensure Alive, Resource Breeze Fruit Beverage, or citrotein.

• For the client with anorexia, who will not eat foods, consider offering 30 mL of a nutritional supplement in a medication cup every hour, often during medication rounds.

• For the client who is malnourished and can eat, offer small quantities of energy-dense and protein-enriched food, served in an appetizing fashion, at frequent intervals. For the client who is able to eat, but has a decreased appetite, try the following activities:

  ■ Offer foods that are familiar to the client and do not offend his/her beliefs.

  ■ Avoid interruptions during mealtimes; meals should be eaten in a calm and peaceful environment. Interruptions have a negative effect on client's nutrition.

  ■ Make food available as desired between early evening and breakfast.

  ■ Use colored trays to identify clients who need help eating or who are at nutritional risk.

• If the client lacks endurance, schedule rest periods before meals, and open packages and cut up food for the client.

• Watch carefully for signs of infection and maintain every action possible to protect the client from infection.

• Provide companionship at mealtime to encourage nutritional intake.

• Monitor state of oral cavity (gums, tongue, mucosa, teeth). Provide good oral hygiene before each meal.

▲ Administer antiemetics and pain medications as ordered and needed before meals.

• If client is nauseated, remove cover of food tray before bringing it into the client's room.

• Work with the client to develop a plan for increased activity.

• = Independent   ▲ = Collaborative

- If the client is anemic, offer foods rich in iron and vitamins B_{12}, C, and folic acid.
- For the agitated, pacing client, offer finger foods (sandwiches, fresh fruit) and fluids
▲ If client has been malnourished for a significant length of time, consult with the dietitian and refeed carefully after correcting electrolyte balance. Watch for heart and respiratory failure.

Critical Care

- Recognize the need to begin enteral feedings within 24 to 48 hours of entrance into the critical care environment, once the client is free of hemodynamic compromise, if the client is unable to eat.
- Recognize that it is important to get the ordered feedings into the client, and that frequently checking for gastric residual, checking placement of the tube, can be a limiting factor to adequate nutrition in the tube-fed client.

Pediatric

- If the client is pregnant, ensure that she is receiving adequate amounts of folic acid by eating a balanced diet and taking prenatal vitamins as ordered.
▲ Utilize a nutritional screening tool designed for nurses such as the Paediatric Yorkhill Malnutrition Score (PYMS) tool, and if the child has a score of 2 or more, make a referral to a dietitian.
- Watch for symptoms of malnutrition in the child including short stature, thin arms and legs, poor condition of skin and hair, visible vertebrae and rib cage, wasted buttocks, wasted facial appearance, lethargy, and in extreme cases, edema.
- Weigh and measure the length (height) of the child and use a growth chart to help determine growth pattern, which reflects nutrition.
▲ Refer to a physician and a dietitian a child who is underweight for any reason.
- Work with the child and parent to develop an appropriate weight gain plan.
- Recognize that a large percentage of girls and teenagers are dieting, which can result in nutritional problems.

• = Independent   ▲ = Collaborative

Geriatric

- Screen for protein-energy malnutrition in elderly clients regardless of setting. Use a screening tool such as the Mini Nutritional Assessment.
- Screen for dysphagia in all elderly clients.
- Recognize that geriatric clients with moderate or severe cognition impairment have a significant risk of developing malnutrition.
▲ Interpret laboratory findings cautiously. Watch the color of urine for an indication of fluid balance; darker urine demonstrates dehydration.
- Recognize that constipation is a common problem with the elderly; therefore, they avoid many types of food for fear of problems with their bowel regimen.
- Consider using dining assistants, trained non-nursing staff, to provide feeding assistance care in extended care facilities to ensure adequate time for feeding clients as needed.
- Consider offering clients healthy snacks twice a day instead of nutritional supplements.
- Encourage client to increase intake of protein, unless medically contraindicated by organ failure. Aim for 1.5 g of protein per kilogram of body weight.
- Encourage physical activity throughout the day.
- Assess intake of components of bone health: calcium intake; the elderly adult needs 1200 mg of calcium and 800 IU of vitamin D.
- Monitor for onset of depression.
- Provide a restful, homelike environment during meals where clients are treated with respect and are encouraged to maintain autonomy as they are able.
- Recommend to families that enteral feedings may or may not be indicated for clients with dementia; instead use hand-feeding assistance, modified food consistency as needed, or environmental alterations.

   NOTE: If the client is unable to feed self, refer to Nursing Interventions for **Feeding Self-Care deficit.** If client has impaired physical function, malnutrition, depression, and cognitive impairment, please refer to care plan on **Adult Failure to Thrive.**

● - Independent   ▲ = Collaborative

Home Care

- The preceding interventions may be adapted for home care use.
- Screen for malnutrition using the Malnutrition Universal Screen Tool (MUST), which is simple and can be done rapidly.
- Monitor food intake. Instruct the client in intake of small frequent meals of foods with increased calories and protein.
- Assess clients' willingness to eat; fashion interventions accordingly.
- ▲ Assess the client for depression. Refer for mental health services as indicated.
- Consider social factors that may interfere with nutrition (e.g., lack of transportation, inadequate income, lack of social support).
- ▲ Monitor the effect of total parenteral nutrition (TPN) as ordered by physician, and appropriate including weight, blood glucose levels, electrolytes, symptoms of fluid overload or deficit, and symptoms of infection at entry site of catheter.

Client/Family Teaching and Discharge Planning

- Help the client/family identify the area to change that will make the greatest contribution to improved nutrition.
- Build on the strengths in the client's/family's food habits. Adapt changes to their current practices.
- Select appropriate teaching aids for the client's/family's background.
- Implement instructional follow-up to answer the client's/family's questions.
- Recommend that clients utilize dietary supplements such as vitamins and minerals only after consulting with their primary care practitioner.
- Suggest community resources as suitable (food sources, counseling, Meals on Wheels, senior centers).
- Teach the client and family how to manage tube feedings or parenteral therapy at home as needed.

Risk for imbalanced Nutrition: more than body requirements

NANDA-I Definition

At risk for intake of nutrients that exceeds metabolic needs

Risk Factors

Concentrating food at the end of day; dysfunctional eating patterns; eating in response to external cues (e.g., time of day, social situation); eating in response to internal cues other than hunger (e.g., anxiety); higher baseline weight at beginning of each pregnancy; observed use of food as comfort measure; observed use of food as reward; pairing food with other activities; parental obesity; rapid transition across growth percentiles in children; reported use of solid food as major food source before 5 months of age

N

Imbalanced Nutrition: more than body requirements

NANDA-I Definition

Intake of nutrients that exceeds metabolic needs

Defining Characteristics

Concentrating food intake at the end of the day; dysfunctional eating pattern (e.g., pairing food with other activities); eating in response to external cues (e.g., time of day, social situation); eating in response to internal cues other than hunger (e.g., anxiety); sedentary activity level; triceps skin fold greater than 25 mm in women, greater than 15 mm in men; weight 20% over ideal for height and frame

Related Factors (r/t)

Excessive intake in relation to metabolic need

Client Outcomes

Client Will (Specify Time Frame):

- State pertinent factors contributing to weight gain
- Identify behaviors that remain under client's control
- Design dietary modifications to meet individual long-term goal of weight control

• = Independent   ▲ = Collaborative

- Lose weight in a reasonable period (1 to 2 lb per week)
- Incorporate increased exercise requiring energy expenditure into daily life

Nursing Interventions

- Ask the client to keep a 1- to 3-day food diary where everything eaten or drunk is recorded.
- Advise the client to measure food periodically. Help the client learn usual portion sizes.
- Help the client determine his or her body mass index (BMI). Use a chart or a website such as http://www.cdc.gov/healthyweight/assessing/bmi/index.html.
- Recommend the client follow the U.S. Dietary Guidelines to determine foods to eat, which can be found at http://www.cnpp.usda.gov/DietaryGuidelines.htm.
- Recommend the client use the Super Tracker, which is available at http://www.choosemyplate.gov/supertracker-tools/supertracker.html, to plan his or her diet, determine the number of calories, evaluate the foods that he/she have eaten, and gain more information on how to eat in a healthy fashion.
- Recommend that clients lose weight slowly, no more than 1 to 2 lb per week, based on a healthy eating pattern and increased exercise.
- Demonstrate the use of food labels to make healthful choices. Alert the client/family to focus on serving size, total fat, and simple carbohydrate. The standardized food label in bold type simplifies the search for information.

Psychological Aspects of Obesity

- Refer the client with binge eating for cognitive-behavioral therapy.
▲ Watch the client for signs of depression: flat affect, poor sleeping habits, lack of interest in life. Refer for counseling/treatment as needed.

Pattern of Dietary Intake

- Recommend the client eat a healthy breakfast every morning.
- Recommend the client avoid eating in fast food restaurants.
- Recommend the client learn about and eat a low glycemic diet.

• = Independent   ▲ = Collaborative

- For information about how to eat healthy and lose weight regarding carbohydrates, protein, and fat, please refer to the care plan **Readiness for enhanced Nutrition.**

Recommended Foods/Fluids

- Encourage the client to increase intake of vegetables and fruits to at least five servings per day, preferably nine servings per day.
- Encourage the client to eat at least three whole grain servings per day, preferably more.
- Encourage the client to stop drinking sugar-sweetened beverages of all kinds, including sodas, lemonade, fruit juice, sweetened tea, vitamin drinks, energy drinks, and sports beverages. Instead encourage the client to drink water, or water with unsweetened fruit in it.
- Evaluate the client's usual intake of fiber. Recommended intake is 25 g per day for women and 38 g per day for men. Increase intake of whole grains, beans, fruits, and vegetables to obtain needed fiber.
- Discuss the possibility of using a primarily plant-based or vegetarian diet to lose weight.
- Recommend client increase intake of water to at least 2000 mL or 2 quarts per day. A guideline is 1 to 1.5 mL of fluid per each calorie needed, so an average intake would be between 2000 and 3000 mL/day, or at least 8 cups of fluid.
- For more information on healthy eating, refer to Nursing Interventions for **Readiness for enhanced Nutrition.**

Behavioral Methods for Weight Loss

- Familiarize the client with the following behavior modification techniques:
  - Self-monitoring of food intake, including keeping a food and exercise diary
  - Graphing weight weekly
  - Controlling stimuli that cause overeating, such as watching television with frequent food-related commercials
  - Limiting food intake to one site in the home
  - Sitting down at the table to eat
  - Planning food intake for each day

N

- Rearranging the schedule to avoid inappropriate eating
- Avoiding boredom that results in eating; keeping a list of activities on the refrigerator
- For a party, eating before arriving, sitting away from the snack foods, and substituting lower-calorie beverages for alcoholic ones
- Deciding beforehand what to order in a restaurant
- Bringing only healthy foods into the house to decrease temptation
- Slowing mealtime by swallowing food before putting more food on the utensil, pausing for a minute during the meal and attempting to increase the number of pauses, and trying to be the last one to finish eating
- Taking fewer bites of food, and chewing food more thoroughly before swallowing.
- Drinking a glass of water before each meal; taking sips of water between bites of food
- Charting one's progress
- Making an agreement with oneself or a significant other for a meaningful reward and not rewarding oneself with food
- Changing one's mindset, as in control of eating behavior
- Practicing relaxation techniques

Physical Activity

▲ Determine reasons why the client would be unable to participate in an exercise program; refer for evaluation by a primary care practitioner as needed.
• Encourage the client to begin an exercise program, walking, swimming, dancing, running, use of the elliptical machine, and more.
• Recommend the client begin a walking program using a pedometer. For further information on a walking program refer to the care plan **Sedentary lifestyle.**
• Encourage the client to engage in both aerobic exercise and strength training.

Pediatric

- Work with parents of the overweight child by encouraging the following behaviors:
  - Emphasize providing good food, not depriving children of food.
  - Accept the child's natural size and shape; the child needs the parents' unconditional love.
  - Make family meals a priority.
  - Involve the child in helping plan menus, and doing cooking and preparation as appropriate for the child's age.
  - Educate parents to participate in activities with children.
  - Encourage children to love their bodies.
- Determine the child's BMI.
- Work with the child and parent to develop an appropriate weight maintenance plan, including behavioral methods of weight loss, as well as increased activity.
- Work with the parent to change the food that is available in the home, eliminating sugary drinks and foods with a high saturated fat or trans fat content.
- Encourage child to increase the amount of walking done per day; if child is willing, ask him or her to wear a pedometer to measure number of steps.
- Recommend that parents do not use food as a reward for good behavior, especially foods that are concentrated sources of sugar or fat.
- Recommend the child decrease television viewing, watching movies, and playing video games. Ask parents to limit television to 1 to 2 hours per day maximum.

Geriatric

- Assess changes in lifestyle and eating patterns.
- Assess fluid intake. Recommend routine drinks of fluids regardless of thirst.
- Observe for socioeconomic factors that influence food choices (e.g., inadequate funds or cooking facilities).
- Recognize that it is generally not appropriate to have an elderly client on a calorie-restrictive diet.

● = Independent ▲ = Collaborative

Multicultural

- Recognize that the BMI's accuracy is different for some ethnic groups.
- Use cultural beliefs, norms, and values of the client when teaching information on nutrition and weight loss.
- Assess for the influence of cultural beliefs, norms, and values on the client's ideal of acceptable body weight and body size.
- Discuss with the client those aspects of his or her diet that will remain unchanged, and work with the client to adapt cultural core foods.

Client/Family Teaching and Discharge Planning

- Utilize the motivational interviewing technique when working with clients to promote healthy eating and weight loss.
- Inform the client about the health risks associated with obesity, which include cancer, diabetes, heart disease, strokes, hypertension, gastroesophageal reflux, gallstones, osteoarthritis, and venous thrombosis.
- Recommend the client weigh self frequently, ideally every day.
- Inform the client and family of the disadvantages of trying to lose weight by dieting alone, and encourage the client to include exercise in the weight loss plan.
- Recommend the client receive adequate amounts of sleep.

Impaired Oral Mucous Membrane

NANDA-I Definition

Disruption of the lips and/or soft tissues of the oral cavity

Defining Characteristics

Bleeding; cheilitis; coated tongue; desquamation; difficult speech; difficulty eating; difficulty swallowing; diminished taste; edema; enlarged tonsils; fissures; geographic tongue; gingival hyperplasia; gingival pallor; gingival recession; halitosis; hyperemia; macroplasia; mucosal denudation; mucosal pallor; nodules; oral discomfort; oral lesions; oral pain; oral ulcers; papules; pocketing deeper than 4 mm; presence of pathogens; purulent drainage; purulent exudates; red or bluish masses

• = Independent   ▲ = Collaborative

(e.g.; hemangiomas); reports bad taste in mouth; smooth atrophic tongue; spongy patches; stomatitis; vesicles; white curd-like exudates; white patches/plaques; xerostomia

Related Factors (r/t)

Barriers to oral self-care; barriers to professional care; chemotherapy; chemical irritants (e.g., alcohol, tobacco, acidic foods, drugs, regular use of inhalers or other noxious agents), cleft lip; cleft palate; decreased platelets; decreased salivation; deficient knowledge of appropriate oral hygiene; dehydration; depression; diminished hormone levels (women); ineffective oral hygiene; infection; immunocompromised; immunosuppression; loss of supportive structures; malnutrition; mechanical factors (e.g.; ill-fitting dentures; braces); tubes (endotracheal/nasogastric); surgery in oral cavity; medication side effects; mouth breathing; NPO for more than 24 hours; radiation therapy; stress; trauma

Client Outcomes

Client Will (Specify Time Frame):

* Maintain intact, moist oral mucous membranes that are free of ulceration, inflammation, infection, and debris
* Demonstrate measures to maintain or regain intact oral mucous membranes

Nursing Interventions

▲ Inspect the oral cavity/teeth at least once daily and note any discoloration, presence of debris, amount of plaque buildup, presence of lesions such as white lesions or patches, edema, or bleeding, and intactness of teeth. Refer to a dentist or periodontist as appropriate.

* If the client does not have a bleeding disorder and is able to swallow, encourage the client to brush the teeth with a soft toothbrush using fluoride-containing toothpaste at least twice per day.

* Recommend the client use a powered toothbrush if desired for removal of dental plaque and prevention of gingivitis.

* Use foam sticks to moisten the oral mucous membranes, clean out debris, and swab out the mouth of the edentulous client. **Do not use foam sticks to clean the teeth** unless the platelet

count is very low and the client is prone to bleeding gums.
Foam sticks are useful for cleansing the oral cavity of a client
who is edentulous.
- If the client does not have a bleeding disorder, encourage the
client to floss once per day or use an interdental cleaner.
- Use an antimicrobial mouthwash as ordered or tap water or
saline only for a mouth rinse. Do not use commercial mouth-
washes containing alcohol or hydrogen peroxide. Also, do not
use lemon-glycerin swabs.
- If the client is unable to care for him- or herself, oral hygiene
must be provided by nursing personnel. The nursing diagnosis
Bathing/Hygiene Self-Care deficit is then applicable.
- If the client is unable to brush own teeth, follow this
procedure:
  - Position the client sitting upright or on side.
  - Use a soft bristle baby toothbrush.
  - Use fluoride toothpaste and tap water or saline as a
  solution.
  - Brush teeth in an up-and-down manner.
  - Suction as needed.
- Monitor the client's nutritional and fluid status to determine
if it is adequate. Refer to the care plan for **Deficient Fluid
Volume** or **Imbalanced Nutrition: less than body require-
ments** if applicable.
- Encourage fluid intake of up to 3000 mL/day if not contrain-
dicated by the client's medical condition.
- Determine the client's usual method of oral care and address
any concerns regarding oral hygiene.
▲ If the client has a dry mouth (xerostomia):
  - Recognize that more than 500 medications may cause xero-
  stomia, and at times the medication can be discontinued to
  increase the client's comfort.
  - Provide saliva substitutes as ordered.
  - Suggest the client chew sugarless gum or sugarless sour
  candy to promote salivary flow.
  - Provide ice chips frequently to keep the mouth moist.
  - Examine the oral cavity for signs of mucositis ulceration
  and oral candidiasis.

- Recommend the client decrease or preferably stop intake of soft drinks.
- If client has halitosis, review good oral care with the client including brushing teeth, using floss, and brushing the tongue.
- Instruct the client with halitosis to clean the tongue when performing oral hygiene; brush tongue with tongue scraper or toothbrush and follow with a mouth rinse.
▲ Assess the client for underlying medical condition that may be causing halitosis.
- Keep the lips well lubricated using a lip balm that is water- or aloe-based.

Client Receiving Chemotherapy/Radiation

- Ensure that the client receives a comprehensive oral examination before initiation of chemotherapy or radiation, with aggressive preventive dental care given as needed.
- Provide instructions both verbal and written about the need for and method of providing frequent oral care to the client before radiation therapy or chemotherapy.
- Assess the condition of the oral cavity daily in the client receiving radiation or chemotherapy.
- For measurement of presence or severity of mucositis, use the Oral Mucositis Assessment Scale (OMAS).
- Use a protocol to prevent/treat mucositis that includes the following:
  - Use of a soft toothbrush that is replaced on a regular basis
  - Use of a validated tool to assess condition of the oral cavity
  - Client teaching of the need for and method of performing oral care
  - Use of a bland rinse to remove debris and moisten the oral cavity
  - Use of a pain assessment tool and treatment of pain as needed.
- Use cryotherapy with ice chips dissolving in client's mouth before, during, and after bolus administration of fluorouracil (5-FU) to reduce the severity of mucositis.
- Help the client use a mouth rinse of normal saline or salt and soda every 1 to 2 hours for prevention and treatment of

stomatitis. A typical mixture is 1 teaspoon of salt or sodium bicarbonate per pint of water. Clients are directed to take a tablespoon of the rinse and swish it in the mouth for 30 seconds, then expectorate.

▲ If the mouth is severely inflamed and it is painful to swallow, contact the physician for a topical anesthetic or analgesic order. Modification of oral intake (e.g., soft or liquid diet) may also be necessary to prevent friction trauma. The nursing diagnosis **Imbalanced Nutrition: less than body requirements** may apply.

• If the client's platelet count is lower than 50,000/mm^3 or the client has a bleeding disorder, use a specially made toothbrush designed for sensitive or diseased tissue, or a toothette that is not soaked in glycerin or flavorings; if the client cannot tolerate a toothbrush or a toothette, a piece of gauze wrapped around a finger can be used to remove plaque and debris.

Critical Care—Client on a Ventilator

• Use a pediatric-sized soft toothbrush to brush teeth; use suction to remove secretions. Recognize that good oral care is paramount in the prevention of ventilator-associated pneumonia (VAP).

▲ Apply chlorhexidine gluconate in the oral cavity by swab or spray early after intubation, and at intervals if ordered.

Geriatric

• Determine the functional ability of the client to provide his or her own oral care. Refer to **Bathing/Hygiene Self-Care deficit.**

• Provide appropriate oral care to the elderly with a self-care deficit, brushing the teeth after breakfast and in the evening.

• If the client has dementia or delirium and exhibits care-resistant behavior such as fighting, biting, or refusing care, utilize the following method:

  ■ Ensure client is in a quiet environment such as own bathroom, sitting or standing at the sink to prime memory for appropriate actions.

- Approach the client at eye level within his or her range of vision.
- Approach with a smile, and begin conversation with a touch of the hand and gradually move up.
- Use mirror-mirror technique, standing behind the client, and brush and floss teeth.
- Use respectful adult speech, not elderspeak—sing-song voice, calling dearie, honey, and so forth.
- Promote self-care where client brushes own teeth if possible.
- Utilize distractors when needed, singing, talking, reminiscing, or use of a teddy bear.
- Carefully observe the oral cavity and lips for abnormal lesions such as white or red patches, masses, ulcerations with an indurated margin, or a raised granular lesion.
- Ensure that dentures are removed and cleaned regularly, preferably after every meal and before bedtime.

Home Care

- The interventions described previously may be adapted for home care use.
- ▲ Instruct the client in ways to soothe the oral cavity (e.g., cool beverages, Popsicles, viscous lidocaine).
- ▲ If necessary, refer for home health aide services to support the family in oral care and observation of the oral cavity.

Client/Family Teaching and Discharge Planning

- Teach the client how to inspect the oral cavity and monitor for signs and symptoms of infection or complications, and when to call the health care practitioner.
- Recommend the client not smoke, use chewing tobacco, or drink excessive amounts of alcohol.
- Teach the client and family if necessary how to perform appropriate mouth care. Utilize the Motivational Interviewing Technique.

Acute Pain

NANDA-I Definition

Unpleasant sensory and emotional experience arising from actual or potential tissue damage or described in terms of such damage; sudden or slow onset of any intensity from mild to severe with an anticipated or predictable end and a duration of less than 6 months

Pain is whatever the experiencing person says it is, existing whenever the person says it does.

Defining Characteristics

Subjective

Pain is a subjective experience, and its presence cannot be proved or disproved. Self-report is the most reliable method of evaluating pain presence and intensity. A client with cognitive ability who is able to speak or provide information about pain in other ways, such as pointing to numbers or words, should use a self-report pain tool (e.g., Numerical Rating Scale [NRS]) to identify the current pain intensity and establish a comfort-function goal.

Objective

Pain is a subjective experience, and objective measurement is impossible. If a client cannot provide a self-report, there is no pain intensity level. Behavioral responses should never serve as the basis for pain management decisions if self-report is possible. However, observation of behavioral responses may be helpful in recognition of pain presence for clients who are unable to provide a self-report. Observable pain responses may include loss of appetite and inability to deep breathe, ambulate, sleep, and perform ADLs. Pain-related behaviors vary widely and are highly individual. They may include guarding, self-protective behavior, and self-focusing; and distraction behavior ranging from crying to laughing, as well as muscle tension or rigidity. Clients may be stoic and lie completely still despite having severe pain. Sudden acute pain may be associated with neurohumoral responses that can lead to increases in heart rate, blood pressure, and respiratory rate. However, physiological responses, such as elevated blood pressure or heart rate, are not sensitive indicators of pain presence and intensity as they do not discriminate pain from other sources of distress, pathological conditions, homeostatic changes, or medications. Behavioral or physiological

• = Independent ▲ = Collaborative

indicators may be used to confirm other findings; however, the absence of these indicators does not mean that pain is absent.

NOTE: The defining characteristics are modified from the work of NANDA-I.

Related Factors (r/t)

Injury agents (biological, chemical, physical, psychological)

Client Outcomes

Client Will (Specify Time Frame):

For the client who is able to provide a self-report:
- Use a self-report pain tool to identify current pain intensity level and establish a comfort-function goal
- Report that pain management regimen achieves comfort-function goal without side effects
- Describe nonpharmacological methods that can be used to help achieve comfort-function goal
- Perform activities of recovery or ADLs easily
- Describe how unrelieved pain will be managed
- State ability to obtain sufficient amounts of rest and sleep
- Notify member of the health care team promptly for pain intensity level that is consistently greater than the comfort-function goal, or occurrence of side effects

For the client who is unable to provide a self-report:
- Decrease in pain-related behaviors
- Perform activities of recovery or ADLs easily as determined by client condition
- Demonstrate the absence of side effects of analgesics
- No pain-related behaviors will be evident in the client who is completely unresponsive; a reasonable outcome is to demonstrate the absence of side effects related to the prescribed pain treatment plan

Nursing Interventions

- Determine if the client is experiencing pain at the time of the initial interview. If pain is present, conduct and document a comprehensive pain assessment and implement or request orders to implement pain management interventions to achieve a satisfactory level of comfort. Components of this

P

• = Independent ▲ = Collaborative

initial assessment include location, quality, onset/duration, temporal profile, intensity, aggravating and alleviating factors, and effects of pain on function and quality of life.

- Assess pain intensity level in a client using a valid and reliable self-report pain tool, such as the 0-10 numerical pain rating scale.

- Assess the client for pain presence routinely; this is often done at the same time as when a full set of vital signs are obtained, and during activity and rest. Also assess for pain with interventions or procedures likely to cause pain.

- Ask the client to describe prior experiences with pain, effectiveness of pain management interventions, responses to analgesic medications including occurrence of side effects, and concerns about pain and its treatment (e.g., fear about addiction, worries, or anxiety) and informational needs.

- Ask the client to identify a comfort-function goal, a pain level, on a self-report pain tool, that will allow the client to perform necessary or desired activities easily. This goal will provide the basis to determine effectiveness of pain management interventions. If the client is unable to provide a self-report, it will not be possible to establish a comfort-function goal.

- Describe the adverse effects of unrelieved pain.

- Use the Hierarchy of Pain Measures as a framework for pain assessment: (1) attempt to obtain the client's self-report of pain; (2) consider the client's condition and search for possible causes of pain (e.g., presence of tissue injury, pathological conditions, or exposure to procedures/interventions that are thought to result in pain); (3) observe for behaviors that may indicate pain presence (e.g., facial expressions, crying, restlessness, and changes in activity); (4) evaluate physiological indicators, with the understanding that these are the least sensitive indicators of pain and may be related to conditions other than pain (e.g., shock, hypovolemia, anxiety); and (5) conduct an analgesic trial.

- Assume that pain is present if the client is unable to provide a self-report and has tissue injury, a pathological condition, or has undergone a procedure that is thought to produce pain.

- Conduct an analgesic trial for clients who are unable to provide self-report and have underlying pathology/condition that is thought to be painful, or who demonstrate behaviors that may indicate pain is present. Administer a nonopioid if pain is thought to be mild and an opioid if pain is thought to be moderate to severe. Reassess the client to evaluate intervention effectiveness within a specific period of time based on pharmacokinetics (intravenous [IV] 15 to 30 minutes, subcutaneous 30 minutes, oral 60 minutes).

- Determine the client's current medication use. Obtain an accurate and complete list of medications the client is taking or has taken.
- Explain to the client the pain management approach, including pharmacological and nonpharmacological interventions, the assessment and reassessment process, potential side effects, and the importance of prompt reporting of unrelieved pain.
- Manage acute pain using a multimodal approach.
- Recognize that the oral route is preferred for pain management interventions. If the client is receiving parenteral analgesia, use an equianalgesic chart to convert to an oral analgesic as soon as possible.
- Provide PCA, perineural infusions, and intraspinal analgesia as ordered, when appropriate and available
- Avoid giving pain medication by the intramuscular (IM) route of administration.
- Obtain a prescription to administer a nonopioid analgesic for mild to moderate pain and an opioid analgesic if indicated for moderate to severe acute pain.
- Treat acute pain in a comprehensive manner.
- Prevent pain by administering analgesia before painful procedures whenever possible (e.g., endotracheal suctioning, wound care, heel puncture, venipunctures, and peripherally inserted IV catheters). Use a topical local anesthetic or IV opioid as determined by individualized client status and severity of associated pain.
- Administer supplemental analgesic doses as ordered to keep the client's pain level at or below the comfort-function goal, or desired outcome based on clinical judgment or behaviors if client is unable to provide a self-report.
- Perform nursing care when the client is comfortable. This is facilitated when the peak time (maximum serum concentration) of the analgesic is considered.

P

• = Independent   ▲ = Collaborative

- Discuss the client's fears of undertreated pain, side effects, and addiction.
- Assess pain level, sedation level, and respiratory status at regular intervals during opioid administration. Assess sedation and respiratory status every 1 to 2 hours during the first 24 hours of opioid therapy, then every 4 hours if respiratory status has been stable without episodes of hypoventilation, or more frequently as determined by individualized client status. Conduct the respiratory assessment before sedation assessment by evaluating the depth, regularity, and noisiness of respiration, and counting respiratory rate for 60 seconds. Awaken sleeping clients for assessment if the respiration is inadequate (e.g., if respirations are shallow, ineffective, irregular, or noisy [snoring], or periods of apnea occur). Snoring indicates respiratory obstruction and warrants prompt arousal, repositioning, and evaluation of respiratory risk factors. Discontinue titration or continuous opioid infusions immediately, and decrease subsequent opioid doses by 25% to 50% if the client develops excessive sedation.
- Ask the client to report side effects, such as nausea and pruritus, and to describe appetite, bowel elimination, and ability to rest and sleep. Administer medications and treatments to prevent and improve these conditions and functions. Obtain a prescription for a combination stool softener plus peristaltic stimulant to prevent opioid-induced constipation.
- Review the client's pain flowsheet and medication administration record to evaluate effectiveness of pain relief, previous 24-hour opioid requirements, and occurrence of side effects.
- Obtain orders to increase or decrease opioid doses as needed; base analgesic and dose on the client's report of pain severity (clinical judgment of effectiveness if the client is unable to provide a self-report), response to the previous dose in terms of pain relief, occurrence of side effects, and ability to perform the activities of recovery or ADLs.
- When the client is able to tolerate oral intake, obtain a prescription to change analgesics to the oral route of administration; use an equianalgesic chart to determine the initial dose and adjust for incomplete cross tolerance.

• = Independent   ▲ = Collaborative

- In addition to administering analgesics, support the client's use of nonpharmacological methods to help control pain, such as distraction, imagery, relaxation, and application of heat and cold.
- Teach and implement nonpharmacological interventions when pain is relatively well controlled with pharmacological interventions.

Pediatric

- Assess for the presence of pain using a valid and reliable pain scale based on age, cognitive development, and the child's ability to provide a self-report.
- Administer analgesics as prescribed.
- Prevent procedural pain in neonates, infants, and children by using opioid analgesics and anesthetics, as indicated, in appropriate dosages.
- Use a topical local anesthetic such as EMLA cream or LMX-4 before performing venipuncture in neonates, infants, and children.
- For the neonate, use oral sucrose and nonnutritional sucking (NNS) or human milk for pain of short duration such as heel stick or venipuncture.
- Recognize that breastfeeding has been shown to reduce behavioral indicators of pain.
- As with adults, use nonpharmacological interventions to supplement, not replace, pharmacological interventions.

Geriatric

- Please refer to the interventions in the care plan for **Chronic Pain**.

Multicultural

- Please refer to the care plan on **Chronic Pain** for multicultural interventions.

Home Care

- Develop the treatment plan with the client and caregivers.
- Develop a full medication profile, including medications prescribed by all physicians and all over-the-counter medications. Assess for drug interactions. Instruct the client to refrain from mixing medications without physician approval.

• = Independent   ▲ = Collaborative

- Assess the client's and family's knowledge of side effects and safety precautions associated with pain medications (e.g., use caution in operating machinery when opioids are first taken or dosage has been increased significantly).
- If medication is administered using highly technological methods, assess the home for the necessary resources (e.g., electricity) and ensure that there will be responsible caregivers available to assist the client with administration.
- Assess the knowledge base of the client and family with regard to highly technological medication administration. Teach as necessary. Be sure the client knows when, how, and whom to contact if analgesia is unsatisfactory.

Client/Family Teaching and Discharge Planning

NOTE: To avoid the negative connotations associated with the words *drugs* and *narcotics*, use the term *pain medicine* when teaching clients.

- Discuss the various discomforts encompassed by the word *pain* and ask the client to give examples of previously experienced pain. Explain the pain assessment process and the purpose of the pain rating scale.
- Teach the client to use the self-report pain tool to rate the intensity of past or current pain. Ask the client to set a comfort-function goal by selecting a pain level on the self-report tool that will allow performance of desired or necessary activities of recovery with relative ease (e.g., turn, cough, deep breathe, ambulate, participate in physical therapy). If the pain level is consistently above the comfort-function goal, the client should take action that decreases pain or notify a member of the health care team so that effective pain management interventions may be implemented promptly. (See information on teaching clients to use the pain rating scale.)
- Provide written materials on pain control that teach how to use a pain rating scale and how to take analgesics.
- Discuss the total plan for pharmacological and nonpharmacological treatment, including the medication plan for around-the-clock administration and supplemental doses, and the use of supplies and equipment. If PCA is ordered, determine the

- client's ability to press the appropriate button. Remind the client and staff that the PCA button is for client use only.
- Reinforce the importance of taking pain medications to maintain the comfort-function goal.
- Demonstrate the use of appropriate nonpharmacological approaches in addition to pharmacological approaches to help control pain, such as application of heat and/or cold, distraction techniques, relaxation breathing, visualization, rocking, stroking, music listening, and television watching).
- Teach nonpharmacological methods when pain is relatively well controlled. Pain interferes with cognition.

Chronic Pain

NANDA-I Definition

Unpleasant sensory and emotional experience arising from actual or potential tissue damage or described in terms of such damage; sudden or slow onset of any intensity from mild to severe, constant or recurring without an anticipated or predictable end. Pain is whatever the experiencing person says it is, existing whenever the person says it does.

Defining Characteristics

Pain is a subjective experience and its presence cannot be proved or disproved. Self-report is the most reliable method of evaluating pain presence and intensity. Please refer to the Defining Characteristics in the **Acute Pain** care plan for further characteristics of pain.

Related Factors (r/t)

Actual or potential tissue damage; tumor progression and related pathology; diagnostic and therapeutic procedures; central or peripheral nerve injury (neuropathic pain)

NOTE: The cause of chronic (persistent) noncancer (nonmalignant) pain may be unknown. It often involves multiple poorly understood underlying mechanisms and includes a complex interaction of physiological, emotional, cognitive, social, and environmental factors. It is the subject of ongoing research.

• = Independent   ▲ = Collaborative

Client Outcomes

Client Will (Specify Time Frame):

For the client who is able to provide a self-report:

- Provide a description of the pain experience including physical, social, emotional, and spiritual aspects
- Use a self-report pain tool to identify current pain level and establish a comfort-function goal
- Report that the pain management regimen achieves comfort-function goal without the occurrence of side effects
- Describe nonpharmacological methods that can be used to supplement, or enhance, pharmacological interventions and help achieve the comfort-function goal
- Perform necessary or desired activities at a pain level less than or equal to the comfort-function goal
- Demonstrate the ability to pace activity, taking rest breaks before they are needed
- Describe how unrelieved pain will be managed
- State the ability to obtain sufficient amounts of rest and sleep
- Notify a member of the health care team for pain level consistently greater than the comfort-function goal or occurrence of side effect

For the client who is unable to provide a self-report:

- Demonstrate decrease or resolved pain-related behaviors
- Perform desired activities as determined by client condition
- Demonstrate the absence of side effects
- No pain-related behaviors will be evident in the client who is completely unresponsive; a reasonable outcome is to demonstrate the absence of side effects related to the prescribed pain treatment plan

Nursing Interventions

- Determine if the client is experiencing pain at the time of the initial interview. If pain is present, conduct and document a comprehensive pain assessment and implement or request orders to implement pain management interventions to achieve a satisfactory level of comfort. Components of this initial assessment include location, quality, onset/duration, temporal profile, intensity, aggravating and alleviating factors, and effects of pain on function and quality of life

● = Independent   ▲ = Collaborative

- Assess pain intensity level in a client using a valid and reliable self-report pain tool, such as the 0-10 numerical pain rating scale.
- Ask the client to describe prior experiences with pain, effectiveness of pain management interventions, responses to analgesic medications including occurrence of side effects, and concerns about pain and its treatment (e.g., fear about addiction, worries, or anxiety) and informational needs.
- Describe the adverse effects of persistent unrelieved pain.
- Ask the client to identify the pain level, on a self-report pain tool, that will allow the client to perform desired activities and achieve an acceptable quality of life. This comfort-function goal will provide the basis to determine effectiveness of the individualized pain management plan. If the client is unable to provide a self-report, it will not be possible to establish a comfort-function goal.
- Assess the client for the presence of pain routinely; this is often done at the same time as when a full set of vital signs are obtained in the inpatient setting. Assess pain during both activity and rest.
- Ask the client to maintain a diary (if able) of pain ratings, timing, precipitating events, medications, and effectiveness of pain management interventions.
- Use the Hierarchy of Pain Measures as a framework for pain assessment: (1) attempt to obtain the client's self-report of pain; (2) consider the client's condition and search for possible causes of pain (e.g., presence of tissue injury, pathological conditions, or exposure to procedures/interventions that are thought to result in pain); (3) observe for behaviors that may indicate pain presence (e.g., facial expressions, crying, restlessness, and changes in activity); (4) evaluate physiological indicators, with the understanding that these are the least sensitive indicators of pain and may be related to conditions other than pain (e.g., shock, hypovolemia, anxiety); and (5) conduct an analgesic trial.
- Assume that pain is present if the client is unable to provide a self-report and has tissue injury or a pathological condition or has undergone a procedure that is thought to produce pain.

P

• = Independent   ▲ = Collaborative

- Conduct an analgesic trial for clients who are unable to provide self-report and have underlying pathology/condition that is thought to be painful, or who demonstrate behaviors that may indicate pain is present. Administer a nonopioid if pain is thought to be mild and an opioid if pain is thought to be moderate to severe. Reassess the client to evaluate intervention effectiveness within a specific period of time based on pharmacokinetics (intravenous [IV] 15 to 30 minutes; subcutaneous 30 minutes; oral 60 minutes).
- Determine the client's current medication use.
- Explain to the client the pain management approach that has been ordered, including therapies, medication administration, side effects, and complications.
- Discuss the client's fears of undertreated pain, addiction, and overdose.
- Manage chronic pain using a multimodal approach.
- Recognize that the oral route is preferred for pain management interventions. If the client is receiving parenteral analgesia, use an equianalgesic chart to convert to an oral analgesic as soon as possible.
- Avoid giving pain medication intramuscularly (IM).
- Recognize that many clients with chronic pain have neuropathic pain. *(Please refer to assessment earlier.)* Treat neuropathic pain with adjuvant analgesics, such as anticonvulsants, antidepressants, and topical local anesthetics.
- Administer a nonopioid analgesic for mild to moderate chronic pain, such as osteoarthritis or cancer pain.
- Recognize that opioid therapy may be indicated for some clients experiencing chronic pain.
- Treat chronic pain in a comprehensive manner.
- Administer supplemental opioid doses for breakthrough pain as needed to keep pain ratings at or below the comfort-function goal.
- Assess pain level, sedation level, and respiratory status at regular intervals during opioid administration in the inpatient setting. Assess sedation and respiratory status every 1 to 2 hours during the first 24 hours of opioid therapy, then every 4 hours if respiratory status has been stable without episodes of hypoventilation, or more frequently as determined by

• = Independent ▲ = Collaborative

individualized client status. Conduct the respiratory assessment before sedation assessment by evaluating the depth, regularity, and noisiness of respiration and counting respiratory rate for 60 seconds. Awaken sleeping clients for assessment if the respiration is inadequate (e.g., if respirations are shallow, ineffective, irregular, or noisy [snoring], or periods of apnea occur). Snoring indicates respiratory obstruction and warrants prompt arousal, repositioning, and evaluation of respiratory risk factors. Discontinue titration or continuous opioid infusions immediately, and decrease subsequent opioid doses by 25% to 50% if the client develops excessive sedation.

- Ask the client to describe appetite, bowel elimination, and ability to rest and sleep. Administer medications and treatments to improve these functions. Obtain a prescription for a combination stool softener plus peristaltic stimulant to prevent opioid-induced constipation.
- Question the client about any disruption in sleep.
- Watch for signs of depression in the clients with chronic pain, including sleeplessness, not eating, flat affect, statements of depression, or suicidal ideation.
- Review the client's pain diary, flow sheet, and medication records to determine the overall degree of pain relief, side effects, and analgesic requirements for an appropriate period (e.g., 1 week).
- Obtain orders to increase or decrease opioid doses as needed; base analgesic and dose on the client's report of pain severity (clinical judgment of effectiveness if the client is unable to provide a self-report), response to the previous dose in terms of pain relief, occurrence of side effects, and ability to perform the activities of recovery or activities of daily living (ADLs).
- In addition to administering analgesics, support the client's use of nonpharmacological methods to help control pain, such as distraction, imagery, relaxation, and application of heat and cold.
- Teach and implement nonpharmacological interventions when pain is relatively well controlled with pharmacological interventions.
- Encourage the client to plan activities around periods of greatest comfort whenever possible. Pain impairs function.

P

● = Independent　　　　　　▲ = Collaborative

- Explore appropriate resources for management of pain on a long-term basis (e.g., hospice, pain care center).
- If the client has progressive cancer pain, assist the client and family with handling issues related to death and dying.

Pediatric

- Assess for the presence of pain using a valid and reliable pain scale based on age, cognitive development, and the child's ability to provide a self-report.
- Administer analgesics as prescribed.
- As with adults, use nonpharmacological interventions to supplement, not replace, pharmacological interventions.

Geriatric

- Always take an older client's report of pain seriously and ensure that the pain is relieved.
- When assessing pain, speak clearly, slowly, and loudly enough for the client to hear, and if the client uses a hearing aid, be sure it is in place; repeat information as needed. Be sure the client can see well enough to read the pain scale (use an enlarged scale) and written materials.
- Handle the client's body gently. Allow the client to move at his or her own speed.
- Use nonopioid analgesics for mild to moderate pain.
- Use opioids cautiously in the older client with moderate to severe pain. Initiate opioid therapy with a low dose, and carefully titrate the dose based on pain and sedation assessment. Titrate the dose using a short-acting opioid, and convert to a long-acting opioid as soon as possible for ongoing continuous pain.
- Avoid the use of meperidine (Demerol) in older clients.
- Use nonpharmacological approaches in addition to analgesics.
- Monitor for signs of depression in older clients and refer to specialists with relevant expertise.

Multicultural

- Assess for pain disparities among racial and ethnic minorities.
- Assess for the influence of cultural beliefs, norms, and values on the client's perception and experience of pain.

● = Independent   ▲ = Collaborative

- Assess for the effect of fatalism on the client's beliefs regarding the current state of comfort.
- Incorporate safe and effective folk health care practices and beliefs into care whenever possible.
- Use a family-centered approach to care.
- Teach information about pain medications and their side effects and how to work with health care providers to manage pain, and encourage use of religious faith as desired to cope with pain.
- Use culturally relevant pain scales to assess pain in the client.
- Ensure that directions for medication use are available in the client's language of choice and are understood by the client and caregiver.

Home Care

- Please refer to the care plan on **Acute Pain** for interventions on home care.

Client/Family Teaching and Discharge Planning

NOTE: To avoid the negative connotations associated with the words *drugs* and *narcotics*, use the term *pain medicine* when teaching clients and *opioids* when speaking with colleagues.

- Discuss the various discomforts encompassed by the word *pain* and ask the client to give examples of previously experienced pain. Explain the pain assessment process and the purpose of the pain rating scale.
- Teach the client to use the self-report pain tool to rate the intensity of past or current pain. Ask the client to set a comfort-function goal by selecting a pain level on the self-report tool that will allow performance of desired or necessary activities of daily living with relative ease (e.g., ambulation, self-care) or achieve acceptable quality of life. If the pain level is consistently above the comfort-function goal, the client should take action that decreases pain or notify a member of the health care team so that effective pain management interventions may be implemented promptly. (See information on teaching clients to use the pain rating scale.)
- Provide written materials on pain control that teach how to use a pain rating scale and how to take analgesics.

● = Independent   ▲ = Collaborative

- Discuss the total plan for pharmacological and nonpharmacological treatment, including the medication plan for ATC administration and supplemental doses, the maintenance of a pain diary, and the use of supplies and equipment. If PCA is ordered, determine the client's ability to press the appropriate button. Remind the client and staff that the PCA button is for client use only.
- Reinforce the importance of taking pain medications to maintain the comfort-function goal.
- Explain that some analgesics (e.g., anticonvulsants, antidepressants) must be titrated over an extended period of time to achieve satisfactory pain relief.
- Reinforce that taking opioids for pain relief is not addiction and that addiction is very unlikely to occur.
- Demonstrate the use of appropriate nonpharmacological approaches in addition to pharmacological approaches for helping to control pain, such as application of heat and/or cold, distraction techniques, relaxation breathing, visualization, rocking, stroking, music listening, and television watching. Teach these methods when pain is relatively well controlled, because pain interferes with cognition.
- Suggest the client with chronic pain try having a massage, with aromatherapy if desired.
- Emphasize to the client the importance of pacing activity and taking rest breaks before they are needed.
- Teach nonpharmacological methods when pain is relatively well controlled.

Impaired Parenting

NANDA-I Definition

Inability of the primary caretaker to create, maintain, or regain an environment that promotes the optimum growth and development of the child

Defining Characteristics

Infant/Child

Behavioral disorders; failure to thrive; frequent accidents; frequent illness; incidence of abuse; incidence of trauma (e.g., physical and

● = Independent ▲ = Collaborative

psychological); lack of attachment; lack of separation anxiety; poor academic performance; poor cognitive development; poor social competence; runaway

Parental
Abandonment; child abuse; child neglect; frequently punitive; hostility to child; inadequate attachment; inadequate child health maintenance; inappropriate caretaking skills; inappropriate child care arrangements; inappropriate stimulation (e.g., visual, tactile, auditory); inconsistent behavior management; inconsistent care; inflexibility in meeting needs of child; little cuddling; maternal-child interaction deficit; negative statements about child; paternal-child interaction deficit; rejection of child; reports frustration; reports inability to control child; reports role inadequacy; statements of inability to meet child's needs; unsafe home environment

Related Factors (r/t)
Infant/Child
Altered perceptual abilities; attention deficit hyperactivity disorder; developmental delay; difficult temperament; handicapping condition; illness; multiple births; not desired gender; premature birth; separation from parent; temperamental conflicts with parental expectations

Knowledge
Deficient knowledge about child development; deficient knowledge about child health maintenance; deficient knowledge about parenting skills; inability to respond to infant cues; lack of cognitive readiness for parenthood; lack of education; limited cognitive functioning; poor communication skills; preference for physical punishment; unrealistic expectations

Physiological
Physical illness

Psychological
Closely spaced pregnancies; depression; difficult birthing process; disability; disturbed sleep pattern; high number of pregnancies; history of mental illness; history of substance abuse; lack of prenatal care; sleep deprivation; young parental age

• = Independent   ▲ = Collaborative

Social

Change in family unit; chronic low self-esteem; economically disadvantaged; father of child not involved; financial difficulties; history of being abused; history of being abusive; inability to put child's needs before own; inadequate child care arrangements; job problems; lack of family cohesiveness; lack of parental role model; lack of resources; lack of social support networks; lack of transportation; lack of valuing of parenthood; legal difficulties; maladaptive coping strategies; marital conflict; mother of child not involved; poor home environment; poor parental role model; poor problem-solving skills; presence of stress (e.g., financial, legal, recent crisis, cultural move); relocations; role strain; single parent; situational low self-esteem; social isolation; unemployment; unplanned pregnancy; unwanted pregnancy

Client Outcomes

Client Will (Specify Time Frame):
- Initiate appropriate measures to develop a safe, nurturing environment
- Acquire and display attentive, supportive parenting behaviors and child supervision
- Identify appropriate strategies to manage a child's inappropriate behaviors
- Identify strategies to protect child from harm and/or neglect and initiate action when indicated

Nursing Interventions

- Use the Parenting Sense of Competence (PSOC) scale to measure parental self-efficacy.
- Examine the characteristics of parenting style and behaviors. Consider dysfunctional child-centered and parent-centered cognitions as potentially critical correlates of abusive behavior.
- ▲ Institute abuse/neglect protection measures if evidence exists of an inability to cope with family stressors or crisis, signs of parental substance abuse are observed, or a significant level of social isolation is apparent.
- ▲ For a mother with a toddler, assess maternal depression. Make appropriate referral.
- Appraise the parent's resources and the availability of social support systems. Determine the single mother's particular sources of support, especially the availability of her own

• = Independent ▲ = Collaborative

mother and partner. Encourage the use of healthy, strong support systems.
- Provide education to at-risk parents on behavioral management techniques such as looking ahead, giving good instructions, providing positive reinforcement, redirecting, planned ignoring, and instituting time-outs.
- Promotion of better-quality relationships between parents and children is an effective strategy that can lead to enhanced learning. Good-quality parenting leads to improved cognitive and social skills for the children.
- Support parents' competence in appraising their infant's behavior and responses.
- Aim supportive interventions at minimizing parents' experience of strain.
- Model age-appropriate and cognitively appropriate caregiver skills by doing the following: communicating with the child at an appropriate cognitive level of development, giving the child tasks and responsibilities appropriate to age or functional age/level, instituting safety considerations such as the use of assistive equipment, and encouraging the child to perform activities of daily living as appropriate. Encourage mothers to understand and capitalize on their infants' capacity to interact, particularly in the early months of life.
- ▲ Provide programs for homeless mothers with severe mental illness who have lost physical custody of their children.
- ▲ Provide a recovery program that includes instruction in parenting skills and child development for mothers who are addicted to cocaine.
- Refer to **Readiness for enhanced Parenting** for additional interventions.

Multicultural

- Acknowledge that value conflicts from acculturation stresses may contribute to increased anxiety and significant conflict with children.
- Approach individuals of color with respect, warmth, and professional courtesy
- Clarify parents' feelings, expectations, perceptions, and availability regarding participation in the care of their sick child.

• = Independent   ▲ = Collaborative

- Carefully assess meaning of terms used to describe health status when working with Native Americans.
- Provide support for Chinese families caring for children with disabilities.
- Facilitate modeling and role playing to help the family improve parenting skills.

Home Care

- The interventions previously described may be adapted for home care use.
- Assess parenting stress at each home visit to provide appropriate support and anticipatory guidance to families of children with a chronic disease.
▲ Assess the single mother's history regarding childhood and partner abuse and current status regarding depressive symptoms, abusive parenting attitudes (lack of empathy, favorable opinion of corporal punishment, parent-child role reversal, and inappropriate expectations). Refer for mental health services as indicated.
- Provide a parenting program of Planned Activities Training (PAT).
- Provide follow-up support for the PAT via cell phone and text messaging.

Client/Family Teaching and Discharge Planning

- Consider individual and/or group-based parenting programs for teenage mothers.
- Consider group-based parenting programs for parents of children younger than 3 years with emotional and behavioral problems.
- Consider group-based parenting programs for parents with anxiety, depression, and/or low self-esteem.
▲ Refer adolescent parents for comprehensive psychoeducational parenting classes.
- Parent training is one of the most effective interventions for behavior problems in young children.
- Encourage positive parenting: respect for children, understanding of normal development, and creative and loving

• = Independent   ▲ = Collaborative

approaches to meet parenting challenges rather than using anger, manipulation, punishment and rewards.

▲ Initiate referrals to community agencies, parent education programs, stress management training, and social support groups. Consider the use of technology and the media.

• Provide information regarding available telephone counseling services and Internet support.

• Refer to the care plans for **Delayed Growth and Development, Risk for impaired Attachment,** and **Readiness for enhanced Parenting** for additional teaching interventions.

Readiness for enhanced Parenting

NANDA-I Definition

A pattern of providing an environment for children or other dependent person(s) that is sufficient to nurture growth and development and can be strengthened

Defining Characteristics

Children report satisfaction with home environment; emotional support of children; emotional support of other dependent persons; evidence of attachment; exhibits realistic expectations of children; exhibits realistic expectations of other dependent person(s); expresses willingness to enhance parenting; needs of children are met (e.g., physical and emotional); needs of other dependent person(s) is/are met (e.g., physical and emotional); other dependent person(s) expresses(es) satisfaction with home environment

Client Outcomes

Client/Family Will (Specify Time Frame):

• Affirm desire to improve parenting skills to further support growth and development of children

• Demonstrate loving relationship with children

• Provide a safe, nurturing environment

• Assess risks in home/environment and takes steps to prevent possibility of harm to children

• Meet physical, psychosocial, and spiritual needs or seek appropriate assistance

• = Independent   ▲ = Collaborative

Nursing Interventions

- Use family-centered care and role modeling for holistic care of families.
- Assess parents' feelings when dealing with a child who has a chronic illness.
- Encourage positive parenting: respect for children, understanding of normal development, and use of creative and loving approaches to meet parenting challenges.
- Promote low-technology interventions, such as massage and multisensory interventions (maternal voice, eye-to-eye contact, and rocking) and music to reduce maternal and infant stress and improve mother-infant relationship.
- Support kangaroo care for infants at risk at birth; keep infants in an upright position in skin-to-skin contact.
- Provide the parent with the opportunity to assist in the newborn's first bath, allowing a flexible bath time.
- When the person who is ill is the parent, use family-centered assessment skills to determine the impact of an adult's illness on the child, and then guide the parent through those topics that are most likely to be of concern.
- Provide practical and psychological assistance for parents of clients with psychiatric diagnoses, such as schizophrenia.
- Refer to the care plan for **Impaired Parenting** for additional interventions.

Multicultural

- Assess the influence of cultural beliefs, norms, and values on the client's perception of parenting.
- Acknowledge racial and ethnic differences at the onset of care and provide appropriate health information and social support.
- Support programs for parents of young children in specific cultural communities.
- Clarify parents' feelings, expectations, perceptions, and availability regarding participation in the care of their sick child.
- Acknowledge and praise parenting strengths noted.

Home Care

- The nursing interventions previously described should be used in the home environment with adaptations as necessary.

• = Independent   ▲ = Collaborative

▲ Refer to a parenting program to facilitate learning of parenting skills.

Client/Family Teaching and Discharge Planning

- Refer to Client/Family Teaching and Discharge Planning for **Impaired Parenting** for suggestions that may be used with minor adaptations.
- Teach parents home safety: reduction of hot water temperature, proper poison storage, use of smoke alarms, and installation of safety gates for stairs.
- Teach parents and young teens conflict resolution by using a hypothetical conflict solution with and without a structured conflict resolution guide. Support self-direction of the families with minimal therapist intervention.
- Refer mothers of children with type 1 diabetes for community support in babysitting, child care, or respite.
- Teach families the importance of monitoring television viewing and limiting exposure to violence.
- Promotion of better-quality relationships between parents and children is an effective strategy that can lead to enhanced learning. Good-quality parenting leads to improved cognitive and social skills for the children.

P

Risk for impaired Parenting

NANDA-I Definition

At risk for inability of the primary caretaker to create, maintain, or regain an environment that promotes the optimum growth and development of the child

Risk Factors

Infant or Child

Altered perceptual abilities; attention deficit hyperactivity disorder; developmental delay; difficult temperament; handicapping condition; illness; multiple births; not gender desired; premature birth; prolonged separation from parent; temperamental conflicts with parental expectation

● = Independent   ▲ = Collaborative

Knowledge

Deficient knowledge about child development; deficient knowledge about child health maintenance; deficient knowledge about parenting skills; inability to respond to infant cues; lack of cognitive readiness for parenthood; low cognitive functioning; low educational level; poor communication skills; preference for physical punishment; unrealistic expectations of child

Physiological

Physical illness

Psychological

Closely spaced pregnancies; depression; difficult birthing process; disability; high number of pregnancies; history of mental illness; history of substance abuse; sleep deprivation; sleep disruption; young parental age

Social

Change in family unit; chronic low self-esteem; economically disadvantaged; father of child not involved; financial difficulties; history of being abused; history of being abusive; inadequate child care arrangements; job problems; lack of access to resources; lack of family cohesiveness; lack of parental role model; lack of prenatal care; lack of resources; lack of social support network; lack of transportation; lack of valuing of parenthood; late prenatal care; legal difficulties; maladaptive coping strategies; marital conflict; mother of child not involved; parent-child separation; poor home environment; poor parental role model; poor problem-solving skills; relocation; role strain; single parent; situational low self-esteem; social isolation; stress; unemployment; unplanned pregnancy; unwanted pregnancy

Client Outcomes, Nursing Interventions, Client/Family Teaching and Discharge Planning

Refer to care plans **Readiness for enhanced Parenting** and **Impaired Parenting**.

Risk for Perioperative Positioning Injury

NANDA-I Definition

At risk for inadvertent anatomical and physical changes as a result of positioning or equipment used during an invasive/surgical procedure

• = Independent   ▲ = Collaborative

Risk Factors

Disorientation; edema; emaciation; immobilization; muscle weakness; obesity; sensory/perceptual disturbances due to anesthesia. High pressure for short periods of time and low pressure for extended periods of time are risk factors for tissue injury.

Client Outcomes

Client Will (Specify Time Frame):

- Demonstrate unchanged skin condition, with exception of the incision, throughout the perioperative experience
- Demonstrate resolution of redness of the skin at points of pressure within 30 minutes after pressure is eliminated
- Remain injury-free related to surgical positioning, including intact skin and absence of pain and/or numbness associated with surgical positioning
- Demonstrate unchanged or improved physical mobility from preoperative status
- Demonstrate unchanged or improved peripheral sensory integrity from preoperative status
- Maintain sense of privacy and dignity

Nursing Interventions

General Interventions for Any Surgical Client

- Recognize that there is a new accountability for perioperative nurses in the need to maintain skin integrity.

Prevention of Pressure Ulcers

- Complete a preoperative assessment to identify physical alterations that may require additional precautions for procedure-specific positioning, to identify specific procedural positioning needs, type of anesthesia, etc.
- Identify risk factors such as length and type of surgery, potential for intraoperative hypotensive episodes, low core temperatures, and decreased mobility on postoperative day 1.
- Recognize that all surgical clients should be considered at high risk for pressure ulcer development, as pressure ulcers can develop in as little as 20 minutes in the operating room.

● = Independent   ▲ = Collaborative

- Recognize that clients undergoing cardiac surgical procedures are at increased risk of developing a pressure ulcer, especially below the waist or in the occiput area.
- Protect the heels during surgery by elevating the heels completely.
- Use pressure-reducing devices and pressure-relieving mattresses as necessary to prevent ulcer formation.
- Use gel pads to provide protection against shearing and friction of superficial tissues.
- Avoid using rolled sheets and towels as positioning devices, as they tend to produce high and inconsistent pressures. Special positioning devices are available for use that redistribute pressure.
- Avoid covering positioning devices or placing extra blankets on top of a pressure-reducing surface.
- Recognize that the nurse must demonstrate knowledge not only of the equipment, but also of anatomy and the application of physiological principles in order to properly position the client.
- Monitor pressure being applied to the client intraoperatively by staff, equipment, and/or instruments.
- Pad all bony prominences.
- Recognize that reddened areas or areas injured by pressure should not be massaged.
- Implement measures to prevent inadvertent hypothermia.
- Utilize pressure-relieving devices for the preoperative and postoperative stretcher.

Positioning the Perioperative Client

- Ensure that linens on the OR table are free of wrinkles.
- Lock the OR table, cart, or bed and stabilize the mattress before transfer/positioning of the client. Monitor the client while on the OR table at all times.
- Lift rather than pull or slide the client when positioning to reduce the incidence of skin injury from shearing and/or friction.
- Ensure that appropriate numbers of personnel are present to assist in positioning the client.
- Recognize that optimally, clients (especially those with limited range of motion/mobility) should be asked to position themselves under the nurse's guidance before induction of anesthesia so that he or she can verify that a position of comfort has been obtained.

• = Independent   ▲ = Collaborative

- Ensure that nerves are protected by positioning extremities carefully.
- Use slow and smooth movements during positioning to allow the circulatory system to readjust.
- Place a pillow under the back of the knees to relieve lower back pressure.
- Reassess the client after positioning and periodically during the procedure for maintenance of proper alignment and skin integrity.
- Frequently assess the eyes and/or monitor intraocular pressure, especially when client is in prone or knee-chest position, when the client is experiencing significant blood loss, or when the procedure lasts 6½ hours or longer.
- Position hips in proper alignment with knees flexed. Unaligned hips can cause pressure to the low back and hip joints.
- Position the arms extended on armboards so that they do not extend beyond a 90-degree angle. Do not position arms at sides unless surgically necessary.
- Prevent pooling of preparative solutions, blood, irrigation, urine, and feces.
- Keep the client appropriately covered during the procedure.
- When positioning the client prone, care should be taken to ensure the head and neck are properly positioned.
- Recognize that clients positioned in lithotomy position should be kept in this position for as short a time as possible.
- The lowest heel position should be used in the lithotomy position.
- Position the client's legs parallel and uncrossed.
- Maintain normal body alignment.
- When applying body supports and restraint straps (safety belt), apply loosely and secure over waist or mid-thigh at least 2 inches above knees, avoiding bony prominences by placing a blanket between the strap and the client.
- Check equipment to verify it is in good working order and is used according to manufacturer's instructions.
- Assess the client's skin integrity immediately postoperatively.
- Remove client jewelry before surgery because it can cause pressure injury, become entangled in bedding, or catch on equipment during transfer and cause injury
- Recognize that complete, concise, accurate documentation of client assessment and use of positioning devices is imperative.

P

• = Independent   ▲ = Collaborative

Risk for Peripheral Neurovascular Dysfunction

NANDA-I Definition

At risk for disruption in circulation, sensation, or motion of an extremity

Risk Factors

Burns; fractures; immobilization; mechanical compression (e.g., tourniquet, cane, cast, brace, dressing, restraint); orthopedic surgery; trauma; vascular obstruction

Client Outcomes

Client Will (Specify Time Frame):

- Maintain circulation, sensation, and movement of an extremity within client's own normal limits
- Explain signs of neurovascular compromise and ways to prevent venous stasis
- Explain and demonstrate low molecular weight heparin or fondaparinux injections which would be expected to be ordered in orthopedic cases and other high-risk conditions unless contraindicated. These injections may be ordered to continue at home after discharge.

Nursing Interventions

▲ Perform neurovascular assessment every 15 minutes to every 4 hours as ordered or needed based on client's condition. Use the six P's of assessment as outlined below.

- **Pain:** Assess severity (on a scale of 1 to 10), quality, radiation, and relief by medications.
- **Pulses:** Check the pulses distal to the injury.
- **Pallor/Poikilothermia:** Check color and temperature changes below the injury site. Check capillary refill.
- **Paresthesia** (change in sensation): Check by lightly touching the skin proximal and distal to the injury. Ask if the client has any unusual sensations such as hypersensitivity, tingling, prickling, decreased feeling, or numbness. Check nerve function (e.g., can the client feel a touch to the area of concern, such as the first web space of the foot [deep peroneal nerve] with tibial fracture).

• = Independent   ▲ = Collaborative

- **Paralysis:** Ask the client to perform appropriate range-of-motion exercises in the unaffected and then the affected extremity.
- **Pressure:** Check by feeling the extremity; note new onset of firmness or swelling of the extremity.
▲ Monitor the client for symptoms of compartment syndrome evidenced by pain greater than expected, pain with passive movement, decreased sensation, weakness, loss of movement, absence of pulse, and tension in the skin that surrounds the muscle compartment.
• Monitor appropriate application and function of corrective device (e.g., cast, splint, traction) every 1 to 4 hours as needed.
• Position the extremity in correct alignment with each position change; check every hour to ensure appropriate alignment.

Prevention of Deep Vein Thrombosis (DVT), Pulmonary Embolism (PE)

Prevention of fatal pulmonary embolism is top priority for prophylaxis programs, as is the prevention of symptomatic DVT, PE, and postphlebitis syndrome.
▲ Get the client out of bed as early possible and ambulate frequently after consultation with the physician.
▲ Monitor for signs of DVT, especially in high-risk populations, including clients of increasing age; clients with immobility or obesity; clients taking estrogen or oral contraceptives; pregnancy and the postpartum period; inherited or acquired thrombophilia (e.g., factor V Leiden); persons with a history of trauma, surgery, or previous DVT; and persons with a cerebrovascular accident, varicose veins, malignancy, or cardiovascular disease.
• Recognize that mechanical methods for DVT prophylaxis, such as graduated compression stockings (GCS), the use of intermittent pneumatic compression (IPC) devices, and the venous foot pump (VFP), increase venous outflow and/or reduce stasis within the leg veins.
▲ Apply graduated compression stockings if ordered; measure carefully to ensure proper fit, removing at least daily to assess circulation and skin condition.
▲ Apply IPC device if ordered.

▲ Watch for and report signs of DVT as evidenced by pain, deep tenderness, swelling in the calf and thigh, and redness in the involved extremity. Take serial leg measurements of the thigh and leg circumferences. In some clients, a tender venous cord can be felt in the popliteal fossa. Do not rely on Homans' sign.

- Help the client perform prescribed exercises every 4 hours as ordered.
- Provide a nutritious diet and adequate fluid replacement.

Geriatric

- Use heat and cold therapies cautiously.
- Recognize that older clients have an increased risk of developing DVTs.

Home Care

- Assess the knowledge base of the client and family after hospitalization.
- Teach about the disease process and care as necessary.
- If risk is related to fractures and cast care, teach the family to complete a neurovascular assessment; it may be performed as often as every 4 hours but is more commonly done two or three times per day.
- If the fracture is peripheral, position the limb for comfort and change position frequently, avoiding dependent positions for extended periods.

▲ Refer to physical therapy services as necessary to establish an exercise program and safety in transfers or mobility within limitations of physical status.

- Establish an emergency plan.

Client/Family Teaching and Discharge Planning

- Teach the client and family to recognize signs of neurovascular dysfunction and report signs immediately to the appropriate person.
- Teach the client and family to recognize side effects of anticoagulant such as irritation, pain, tenderness, and redness that may occur at the site of injection.
- Teach the client and family to notify the doctor if the client experiences increased bruising, bleeding, or black stools.

• = Independent   ▲ = Collaborative

- Emphasize proper nutrition to promote healing.
▲ If necessary, refer the client to a rehabilitation facility for instruction in proper use of assistive devices and measures to improve mobility without compromising neurovascular function.
- See **Ineffective peripheral Tissue Perfusion** (venous insufficiency) for further interventions to prevent DVT.

Risk for Poisoning

NANDA-I Definition

Accentuated risk of accidental exposure to, or ingestion of, drugs or dangerous products in doses sufficient to cause poisoning

Risk Factors

External

Availability of illicit drugs potentially contaminated by poisonous additives; dangerous products placed within reach of children; dangerous products placed within reach of confused individuals or children; large supplies of drugs in house; medicines stored in unlocked cabinets; medicines stored in unlocked cabinets accessible to confused individuals or children; medications not maintained in original containers; breastfeeding mothers who are drug addicted; use of over-the-counter cold and cough medication for children

Internal

Cognitive difficulties; emotional difficulties; lack of drug education; lack of proper precaution; lack of safety education; reduced vision; verbalization that occupational setting is without adequate safeguards

Client Outcomes

Client Will (Specify Time Frame):

- Prevent inadvertent ingestion of or exposure to toxins or poisonous substances
- Explain and undertake appropriate safety measures to prevent ingestion of or exposure to toxins or poisonous substances
- Verbalize appropriate response to apparent or suspected toxic ingestion or poisoning

● = Independent   ▲ = Collaborative

Nursing Interventions

- When a client comes to the hospital with possible poisoning, begin care following the ABCs and administer oxygen if needed.
- ▲ It is important for the triage nurse to call the poison control center.
- Obtain a thorough history of what was ingested, how much, and when, and ask to look at the container. Note the client's age, weight, medications, any medical conditions, and any history of vomiting, choking, coughing, or change in mental status. Also take note of any interventions performed before seeking treatment.
- Carefully inspect for signs of ingestion of poisons, including an odor on the breath, a trace of the substance on the clothing, burns, or redness around the mouth and lips, as well as signs of confusion, vomiting, or dyspnea.
- ▲ Note results of toxicology screens, arterial blood gases, blood glucose levels, and any other ordered laboratory tests.
- ▲ Initiate any ordered treatment for poisoning quickly.

Safety Guidelines for Medication Administration

- Prevent iatrogenic harm to the hospitalized client by following these guidelines for administering medications:
  - Use at least two methods to identify the client before administering medications or blood products, such as the client's name and medical record number or birth date. Do not use the client's room number.
  - When taking verbal or telephone orders, the orders should be written down and then read back for verification to the individual giving the order. The person who gave the orders for the medication then needs to confirm the information that was read back.
  - Standardize use of abbreviations, acronyms, symbols, and dose designations and eliminate those that are prone to cause errors. (Please refer to The Joint Commission, Critical Access Hospital National Patient Safety goals for list of abbreviations, acronyms, symbols and dose designations that should not be used.)

P

• = Independent   ▲ = Collaborative

- Be aware of the medications that look/sound alike and ensure that the correct medication is ordered.
- Take high-alert medications off the nursing unit, such as potassium chloride. Standardize concentrations of medications such as morphine in PCA pumps.
- Label all medications and medication containers or other solutions that are on or off a sterile field for a procedure. Label them when they are first taken out of the original packaging to another container. Label with medication name, strength, amount, and expiration date/time. Review the labels whenever there is a change of personnel.
- Use only IV pumps that prevent free flow of IV solution when the tubing is taken out of the pump.
- Identify all the client's current medications on admission to a health care facility and compare the list with the current ordered medications. Reconcile any differences in medications. Reconcile the list of medications if the client is transferred from one unit to another, when there is a handoff to the next provider of care, and when the client is discharged
▲ Detect possible interactions and cumulative or other adverse effects among prescribed medications, self-administered over-the-counter products, culturally based home treatments, herbal remedies, and foods.

Pediatric

▲ Evaluate lead exposure risk and consult the health care provider regarding lead screening measures as indicated (public/ambulatory health).
- Provide guidance for parents and caregivers regarding age-related safety measures, including the following:
  - Store prescription and over-the-counter medications, vitamins, herbs, and alcohol in a locked cabinet far from children's reach.
  - Do not take medications in front of children.
  - Store cleaning products including things like dishwashing liquids in a high cabinet, out of children's reach.
  - Use safety latches on cabinets that contain poisonous substances.

• = Independent   ▲ = Collaborative

- Store potentially harmful substances in the original containers with safety closures intact.
- Recognize that no container is completely childproof.
- Do not store medications or toxic substances in food containers.
- Do not leave alcoholic drinks, cosmetics, or toiletries where children can reach them.
- Remove poisonous houseplants from the home. Teach children not to put leaves or berries in their mouths.
- Do not suggest that medications are candy.
- If interrupted when using a harmful product, take it with you; children can get into it within seconds.
- Store poisonous automotive or gardening supplies in a locked area.
- Use extreme caution with pesticides and gardening materials close to children's play areas.
- When visitors enter the home, place their handbags or backpacks up high where children are unable to reach them, and obtain poisonous substances.

▲ Advise families that syrup of ipecac is no longer recommended to be kept and used in the home. Vomiting should not be induced following poisoning in the home.

▲ Advise families that over-the-counter cough and cold suppressant medications are not recommended and are no longer considered safe for young children 4 or younger.

• Recognize that some children may have been exposed to methamphetamines or the components used to make methamphetamines.

Geriatric

• Caution the client and family to avoid storing medications with similar appearances close to one another (e.g., nitroglycerin ointment near toothpaste or denture creams).

• Remind the older client to store medications out of reach when young children come to visit.

• Perform medication reconciliation on all elderly clients entering the health care system as well as on discharge.

• = Independent   ▲ = Collaborative

Home Care

- The interventions previously described may be adapted for home care use.
- Provide the client and/or family with a poison control poster to be kept on the refrigerator or a bulletin board. Ensure that the telephone number for local poison control information is readily available.
- Pre-pour medications for a client who is at risk of ingesting too much of a given medication because of mistakes in preparation. Delegate this task to the family or caregivers if possible.
- Identify poisonous substances in the immediate surroundings of the home, such as a garage or barn, including paints and thinners, fertilizers, rodent and bug control substances, animal medications, gasoline, and oil. Label with the name, a poison warning sign, and a poison control center number. Lock out of the reach of children.
- Identify the risk of toxicity from environmental activities such as spraying trees or roadside shrubs. Contact local departments of agriculture or transportation to obtain material safety data sheets or to prevent the activity in desired areas.
- To prevent carbon monoxide poisoning, instruct the client and family in the importance of using a carbon monoxide detector in the home, having the chimney professionally cleaned each year, having the furnace professionally inspected each year, ensuring that all combustion equipment is properly vented, and installing a chimney screen and cap to prevent small animals from moving into the chimney.

Multicultural

- Assess housing for pathways of lead poisoning.
- Prompt caregivers to take action to prevent lead poisoning.
  - If children live in a high-lead environment, teach the need for handwashing before each meal, annual blood testing for lead levels, and avoidance of high lead areas as possible.
- Work with immigrant Mexican families to implement medication, household cleaners, and carbon monoxide safety interventions in the home to prevent accidental poisoning in children. Use the Hispanic social network.

● = Independent   ▲ = Collaborative

Client/Family Teaching and Discharge Planning

- Teach parents that poison is any substance that is harmful when it enters the body through ingestion, inhalation, injection, or absorption through the skin or mucous membranes. The list of possible poisons is long, including laundry detergent, floor cleaners, antifreeze, fuel, silica gel, and glow-in-the-dark products; drugs; and venom from spider and snake bites.
- Counsel the client and family members regarding the following points of medication safety:
  - Avoid sharing prescriptions.
  - Always use good light when preparing medication. Do not dispense medication during the night without a light on.
  - Read the label before you open the bottle, after you remove a dose, and again before you give it.
  - Always use child-resistant caps and lock all medications away from your child or confused elder.
  - Give the correct dose. *Never* guess.
  - Do not increase or decrease the dose without calling the physician.
  - Always follow the weight and age recommendations on the label.
  - Avoid making conversions. If the label calls for 2 tsp and you have a dosing cup labeled only with ounces, do not use it.
  - Be sure the physician knows if you are taking more than one medication at a time.
  - Never let young children take medication by themselves.
  - Read and follow labeling instructions on all products; adjust dosage for age.
  - Avoid excessive amounts and/or frequency of doses. ("If a little does some good, a lot should do more.")
- Advise the family to post first-aid charts and poison control center instructions in an accessible location. Poison control center telephone numbers should be posted close to each telephone and the number programmed into cell phones.
- Advise family when calling the poison control center to do the following:
  - Give as much information as possible, including your name, location, and telephone number, so that the poison control

operator can call back in case you are disconnected or summon help if needed.

- Give the name of the potential poison ingested and, if possible, the amount and time of ingestion. If the bottle or package is available, give the trade name and ingredients if they are listed.
- Be prepared to tell the person the child's height, weight, and age.
- Describe the state of the poisoning victim. Is the victim conscious? Does he or she have any symptoms? What is the person's general appearance, skin color, respiration, breathing difficulties, mental status (alert, sleepy, unusual behavior)? Is the person vomiting? Having convulsions?
- Encourage the client and family to take first-aid and other types of safety-related programs.
▲ Initiate referrals to peer group interventions, peer counseling, and other types of substance abuse prevention/rehabilitation programs when substance abuse is identified as a risk factor.
- Teach parents and other caregivers that cough and cold medication bought over-the-counter are not safe for a child under 2 unless specifically ordered by a health care provider.
- Teach parents that bring in a child to ER for possible or actual poisoning, methods to prevent poisoning of the child in the future.
- Teach parents that if a parent is employed in a lead-related occupation, lead contamination as a dust can be transported to the home via worksite clothing, shoes, tools, or vehicles. The dust must be kept away from children.

Post-Trauma Syndrome

NANDA-I Definition

Sustained maladaptive response to a traumatic, overwhelming event

Defining Characteristics

Aggression; alienation; altered mood state; anger; anxiety; avoidance; compulsive behavior; denial; depression; detachment; difficulty concentrating; enuresis (in children); exaggerated startle response; fear; flashbacks;

• = Independent   ▲ = Collaborative

gastric irritability; grieving; guilt; headaches; hopelessness; horror; hypervigilance; intrusive dreams; intrusive thoughts; irritability; neurosensory irritability; nightmares; palpitations; panic attacks; psychogenic amnesia; rage; rape; reports feeling numb; repression; shame; substance abuse

Related Factors (r/t)

Being held prisoner of war; criminal victimization; disasters; epidemics; events outside the range of usual human experience; physical abuse; psychological abuse; serious accidents (e.g., industrial, motor vehicle); serious injury to loved ones; serious injury to self; serious threat to loved ones; serious threat to self; sudden destruction of one's community; sudden destruction of one's home; torture; tragic occurrence involving multiple deaths; war witnessing mutilation; witnessing violent death

Client Outcomes

Client Will (Specify Time Frame):

- Return to pre-trauma level of functioning as quickly as possible.
- Acknowledge traumatic event and begin to work with the trauma by talking about the experience and expressing feelings of fear, anger, anxiety, guilt, and helplessness.
- Identify support systems and available resources and be able to connect with them.
- Return to and strengthen coping mechanisms used in previous traumatic event.
- Acknowledge event and perceive it without distortions.
- Assimilate event and move forward to set and pursue life goals.

Nursing Interventions

- Observe for a reaction to a traumatic event in all clients regardless of age or sex.
- After a traumatic event assess for intrusive memories, avoidance and numbing, and hyperarousal.
- Remain with the client and provide support during periods of overwhelming emotions.
- Help the individual try to comprehend the trauma if possible.
- Use touch with the client's permission (e.g., a hand on the shoulder, holding a hand).
- Explore and enhance available support systems.
- Help the client regain previous sleeping and eating habits.

• = Independent ▲ = Collaborative

▲ Provide the client pain medication if he or she has physical pain.

▲ Assess the need for pharmacotherapy.

▲ Refer for appropriate psychotherapy: cognitive therapy, exposure therapy, eye movement desensitization and reprocessing (EMDR), cognitive-behavioral therapy.

• Help the client use positive cognitive restructuring to reestablish feelings of self-worth

• Provide the means for the client to express feelings through therapeutic drawing.

• Encourage the client to return to the normal routine as quickly as possible.

• Talk to and assess the client's social support after a traumatic event.

Pediatric

• Refer to nursing care plan **Risk for Post-Trauma Syndrome.**

▲ Carefully assess children exposed to disasters and trauma. Note behavior specific to developmental age. Refer for therapy as needed.

Geriatric

• Carefully screen elderly for signs of PTSD, especially after a disaster.

• Consider using the Horwitz Impact of Event Scale, an appropriate instrument to measure the subjective response to stress in the senior population

▲ Monitor the client for clinical signs of depression and anxiety; refer to a physician for medication if appropriate.

• Instill hope.

Multicultural

• Assess the influence of cultural beliefs, norms, and values on the client's ability to cope with a traumatic experience.

• Acknowledge racial and ethnic differences at the onset of care.

▲ Carefully assess refugees for PTSD and refer for treatment as appropriate; encourage them to learn the language of their new residence.

• Use a family-centered approach when working with Latino, Asian, African American, and Native American clients.

• = Independent   ▲ = Collaborative

- When working with Asian American clients, provide opportunities by which the family can save face.
- Incorporate cultural traditions as appropriate.

Home Care

▲ Assess family support and the response to the client's coping mechanisms. Refer the family for medical social services or other counseling as necessary.
- Assess the impact of the trauma on significant others (e.g., a father may have to take over his partner's parenting responsibility after she has been raped and injured). Provide empathy and caring to significant others. Refer for additional services as necessary.

Client/Family Teaching and Discharge Planning

- Teach positive coping skills and avoidance of negative coping skills.
- Teach stress reduction methods such as deep breathing, visualization, meditation, and physical exercise. Encourage their use especially when intrusive thoughts or flashbacks occur
- Encourage other healthy living habits of proper diet, adequate sleep, regular exercise, family activities, and spiritual pursuits.
- Refer the client to peer support groups.
- Consider the use of complementary and alternative therapies.

Risk for Post-Trauma Syndrome

NANDA-I Definition

At risk for sustained maladaptive response to a traumatic, overwhelming event

Risk Factors

Diminished ego strength; displacement from home; duration of event; exaggerated sense of responsibility; inadequate social support; occupation (e.g., police, fire, rescue, corrections, emergency room staff, mental health worker); perception of event; survivor's role in the event; unsupportive environment

● = Independent   ▲ = Collaborative

Client Outcomes

Client Will (Specify Time Frame):

- Identify symptoms associated with PTSD and seek help
- Acknowledge event and perceive it without distortions
- Identify support systems and available resources and be able to connect with them
- State that he or she is not to blame for the event

Nursing Interventions

- Assess for PTSD in a client who has chronic/critical illness, anxiety, or personality disorder; was a witness to serious injury or death; or experienced sexual molestation.
- Consider the use of a self-reported screening questionnaire.
- Assess for ongoing symptoms of dissociation, avoidant behavior, hypervigilance, and reexperiencing.
- Assess for past experiences with traumatic events.
- Consider screening for PTSD in a client who is a high user of medical care.
- ▲ Provide deployed combat veterans with previous history of low mental or physical health status before deployment with appropriate referral after deployment.
- Provide peer support to contact co-workers experiencing trauma to remind them that others in the organization are concerned about their welfare.
- Consider implementation of a school-based program for children to decrease PTSD after catastrophic events.

Geriatric and Multicultural

- Refer to the care plan for **Post-Trauma Syndrome.**

Home Care

- ▲ Evaluate the client's response to a traumatic event. If screening warrants, refer to a therapist for counseling/treatment.
- Refer to the care plan for **Post-Trauma Syndrome.**

Client/Family Teaching and Discharge Planning

- Instruct family and friends to use the following critical incident stress management techniques:
  - Listen carefully; Spend time with the traumatized person; Offer your assistance and a listening ear, even if the person

• = Independent ▲ = Collaborative

has not asked for help; Help the person with everyday
tasks such as cleaning, cooking, caring for the family, and
minding children; Give the person some private time; Do
not take the individual's anger or other feelings personally,
and do not tell the person that he or she is "lucky it wasn't
worse"; such statements do not console traumatized people.
Instead, tell the person that you are sorry such an event has
occurred and you want to understand and assist him or her.

▲ After exposure to trauma teach the client and family to recognize symptoms of PTSD and seek treatment for "recurrent
and intrusive distressing recollections of the traumatic event,"
insomnia, irritability, difficulty concentrating, hypervigilance.

• Provide education to explain that acute stress disorder symptoms
are normal when preparing combatants for their role in deployment. Instruct clients to seek help if the symptoms persist.

• Provide post-trauma debriefings. Effective post-trauma coping skills are taught, and each participant creates a plan for his
or her recovery. During the debriefing, the facilitators assess
participants to determine their needs for further services in the
form of post-trauma counseling. For maximal effectiveness, the
debriefing should occur within 2 to 5 days of the incident.

• Provide post-trauma counseling. Counseling sessions are
extensions of debriefings and include continued discussion of
the traumatic event and post-trauma consequences and the
further development of coping skills.

• Consider exposure therapy for civilian trauma survivors following a nonsexual assault or motor vehicle crash.

Things to Try: Critical Incident Stress Debriefing

• Instruct the client to use the following critical incident stress
management techniques:

■ Within the first 24 to 48 hours, engaging in periods of
appropriate physical exercise alternated with relaxation to
alleviate some of the physical reactions; Structure your time;
keep busy; You are normal and are having normal reactions;
do not label yourself as "crazy"; Talk to people; talk is the
most healing medicine; Be aware of numbing the pain with
overuse of drugs or alcohol; you do not need to complicate
the stress with a substance abuse problem; Reach out; people

do care; Maintain as normal a schedule as possible; Spend time with others; Help your co-workers as much as possible by sharing feelings and checking out how they are doing; Give yourself permission to feel rotten and share your feelings with others; Keep a journal; write your way through those sleepless hours; Do things that feel good to you; Realize that those around you are under stress; Do not make any big life changes; Do make as many daily decisions as possible to give you a feeling of control over your life (e.g., if someone asks you what you want to eat, answer the person even if you are not sure); Get plenty of rest; Recurring thoughts, dreams, or flashbacks are normal; do not try to fight them because they will decrease over time and become less painful; Eat well-balanced and regular meals (even if you do not feel like it).

▲ Assess for a history of life-threatening illness such as cancer and provide appropriate counseling. The physical and psychological impact of having a life-threatening disease, undergoing cancer treatment, and living with recurring threats to physical integrity and autonomy constitute traumatic experiences for many cancer clients.

Pediatric

* Children with cancer should continue to be assessed for PTSD into adulthood.
* Provide protection for a child who has witnessed violence or who has had traumatic injuries. Help the child acknowledge the event and express grief over the event.
* Assess for a medical history of anxiety disorders.
▲ Assess children of deployed parents for PTSD and provide appropriate referrals.
* Consider implementation of a school-based program for children to decrease PTSD after catastrophic events.

Geriatric and Multicultural

* Refer to the care plan for **Post-Trauma Syndrome.**

Home Care

▲ Evaluate the client's response to a traumatic or critical event. If screening warrants, refer to a therapist for counseling/treatment.

● = Independent   ▲ = Collaborative

- Refer to the care plan for **Post-Trauma Syndrome.**

Client/Family Teaching and Discharge Planning

- Instruct family and friends to use the following critical incident stress management techniques:
  - Listen carefully; Spend time with the traumatized person; Offer your assistance and a listening ear, even if the person has not asked for help; Help the person with everyday tasks such as cleaning, cooking, caring for the family, and minding children; Give the person some private time; Do not take the individual's anger or other feelings personally, and do not tell the person that he or she is "lucky it wasn't worse"; such statements do not console traumatized people. Instead, tell the person that you are sorry such an event has occurred and you want to understand and assist him or her.
- ▲ After exposure to trauma teach the client and family to recognize symptoms of PTSD and seek treatment for "recurrent and intrusive distressing recollections of the traumatic event," insomnia, irritability, difficulty concentrating, hypervigilance.
- Provide education to explain that acute stress disorder symptoms are normal when preparing combatants for their role in deployment. Instruct clients to seek help if the symptoms persist.

Readiness for enhanced Power

NANDA-I Definition

A pattern of participating knowingly in change that is sufficient for well-being and can be strengthened

Defining Characteristics

Expresses readiness to enhance awareness of possible changes to be made; expresses readiness to enhance freedom to perform actions for change; expresses readiness to enhance identification of choices that can be made for change; expresses readiness to enhance involvement in creating change; expresses readiness to enhance knowledge for participation in change; expresses readiness to enhance participation in choices

• = Independent ▲ = Collaborative

for daily living; expresses readiness to enhance participation in choices for health; expresses readiness to enhance power

Client Outcomes

Client Will (Specify Time Frame):
- Describe power resources
- Identify realistic perceptions of control
- Develop a plan of action based on power resources
- Seek assistance as needed

Nursing Interventions

- Develop partnerships for shared power.
- Focus on the positive aspects of power, rather than prevention of powerlessness.
- Listen with intent.
- Collaborate with the person to identify resources to put a plan into action.
- Assess the meaning of the event to the person.
- Identify the client's health literacy in decision-making.
- Facilitate trust in self and others.
- Help client to mobilize social supports, a power resource.
- Support beliefs of power and perceptions of behavioral control.
- Promote the client's optimum level of physical functioning.
- Reframe professional image, role, and values to incorporate a vision of clients as the experts in their own care.

Home Care

- The preceding interventions may be adapted for home care use.

Client/Family Teaching and Discharge Planning

- Assess motivation to learn specific content.

Powerlessness

NANDA-I Definition

The lived experience of lack of control over a situation, including a perception that one's actions do not significantly affect an outcome

• = Independent   ▲ = Collaborative

Defining Characteristics

Dependence on others; depression over physical deterioration; non-participation in care; reports alienation; reports doubt regarding role performance; reports frustration over inability to perform previous activities; reports lack of control; reports shame

Related Factors (r/t)

Illness-related regimen; institutional environment; unsatisfying interpersonal interactions

Client Outcomes

Client Will (Specify Time Frame):

- State feelings of powerlessness and other feelings related to powerlessness (e.g., anger, sadness, hopelessness)
- Identify factors that are uncontrollable
- Participate in planning and implementing care; make decisions regarding care and treatment when possible
- Ask questions about care and treatment
- Verbalize hope for the future and sense of participation in planning and implementing care

Nursing Interventions

NOTE: Before implementation of interventions in the face of client powerlessness, nurses should examine their own philosophies of care to ensure that control issues or lack of faith in client capabilities will not bias the ability to intervene sincerely and effectively.

- Observe for factors contributing to powerlessness (e.g., immobility, hospitalization, unfavorable prognosis, lack of support system, misinformation about situation, inflexible routine, chronic illness). Help clients channel their behaviors in an effective manner.
- Assess the client's locus of control related to his or her health.
- Establish a therapeutic relationship with the client by spending one-on-one time with him or her, assigning the same caregiver, keeping commitments (e.g., saying, "I will be back to answer your questions in the next hour"), providing encouragement and support, and being empathetic.

• = Independent   ▲ = Collaborative

- Encourage the client to share his or her beliefs, thoughts, and expectations about his or her illness.
- Help the client assist in planning care and specify the health goals he or she would like to achieve, prioritizing those goals with regard to immediate concerns and identifying actions that will achieve the goals. Goals may need to be small to be attainable (e.g., dangle legs at bedside for 2 days, then sit in chair 10 minutes for 2 days, then walk to window).
- Encourage the client in goal-directed activities that promote a sense of accomplishment, especially regular exercise.
- Recognize the client's need to experience a sense of reciprocity in dealing with others. Negotiate actions that the client can contribute to the caregiving partnership with both family and nurse (e.g., have the client prepare a cup of tea for the nurse during visits if the client is able.)
- Allow time for questions (15 to 20 minutes each shift). Have the client write down questions, and encourage the client to record a summary of answers received, or provide written material that reinforces answers.
- Encourage the client to take control of as many ADLs as possible; keep the client informed of all care that will be given. Keep items the client uses and needs within reach (e.g., a urinal, tissues, telephone, and television controls).
- Give realistic and sincere praise for accomplishments.
- Consider using one of the measures of powerlessness that are available for general and specific client groups:
  - Measure of Powerlessness for Adult Patients
  - Spreitzer's Psychological Empowerment Questionnaire
  - Personal Progress Scale— Revised, tested with women
  - Life Situation Questionnaire—Powerlessness subscale, tested with stroke caregivers
  - Making Decisions Scale, tested in clients with mental illness
- Refer to the care plans for **Hopelessness** and **Spiritual Distress.**

Pediatric

- Two key issues that lead to powerlessness for children and their families are hospitalization and peer victimization or bullying.

- Encourage emotional expression through processes that are appropriate to the child's level of development.
- Recognize that a sense of powerlessness can prevent children and adolescents from reporting peer victimization. Be supportive, encourage disclosure without pressure, and help the child or adolescent problem solve options to deal with their stressors.
- Provide instruction and visual aids to family members so they may better understand a child's illness and how the family members can help.

Geriatric

- In addition to the preceding interventions as appropriate:
  - Initiate focused assessment questioning and education of client and caregivers regarding syndromes common in the elderly, including dementia.
  - Assess for the presence of elder abuse. Initiate referral to Adult Protective Services and help client regain a sense of safety and control.

Multicultural

- In addition to the preceding interventions as appropriate:
  - Assess the influence of cultural beliefs, norms, and values on the client's feelings of powerlessness

Home Care

- In addition to the preceding interventions as appropriate:
  - Develop a therapeutic relationship in the home setting that respects the client's domain.
  - Empower the client by encouraging the client to guide specifics of care such as wound care procedures and dressing and grooming details. Confirm the client's knowledge and document in the chart that the client is able to guide procedures. Document in the home and in the chart the preferred approach to procedures. Orient the family and caregivers to the client's role.
  - Assess the affective climate within the family and family support system, including other caregivers. Instruct the

• = Independent   ▲ = Collaborative

family in appropriate expectations of the client and in the specifics of the client's illness. Encourage the family and client in efforts toward educating friends and co-workers regarding appropriate expectations for the client.

- Evaluate the powerlessness of caregivers to ensure they continue their ability to care for the client. Provide assistance using interventions from this care plan.

• Be aware of and assist clients with potential needs for help in negotiating the health care system.

• Teach stress reduction, relaxation, and imagery. Many audio recordings are available on relaxation and meditation.

• Teach cognitive-behavioral activities, such as active problem solving, reframing (reappraising the situation from a different perspective), or thought stopping (in response to a negative thought, such as picturing a large stop sign and replacing the image with a prearranged positive alternative). Teach the client to confront his or her own negative thought patterns (cognitive distortions).

• Identify the strengths of the caregiver and efforts to gain control of unpredictable situations. Help the caregiver stay connected with a client who may be behaving differently than usual to make life as routine as possible, help the client set goals and sustain hope, and allow the client space to experience progress.

▲ Refer the client to support groups, pastoral care, or social services. These services help decrease levels of stress, increase levels of self-esteem, and reassure clients that they are not alone.

Client/Family Teaching and Discharge Planning

• The preceding interventions may be adapted for home care use.

Risk for Powerlessness

NANDA-I Definition

At risk for the lived experience of lack of control over a situation including a perception that one's actions do not significantly affect an outcome

• = Independent   ▲ = Collaborative

Risk Factors (r/t)

Anxiety; caregiving; chronic low self-esteem; deficient knowledge; economically disadvantaged; illness; ineffective coping patterns; lack of social support; pain; progressive debilitating disease; situational low self-esteem; social marginalization; stigmatized condition; stigmatized disease; unpredictable course of illness

Client Outcomes, Nursing Interventions, Client/Family Teaching and Discharge Planning

Refer to care plans **Powerlessness** and **Readiness for enhanced Power.**

Ineffective Protection

NANDA-I Definition

Decrease in the ability to guard self from internal or external threats such as illness or injury

Defining Characteristics

Altered clotting; anorexia; chilling; cough; deficient immunity; disorientation; dyspnea; fatigue; immobility; impaired healing; insomnia; itching; maladaptive stress response; neurosensory alteration; perspiring; pressure ulcers; restlessness; weakness

Related Factors (r/t)

Abnormal blood profiles (e.g., leukopenia, thrombocytopenia, anemia, coagulation); cancer; extremes of age; immune disorders; inadequate nutrition; pharmaceutical agents (e.g., antineoplastic, corticosteroid, immune, anticoagulant, thrombolytic) substance abuse; treatment-related side effects (e.g., surgery, radiation)

Patient Outcomes

Patient Will (Specify Time Frame):

* Remain free of infection
* Remain free of any evidence of new bleeding
* Explain precautions to take to prevent infection
* Explain precautions to take to prevent bleeding

Nursing Interventions

- Take temperature, pulse, and blood pressure (e.g., every 1 to 4 hours)
- ▲ Observe nutritional status (e.g., weight, serum protein and albumin levels, muscle mass, and usual food intake). Work with the dietitian to improve nutritional status if needed.
- Observe the client's sleep pattern; if altered, see Nursing Interventions for **Disturbed Sleep Pattern.**
- Identify stressors in the client's life. If stress is uncontrollable, see Nursing Interventions for **Ineffective Coping.**

Prevention of Infection

- ▲ Monitor for and report any signs of infection (e.g., fever, chills, flushed skin, drainage, edema, redness, abnormal laboratory values, and pain) and notify the physician promptly.
- ▲ If the client's immune system is depressed, notify the physician of elevated temperature, even in the absence of other symptoms of infection.
- If white blood cell count is severely decreased (i.e., absolute neutrophil count of less than 1000/mm^3), initiate the following precautions:
  - ▲ Take vital signs every 2 to 4 hours.
  - ▲ Complete a head-to-toe assessment twice daily, including inspection of oral mucosa, invasive sites, wounds, urine, and stool; monitor for onset of new reports of pain.
  - ▲ Avoid any invasive procedures, including catheterization, injections, or rectal or vaginal procedures unless absolutely necessary.
- Consider warming the client before elective surgery.
- ▲ Administer granulocyte growth factor as ordered.
- Take meticulous care of all invasive sites; use chlorhexidine gluconate for cleansing.
- Provide frequent oral care.
- ▲ Follow Standard Precautions, especially performing hand hygiene to prevent health care–associated infections.
- ▲ Refer for appropriate prophylactic antifungal treatment and avoid pathogen exposure (through air filtration, regular hand hygiene, and avoidance of plants and flowers).

P

● = Independent   ▲ = Collaborative

- Have the client wear a mask when leaving the room.
- Limit and screen visitors to minimize exposure to contagion.
- Help the client bathe daily.
- Practice food safety; a neutropenic diet may not be necessary.
▲ Ensure that the client is well nourished. Provide food with protein, and consider vitamin supplements. If appetite is suppressed, institute a dietary referral. Keep track of serum albumin levels, as well as transferrin and prealbumin levels.
- Help the client to cough and practice deep breathing regularly. Maintain an appropriate activity level.
- Obtain a private room for the client. Use high-energy particulate air filters if available and appropriate. Protective isolation is not recommended. Recognize that cotton cover gowns may not be effective in decreasing infection.
▲ Watch for signs of sepsis, including change in mental status, fever, shaking, chills, and hypotension. If present, notify the physician promptly.
- Refer to care plan for **Risk for Infection.**
- Refer to care plan for **Readiness for enhanced Nutrition** for additional interventions.

Pediatric

- Suggest kangaroo care, frequent and exclusive or nearly exclusive breastfeeding, and early discharge from hospital for low-birth-weight infants.
- Assess postoperative fever in pediatric oncology clients promptly.
- For hand hygiene with low-birth-weight infants, use alcohol hand rub and gloves

Geriatric

- If not contraindicated, promote exercise to promote improved quality of life in the elderly.
- Give elderly clients with imbalanced nutrition a vitamin D supplement to reduce risk of fracture.
- Refer to the care plan for **Risk for Infection** for more interventions related to the prevention of infection.

Prevention of Bleeding

- Monitor the client's risk for bleeding; evaluate results of clotting studies and platelet counts.
- Watch for hematuria, melena, hematemesis, hemoptysis, epistaxis, bleeding from mucosa, petechiae, and ecchymoses.
- ▲ Give medications orally or IV only; avoid giving them IM, subcutaneously, or rectally.
- Apply pressure for a longer time than usual to invasive sites, such as venipuncture or injection sites.
- Take vital signs often; watch for changes associated with fluid volume loss. Excessive bleeding causes decreased blood pressure and increased pulse and respiratory rates.
- Monitor menstrual flow if relevant; have the client use pads instead of tampons.
- ▲ Have the client use a moistened toothette or a very soft child's toothbrush instead of an adult toothbrush. Follow the dentist's recommendation for flossing and appropriate rinses to use. Control gum bleeding by applying pressure to gums with gauze pad soaked in ice water.
- Ask the client either to not shave or to use only an electric razor.
- To decrease risk of bleeding, avoid administering salicylates or nonsteroidal antiinflammatory drugs (NSAIDs) if possible.

Home Care

- Some of the interventions previously described may be adapted for home care use.
- ▲ Consider using a nurse-led patient-centered medical home (PCMH) for monitoring anticoagulant therapy.
- ▲ For terminally ill clients, teach and institute all of the aforementioned noninvasive precautions that maintain quality of life. Discuss with the client, family, and physician the consequences of contracting infection. Determine which precautions do not maintain quality of life and should not be used (e.g., physical assessment twice daily or multiple vital sign assessments).

P

Client/Family Teaching and Discharge Planning

Depressed Immune Function

- Teach the client and family how to take a temperature. Encourage the family to take the client's temperature between 3 PM and 7 PM at least once daily.
- Teach precautions to use to decrease the chance of infection (e.g., avoiding uncooked fruits and vegetables, using appropriate self-care including good hand hygiene, and ensuring a safe environment). Teach the client to avoid crowds and contact with persons who have infections. Teach the need for good nutrition, avoidance of stress, and adequate rest to maintain immune system function.

Bleeding Disorder

- ▲ Teach the client to wear a medical alert bracelet and notify all health care personnel of the bleeding disorder.
- ▲ Teach the client and family the signs of bleeding, precautions to take to prevent bleeding, and action to take if bleeding begins. Caution the client to avoid taking over-the-counter medications without the permission of the physician.
- Teach the client to wear loose-fitting clothes and avoid physical activity that might cause trauma.

Rape-Trauma Syndrome

NANDA-I Definition

Sustained adaptive response to a forced, violent sexual penetration against the victim's will and consent

Defining Characteristics

Aggression; agitation; anger; anxiety; change in relationships; confusion; denial; dependence; depression; disorganization; dissociative disorders; embarrassment; fear; guilt; helplessness; humiliation; hyperalertness; impaired decision-making; loss of self-esteem; mood swings; muscle spasms; muscle tension; nightmares; paranoia; phobias; physical trauma;

• = Independent   ▲ = Collaborative

powerlessness; revenge; self-blame; sexual dysfunction; shame; shock; sleep disturbances; substance abuse; suicide attempts; vulnerability

Related Factors (r/t)

Rape

Client Outcomes

Client Will (Specify Time Frame):

- Share feelings, concerns, and fears
- Recognize that the rape or attempt was not client's own fault
- State that, no matter what the situation, no one has the right to assault another
- Describe medical/legal treatment procedures and reasons for treatment
- Report absence of physical complications or pain
- Identify support resources and attend psychotherapy/group assistance in coping with the trauma and effects of the traumatic experience
- Function at same level as before crisis, including sexual functioning
- Recognize that it is normal for full recovery to take a minimum of 1 year

Nursing Interventions

- Escort the client to a treatment room immediately on arrival to the emergency department. Avoid interruptions during contact with the client. Stay with (or have a trusted person stay with) the client initially.
- Provide a sexual assault response team (SART), if available, that includes a sexual assault nurse examiner (SANE), rape counseling advocate, and representative of law enforcement for best possible outcomes
- Observe for signs of physical injury.
- Ask the client if she/he is in pain. If further clarification is needed, ask the client to point to areas that were injured or touched.
- Document the client's chief complaint and request an event history of the sexual assault in her/his own words.
- Monitor the client's verbal and nonverbal affect. Encourage the client to verbalize his/her feelings.
- Explain everything you are doing.

● = Independent ▲ = Collaborative

- Explain to the client that all or some of the client's clothing may be kept for evidential purposes and photographs may be taken (with consent) to document the client's injuries.
- If a law enforcement interview is permitted, provide support by staying with the client on her/his request.
- Utilize the sexual assault evidence collection kits that have been reviewed by the SART members and provided by your state to collect adequate and accurate evidence for analysis by a forensic laboratory.
- Discuss the possibility of pregnancy and sexually transmitted infections (STIs) and the treatments available.
- Encourage the client to report the rape to a law enforcement agency.
- Involve the support system if appropriate and if the client grants permission.
- For those interested in a spiritual connection, make the appropriate recommendation.
- Stress the necessity of follow-up care with a mental health professional to recognize and intervene with problems associated with the effects of rape-trauma.
- Stress the importance of awareness throughout the community of the scope and severity of the effects of sexual abuse as a means of additional healing empowerment.

Geriatric

- Build a trusting relationship with the client.
- All examinations should be done on the elderly as they would be done on any adult client after sexual assault with modifications for comfort if necessary.
- Assess for mobility limitations and cognitive impairment.
- Explain and encourage the client to report sexual abuse.
- Observe for psychosocial distress.
- Consider arrangements for temporary housing.

Male Rape

- Encourage men who are raped to report the assault.

• = Independent ▲ = Collaborative

Multicultural

- Assess for the influence of cultural beliefs, norms, and values on the client's ability to cope with the trauma of the rape experience.
- Assure the client of confidentiality.

Home Care

- Some of the interventions described previously may be adapted for home care use.
- Corroborate the client's feelings of self-worth.
- Assist the client with realistically assessing the home setting for safety and/or selecting a safe environment in which to live.
- ▲ Ensure that the client has systems in place for long-term support.
- ▲ Design a practical discharge plan to include a safe shelter if needed, follow-up care for physical injury and follow-up referral for psychological support.
- ▲ Assess for other client vulnerabilities such as mental health issues or addiction and refer client to social agencies for implementation of a therapeutic regimen.

Client/Family Teaching and Discharge Planning

- ▲ Discuss the need for prophylactic antibiotic therapy, hepatitis B vaccination, tetanus prophylaxis, and emergency contraception as needed.
- Emphasize the client's needs for safety and to decrease the opportunities for repeat attacks.
- Recognize the vulnerability of the client.

NOTE: Post-traumatic stress (PTSD) disorder has a high probability of being a psychological sequela to rape. Research demonstrated two effective treatments for improvement of PTSD in rape victims—prolonged exposure and stress inoculation training. Prolonged exposure involves reliving the rape experience by imagining it as vividly as possible, describing it aloud in the present tense, taping this description, and listening to the tape at least once daily. Stress inoculation training uses breathing exercises to diminish anxiety and instruction in coping skills, thought stopping, cognitive restructuring,

R

• = Independent   ▲ = Collaborative

self-dialogue, and role playing. Research suggests that a combination of both treatments may provide the optimal effect. Furthermore, for those who reported the assault to police, lower levels of legal system success and satisfaction were linked to higher levels of perceived control over present recovery.

Ineffective Relationship

NANDA-I Definition

A pattern of mutual partnership that is insufficient to provide for each other's needs

Defining Characteristics

Does not identify partner as a key person; does not meet developmental goals appropriate for family life-cycle stage; inability to communicate in a satisfying manner between partners; no demonstration of mutual respect between partners; no demonstration of mutual support in daily activities between partners; no demonstration of understanding of partner's insufficient (physical, social, psychological) functioning; no demonstration of well-balanced autonomy between partners; no demonstration of well-balanced collaboration between partners; reports dissatisfaction with complementary relation between partners; reports dissatisfaction with fulfilling physical needs between partners; reports dissatisfaction with sharing of ideas between partners; reports dissatisfaction with sharing of information between partners

Related Factors

Cognitive changes in one partner; developmental crises; history of domestic violence; incarceration of one partner; poor communication skills; stressful life events; substance abuse; unrealistic expectations

Client Outcomes, Nursing Interventions, Client/ Family Teaching and Discharge Planning

Refer to care plan **Readiness for enhanced Relationship.**

• = Independent   ▲ = Collaborative

Readiness for enhanced Relationship

NANDA-I Definition

A pattern of mutual partnership that is sufficient to provide for each other's needs and can be strengthened

Defining Characteristics

Demonstrates mutual respect between partners; demonstrates mutual support in daily activities between partners; demonstrates understanding of partner's insufficient (physical, social, psychological) function; demonstrates well-balanced autonomy between partners; demonstrates well-balanced collaboration between partners; identifies each other as a key person; meets developmental goals appropriate for family life-cycle stage; reports desire to enhance communication between partners; reports satisfaction with complementary relationship between partners; reports satisfaction with fulfilling emotional needs by one's partner; reports satisfaction with fulfilling physical needs by one's partner; reports satisfaction with sharing of ideas between partners; reports satisfaction with sharing of information between partners.

Client Outcomes

Family/Client Will (Specify Time Frame):
- Share thoughts and feelings with each other
- Communicate openly with each other
- Assist in performing family roles and tasks
- Provide support for each other
- Obtain appropriate assistance

Nursing Interventions

- ▲ Assess for signs of depression in the family when one partner is depressed, and make appropriate referrals.
- • Support "relationship talk" between couples (talking with a partner about the relationship, what one needs from one's partner, and/or the relationship implications of a shared stressor).
- • Encourage couples to participate and share in exciting and satisfying leisure activities and to share stories.

• = Independent   ▲ = Collaborative

- Assist couples in establishing boundaries between work and home.
- Assist couples in regulating negative emotions.
- Assist couples in dealing with anger and communication when the diagnosis is cancer.
- Refer to care plans **Readiness for enhanced Family Processes** and **Readiness for enhanced family Coping.**

Pediatric

- Provide guidance and information on communication techniques for teenagers, especially those involved in intimate relationships.
- Encourage supportive relationships among parents and teenagers.

Geriatric

- ▲ Assess for spousal depression when one partner has cardiovascular disease, and make appropriate referrals.
- ▲ Assess for depression and anxiety and make appropriate referrals for "prewidows" caring for spouses with chronic life-limiting conditions.
- Support older couples' positive collaborative communication.
- Encourage collaborative coping (i.e., spouses pooling resources and problem solving jointly) among older adults.

Multicultural

- Provide culturally tailored community-level interventions to raise awareness about HIV and bisexuality, and decrease HIV and sexual orientation stigma.

Home Care

- Provide home-based psychoeducation to assist new parent couples with parenting and their couple relationship.

Client/Family Teaching and Discharge Planning

- Encourage clients and spouses to participate together in interventions to lower low-density lipoprotein cholesterol (LDL-C). Teach spouses how to provide emotional and instrumental support, allow clients to decide which component of the intervention they would like to receive, and have clients determine their own goals and action plans. Provide telephone calls to clients and spouses separately. During each client telephone call, client progress is reviewed, and clients create goals and action plans for the upcoming month. During spouse telephone calls, which occur within 1 week of client calls, spouses are informed of clients' goals and action plans and devise strategies to increase emotional and instrumental support.

Risk for ineffective Relationship

NANDA-I Definition

Risk for a pattern of mutual partnership that is insufficient to provide for each other's needs

Risk Factors

- Cognitive changes in one partner
- Developmental crises
- History of domestic violence
- Incarceration of one partner
- Poor communication skills
- Stressful life events
- Substance abuse
- Unrealistic expectations

Client Outcomes, Nursing Interventions, Client/ Family Teaching and Discharge Planning

Refer to care plan **Readiness for enhanced Relationship.**

Impaired Religiosity

NANDA-I Definition

Impaired ability to exercise reliance on beliefs and/or participate in rituals of a particular faith tradition

• = Independent ▲ = Collaborative

Defining Characteristics

Difficulty adhering to prescribed religious beliefs; difficulty adhering to prescribed religious rituals (e.g., religious ceremonies, dietary regulations, clothing, prayer, worship/religious services, private religious behaviors/reading religious materials/media, holiday observances, meetings with religious leaders); questions religious belief patterns; questions religious customs; reports a need to reconnect with previous belief patterns; reports a need to reconnect with previous customs; reports emotional distress because of separation from faith community

Related Factors (r/t)

Developmental and Situational
Aging; end-stage life crises; life transitions

Physical
Illness; pain

Psychological
Anxiety; fear of death; ineffective coping; ineffective support; lack of security; personal crisis; use of religion to manipulate

Sociocultural
Cultural barriers to practicing religion; environmental barriers to practicing religion; lack of social integration; lack of sociocultural interaction

Spiritual
Spiritual crises; suffering

Client Outcomes

Client Will (Specify Time Frame):
Express satisfaction with the ability to express religious practices

Express satisfaction with access to religious materials and rituals

Demonstrate balance between religious practices and healthy lifestyles

Avoid high-risk, controlling religious relationships that inflict physical, sexual, or emotional harm and/or exploitation

• = Independent   ▲ = Collaborative

Nursing Interventions

- Recognize when clients integrate religious practices in their life.
- Encourage and/or coordinate the use of and participation in usual religious rituals or practices that support coping.
- Encourage the use of prayer or meditation as appropriate.
- Promote family coping using religious practices to help cope with loss, as appropriate.
- ▲ Refer to religious leader, professional counseling, or support group as needed.

Geriatric

- Promote established religious practices in the elderly.

Multicultural

- Promote religious practices that are culturally appropriate:
  - African American
  - Hawaiian women
  - African
  - Aborigine

R

Readiness for enhanced Religiosity

NANDA-I Definition

A pattern of reliance on religious beliefs and/or participation in rituals of a particular faith tradition that is sufficient for well-being and can be strengthened

Defining Characteristics

Expresses desire to strengthen belief patterns that have provided religion in the past; expresses desire to strengthen religious belief patterns that have provided comfort in the past; expresses desire to strengthen religious customs that have provided comfort in the past; questions belief patterns that are harmful; questions customs that are harmful; rejects belief patterns that are harmful; rejects customs that are harmful; requests assistance to expand religious options; request assistance to increase participation in prescribed religious

• = Independent ▲ = Collaborative

beliefs (e.g., religious ceremonies, dietary regulations/rituals, clothing, prayer, worship/religious services, private religious behaviors, reading religious materials/media, holiday observances); requests forgiveness; requests meeting with religious leaders/facilitators; requests reconciliation; requests religious experiences; requests religious materials

Nursing Interventions

- Provide spiritual care for children based on developmental level.
  - **Infants:** Have the same nurse care for the child on a daily basis. Encourage holding, cuddling, rocking, playing with, and singing to the infant.
  - **Toddlers:** Provide consistency in care and familiar toys, music, stories, clothing blankets, pillows, and any other individual object of contentment. Schedule home religious routines into the plan of care, and support home routines regarding good and bad behavior.
  - **School-age children and adolescents:** Encourage both groups to express their feelings regarding spirituality. Ask them, "Do you wish to pray, and what do want to pray about?" Offer age-appropriate complementary therapies such as music, art, videos, and connectedness with peers through cards, letters, and visits.

Risk for impaired Religiosity

NANDA-I Definition

At risk for an impaired ability to exercise reliance on religious beliefs and/or participate in rituals of a particular faith tradition

Related Factors (r/t)

Developmental
Life transitions

Environmental
Barriers to practicing religion; lack of transportation

     ● = Independent   ▲ = Collaborative

Physical
Hospitalization; illness; pain

Psychological
Depression; ineffective caregiving; ineffective coping; ineffective support; lack of security

Sociocultural
Cultural barrier to practicing religion; lack of social interaction; social isolation

Spiritual
Suffering

Client Outcomes, Nursing Interventions, Client/Family Teaching and Discharge Planning

Refer to care plan **Impaired Religiosity**.

Relocation Stress Syndrome

NANDA-I Definition

Physiological and/or psychosocial disturbances that result from transfer from one environment to another

Defining Characteristics

Alienation; aloneness; anger; anxiety (e.g., separation); concern over relocation; dependency; depression; fear; frustration; increased illness; increased physical symptoms; increased verbalization of needs; insecurity; loneliness; loss of identity; loss of self-esteem; loss of self-worth; pessimism; sleep disturbance; verbalizes unwillingness to move; withdrawal; worry

Related Factors (r/t)

Decreased health status; feelings of powerlessness; unpredictability of experience; impaired psychosocial health; isolation; lack of adequate support system; lack of predeparture counseling; language barrier; losses; move from one environment to another; passive coping

Client Outcomes

Client Will (Specify Time Frame):
- Recognize and know the name of at least one staff member

• = Independent   ▲ = Collaborative

- Express concern about move when encouraged to do so during individual contacts
- Carry out activities of daily living (ADLs) in usual manner
- Maintain previous mental and physical health status (e.g., nutrition, elimination, sleep, social interaction, physical activity)

Nursing Interventions

- Be aware that relocation to supportive housing may be a positive change.
- Begin relocation planning as early in the decision process as possible.
- Obtain a history, including the reason for the move, the client's usual coping mechanisms, history of losses, and family support for the client.
- Identify to what extent the client can participate in the relocation decisions and advocate for this participation.
- Assess client's readiness to relocate and relocation self-efficacy.
- Consult an evidence-based practice guide for relocation.
- Assess family members' perceptions of clients' ability to participate in relocation decisions. Particularly in cases of dementia, be alert to care worker's involvement in making the decision to relocate. They may need support and encouragement through the process.
- Consider the clients' and families' cultural and ethnic values as much as possible when choosing roommates, foods, and other aspects of care.
- Promote clear communication between all participants in the relocation process.
- Observe the following procedures if the client is being transferred to an extended care facility or assisted living facility:
  - Facilitate the client's participation in decisions and choice of placement and arrange a preadmission visit if possible
  - If the client cannot visit the new facility, arrange for a visit or telephone call by a member of the staff to welcome the client and show a videotape or at least provide pictures of the new care facility.
  - Have a familiar person accompany the client to the new facility.
  - Recommend that the caregiver write a journal of thoughts and feelings regarding the relocation of his or her loved one.
  - Continue to assess caregiver psychological distress during a 6-month period following relocation.

● = Independent   ▲ = Collaborative

- Identify previous routines for ADLs. Try to maintain as much continuity with the previous schedule as possible.
- Bring in familiar items from home (e.g., pictures, clocks, afghans).
- Establish the way the client would like to be addressed (Mr., Mrs., Miss, first name, nickname).
- Thoroughly orient the client and the family to the new environment and routines; repeat directions as needed.
- Spend one-to-one time with the client. Allow the client to express feelings and convey acceptance of them; emphasize that the client's feelings are real and individual and that it is acceptable to be sad or angry about moving.
- Allocate a caring staff member to help the client adjust to the move. Assign the same staff members to the client for care if compatible with client; maintain consistency in the personnel the client interacts with.
- Ask the client to state one positive aspect of the new living situation each day.
- Monitor the client's health status and provide appropriate interventions for problems with social interaction, nutrition, sleep, new onset of infection, or elimination problems.
- If the client is being transferred within a facility, have staff members from the new unit visit the client before transfer.
- Work with the caregivers and family members helping them deal with stages of "making the best of it," "making the move," and "making it better."
- If a client is being transferred from the intensive care unit (ICU), have previous staff make occasional visits until the client is comfortable in the new surroundings. Ensure that the family is told relevant information.
- Watch for coping problems (e.g., withdrawal, regression, angry behavior, impaired sleeping, refusal to eat, flat affect) and intervene immediately.
- Encourage the client to express grief for the loss of the old situation; explain that it is normal to feel sadness over change and loss.
- Pay special attention to assessing and giving psychosocial care.
- Encourage the client to participate in care as much as possible and make own decisions when possible (e.g., placement of the bed, choice of roommate, bathing routines).

• = Independent   ▲ = Collaborative

Pediatric

- Assess family history and contact information from children relocated to rescue shelters.
- Be aware that community relocation may be beneficial for children, and assess community resources of new location.
- Provide support for a child and family who must relocate to be near a transplant center.
- In divorce situations, recommend alternative dispute resolution versus traditional litigated settlement.
- Encourage child to verbalize concerns in divorce situations when they and/or a parent relocate.
- Assess presence of allergies before and after relocation.
- If the client is an adolescent, try to avoid a move in the middle of the school year, find a newcomers' club for the adolescent to join, and refer for counseling if needed.
- Assess adolescents' perceptions of their acceptance by peers.
- Help parents recognize that relocation stress syndrome may persist for prolonged periods (e.g., 2 years) in adolescents.

Geriatric

- Monitor the need for transfer and transfer only when necessary.
- Implement discharge planning early so that it is not rushed.
- Protect the client from injuries such as falls.
- After the transfer, determine the client's mental status.
- Facilitate visits from companion animals.
- Encourage reminiscence of happy times.
- Refer for music therapy.
- Monitor for neuroleptic prescriptions.

Client/Family Teaching and Discharge Planning

- Teach family members and remind direct care staff about relocation stress syndrome. Encourage them to monitor for signs of the syndrome
- Help significant others learn how to support the client in the move by setting up a schedule of visits, arranging for holidays, bringing familiar items from home, and establishing a system for contact when the client needs support.
- Assist family members and the relocating older adult to use webcam technology for interaction to supplement in-person visits.

• = Independent ▲ = Collaborative

Risk for Relocation Stress Syndrome

NANDA-I Definition

At risk for physiological and/or psychosocial disturbances following transfer from one environment to another

Risk Factors

Decreased health status; lack of adequate support system; lack of predeparture counseling; losses; moderate to high degree of environmental change; moderate mental competence; move from one environment to another; passive coping; reports powerlessness; unpredictability of experiences

Client Outcomes, Nursing Interventions, Client/ Family Teaching and Discharge Planning

Refer to care plan for **Relocation Stress Syndrome.**

Risk for ineffective Renal Perfusion

NANDA-I Definition

At risk for a decrease in blood circulation to the kidney that may compromise health

Risk Factors

Abdominal compartment syndrome; advanced age; bilateral cortical necrosis; burns; cardiac surgery; cardiopulmonary bypass; diabetes mellitus; exposure to toxins; female glomerulonephritis; hyperlipidemia; hypertension; hypovolemia; hypoxemia; hypoxia; infection (e.g., sepsis, localized infection); malignancy; malignant hypertension; metabolic acidosis; multitrauma; polynephritis; renal artery stenosis; renal disease (polycystic kidney); smoking; systemic inflammatory response syndrome; treatment-related side effects (medications); vascular embolism; vasculitis

Client Outcomes

Client Will (Specify Time Frame):

- Maintain normal blood urea nitrogen and serum creatinine levels
- Maintain urine output of 0.5 mL/kg/hr
- Maintain urine output that is yellow and clear
- Maintain serum electrolytes (K^+, PO_4, Na^+) within normal limits
- Maintain glomerular filtration rate (GFR) of 60 to 89 mL/min/1.73 m^2

● = Independent ▲ = Collaborative

Nursing Interventions

- Measure intake and output on a regular basis. Calculate intake against the output to monitor fluid retention.
- Monitor for edema.
- Assess client for history of risk factors for decreased renal perfusion, which can result in renal insufficiency, renal artery stenosis, and acute renal failure. These factors can be classified into three categories:
  - **Prerenal:** The cause of renal damage comes before the kidneys, from decreased renal perfusion. Causes include renal arterial disease, shock states, cardiac and thoracoabdominal surgeries, hypovolemia, heart failure, and decreased cardiac output.
  - **Intrinsic (Intrarenal):** There is structural damage to the kidney, something directly toxic to the kidney. Causes include hypertension, diabetes, glomerulonephritis, kidney infection, lupus, Goodpasture syndrome, nephrotoxic drugs, and IV contrast.
  - **Postrenal:** The cause of renal disease is a mechanical obstruction of the urinary collecting system. Causes include benign prostatic hypertrophy, cancer of the kidney, obstruction of ureters and the urethra, and strictures.
- Assess for signs of dehydration. Refer to care plan for **Deficient Fluid Volume.**
- Ensure that clients are receiving appropriate amounts of fluids to prevent dehydration.
- Monitor vital signs carefully. Especially note new onset of hypertension from onset of kidney dysfunction, or decreased mean arterial pressure (MAP).
- ▲ Utilize continuous cardiac monitoring as needed. Monitor for dysrhythmias due to possible increased serum potassium and phosphorus, or low hemoglobin due to poor kidney function.
- Listen to lung sounds, noting presence of adventitious lung sounds. Refer to care plan for **Excess Fluid Volume.**
- Monitor for changes in mental status and headache.
- Weigh the client daily.
- ▲ Monitor peak and trough blood levels carefully in clients receiving nephrotoxic antibiotics, including vancomycin and aminoglycosides.

• = Independent   ▲ = Collaborative

▲ Ensure that clients having diagnostic testing with contrast are well hydrated with IV saline as ordered before and after the examination. Refer to care plan **Risk for adverse reaction to iodinated Contrast media.**

▲ Collect a 24-hour urine specimen for examination as ordered; place on ice to preserve the quality of the urine.

▲ Note the results of diagnostic studies as available: renal ultrasound, radionuclide scanning, abdominal/pelvic CT, MRA, arteriography.

▲ Perform a complete pain assessment. Assess and document the onset, intensity, character, location, duration, aggravating factors, and relieving factors. Notify the provider of any increase in pain or discomfort or if comfort measures are not effective.

▲ Monitor laboratory data as ordered or per protocol. Laboratory data could include BUN, serum creatinine, inulin clearance, glomerular filtration rate, serum and urine electrolytes, calcium, phosphate, complete blood count, urine total protein, albumin, alkaline phosphatase, and urinalysis. Report abnormalities to attending provider.

Client/Family Teaching and Discharge Planning

• Provide client teaching related to risk factors for renal insufficiency or acute renal failure, including signs and symptoms of acute renal failure, and lifestyle changes that can improve renal function.

▲ Teach client about any medications prescribed.

▲ Stress the importance of stopping smoking.

Impaired individual Resilience

NANDA-I Definition

Decreased ability to sustain a pattern of positive responses to an adverse situation or crisis

Defining Characteristics

Decreased interest in academic activities; decreased interest in vocational activities; depression; guilt; isolation; lower perceived health status; low

• = Independent   ▲ = Collaborative

self-esteem; renewed elevation of distress; shame; social isolation; using maladaptive coping skills (i.e., drug use, violence, etc.)

Related Factors (r/t)

Demographics that increase chance of maladjustment; gender; inconsistent parenting; large family size; low intelligence; low maternal education; minority status; neighborhood violence; parental mental illness; poor impulse control; poverty; psychological disorders; substance abuse; violence; vulnerability factors which encompass indices that exacerbate the negative effects of the risk condition

Client Outcomes

Client Will (Specify Time Frame):
- Demonstrate reduced or cessation of drug and alcohol usage
- State effective life events on feelings about self
- Will seek help when necessary
- Verbalize or demonstrate cessation of abuse
- Adapt to unexpected crises or challenges
- Verbalize positive outlook on illness, family, situation, and life
- Use available resources to meet coping needs
- Identify role models
- Identify available assets and resources
- Able to verbalize meaning of one's life

Nursing Interventions

- Encourage positive, health-seeking behaviors.
- Ensure access to biological, psychological, and spiritual resources.
- Foster communication skills through basic communication skill training.
- Foster cognitive skills in decision-making.
- Assist client in cognitive restructuring of negative thought processes.
- Facilitate supportive family environments and communication.
- Promote engagement in positive social activities.
- Assist client to identify strengths, and reinforce these.
- Help the client to identify positive emotions in the midst of adverse situations.
- Build on supportive counseling and therapy.

● = Independent   ▲ = Collaborative

- Identify protective factors such as assets and resources to enhance coping.
- Provide positive reinforcement and emotional support during the learning process.
- Encourage mindfulness, a conscious attention and awareness of self.
- Assist the client to have an optimistic worldview.

Pediatric

- The preceding interventions may be adapted for the pediatric client.
- Support the seeking of opportunities to improve cognitive abilities, such as tutoring and other resources; the development of positive and supportive relations such as family, community members, or mentors; and the improvement of general health.
- Promote the development of positive mentor relationships.

Readiness for enhanced Resilience

R

NANDA-I Definition

A pattern of positive responses to an adverse situation or crisis that is sufficient for optimizing human potential and can be strengthened

Defining Characteristics

Access to resources; demonstrates positive outlook; effective use of conflict management strategies; enhances personal coping skills; expressed desire to enhance resilience; identifies available resources; identifies support systems; increases positive relationships with others; involvement in activities; makes progress toward goals; presence of a crisis; reports enhanced sense of control; reports self-esteem; safe environment is maintained; sets goals; takes responsibilities for actions; use of effective communication skills

Client Outcomes

Client Will (Specify Time Frame):

- Adapt to adversities and challenges
- Communicate clearly and appropriately for age

• = Independent ▲ = Collaborative

- Take responsibility for own actions
- Make progress towards goals
- Use effective coping strategies
- Express emotions

Nursing Interventions

- Listen to and encourage expressions of feelings and beliefs.
- Establish a therapeutic relationship based on trust and respect.
- Assist client to identify strengths and reinforce these.
- Provide positive reinforcement and emotional support during implementation of care.
- ▲ Facilitate the development of mentorship opportunities.
- Determine how family behavior affects the client.
- Provide assistance in decision-making.
- Establish individual/family/community goals.

Pediatric

- The preceding interventions may be adapted for the pediatric client.
- Encourage the promotion of protective factors by fostering the seeking of opportunities to improve cognitive abilities such as tutoring and other resources; the development of positive and supportive relations such as family, community members, or mentors; and the improvement of general health.

Multicultural

- Use teaching strategies that are culturally and age appropriate.

Risk for compromised Resilience

NANDA-I Definition

At risk for decreased ability to sustain a pattern of positive responses to an adverse situation or crisis

Risk Factors

Chronicity of existing crises; multiple coexisting adverse situations; presence of an additional new crisis (e.g., unplanned pregnancy, death of a spouse, loss of job, illness; loss of housing, death of family member)

● = Independent   ▲ = Collaborative

Client Outcomes

Client Will (Specify Time Frame):

- Identify available community resources
- Propose practical, constructive solutions for disputes
- Identify and access community resources for assistance
- Accept assistance with activities of daily living from family and friends
- Verbalize an enhanced sense of control
- Verbalize meaningfulness of one's life

Nursing Interventions

- Determine how family behavior affects client.
- Help to identify personal rights, responsibilities, and conflicting norms.
- Encourage consideration of values underlying choices and consequences of the choice.
- Help client to practice conversational and social skills.
- Assist client to prioritize values.
- Create an accepting, nonjudgmental atmosphere.
- Help identify self-defeating thoughts.
- ▲ Refer to community resources as appropriate.
- Help clarify problem areas in interpersonal relationships.
- Identify and enroll high-risk families in follow-up programs.

Parental Role Conflict

NANDA-I Definition

Parent's experience of role confusion and conflict in response to crisis

Defining Characteristics

Anxiety; demonstrated disruption in caretaking routines; fear; reluctant to participate in usual caretaking activities; reports concern about changes in parental role; reports concern about family (e.g., functioning, communication, health); reports concern about perceived loss of control over decisions relating to child; reports feelings of frustration; reports feelings of guilt; reports feeling of inadequacy to provide for child's needs (e.g., physical, emotional)

● = Independent   ▲ = Collaborative

Related Factors (r/t)

Change in marital status; home care of a child with special needs; interruptions of family life due to home care regimen (e.g., treatments, caregivers, lack of respite); intimidation with invasive modalities (e.g., intubation); intimidation with restrictive modalities (e.g., isolation); parent-child separation due to chronic illness; specialized care center

Client Outcomes

Client Will (Specify Time Frame):

- Express feelings and perceptions regarding impacts of illness, disability, and/or hospitalization on parental role
- Participate in hospital and home care as much as able given the availability of resources and support systems
- Exhibit assertiveness and responsibility in active family decision-making regarding care of the child
- Describe and select available resources to support parental management of the child's and family's needs

Nursing Interventions

- Assess and support parents' previous coping behaviors.
- Determine parent/family sources of stress, usual methods of coping, and perceptions of illness/condition. Maximize on the strengths identified.
- Evaluate the family's perceived strength of its social support system, including religious beliefs. Encourage the family to use social support.
- Determine the older childbearing woman's support systems and expectations for motherhood.
- Consider the use of family-centered theory as the conceptual foundation to help guide interventions.
- Be available to accept and support parents, listening and discussing concerns.
- ▲ Maintain parental involvement in shared decision-making with regard to care by using the following steps: Incorporate parents' information concerning the child's typical routines, behaviors, fears, likes, and dislikes; provide clear and direct firsthand information concerning the child's condition and progress; normalize the home/hospital environment as much as possible; collaborate in care by providing choices when possible.

• = Independent   ▲ = Collaborative

- Seek and support parental participation in care.
- Provide support for each parent's primary coping strategies and needs.
▲ Inform parents of financial resources, respite care, and home support to assist them in maintaining sufficient energy and personal resources to continue caregiving responsibilities.
- Encourage the parent to meet his or her own needs for rest, nutrition, and hygiene. Provide parent bed spaces so that the parent may stay with the sick child.
- Provide family-centered care: allowing parents to touch and talk to the child, assisting in the handling of medical equipment, and offering a comfortable chair, preferably a rocking chair. Provide opportunities and offer praise for successful caregiving.
- Refer parents to available telephone and/or Internet support groups.
- Involve new mothers' partners or parents in clinical encounters and invite family members to discuss their expectations and parenting experiences.

Multicultural

- Acknowledge racial/ethnic differences at the onset of care.
- Assess for the influence of cultural beliefs, norms, and values on the client's perceptions of the parental role.
- Acknowledge that value conflicts arising from acculturation stresses may contribute to increased anxiety and significant conflict with the parental role.
- Promote the female parenting role by providing a treatment environment that is culturally based and woman-centered.
- Support the client's parenting role in her usual setting via social exchange.

Home Care

- The interventions described previously may be adapted for home care use.
- Assess family adjustment prenatally and postpartum; assist new parents to renegotiate parenting roles and responsibilities with co-parenting. Encourage the father to take an active role in infant care with the mother's support.

● = Independent   ▲ = Collaborative

Client/Family Teaching and Discharge Planning

- Offer family-led education interventions to improve participants' knowledge about their condition and its treatment and
decreasing their information needs.
- For children and their parents involved in bereavement support groups, identify the family's positive way of coping.
▲ Refer parents of children with behavioral problems to parenting programs.
- Involve parents in formal and/or informal social support situations, such as Internet support groups.
- Teach the client about available community resources (e.g.,
therapists, ministers, counselors, self-help groups).
- Encourage parents with human immunodeficiency virus/
acquired immunodeficiency syndrome (HIV/AIDS) to implement custody plans for their children.

R   Ineffective Role Performance

NANDA-I Definition

Patterns of behavior and self-expression that do not match the environmental context, norms, and expectations

Defining Characteristics

Altered role perceptions; anxiety; change in capacity to resume role;
change in other's perception of role; change in self-perception of role;
change in usual patterns of responsibility; deficient knowledge; depression; discrimination; domestic violence; harassment; inadequate adaptation to change; inadequate confidence; inadequate external support
for role enactment; inadequate motivation; inadequate opportunities
for role enactment; inadequate self-management; inadequate skills;
inappropriate developmental expectations; ineffective coping; ineffective role performance; pessimism; powerlessness; role ambivalence; role
conflict; role confusion; role denial; role dissatisfaction; role overload;
role strain; system conflict; uncertainty

● = Independent   ▲ = Collaborative

Related Factors (r/t)

Knowledge

Inadequate role model; inadequate role preparation (e.g., role transition, skill rehearsal, validation); lack of education; lack of role model; unrealistic role expectations

Physiological

Body image alteration; chronic low self-esteem; cognitive deficits; depression; fatigue; mental illness; neurological defects; pain; physical illness; situational low self-esteem; substance abuse

Social

Conflict; developmental level; domestic violence; economically disadvantaged; inadequate role socialization; inadequate support system; inappropriate linkage with the health care system; job schedule demands, lack of resources; lack of rewards; stress; young age

Client Outcomes

Client Will (Specify Time Frame):

- Identify realistic perception of role
- State personal strengths
- Acknowledge problems contributing to inability to carry out usual role
- Accept physical limitations regarding role responsibility and consider ways to change lifestyle to accomplish goals associated with role performance
- Demonstrate knowledge of appropriate behaviors associated with new or changed role
- State knowledge of change in responsibility and new behaviors associated with new responsibility
- Verbalize acceptance of new responsibility

Nursing Interventions

Social

- Ask the client direct questions regarding new roles and how the health care system can help him or her continue in roles
- ▲ Allow the client to express feelings regarding the role change; refer for support as needed.

• = Independent   ▲ = Collaborative

▲ Refer for support as needed for home caregivers of military families during the deployment of spouses.

• Reinforce the client's strengths and internalized values.

• Have the client make a list of strengths that are needed for the new role. Acknowledge which strengths the client has and which strengths need to be developed. Work with the client to set goals for desired role.

• Support the client's religious practices.

Physiological

• Identify ways to compensate for physical disabilities (e.g., have a ramp built to provide access to house, put household objects within the client's reach from wheelchair) and provide technological assistance when available.

• Refer to the care plans for **Readiness for enhanced family Coping, Readiness for enhanced Decision-Making, Impaired Home Maintenance, Impaired Parenting, Risk for Loneliness, Readiness for enhanced community Coping, Readiness for enhanced Self-Care,** and **Ineffective Sexuality Pattern.**

Pediatric

• Assist new parents to adjust to changes in workload associated with childbirth. Mothers may need additional support.

▲ Refer teen parents and families to a community-based, multi-family group (MFG) intervention strategy (e.g., Families and Schools Together [FAST] babies).

▲ Refer to home health agency for home visits when there is an infant who has excessive crying.

• Provide parents with coping skills when the role change is associated with a critically and chronically ill child.

▲ Assist families how to manage day-to-day needs of a child with cerebral palsy (CP). Teach family members to value the small things children do, connect with other families, locate community resources, and understand the short- and long-term needs of the child.

• Consider the use of media-based behavioral treatments for children with behavioral disorders.

• = Independent   ▲ = Collaborative

Geriatric

- Assess older adults' choices regarding their care and enable them to live as they wish and receive the help they want by carefully listening to their stories.
- Provide support and practice for the elderly to use assistive devices.
- Support the client's religious beliefs and activities and provide appropriate spiritual support persons.
- Explore community needs after assessing the client's strengths. Encourage elders to participate in volunteer programs.
- Provide educational materials for older clients who are recovering from hip surgery or fractures to promote early mobility.
▲ Refer to appropriate support groups for mental stress related to role changes.
▲ Refer clients to therapeutic recreation programs that use humor.
▲ Refer to therapy to improve memory for clients with Alzheimer's disease.
- Provide music of choice for clients with Alzheimer's.
- Provide support for grandparents raising grandchildren.

Multicultural

- Assess for the influence of cultural beliefs, norms, values, and expectations on the individual's role.
- Assess for conflicts between the caregiver's cultural role obligations and competing factors such as employment or school.
- Negotiate with the client regarding the aspects of their role that can be modified and still honor cultural beliefs.
- Encourage family to use support groups or other service programs to assist with role changes.
- Refer new moms to a new mothers' Internet-based social support network.

Home Care

- The preceding interventions may be adapted for home care use.
▲ Offer a referral to medical social services to assist with assessing the short- and long-term impacts of role change.

● = Independent ▲ = Collaborative

Client/Family Teaching and Discharge Planning

- Provide educational materials to family members on client behavior management plus caregiver stress-coping management.
- Help the client identify resources for assistance in caring for a disabled or aging parent (e.g., adult day care, nursing home placement).
- ▲ Refer to appropriate community agencies to learn skills for functioning in the new or changed role (e.g., vocational rehabilitation, parenting classes, hospice, respite care).
- Consider pet therapy for college students in a new role, their first semester away from home.

Sedentary lifestyle

NANDA-I Definition

Reports a habit of life that is characterized by a low physical activity level

Defining Characteristics

Chooses a daily routine lacking physical exercise; demonstrates physical deconditioning; verbalizes preference for activities low in physical activity

Related Factors (r/t)

Deficient knowledge of health benefits of physical exercise; lack of training for accomplishment of physical exercise; lack of resources (time, money, companionship, facilities); lack of motivation; lack of interest

Client Outcomes

Client Will (Specify Time Frame):

- Engage in purposeful moderate-intensity cardiorespiratory (aerobic) exercise for 30 to 60 minutes per day on greater/equal to 5 days per week for a total of 2 hours and 30 minutes (150 minutes) per week.
- Increase exercise to 20 minutes per day (less than 150 minutes per week). Light to moderate intensity exercise may be beneficial in deconditioned persons.

• = Independent   ▲ = Collaborative

- Increase pedometer step counts by 1000 steps per day every 2 weeks to reach a daily step count of at least 7000 steps per day, with a daily goal for most healthy adults of 10,000 steps per day.
- Perform resistance exercises that involve all major muscle groups (legs, hips, back, chest, abdomen, shoulders, and arms) performed on 2 to 3 days per week.
- Perform flexibility exercise (stretching) for each of the major muscle-tendon groups 2 days per week for 10 to 60 seconds to improve joint range of motion; greatest gains occur with daily exercise.
- Engage in neuromotor exercise 20 to 30 minutes per day including motor skills (e.g., balance, agility, coordination, and gait), proprioceptive exercise training, and multifaceted activities (e.g., tai chi and yoga) to improve and maintain physical function and reduce falls in those at risk for falling (older persons).
- Meet mutually defined goals of exercise that include individual choice, preference and enjoyment in the exercise prescription

Nursing Interventions

- Observe the client for cause of sedentary lifestyle. Determine whether cause is physical, psychological, social, or ecological. See care plans for **Ineffective Coping** or **Hopelessness.**
- ▲ Assess for reasons why the client would be unable to participate in an exercise program; refer for evaluation by a primary care provider as needed.
- Use the Self-Efficacy for Exercise Scale and the Outcome Expectation for Exercise Scale to determine client's self-efficacy and outcome expectations toward exercise.
- Recommend the client enter an exercise program with a person who supports exercise behavior (e.g., friend or exercise buddy).
- Recommend using fitness smartphone applications for customizing, cueing, tracking, and analyzing an exercise program.
- Recommend the client begin a walking program using the following criteria:
  - Obtain a pedometer by purchase or from community/public health resources
  - Determine common times when brisk walking for at least 10-minute intervals can be incorporated into lifestyle and daily activities.

• = Independent   ▲ = Collaborative

- Set incremental walking goal and increase it by 1000 steps per day every 2 weeks for a minimum of 7000 steps per day with a daily goal for most healthy adults of 10,000 steps per day (approximately 5 miles).
- Toward the end of day, if have not met walking goal, look for opportunities to increase activity level (e.g., park further from destination; use stairs) or go for a walk indoors or outdoors until reach designated goal of 7000 to 10,000 steps per day.

• Recommend client begin performing resistance exercises for additional health benefits of increased bone strength and muscular fitness.

- Encourage prescriptive resistance exercise of each major muscle group (hips, thighs, legs, back, chest, shoulders, and abdomen) using a variety of exercise equipment such as free weights, bands, stair climbing, or machines 2 to 3 days per week. Involve the major muscle groups for 8 to 12 repetitions to improve strength and power in most adults; 10 to 15 repetitions to improve strength in middle-aged and older persons starting exercise; 15 to 20 repetitions to improve muscular endurance. Intensity should be between moderate (5 to 6) and hard (7 to 8) on a scale of 0 to 10
- Encourage to use a gradual progression of greater resistance, and/or more repetitions per set, and/or increasing frequency using concentric, eccentric, and isometric muscle actions. Perform bilateral and unilateral single and multiple joint exercises. Optimize exercise intensity by working large before small muscle groups, multiple joint exercises before single-joint exercises, and higher intensity before lower intensity exercises.

Pediatric

• Encourage child to increase the amount of walking done per day; if child is willing, ask him or her to wear a pedometer to measure number of steps.

• Recommend the child decrease television viewing, watching movies, and playing video games. Ask parents to limit television to 1 to 2 hours per day maximum.

• = Independent   ▲ = Collaborative

Geriatric

- Use valid and reliable criterion-referenced standards for fitness testing (e.g., Senior Fitness Test) designed for older adults that can predict the level of capacity associated with maintaining physical independence into later years of life (e.g., get up and go test).
- Recommend the client begin a regular exercise program, even if generally active.
▲ Refer the client to physical therapy for resistance exercise training as able involving all major muscle groups.
- Use the Function-Focused Care (FFC) rehabilitative philosophy of care with older adults in residential nursing facilities to prevent avoidable functional decline.
- Recommend the client begin a tai chi practice.
- If client is scheduled for an elective surgery that will result in admission into the intensive care unit (ICU) and immobility, or recovery from a joint replacement, for example, initiate a prehabilitation program that includes a warm-up followed by aerobic, strength, flexibility, neuromotor, and functional task work.

Home Care

- The preceding interventions may be adapted for home care use.
▲ Assess home environment for factors that create barriers to mobility. Refer to physical and occupational therapy services if needed to assist the client in restructuring home environment and daily living patterns. Use home safety assessment tool to prevent falls and improve mobility and function such as the tool found at http://agingresearch.buffalo.edu/hssat/index.htm.

Client/Family Teaching and Discharge Planning

- Work with the client using theory-based interventions (e.g., social cognitive theoretical components such as self-efficacy; transtheoretical model).
- Recommend the client use the Exercise Assessment and Screening for You (EASY) tool to help determine appropriate exercise for the older adult client. This tool is available online at http://www.easyforyou.info.
- Consider using motivational interviewing techniques when working with both children and adult clients to increase their activity.

• = Independent   ▲ = Collaborative

Readiness for enhanced Self-Care

NANDA-I Definition

A pattern of performing activities for oneself that helps to meet health-related goals and can be strengthened

Defining Characteristics

Expresses desire to enhance independence in maintaining health; expresses desire to enhance independence in maintaining life; expresses desire to enhance independence in maintaining personal development; expresses desire to enhance independence in maintaining well-being; expresses desire to enhance knowledge of strategies for self-care; expresses desire to enhance responsibility for self-care; expresses desire to enhance self-care

Client Outcomes

Client Will (Specify Time Frame):

- Evaluate current levels of self-care as optimum for abilities
- Express the need or desire to continue to enhance levels of self-care
- Seek health-related information as needed
- Identify strategies to enhance self-care
- Perform appropriate interventions as needed
- Monitor level of self-care
- Evaluate the effectiveness of self-care interventions at regular intervals

Nursing Interventions

- For assessment of self-care, use a valid and reliable screening tool if available for specific characteristics of the person, such as arthritis, diabetes, stroke, heart failure, or dementia.
- Conduct mutual goal setting with the person.
- Support the person's awareness that enhanced self-care is an achievable, desirable, and positive life goal.
- Show respect for the person, regardless of characteristics and/or background.
- Promote trust and enhanced communication between the person and health care providers.

• = Independent ▲ = Collaborative

- Promote opportunities for spiritual care and growth.
- Promote social support through facilitation of family involvement.
- Provide opportunities for ongoing group support through establishment of self-help groups on the Internet.
- Help the person identify and reduce the barriers to self-care.
- Provide literacy-appropriate education for self-care activities.
- Facilitate self-efficacy by ensuring the adequacy of self-care education.
- Conduct demonstrations and evaluate return demonstrations of self-care procedures such as use of an inhaler for asthma.
- Provide alternative mind-body therapies such as reiki, guided imagery, yoga, and self-hypnosis.
- Promote the person's hope to maintain self-care.

Pediatric

- Assess and evaluate a child's level of self-care and adjust strategies as needed.
- Assist families to engage in and maintain social support networks.
- Encourage activities that support or enhance spiritual care.

Multicultural

- Identify cultural beliefs, values, lifestyle practices, and problem-solving strategies when assessing the client's level of self-care.
- Enhance cultural knowledge by seeking out information regarding different cultural or ethnic groups.
- Recognize the impact of culture on self-care behaviors.
- Provide culturally competent care.
- Support independent self-care activities.

Home Care

- The nursing interventions described previously may also be used in home care settings.
- Support the new sense of self that may occur with complex health problems.
- Assist individuals and families to prevent exacerbations of chronic illness symptoms so rehospitalization is not necessary.

● = Independent ▲ = Collaborative

- In complex chronic illnesses such as heart failure, help individuals and families to accept continued functional disabilities and work toward maintenance of optimum functional status, considering the reality of illness status.
- Use educational guidelines for stroke survivors.
- Ensure appropriate interdisciplinary communication to support client safety.
- Enhance individual and family coping with chronic illnesses.
- Implement a community care management program

Client/Family Teaching and Discharge Planning

- Teach clients how to regularly assess their level of self-care.
- Instruct clients that a variety of interventions may be needed to enhance self-care.
- Help clients to understand that enhanced self-care is an achievable goal.
- Empower clients.
- Teach clients about the decision-making process and self-care activities needed to manage their illness state and promote well-being.
- Continuously stress that all self-care activities must be regularly evaluated to ensure that enhanced levels of self-care can be maintained.

Bathing Self-Care deficit

NANDA-I Definition

Impaired ability to perform or complete bathing/hygiene activities for self

Defining Characteristics

Inability to access bathroom; inability to dry body; inability to get bath supplies; inability to obtain water source; inability to regulate bath water; inability to wash body

Related Factors (r/t)

Cognitive impairment; decreased motivation; environmental barriers; inability to perceive body part; inability to perceive spatial relationship;

• = Independent   ▲ = Collaborative

musculoskeletal impairment; neuromuscular impairment; pain; perceptual impairment; severe anxiety; weakness

NOTE: Specify level of independence using a standardized functional scale.

Client Outcomes

Client Will (Specify Time Frame):

* Remain free of body odor and maintain intact skin
* State satisfaction with ability to use adaptive devices to bathe
* Use methods to bathe safely with minimal difficulty
* Bathe with assistance of caregiver as needed and report satisfaction, and dignity maintained during bathing experience
* Bathe with assistance of caregiver as needed without exhibiting defensive (aggressive) behaviors

Nursing Interventions

* QSEN (Safety): Warm bathing area above 25.1° C (77.18° F) while bathing, especially on cold days.
* QSEN (Safety): Consider using chlorhexidine-impregnated cloths rather than soap and water for daily client bathing.
* QSEN (Safety): Consider using a prepackaged bath, especially for high-risk clients (elderly, immunocompromised, invasive procedures, wounds, catheters, drains), to avoid client exposure to pathogens from contaminated bath basin, water source, and release of skin flora into bath water.
* Establish the goal of client's bathing as being a pleasant experience, especially for cognitively impaired clients, without the symptoms of unmet needs—hitting, biting, kicking, screaming, resisting—and plan for client preferences in timing, type and length of bathing, water temperature, and with silence or music.
* QSEN (Patient-Centered): Role model and teach the sequence of behaviors for client-centered care: greet client, orient client to task, offer client choices and input, converse with client, and exhibit interest in client and convey approval of client as a person.
* QSEN (Patient-Centered): Use client-centered bathing interventions: plan for client's comfort and bathing preferences, show respect in communications, critically think to solve issues that arise, and use a gentle approach.

● = Independent   ▲ = Collaborative

- Provide a 41° C footbath for 40 minutes before bedtime.
▲ Provide pain relief measures, such as ice packs, heat, and analgesics for sore joints 45 minutes before bathing; move extremities slowly and carefully; and inform the client before movements associated with pain occur (walking; transferring to a new location; moving joints; and washing genitals, face, and between toes and under arms). Have the client wash painful areas, recognize indicators of pain, and apologize for any pain caused.
- Consider environmental and human factors that may limit bathing ability, such as bending to get into the tub, reaching for bathing items, grasping faucets, and lifting oneself. Adapt environment by placing items within easy reach, installing grab bars, lowering faucets, and using a handheld shower.
- Use a comfortable padded shower chair with foot support, or adapt a chair: pad it with towels/washcloths, cover the cold back with dry towels, and cover the arms with foam pipe insulation.
- Ensure that bathing assistance preserves client dignity through use of privacy with a traffic-free bathing area and posted privacy signs, timeliness of personal care, and conveyance of honor and recognition of the deservedness of respect and esteem of all persons.
- QSEN (Safety): If the client is bathing alone, place the assistance call light within reach.
- For cognitively impaired clients, avoid upsetting factors associated with bathing: instead of using the terms *bath*, *shower*, or *wash*, use comforting words, such as *warm*, *relaxing*, or *massage*. Start at the client's feet and bathe upward; bathe the face last after washing hands and using a clean cloth. Use a beautician/barber or wash hair at another time to avoid water dripping in the face.
- Use towel bathing to bathe client in bed, a bath blanket, and warm towels to keep the client covered the entire time. Warm and moisten towels/washcloths and place in plastic bags to keep them warm. Use the towels to massage large areas (front, back) and one washcloth for facial areas and another one for genital areas. No rinsing or drying is needed as is commonly thought for bathing.

- QSEN (Patient-Centered): For shower bathing: use client-centered techniques, keep client covered with towels and cleanse under the towels, use no-rinse products, use favorite bathing items, and use a handheld shower with adjustable spray.

Geriatric

- QSEN (Patient-Centered): Assess older clients' preferences for bathing and their responses to bathing difficulties.
- Design the bathing environment for comfort: **Visual.** Reduce clutter and use partitions to hide equipment storage. Laminate and put artwork or decorative objects in bather's view, or place cue cards to bathing process (wall, ceiling, shower). Stand or sit in bather's position to experience what he/she sees. Decrease glare from tiles, white walls, and artificial lights. Use contrasting colors and soft but adequate lighting on a dimming switch for adjustment.
- Arrange the bathing environment to promote sensory comfort: **Auditory.** Reduce noise of voices and water. Do not allow traffic into bathing room. Add fabric to absorb sound (three to four times the width of the opening for sound-absorbing folds). Play soft music.
- Design the bathing environment for comfort: **Tactile.** Use heat lamps or radiant heat panels to keep the room warm. Use powder-coated grab bars in decorative colors with nonslip grip. Provide a soft rug to stand on. Ensure that flooring is not slippery (a high coefficient of friction, ideally above 80, is desired and obtained through flooring coatings).
- When bathing a cognitively impaired client, have all bathing items ready for the client's needs before bathing begins.
- Train caregivers bathing clients with dementia to avoid behaviors that can trigger assault: confrontational communication, invalidation of the resident's feelings, failure to prepare a resident for a task, initiating shower spray or touch during bathing without verbal prompts beforehand, washing the hair/face, speaking disrespectfully to the client, and hurrying the pace of the bath.
- QSEN (Safety): Test water temperature before use with a thermometer to prevent scalding.
- Use a prepackaged bath for older adults to prevent skin dryness.

S

• = Independent   ▲ = Collaborative

- Focus on the abilities of the client with dementia to obtain client's participation in bathing.
- Encourage client to perform bathing tasks and allow adequate time for performance of tasks.

Multicultural

- QSEN (Patient-Centered): Ask the client for input on bathing habits and cultural bathing preferences.

Home Care

- If in a typical bathing setting for the client, assess the client's ability to bathe self via direct observation using physical performance tests for ADLs.
- ▲ Request referrals for occupational therapy for clients who have experienced a stroke.
- ▲ Based on functional assessment and rehabilitation capacity, refer for home health aide services to assist with bathing and hygiene.
- QSEN (Safety): Turn down temperature of water heater and recommend use of a water temperature–sensing shower valve to prevent scalding.

Client/Family Teaching and Discharge Planning

- Teach the client and family a client-centered bathing routine that includes a frequency schedule, privacy, skin inspection, no-rinse products, skin lubricants, chill prevention, bathing options such as sponge or towel, and safety methods such as checking water temperature.

Dressing Self-Care deficit

NANDA-I Definition

Impaired ability to perform or complete dressing activities for self

Defining Characteristics

Impaired ability to fasten clothing; impaired ability to obtain clothing; impaired ability to put on necessary items of clothing; impaired ability to put on shoes; impaired ability to put on socks; impaired ability to take off necessary items of clothing; impaired ability to take off shoes; impaired ability to take off socks; inability to choose clothing; inability to maintain appearance at a satisfactory level; inability to pick up clothing; inability to put clothing on lower body; inability to put clothing on upper body; inability to put on shoes; inability to put on socks; inability to remove clothes; inability to remove shoes; inability to remove socks; inability to use assistive devices; inability to use zippers

Related Factors (r/t)

Cognitive impairment; decreased motivation; discomfort; environmental barriers; fatigue; musculoskeletal impairment; neuromuscular impairment; pain; perceptual impairment; severe anxiety; weakness

Note: Specify level of independence using a standardized functional scale.

Client Outcomes

Client Will (Specify Time Frame):

- Dress and groom self to optimal potential
- Use assistive technology to dress and groom
- Explain and use methods to enhance strengths during dressing and grooming
- Dress and groom with assistance of caregiver as needed

Nursing Interventions

- Assess a client's range of movement, upper limb strength, balance, coordination, functional grip, dexterity, sensation, and ability to detect limb position.
- ▲ Provide pain medication 45 minutes before dressing and grooming as needed.
- Select adaptive clothing: loose clothing; elastic waistbands and cuffs; square, large arm holes; no seam lines; dresses that open down the back and short coats (for wheelchair users); Velcro fasteners; larger or magnetic buttons; zipper pulls for grasping; and for drooling, absorbent scarves that can be easily changed.
- For clients with limited arm and shoulder movement, use clothing that fastens at the front, such as for blouses, bras, and shirts.
- QSEN (Safety): Allow client with poor balance or postural hypotension to sit rather than stand when dressing, for safety.

● = Independent ▲ = Collaborative

- Dress the affected side first, then the unaffected side; undressing the affected side is done last.
- Use adaptive dressing and grooming equipment as needed (e.g., long-handled brushes, long grasping devices, button hooks, elastic shoelaces, Velcro shoes, soap-on-a-rope, suction holders).
- For clients with a fine hand tremor, use weighted handles on grooming items or stabilize the client's arm on a table; for a weak or painful grip, use lightweight, large-grip handles.
- Maintain individuality with hairstyle, jewelry, and clothing.

Geriatric

- QSEN (Patient-Centered): Determine the client's personal preferences for dressing and grooming by using the Self-maintenance Habits and Preferences in Elderly (SHAPE) questionnaire and focus on items most preferred by the client.
- Assist residents with goal setting and their highest ADL performance level rather than providing the care for them.
- Ensure clients can see clothing to select what to wear by administering annual vision testing and having client wear clean glasses.
- Consider individualized smart machine-based prompting for dressing task completion for dementia clients.
- Use clocks, routines, and explanations for the client with dementia to convey that it is morning and time to get ready for the day's activities by dressing.
- Lay clothing out (with label in back facing up) in the order that it will be put on by the client, either one item at a time or in piles with first item on top of pile (dress bottom half first: underwear, then slacks, socks; then dress top half: bra, shirt, sweater).
- ▲ Request referral for physical therapy.

Multicultural

- Consider use of assistive technology versus personal care assistance for Native Americans.

Home Care

- ▲ Involve the client in planning of informal care and provide access to health professionals and financial support for the care.

● = Independent   ▲ = Collaborative

Client/Family Teaching and Discharge Planning

- Teach caregivers to see dressing as an opportunity to promote independence and a better quality of life for clients who are able, and as a time to increase social talk for others.
- ▲ Consider referral for use of assistive technology to prompt independent learning of self-care skills such as dressing.

Feeding Self-Care deficit

NANDA-I Definition

Impaired ability to perform or complete self-feeding activities

Defining Characteristics

Inability to bring food from a receptacle to the mouth; inability to chew food; inability to complete a meal; inability to get food onto utensil; inability to handle utensils; inability to ingest food in a socially acceptable manner; inability to ingest food safely; inability to ingest sufficient food; inability to manipulate food in mouth; inability to open containers; inability to pick up cup or glass; inability to prepare food for ingestion; inability to swallow food; inability to use assistive device

Related Factors (r/t)

Cognitive impairment; decreased motivation; discomfort; environmental barriers; fatigue; musculoskeletal impairment; neuromuscular impairment; pain; perceptual impairment; severe anxiety; weakness

NOTE: Specify level of independence using a standardized functional scale.

Client Outcomes

Client Will (Specify Time Frame):

- Feed self safely
- State satisfaction with ability to use adaptive devices for feeding
- Use assistance with feeding when necessary (caregiver)

Nursing Interventions

- QSEN (Safety): Assess for choking and swallowing risk for clients with learning disability and note condition of teeth, medication side effects, and abnormal eating behaviors.
- ▲ QSEN (Safety): Consult speech-language therapist to assess swallowing and identify safe feeding plan for client with a stroke.
- QSEN (Safety): Consider assessment of ICU and stepdown clients' readiness for an oral diet with a 3-oz water swallow challenge by a trained provider.
- QSEN (Patient-Centered): Individualize assisted feeding for those who are completely dependent.
- QSEN (Teamwork and Collaboration): Give priority to continuity in the cooperation between the parties involved in assisted feeding for those who are completely dependent.
- QSEN (Patient-Centered): Consult client on the benefit or desire to use assistive devices for feeding.
- QSEN (Safety): Presentation of feeding: provide 1 teaspoon of solid food or 10 to 15 mL of liquid at a time; wait until client has swallowed prior food/liquid.
- QSEN (Safety): Individualize nutritional plan to promote a positive mealtime experience for clients after surgical and radiotherapy treatment for tongue cancer.
- QSEN (Patient-Centered): Assist clients with cancer to plan self-care strategies to promote control (choosing foods), self-worth (food value for survival), and positive relationships (family meal interactions), and use distraction (humor) to manage eating problems.
- QSEN (Safety): Ensure oral care is provided to all clients regardless of type of feeding.

Geriatric

- QSEN (Patient-Centered): Obtain and incorporate the client's view of the agency's food selection and presentation into agency food service.
- QSEN (Patient-Centered): Assess the ability of clients with dementia to self-feed, and supervise the feeding of those with moderate dependency by providing verbal or physical assistance.
- QSEN (Patient-Centered): Use the Edinburgh Feeding Evaluation in Dementia scale to assess eating and feeding problems in clients with late-stage dementia.

● = Independent   ▲ = Collaborative

- QSEN (Patient-Centered): Consider "comfort-only feeding" for clients with dementia using careful hand feeding.
- QSEN (Patient-Centered): Allow a resident an average of 42 minutes of staff time per meal and 13 minutes per between-meal snack to improve oral intake.
- QSEN (Patient-Centered): Promote family visits at mealtimes for clients with dementia to encourage eating.
- QSEN (Patient-Centered): Play familiar music during meals for clients with Alzheimer's disease.
- Use aromatherapy with the smell of baking bread for those with dementia.
▲ QSEN (Safety): Provide targeted feeding with trained feeding assistants to older clients with dysphagia who are on texture modified diets.
▲ QSEN (Safety): Provide CNAs with information on techniques to feed clients with dementia.
- QSEN (Patient-Centered): Provide individualized dining experience for those with dementia through consistent routine, such as same seat placed for limited distractions, preferred dining companions, presentation of one food item at a time, use of a Plexiglas barrier around place setting to prevent reaching.

Multicultural

- QSEN (Patient-Centered): For those who use chopsticks with impaired hand function, suggest adapted chopsticks.
- Avoid wasting food with those of Chinese culture.

Home Care

▲ QSEN (Teamwork and Collaboration): Request referral for occupational therapy to provide client and caregiver support with feeding.

Client/Family Teaching and Discharge Planning

- QSEN (Patient-Centered): Provide clients with nutritional food tasting samples and recipes.
- QSEN (Patient-Centered): Educate family members about the benefits of hand feeding as long as possible, and the risks versus benefits of tube feeding for clients with dementia.

• = Independent   ▲ = Collaborative

Toileting Self-Care deficit

NANDA-I Definition

Impaired ability to perform or complete toileting activities for self

Defining Characteristics

Inability to carry out proper toilet hygiene; inability to flush toilet or commode; inability to get to toilet or commode; inability to manipulate clothing for toileting; inability to rise from toilet or commode; inability to sit on toilet or commode

Related Factors (r/t)

Cognitive impairment; decreased motivation; environmental barriers; fatigue; impaired mobility status; impaired transfer ability; musculoskeletal impairment; neuromuscular impairment; pain; perceptual impairment; severe anxiety; weakness

Client Outcomes

Client Will (Specify Time Frame):

- Remain free of incontinence and impaction with no urine or stool on skin
- State satisfaction with ability to use adaptive devices for toileting
- Explain and use methods to be safe and independent in toileting

Nursing Interventions

- QSEN (Patient-Centered): Assess client's usual toileting patterns and preferences, and factors contributing to impaired toileting leading to constipation or urinary incontinence.
- QSEN (Patient-Centered): Ask client to participate in recovery preference exploration (RPE) to assist in defining client's recovery preferences and treatment goals.
- QSEN (Patient-Centered): Before use of a bedpan, discuss its use with clients.
- QSEN (Patient-Centered): Use necessary assistive toileting equipment (e.g., raised toilet seat, bedside commode, suction mats, spill-proof urinals, support rails next to toilet, toilet safety frames, female urinal, fracture bedpans, long-handled toilet paper holders).

● = Independent   ▲ = Collaborative

- QSEN (Patient-Centered): Assess client's prior use of incontinence briefs and avoid use for hospitalized continent but limited mobility client.
- QSEN (Safety): Make assistance call button readily available to the client and answer call light promptly.
- QSEN (Safety): Provide folding commode chairs in patient bathrooms.

Geriatric

- QSEN (Patient-Centered): For residents who show occasional/frequent bowel/bladder incontinence on the Minimum Data Set, plan an individualized toileting schedule.
- QSEN (Patient-Centered): Assess the client's functional ability to manipulate clothing for toileting, and if necessary modify clothing with Velcro fasteners, elastic waists, dropfront underwear, or slacks.
- QSEN (Safety): Avoid the use of indwelling catheters if possible, and use condom catheters in men without dementia.
- QSEN (Patient-Centered): Provide clients with dementia access to regular exercise.

Multicultural

- QSEN (Patient-Centered): Remove barriers to toileting, support client's cultural beliefs, and preserve dignity.

Home Care

- ▲ QSEN (Teamwork and Collaboration): Request referral for home physical therapy when client is recovering from illness or surgery.
- QSEN (Patient-Centered): To design a bathroom for an older adult, consider adaptable bath fixtures/furniture and safety needs.

Client/Family Teaching and Discharge Planning

- Teach client and family to wash hands after toileting.
- Have the family install a toilet seat of a contrasting color.

• = Independent   ▲ = Collaborative

Readiness for enhanced Self-Concept

NANDA-I Definition

A pattern of perceptions or ideas about the self that is sufficient for well-being and can be strengthened

Defining Characteristics

Accepts limitations; accepts strengths; actions are congruent with verbal expression; expresses confidence in abilities; expresses satisfaction with body image; expresses satisfaction with personal identity; expresses satisfaction with role performance; expresses satisfaction with sense of worthiness; expresses satisfaction with thoughts about self; expresses willingness to enhance self-concept

Client Outcomes

Client Will (Specify Time Frame):

- State willingness to enhance self-concept
- State satisfaction with thoughts about self, sense of worthiness, role performance, body image, and personal identity
- Demonstrate actions that are congruent with expressed feelings and thoughts
- State confidence in abilities
- Accept strengths and limitations

Nursing Interventions

- Assess and support activities that promote self-concept developmentally.
- Refer to nutritional and exercise programs to support weight loss.
- Refer clients to massage therapy as an adjunct treatment.
- Support establishing church-based community health promotion programs (CBHPPs) with the following key elements: partnerships, positive health values, availability of services, access to church facilities, community-focused interventions, health behavior change, and supportive social relationships.
- Offer client choices in clothing when client is hospitalized.
- ▲ Refer clients with history of childhood sexual abuse for intensive therapy that uses narrative life stories to promote positive sense of self.

● = Independent   ▲ = Collaborative

Pediatric

- Consider the development of a Healthy Kids Mentoring Program that has four components: (1) relationship building, (2) self-esteem enhancement, (3) goal setting, and (4) academic assistance (tutoring). Mentors met with students twice each week for 1 hour each session on school grounds. During each meeting, mentors devoted time to each program component.
- ▲ Assess and provide referrals to mental health professionals for clients with unresolved worries associated with terrorism.
- Provide an alternative school-based program for pregnant and parenting teenagers.

Geriatric

- Encourage clients to consider a web-based support program when they are in a caregiving situation.
- Encourage activity and a strength, mobility, balance, and endurance training program.
- Provide opportunities for clients to engage in life skills (themed collections of everyday items based upon general activities that residents may have previously carried out).
- Provide information on advance directives.

Multicultural

- Carefully assess each client and allow families to participate in providing care that is acceptable based on the client's cultural beliefs.
- Provide education and support for health-promoting behaviors and self-concept for clients from diverse cultures.
- Refer to the care plans **Disturbed Body Image, Readiness for enhanced Coping, Chronic low Self-Esteem,** and **Readiness for enhanced Spiritual Well-Being.**

Home Care

- Previously discussed interventions may be used in the home care setting.

• = Independent   ▲ = Collaborative

Chronic low Self-Esteem

NANDA-I Definition

Long-standing negative self-evaluating/feelings about self or self-capabilities

Defining Characteristics

Dependent on others' opinions; evaluation of self as unable to deal with events; exaggerates negative feedback about self; excessively seeks reassurance; frequent lack of success in life events; hesitant to try new situations; hesitant to try new things; indecisive behavior; lack of eye contact; nonassertive behavior; overly conforming; passive; rejects positive feedback about self; reports feelings of guilt; reports feelings of shame

Related Factors (r/t)

Ineffective adaptation to loss; lack of affection; lack of approval; lack of membership in group; perceived discrepancy between self and cultural norms; perceived discrepancy between self and spiritual norms; perceived lack of belonging; perceived lack of respect from others; psychiatric disorder; repeated failures; repeated negative reinforcement; traumatic event; traumatic situation

Client Outcomes

Client Will (Specify Time Frame):

- Demonstrate improved ability to interact with others (e.g., maintains eye contact, engages in conversation, expresses thoughts/feelings)
- Verbalize increased self-acceptance through positive self-statements about self
- Identify personal strengths, accomplishments, and values
- Identify and work on small, achievable goals
- Improve independent decision-making and problem-solving skills

• = Independent   ▲ = Collaborative

Nursing Interventions

- Actively listen to and respect the client.
- Assess the client's environmental and everyday stressors, including physical health concerns and the potential for abusive relationships.
- Assess existing strengths and coping abilities, and provide opportunities for their expression and recognition.
- Reinforce the personal strengths and positive self-perceptions that a client identifies.
- Identify client's negative self-assessments.
- Encourage realistic and achievable goal setting and resources and identify impediments to achievement.
- Demonstrate and promote effective communication techniques; spend time with the client.
- Encourage independent decision-making by reviewing options and their possible consequences with client.
- Assist client to challenge negative perceptions of self and performance.
- Use failure as an opportunity to provide valuable feedback.
- Promote maintaining a level of functioning in the community.
- Assist client with evaluating the effect of family and peer group on feelings of self-worth.
- Support socialization and communication skills.
- Encourage journal/diary writing as a safe way of expressing emotions.

Pediatric

▲ Provide bully prevention programs and include information on cyberbullying.

Geriatric

- Support client in identifying and adapting to functional changes.
- Use reminiscence therapy to identify patterns of strength and accomplishment.
- Encourage participation in peer group activities.
- Encourage activities in which a client can support/help others.

● = Independent   ▲ = Collaborative

Multicultural

- Assess for the influence of cultural beliefs, norms, and values on the client's sense of self-esteem.
- Assess socioeconomic issues.
- Validate the client's feelings regarding ethnic or racial identity.

Home Care

- Assess a client's immediate support system/family for relationship patterns and content of communication.
- ▲ Refer to medical social services to assist the family in pattern changes that could benefit the client.
- ▲ If a client is taking prescribed psychotropic medications, assess for knowledge of medication side effects and reasons for taking medication. Teach as necessary.
- ▲ Assess medications for effectiveness and side effects and monitor client for compliance.

Client/Family Teaching and Discharge Planning

- ▲ Refer to community agencies for psychotherapeutic counseling.
- ▲ Refer to psychoeducational groups on stress reduction and coping skills.
- ▲ Refer to self-help support groups specific to needs.

S

Situational low Self-Esteem

NANDA-I Definition

Development of a negative perception of self-worth in response to a current situation

Defining Characteristics

Evaluation of self as unable to deal with events; evaluation of self as unable to deal with situations; indecisive behavior; nonassertive behavior; reports current situational challenge to self-worth; reports helplessness; reports uselessness; self-negating verbalizations

• = Independent   ▲ = Collaborative

Related Factors (r/t)

Behavior inconsistent with values; developmental changes; disturbed body image; failures; functional impairment; lack of recognition; loss; rejections; social role changes

Client Outcomes

Client Will (Specify Time Frame):

- State effect of life events on feelings about self
- State personal strengths
- Acknowledge presence of guilt and not blame self if an action was related to another person's appraisal
- Seek help when necessary
- Demonstrate self-perceptions are accurate given physical capabilities
- Demonstrate separation of self-perceptions from societal stigmas

Nursing Interventions

▲ Assess the client for signs and symptoms of depression and potential for suicide and/or violence. If present, immediately notify the appropriate personnel of symptoms. See care plans for **Risk for other-directed Violence** and **Risk for Suicide.**

- Assess the client's environmental and everyday stressors, including evidence of abusive relationships.
- Assist in the identification of problems and situational factors that contribute to problems, offering options for resolution.
- Mutually identify strengths, resources, and previously effective coping strategies.
- Have client list strengths.
- Accept client's own pace in working through grief or crisis situations.
- Accept the client's own defenses in dealing with the crisis.
- Provide information about support groups of people who have common experiences or interests.
- Teach the client mindfulness techniques to cope more effectively with strong emotional responses.
- Support client's decisions in health care treatment.
- Encourage objective appraisal of self and life events and challenge negative or perfectionist expectations of self.

S

- Provide psychoeducation to client and family.
- Validate confusion when feeling ill but looking well.
- Acknowledge the presence of societal stigma. Teach management tools.
- Validate the effect of negative past experiences on self-esteem and work on corrective measures.
- See care plan for **Chronic low Self-Esteem.**

Geriatric and Multicultural

- See care plan for **Chronic low Self-Esteem.**

Home Care

- Establish an emergency plan and contract with the client for its use.
- Access supplies that support a client's success at independent living.
- See care plan for **Chronic low Self-Esteem.**

Client/Family Teaching and Discharge Planning

- Assess the person's support system (family, friends, and community) and involve them if desired.
- Educate client and family regarding the grief process.
- Teach client and family that the crisis is temporary.
- ▲ Refer to appropriate community resources or crisis intervention centers.
- ▲ Refer to resources for handicap and/or disability services.
- Refer to illness-specific consumer support groups.
- See care plan for **Chronic low Self-Esteem.**

Risk for chronic low Self-Esteem

NANDA-I Definition

At risk for long-standing negative self-evaluating/feelings about self or self-capabilities

Risk Factors

Ineffective adaptation to loss; lack of affection; lack of membership in group; perceived discrepancy between self and cultural norms; perceived

● = Independent ▲ = Collaborative

discrepancy between self and spiritual norms; perceived lack of belonging; perceived lack of respect from others; psychiatric disorder; repeated failures; repeated negative reinforcement; traumatic event; traumatic situation

Client Outcomes, Nursing Interventions, Client/Family Teaching and Discharge Planning

Refer to Care Plan **Chronic low Self-Esteem.**

Risk for situational low Self-Esteem

NANDA-I Definition

At risk for developing negative perception of self-worth in response to a current situation

Risk Factors

Behavior inconsistent with values; decreased control over environment; developmental changes; disturbed body image; failures; functional impairment; history of abandonment; history of abuse; history of learned helplessness; history of neglect; lack of recognition; loss; physical illness; rejections; social role changes; unrealistic self-expectations

Client Outcomes

Client Will (Specify Time Frame):
- State accurate self-appraisal
- Demonstrate the ability to self-validate
- Demonstrate the ability to make decisions independent of primary peer group
- Express effects of media on self-appraisal
- Express influence of substances on self-esteem
- Identify strengths and healthy coping skills
- State life events and change as influencing self-esteem

Nursing Interventions

- Identify environmental and/or developmental factors that increase risk for low self-esteem, especially in children/adolescents, to make needed referrals.
- Assess the client's previous experiences with health care and coping with illness to determine the level of education and support needed.
- Assess for low and negative affect (expression of feelings).

• = Independent   ▲ = Collaborative

- Encourage client to maintain highest level of community functioning.
- Treat the client with respect and as an equal to maintain positive self-esteem.
- Help the client to identify the resources and social support network available at this time. Encourage the client to find a self-help or therapy group that focuses on self-esteem enhancement.
- Encourage the client to create a sense of competence through short-term goal setting and goal achievement.
▲ Assess the client for symptoms of depression and anxiety. Refer to specialist as needed. Prompt and effective treatment can prevent exacerbation of symptoms or safety risks.
- See care plans for **Disturbed personal Identity, Situational low Self-Esteem,** and **Chronic low Self-Esteem.**

Pediatric

▲ Provide support for children who do not have supportive families, and provide a haven outside of the home.

Geriatric

- Support humor as a coping mechanism.
- Assist the client in life review and identifying positive accomplishments.
- Help client to establish a peer group and structured daily activities.
- See care plans for **Situational low Self-Esteem** and **Chronic low Self-Esteem.**

Home Care

- Assess current environmental stresses and identify community resources.
- Encourage family members to acknowledge and validate the client's strengths.
- Assess the need for establishing an emergency plan.
- See care plans for **Situational low Self-Esteem** and **Chronic low Self-Esteem.**

Client/Family Teaching and Discharge Planning

▲ Refer the client/family to community-based self-help and support groups.

● = Independent   ▲ = Collaborative

▲ Refer the client to educational classes on stress management, relaxation training, and so on.

▲ Refer the client to community agencies that offer support and environmental resources.

• See care plans for **Situational low Self-Esteem** and **Chronic low Self-Esteem.**

Ineffective Self-Health Management

NANDA-I Definition

Pattern of regulating and integrating into daily living a therapeutic regimen for treatment of illness and its sequelae that is unsatisfactory for meeting specific health goals

Defining Characteristics

Failure to include treatment regimens in daily living; failure to take action to reduce risk factors; ineffective choices in daily living for meeting health goals; reports desire to manage the illness; reports difficulty with prescribed regimens

Related Factors (r/t)

Complexity of health care system; complexity of therapeutic regimen; decisional conflicts; deficient knowledge; economic difficulties; excessive demands made (e.g., individual, family); family conflict; family patterns of health care; inadequate number of cues to action; perceived barriers; perceived benefits; perceived seriousness; perceived susceptibility; powerlessness; regimen; social support deficit

Client Outcomes

Client Will (Specify Time Frame):

• Describe daily food and fluid intake that meets therapeutic goals
• Describe activity/exercise patterns that meet therapeutic goals
• Describe scheduling of medications that meets therapeutic goals
• Verbalize ability to manage therapeutic regimens
• Collaborate with health providers to decide on a therapeutic regimen that is congruent with health goals and lifestyle

• = Independent ▲ = Collaborative

Nursing Interventions

NOTE: This diagnosis does not have the same meaning as the diagnosis **Noncompliance.** This diagnosis is made with the client, so if the client does not agree with the diagnosis, it should not be made. The emphasis is on helping the client direct his or her own life and health, not on the client's compliance with the provider's instructions.

- Establish a collaborative partnership with the client for purposes of meeting health-related goals.
- Listen to the person's story about his or her illness self-management.
- Explore the meaning of the person's illness experience and identify uncertainties and needs through open-ended questions.
- Help the client enhance self-efficacy or confidence in his or her own ability to manage the illness.
- Involve family members in knowledge development, planning for self-management, and shared decision-making.
- Review factors of the Health Belief Model (individual perceptions of seriousness and susceptibility, demographic and other modifying factors, and perceived benefits and barriers) with the client.
- Use various formats to provide information about the therapeutic regimen, including group education, brochures, videotapes, written instructions, computer-based programs, and telephone contact.
- Help the client identify and modify barriers to effective self-management.
- Help the client self-manage his or her own health through teaching about strategies for changing habits such as overeating, sedentary lifestyle, and smoking.
- Develop a contract with the client to maintain motivation for changes in behavior.
- Use focus groups to evaluate the implementation of self-management programs.
- Refer to the care plan **Ineffective family Therapeutic Regimen Management.**

• = Independent   ▲ = Collaborative

Geriatric

- Identify the reasons for actions that are not therapeutic and discuss alternatives.

Multicultural

- Assess the influence of cultural beliefs, norms, and values on the individual's perceptions of the therapeutic regimen.
- Discuss all strategies with the client in the context of the client's culture.
- Provide health information that is consistent with the health literacy of clients.
- Assess for barriers that may interfere with client follow-up of treatment recommendations.
- Use electronic monitoring to improve management of medications.
- Validate the client's feelings regarding the ability to manage his or her own care and the impact on current lifestyle.

Home Care

- Prepare and instruct clients and family members in the use of a medication box. Set up an appropriate schedule for filling of the medication box, and post medication times and doses in an accessible area (e.g., attached by a magnet to the refrigerator).
- Monitor self-management of the medical regimen.
- ▲ Refer to health care professionals for questions and self-care management.

Client/Family Teaching and Discharge Planning

- Identify what the client and/or family know and adjust teaching accordingly. Teach the client and family about all aspects of the therapeutic regimen, providing as much knowledge as the client and family will accept, in a culturally congruent manner.
- Teach ways to adjust ADLs for inclusion of therapeutic regimens.
- Teach safety in taking medications.
- Teach the client to act as a self-advocate with health providers who prescribe therapeutic regimens.

• = Independent   ▲ = Collaborative

Readiness for enhanced Self-Health Management

NANDA-I Definition

A pattern of regulating and integrating into daily living a therapeutic regimen for treatment of illness and its sequelae that is sufficient for meeting health-related goals and can be strengthened

Defining Characteristics

Choices of daily living are appropriate for meeting goals (e.g., treatment, prevention); describes reduction of risk factors; expresses desire to manage the illness (e.g., treatment, prevention of sequelae); expresses little difficulty with prescribed regimens; no unexpected acceleration of illness symptoms

Client Outcomes

Client Will (Specify Time Frame):

- Describe integration of therapeutic regimen into daily living
- Demonstrate continued commitment to integration of therapeutic regimen into daily living routines

Nursing Interventions

- Acknowledge the expertise that the client and family bring to self-health management.
- Review factors that contribute to the likelihood of health promotion and health protection. Use Pender's Health Promotion Model and Becker's Health Belief Model to identify contributing factors.
- Further develop and reinforce contributing factors that might change with ongoing management of the therapeutic regimen (e.g., knowledge, self-efficacy, self-esteem, and perceived benefits).
- Support all efforts to self-manage therapeutic regimens.
- Review the client's strengths in the management of the therapeutic regimen.
- Collaborate with the client to identify strategies to maintain strengths and develop additional strengths as indicated.
- Identify contributing factors that may need to be improved now or in the future.

● = Independent   ▲ = Collaborative

- Provide knowledge as needed related to the pathophysiology of the disease or illness, prescribed activities, prescribed medications, and nutrition.
- Support positive health-promotion and health-protection behaviors.
- Help the client maintain existing support and seek additional supports as needed.

Geriatric

- Facilitate the client and family to obtain health insurance and drug payment plans whenever needed and possible.

Multicultural

- Assess client's perspectives on self-management.
- Assess health literacy in clients of diverse backgrounds.
- Validate the client's feelings regarding the ability to manage his or her own care and the impact on current lifestyle.
- Facilitate the client and family to obtain health insurance and drug payment plans whenever needed and possible.
- Use electronic monitoring to improve medication adherence.
- Discuss with clients their beliefs about medication and treatment to enhance medication and treatment adherence.

Community Teaching

- Review therapeutic regimens and their optimal integration with daily living routines.
- Teach disease processes and therapeutic regimens for management of these disease processes. Suggest peer support groups for clients with schizophrenia.

Risk for Self-Mutilation

NANDA-I Definition

At risk for deliberate self-injurious behavior causing tissue damage with the intent of causing nonfatal injury to attain relief of tension

Risk Factors

Adolescence; autistic individuals; battered child; borderline personality disorders; character disorders; childhood illness; childhood sexual abuse; childhood surgery; depersonalization; developmentally delayed individuals; dissociation; disturbed body image; disturbed interpersonal relationships; eating disorders; emotional disorder; family divorce; family history of self-destructive behaviors; family substance abuse; feels threatened with loss of significant relationship; history of inability to plan solutions; history of inability to see long-term consequences; history of self-directed violence; impulsivity; inability to express tension verbally; inadequate coping; incarceration; irresistible urge for self-directed violence; isolation from peers; living in nontraditional setting (e.g., foster group, or institutional care); loss of control over problem-solving situations; loss of significant relationship(s); low self-esteem; mounting tension that is intolerable; need for quick reduction of stress; peers who self-mutilate; perfectionism; psychotic state (e.g., command hallucinations); reports negative feelings (e.g. depression, rejection, self-hatred, separation anxiety, guilt); sexual identity crisis; substance abuse; unstable self-esteem; use of manipulation to obtain nurturing relationship with others; violence between parental figures

Client Outcomes

Client Will (Specify Time Frame):

- Refrain from self-injury
- Identify triggers to self-mutilation
- State appropriate ways to cope with increased psychological or physiological tension
- Express feelings
- Seek help when having urges to self-mutilate
- Maintain self-control without supervision
- Use appropriate community agencies when caregivers are unable to attend to emotional needs

Nursing Interventions

NOTE: Before implementing interventions in the face of self-injury, nurses should examine their own emotional responses to incidents of self-injury to ensure that interventions will not be based on countertransference reactions.

- Assess client's ability to regulate his or her own emotional states.
- Assess client's degree of self-criticism and use of effective coping skills. Self-harm serves as a coping mechanism for clients.
- Assess client's perception of powerlessness. Refer to the care plan for **Powerlessness.**

• = Independent   ▲ = Collaborative

- Assessment data from the client and family members may have to be gathered at different times; allowing a family member or trusted friend with whom the client is comfortable to be present during the assessment may be helpful.
- Assess for risk factors of self-mutilation, including categories of psychiatric disorders (particularly borderline personality disorder, psychosis, eating disorders, autism); psychological precursors (e.g., low tolerance for stress, impulsivity, perfectionism); psychosocial dysfunction (e.g., presence of sexual abuse, divorce or alcoholism in the family, manipulative behavior to gain nurturing, chaotic interpersonal relationships); coping difficulties (e.g., inability to plan solutions or see long-term consequences of behavior); personal history (e.g., childhood illness or surgery, past self-injurious behavior); and peer influences (e.g., friends who mutilate, isolation from peers).
- Assess for co-occurring disorders that require response, specifically childhood abuse, substance abuse, and suicide attempts. Implement reporting or referral as indicated.
- Assess family dynamics and the need for family therapy and community supports.
- Assess for the presence of medical disorders, mental retardation, medication effects, or disorders such as autism that may include self-mutilation. Initiate referral for evaluation and treatment as appropriate.
- Be alert to other risk factors of self-mutilation in clients with psychosis, including acute intoxication, dramatic changes in body appearance, preoccupation with religion and sexuality, and anticipated or perceived object loss.
- Monitor the client's behavior closely, using engagement and support as elements of safety checks while avoiding intrusive overstimulation. Offer activities that will serve as a distraction.
- Assess the client's ability to enter into a no-suicide or no-self-harm contract. Secure a written or verbal contract from the client to notify staff when experiencing the desire to self-mutilate.
- Establish trust, listen to client, convey safety, and assist in developing positive goals for the future.
- ▲ Refer to mental health counseling. Multiple therapeutic modalities are available for treatment.

• = Independent   ▲ = Collaborative

- When working with self-mutilative clients who have borderline personality disorder, develop an effective therapeutic relationship by avoiding labeling, seeking to understand the meaning of the self-mutilation, and advocating for adequate opportunities for care.
- Maintain a consistent relational distance from the client with borderline personality disorder who self-mutilates: neither too close nor too distant, neither rewarding unacceptable behavior nor trying to control or avoid the client.
- Inform the client of expectations for appropriate behavior and consequences within the unit. Emphasize that the client must comply with the rules. Give positive reinforcement for compliance and minimize attention paid to disruptive behavior while setting limits.
- Clients need to learn to recognize distress as it occurs and express it verbally rather than as a physical action against the self.
- Assist the client to identify the motives/reasons for self-mutilation that have been perceived as positive. Self-harm serves as a defense mechanism.
- Help the client identify cues that precede impulsive behavior.
- Assist clients to identify ways to soothe themselves and generate hopefulness when faced with painful emotions.
- Reinforce alternative ways of dealing with depression and anxiety, such as exercise, engaging in unit activities, or talking about feelings.
- Keep the environment safe; remove all harmful objects from the area. Use of unbreakable glass is recommended for the client at risk for self-injury.
- Anticipate trigger situations and intervene to assist the client in applying alternatives to self-mutilation.
- If self-mutilation does occur, use a calm, nonpunitive approach. Whenever possible, assist the client to assume responsibility for consequences (e.g., dress self-inflicted wound). Refer to the care plan for **Self-Mutilation.**
- If the client is unable to control self-mutilation behavior, provide interactive supervision, not isolation.
- Involve the client in planning his or her care and problem solving, and emphasize that the client makes choices.

• = Independent   ▲ = Collaborative

▲ Use group therapy to exchange information about methods of coping with loneliness, self-destructive impulses, and interpersonal relationships as well as housing, employment, and health care system issues directly and do not interpret.

• Internet groups may provide additional support.

▲ Refer to protective services if evidence of abuse exists.

• Refer to the care plan for **Self-Mutilation.**

Pediatric

• The same dynamics described previously apply to adolescents.

• Conduct a thorough physical examination, being alert for superficial scars that may be patterned, although in most cases scabbing or infection is not evident. This should be done also with children and adolescents who have a chronic medical condition.

• Maintaining a therapeutic relationship with teens requires explicit assurances of confidentiality, consistency of clinical routines, and a nonjudgmental communication style.

• Attend to behavioral clues of self-mutilation; a brief self-report assessment can be useful.

• Encourage expression of painful experiences and provide supportive counseling.

• Multiple treatment modalities may be used in addressing the themes of young people who self-harm.

• Teaching coping skills can be an important intervention for adolescents.

• Assess for the presence of an eating disorder or substance abuse. Attend to the themes that preoccupy teens with eating disorders who self-mutilate.

• Evaluate for suicidal ideation/suicide risk. Refer to the care plan for **Risk for Suicide** for additional information.

• Be aware that there is not complete overlap between self-mutilation and suicidal behavior. The motivation may be different (coping with difficult feelings rather than ending life), and the method is usually different.

• Use treatment approaches detailed previously, with modifications as appropriate for this age group.

S

• = Independent   ▲ = Collaborative

Geriatric

- Provide hand or back rubs and calming music when elderly clients experience anxiety.
- Provide soft objects for elderly clients to hold and manipulate when self-mutilation occurs as a function of delirium or dementia. Apply mitts, splints, helmets, or restraints as appropriate.
- Older adults who show self-destructive behaviors should be evaluated for dementia.

Home Care

- Communicate degree of risk to family/caregivers; assess the family and caregiving situation for ability to protect the client and to understand the client's self-mutilative behavior. Provide family and caregivers with guidelines on how to manage self-harm behaviors in the home environment.
- Establish an emergency plan, including when to use hotlines and 911. Develop a contract with the client and family for use of the emergency plan. Role-play access to the emergency resources with the client and caregivers.
- Assess the home environment for harmful objects. Have family remove or lock objects as able.
- ▲ If client behaviors intensify, institute an emergency plan for mental health intervention.
- ▲ Refer for homemaker or psychiatric home health care services for respite, client reassurance, and implementation of therapeutic regimen.
- ▲ If the client is on psychotropic medications, assess client and family knowledge of medication administration and side effects.
- ▲ Evaluate the effectiveness and side effects of medications.

Client/Family Teaching and Discharge Planning

- Explain all relevant symptoms, procedures, treatments, and expected outcomes for self-mutilation that is illness based (e.g., borderline personality disorder, autism).
- Assist family members to understand the complex issues of self-mutilation. Provide instruction on relevant developmental issues and on actions parents can take to avoid media that glorify self-harm behaviors.

• = Independent   ▲ = Collaborative

- Provide written instructions for treatments and procedures for which the client will be responsible.
- Instruct the client in coping strategies (assertiveness training, impulse control training, deep breathing, progressive muscle relaxation).
- Role play (e.g., say, "Tell me how you will respond if someone ignores you").
- Teach cognitive-behavioral activities, such as active problem solving, reframing (reappraising the situation from a different perspective), or thought-stopping (in response to a negative thought, picture a large stop sign and replace the image with a prearranged positive alternative). Teach the client to confront his or her own negative thought patterns (or cognitive distortions), such as catastrophizing (expecting the very worst), dichotomous thinking (perceiving events in only one of two opposite categories), or magnification (placing distorted emphasis on a single event).
▲ Provide the client and family with phone numbers of appropriate community agencies for therapy and counseling.
▲ Give the client positive things on which to focus by referring to appropriate agencies for job-training skills or education.

Self-Mutilation

NANDA-I Definition

Deliberate self-injurious behavior causing tissue damage with the intent of causing nonfatal injury to attain relief of tension

Defining Characteristics

Abrading; biting; constricting a body part; cuts on body; hitting; ingestion of harmful substances; inhalation of harmful substances; insertion of object into body orifice; picking at wounds; scratches on body; self-inflicted burns; severing

Related Factors (r/t)

Adolescence; autistic individual; battered child; borderline personality disorder; character disorder; childhood illness; childhood sexual abuse; childhood surgery; depersonalization; developmentally delayed

● = Independent   ▲ = Collaborative

individual; dissociation; disturbed body image; disturbed interpersonal relationships; eating disorders; emotional disorder; family divorce; family history of self-destructive behaviors; family substance abuse; feels threatened with loss of significant relationship; history of inability to plan solutions; history of inability to see long-term consequences; history of self-directed violence; impulsivity; inability to express tension verbally; incarceration; ineffective coping; irresistible urge to cut self; irresistible urge for self-directed violence; isolation from peers; labile behavior; lack of family confidant; living in nontraditional setting (e.g., foster, group institutional care); low self-esteem; mounting tension that is intolerable; needs quick reduction of stress; peers who self-mutilate; perfectionism; poor communication between parent and adolescent; psychotic state (e.g., command hallucinations); report negative feelings (e.g., depression, rejection, self-hatred, separation anxiety, guilt, depersonalization); sexual identity crisis; substance abuse; unstable body image; unstable self-esteem; use of manipulation to obtain nurturing relationship with others; violence between parental figures

Client Outcomes

Client Will (Specify Time Frame):

- Have injuries treated
- Refrain from further self-injury
- State appropriate ways to cope with increased psychological or physiological tension
- Express feelings
- Seek help when having urges to self-mutilate
- Maintain self-control without supervision
- Use appropriate community agencies when caregivers are unable to attend to emotional needs

Nursing Interventions

NOTE: Before implementing interventions in the face of self-mutilation, nurses should examine their own emotional responses to incidents of self-harm to ensure that interventions will not be based on countertransference reactions.

▲ Provide medical treatment for injuries. Use careful aseptic technique when caring for wounds. Care for the wounds in a matter-of-fact manner.
- Assess for risk of suicide or other self-damaging behaviors. Refer to the care plan for **Risk for Suicide.**

• = Independent   ▲ = Collaborative

- Assess for signs of psychiatric disorders, including depression, anxiety, borderline personality disorder, dissociative disorders, eating disorders, and impulsivity.
- Assess for presence of hallucinations. Ask specific questions such as, "Do you hear voices that other people do not hear? Are they telling you to hurt yourself?"
▲ Assure the client that he or she will be safe during hallucinations, and engage supportively. Provide referrals for medication.
▲ Assess for the presence of medical disorders, mental retardation, medication effects, or disorders such as autism that may include self-mutilation. Initiate referral for evaluation and treatment as appropriate.
▲ Case finding and referral by school nurses for psychological or psychiatric treatment is critical.
- Monitor the client's behavior closely, using engagement and support as elements of safety checks while avoiding intrusive overstimulation.
- Establish trust, listen to client, convey safety, and assist in developing positive goals for the future.
- Recognize that self-mutilation may serve a variety of functions for the person.
- Assess the client's ability to enter into a no-suicide or no-self-harm contract. Secure a written or verbal contract from the client to notify staff when experiencing the desire to self-mutilate.
▲ Use a collaborative approach for care.
- Refer to the care plan for **Risk for Self-Mutilation** for additional information.

Home Care and Client/Family Teaching and Discharge Planning

- See the care plan for **Risk for Self-Mutilation**.

● = Independent ▲ = Collaborative

Self-Neglect

NANDA-I Definition

A constellation of culturally framed behaviors involving one or more self-care activities in which there is a failure to maintain a socially accepted standard of health and well-being

Defining Characteristics

Inadequate environmental hygiene; inadequate personal hygiene; non-adherence to health activities

Related Factors (r/t)

Capgras syndrome; cognitive impairment (e.g., dementia); depression; executive processing ability; fear of institutionalization; frontal lobe dysfunction; functional impairment; learning disability; lifestyle choice; maintaining control; major life stressor; malingering; obsessive-compulsive disorder; paranoid personality disorders; schizotypal personality disorders; substance abuse

Client Outcomes

Client Will (Specify Time Frame):
- Show improvement in mental health problems
- Show improvement in chronic medical problems
- Reveal improvement in cognition (e.g., if reversible and treatable)
- Demonstrate improvement in functional status (e.g., basic and instrumental activities of daily living)
- Demonstrate adherence to health activities
- Exhibit improved personal hygiene
- Exhibit improved environmental hygiene
- Have fewer hospitalizations and emergency room visits
- Increase safety of client
- Increase safety of community in which client lives
- Agree to necessary personal and environmental changes that eliminate risk/endangerment to self or others (i.e., neighbors)

NOTE: Because self-neglect is a culturally framed and socially defined phenomenon, change in a client's status must occur in such a way that it respects individual rights while ensuring individual health and well-being. This is accomplished through client-nurse partnership, but in some instances, assistance of next of kin and/or

● = Independent   ▲ = Collaborative

adult protective services may be needed (e.g., a state agency or local social services program).

Nursing Interventions

- Monitor individuals with acute or chronic mental and complex physical illness for defining characteristics for self-neglect.
- Assist individuals with complex mental and physical health issues to adopt positive health behaviors so that they may maintain their health status.
- Assess persons with complex health issues for adequate coping abilities, and assist those with coping problems to maintain their health and well-being in the community.
- Assist individuals whose self-care is failing with managing their medication regimen.
- Assess individuals with failing self-care for noncompliance (i.e., diagnostic testing, medication regimen, therapeutic regimen, and safety precautions).
- Assist persons with self-care deficits due to ADL or IADL impairments.
- Assess persons with failing self-care for changes in cognitive function (i.e., dementia or delirium).
- ▲ Refer persons with failing self-care to appropriate specialists (i.e., psychologist, psychiatrist, social work) and therapists (i.e., physical therapy, occupational therapy, etc.).
- Utilize behavioral modification as appropriate to bring about client changes that lead to improvement in personal hygiene, environmental hygiene, and adherence to medical regimen.
- Monitor persons with substance abuse problems (i.e., drugs, alcohol, smoking) for adequate safety.
- ▲ Refer persons with failing self-care who are significantly impaired cognitively or functionally and who are suspected victims of abuse to APS.
- Monitor clients with changes in cognitive function for adequate safety.
- Monitor clients with functional impairments for adequate safety.
- Assist individuals with complex mental and physical health needs with maintaining their health and well-being in the community.

• = Independent   ▲ = Collaborative

Geriatric

▲ Assess client's socioeconomic status and refer for appropriate support.

▲ Refer persons demonstrating a significant decline in self-care abilities (i.e., posing a threat to themselves or to their community) for evaluation of capacity and executive function.

▲ Obtain the assistance of APS in the case of refusal of professional health care services when there is a clear indication of self-endangerment.

Multicultural

• Deliver health care that is sensitive to the culture and philosophy of individuals whose self-care appears inadequate.

• Awareness that racial differences for self-neglect may exist, putting some older adults more at risk than others.

Sexual Dysfunction

S **NANDA-I** Definition

The state in which an individual experiences a change in sexual function during the sexual response phases of desire, excitation, and/or orgasm, which is viewed as unsatisfying, unrewarding, or inadequate

Defining Characteristics

Actual limitations imposed by disease; actual limitations imposed by therapy; alterations in achieving perceived sex role; alterations in achieving sexual satisfaction; change of interest in others; change of interest in self; inability to achieve desired satisfaction; perceived alteration in sexual excitation; perceived deficiency of sexual desire; perceived limitations imposed by disease; perceived limitations imposed by therapy; seeking confirmation of desirability; verbalization of problem

Related Factors (r/t)

Absent role models; altered body function (e.g., pregnancy, recent childbirth, drugs, surgery, anomalies, disease process, trauma, radiation); altered body structure (e.g., pregnancy, recent childbirth, surgery, anomalies, disease process, trauma, radiation); biopsychosocial alteration of sexuality; deficient knowledge; ineffectual role models; lack of privacy; lack of significant other; misinformation; physical abuse; psychosocial abuse (e.g., harmful relationships); values conflict; vulnerability

Client Outcomes

Client Will (Specify Time Frame):

- Identify individual cause of sexual dysfunction
- Identify stressors that contribute to dysfunction
- Discuss alternative, satisfying, and acceptable sexual practices for self and partner
- Identify the degree of sexual interest by the client and partner
- Adapt sexual technique as needed to cope with sexual problems
- Discuss with partner concerns about body image and sex role

Nursing Interventions

- Gather the client's sexual history, noting normal patterns of functioning and the client's vocabulary.
- Assess duration of sexual dysfunction and explore potential causes such as medications, medical problems, or psychosocial issues. Evaluate sexual dysfunction related to either psychological or medical causes.
- Assess for problems of sexual desire.
- Assess for history of sexual abuse.
- Determine the client and partner's current knowledge and understanding.
- Assess and provide treatment for sexual dysfunction, involving the person's partner in the process, and evaluating pharmacological and nonpharmacological interventions.
- Evaluate symptoms of sexual dysfunction as predictors of other illnesses.
- Assess risk factors for sexual dysfunction especially with varying sexual partners.
- Observe for stress and anxiety as possible causes of dysfunction.
- Assess for depression as a possible cause of sexual dysfunction. Sexual problems and depression are common in chronic disease and chronic pain.
- Observe for grief related to loss (e.g., amputation, mastectomy, ostomy).

● = Independent   ▲ = Collaborative

- Explore physical causes such as diabetes, cardiovascular disease, arthritis, or benign prostatic hypertrophy (BPH).
- Certain chronic diseases such as cancer often have significant effects on sexual function, and both the disease process and treatment can contribute to sexual dysfunction.
- Consider that neurological diseases such as multiple sclerosis (MS) affect sexual function directly, but with secondary effects due to disability related to the illness, social, and emotional effects.
- Explore behavioral causes of sexual dysfunction, such as smoking.
- Consider medications as a cause of sexual dysfunction.
- Provide privacy and be verbally and nonverbally nonjudgmental.
- Provide privacy to allow sexual expression between the client and partner (e.g., private room, "Do Not Disturb" sign for a specified length of time).
- Explain the need for the client to share concerns with partner.
- Validate the client's feelings, let the client know that he or she is normal, and correct misinformation.
- Refer to appropriate medical providers for consideration of medication for premature ejaculation, erectile dysfunction, or orgasmic problems.
- Refer women for possible pharmacological intervention for sexual dysfunction.

Geriatric

- Carefully assess the sexuality needs of the elderly client and refer for counseling if needed. Carefully assess sexual functioning needs of clients with dementia and provide privacy for them and their spouse.
- Teach about normal changes that occur with aging: female—reduction in vaginal lubrication, decrease in the degree and speed of vaginal expansion, reduction in duration and resolution of orgasm; male—increased time required for erection, increased erection time without ejaculation, less firm erection, decreased volume of seminal fluid, increased time before subsequent erection (12 to 24 hours).

• = Independent   ▲ = Collaborative

- To enhance sexual functioning suggest: female—use water-based vaginal lubricant, increase foreplay time, avoid direct stimulation of the clitoris if painful (clitoris may be exposed because of atrophy of the labia), practice Kegel exercises (alternately contracting and relaxing the muscles in the pelvic area), urinate immediately after coitus to prevent irritation of the urethra and bladder, and consult with a physician about use of systemic or topical estrogen therapy; male—have female partner try a new coital position by bending her knees and placing a pillow under her hips to elevate pelvis to more easily accommodate a partially erect penis; massage penis downward using pressure at base to keep blood in the penis; ask the female partner to push the penis into the vagina herself and flex her vaginal muscles that have been strengthened by Kegel exercises, and if a partner has a protruding abdomen, experiment to find a position that allows the penis to reach the vagina (e.g., woman lies on her back with legs apart and knees sharply bent while the man places himself over her with his hips under the angle formed by the raised knees).
- Explore various sexual gratification alternatives (e.g., caressing, sharing feelings) with the client and partner.
- Discuss the difference between sexual function, sexuality, and sexual dysfunction, including that all individuals possess sexuality from birth to death, regardless of changes occurring over the life span.
- If prescribed, instruct clients with chronic pain to take pain medication before sexual activity.
- See care plan for **Ineffective Sexuality Pattern.**

Multicultural

- Assess for the influence of cultural beliefs, norms, and values on the client's perceptions of normal sexual functioning.
- Discuss with the client those aspects of sexual health/lifestyle that remain unchanged by his or her health status.
- Evaluate culturally influenced risk factors for sexual dysfunction.
- Validate client feelings and emotions regarding the changes in sexual behavior, letting the client know that the nurse heard and understands what was said, and promoting the nurse-client relationship.

• = Independent   ▲ = Collaborative

Home Care

- Previously discussed interventions may be adapted for home care use.
- Identify specific sources of concern about sexual activity and provide reassurance and instruction on appropriate expectations as indicated.
- Confirm that physical reasons for dysfunction have been addressed. Encourage participation in support groups or therapy if appropriate.
- Reinforce or teach the client about sexual functioning, alternative sexual practices, and necessary sexual precautions. Update teaching as client status changes.

Client/Family Teaching and Discharge Planning

- Provide accurate information for clients concerning sexual activity after a cardiac event; consider using cognitive and behavioral strategies.
- Include the partner/family in discharge instructions, as partner concerns are often overlooked in regard to sexual issues.
- Teach the client and partner about condom use, for those at risk.
- Teach the client with cardiovascular disease that sexual activity can be resumed within a few weeks for those with minimal symptoms with routine activities.
- For cardiac clients, discuss being well rested, reporting any cardiac warning signs, using foreplay to determine tolerance for sexual activity, not using alcohol or eating heavy meals before sex, and having sex with a familiar partner and in the usual setting to decrease any stress the couple might feel.
- Provide written educational materials that address sexual issues for clients and families of clients with implantable cardiac defibrillators (ICDs).
- Discuss sexual problems and adaptations needed for sexual activity with spinal cord injury.
- Refer to appropriate community resources, such as a clinical specialist, family counselor, or cardiac rehabilitation, including the partner if appropriate; for complex issues, a referral to a sex counselor, urologist, gynecologist, or other specialist may be needed.

● = Independent ▲ = Collaborative

- Teach how drug therapy affects sexual response and potential side effects.
- Teach the importance of diabetic control and its effect on sexuality to clients with diabetes.
- Refer for medical advice for ED that lasts longer than 2 months or is recurring.
- Teach the following interventions to decrease the likelihood of ED: limit or avoid the use of alcohol, stop smoking, exercise regularly, reduce stress, get enough sleep, deal with anxiety or depression, and see a physician/health care provider for regular checkups and medical screening tests.
- Refer for medication to treat ED if necessary.

Ineffective Sexuality Pattern

NANDA-I Definition

Expressions of concern regarding own sexuality

Defining Characteristics

Alterations in achieving perceived sex role; alteration in relationship with significant other; reports changes in sexual activities; reports changes in sexual behaviors; reports difficulties with sexual activities; reports difficulties in sexual behaviors; reports limitations in sexual activities; reports limitations in sexual behaviors; values conflict

Related Factors (r/t)

Absent role model; conflicts with sexual orientation; conflicts with variant preferences; deficient knowledge about alternative responses to health-related transitions, altered body function or structure, illness or medical treatment; fear of acquiring a sexually transmitted infection; fear of pregnancy; impaired relationship with a significant other; ineffective role model; lack of privacy; lack of significant other; skill deficit about alternative responses to health-related transitions, altered body function or structure, illness, or medical treatment

Client Outcomes

Client Will (Specify Time Frame):
- State knowledge of difficulties, limitations, or changes in sexual behaviors or activities

● = Independent   ▲ = Collaborative

- State knowledge of sexual anatomy and functioning
- State acceptance of altered body structure or functioning
- Describe acceptable alternative sexual practices
- Identify importance of discussing sexual issues with significant other
- Describe practice of safe sex with regard to pregnancy and avoidance of STDs

Nursing Interventions

- After establishing rapport or therapeutic relationship, give the client permission to discuss issues dealing with sexuality, for example: "Have you been or are you concerned about functioning sexually because of your health status?"
- Use assessment questions and standardized instruments to assess sexual problems, where possible.
- Include the client's partner in discussing sexual concerns and in providing sexual counseling.
- Encourage the client to discuss concerns with his or her partner.
- Explore attitudes about sexual intimacy and changes in sexuality patterns.
- Assess psychosocial function such as anxiety, fear, depression, and low self-esteem.
- Discuss alternative sexual expressions for altered body functioning or structure, including closeness and touching as other forms of expression.
- Some clients choose masturbation for sexual release, an acceptable form of sexual expression, and for some with chronic illnesses, it may be an alternative to sexual intercourse when exercise tolerance is low.
- Assess the client's sexual orientation and usual pattern of sexual activities, and discuss prevention of illnesses for which the client may be at increased risk (e.g., anorectal cancer).
- Specific guidelines for sexual activity for clients who have had total hip replacement (THR) surgery include: Avoid bending the affected leg more than 90 degrees at the hip; when lying on one's back, turning or rolling the affected leg or turning the toes toward the other leg should be avoided. When side-lying, legs are separated with pillows, avoiding knees

● = Independent ▲ = Collaborative

touching and toes of the affected leg pointing downward. In an on-bottom sexual position, pillows should be used under the affected thigh for support, with toes pointed upward and slightly outward. Lying on the unaffected side is a preferred position for men with both partners facing the same direction, the man behind the woman in a "spooning" position, with pillows between her legs and the man's leg resting on top of hers during intercourse. The woman in a side-lying position should place pillows between her legs to support the affected hip, taking care not to bend the affected hip more than 90 degrees or letting toes dangle downward, and with the partner in the "spooning" position behind her. *Caution:* Hip dislocation during sexual intercourse results in pain; the affected leg will appear shorter, and the foot will turn inward, so direct the client to lie down, not move, and have the partner call an ambulance.

- Specific guidelines for those who have had a myocardial infarction (MI) include: Sexual activity can generally be resumed within a few weeks after MI unless complications are experienced such as arrhythmias or cardiac arrest or if exercise testing reveals that sexual activity is not safe. Sex should occur in familiar surroundings, a comfortable room temperature, with the usual partner, when well rested to minimize cardiac stress, as well as avoiding heavy meals or alcohol for 2 to 3 hours before sexual activity, and choosing a position of comfort to minimize stress of the cardiac client.
- Specific guidelines for those who have had coronary artery bypass grafting (CABG) are similar to those after MI with the following additions: Incisional pain with sexual activity is generally a dull ache in the midsternal area and does not radiate (unlike prior experiences with chest pain); therefore, reassure the client and partner that sexual activity will not harm the sternum; sexual activity can be generally resumed in 3 to 6 weeks following CABG.
- Specific guidelines for those with an ICD include assuring the client and partner that fears about being shocked during sexual activity are normal, and sex can be resumed after the ICD is placed as long as strain on the implant site is avoided; if the ICD discharges with sexual activity, the client should

stop, rest, and later notify the physician that the device fired so that a determination can be made if this was an appropriate shock or not; and the client should be instructed to report any dyspnea, chest pain, or dizziness with sexual activity.

- Specific guidelines for those with chronic lung disease include planning for sexual activity when energy level is highest; using positions that minimize shortness of breath, such as a semireclining position; engaging in sexual activity when medications are at peak effectiveness; and use of an oxygen cannula, if prescribed, to provide oxygen before, during, or after sex. Also, pulmonary rehabilitation, including exercise and respiratory muscle training, may improve physical and sexual function.
- Specific guidelines for those with multiple sclerosis include treatment of symptoms with prescribed medications and supportive therapies to assist with a more satisfying sexual experience.
- Those with osteoarthritis, rheumatoid arthritis, or fibromyalgia may fear being in pain or causing pain to their partner; therefore, sexual intercourse may be difficult and may take practice to determine the position of least discomfort, discussing the type of stimulation preferred or trying new positions, allowing plenty of time for sexual foreplay and intercourse, and using touch for sexual stimulation.
- Refer to the care plan **Sexual Dysfunction** for additional interventions.

Pediatric

- Provide age-appropriate information for adolescents regarding human immunodeficiency virus (HIV) or the acquired immunodeficiency syndrome (AIDS) and sexual behavior. For all adolescents, discuss sexually transmitted infections, particularly human papillomavirus, including the risks of perinatal transmission and methods to reduce risks among HIV-infected adolescents.
- Encourage client and partner communication in HIV prevention strategies.
- Provide age-appropriate information regarding potential for sexual abuse.

• = Independent ▲ = Collaborative

Geriatric

- Carefully assess the sexuality needs of the elderly client and refer for counseling if needed; the ability to form satisfying social relationships and to be intimate with others, including building strong emotional intimate connections, contributes to adaptation and successful aging.
- Explore possible changes in sexuality related to health status, menopause, and medications, and make appropriate referrals.
- Allow the client to verbalize feelings regarding loss of sexual partner, and acknowledge problems such as disapproving children, lack of available partner for women, and environmental variables that make forming new relationships difficult.
- Provide a milieu that allows for discussion of sexual issues and a higher level of sexual satisfaction, including allowing couples to room together and bring in double beds from home, and the provision of privacy.
- See care plan for **Sexual Dysfunction.**

Multicultural

- Assess for the influence of cultural beliefs, norms, and values on client's perceptions of normal sexual behavior.

Home Care

- Previously discussed interventions may be adapted for home care use. Also see care plan for **Sexual Dysfunction.**
- Help the client and significant other identify a place and time in the home and daily living for privacy in sharing sexual or relationship activity, and if necessary, help the client communicate the need for privacy to family members.
- Confirm that physical reasons for dysfunction have been addressed, and provide support for coping behaviors, including participation in support groups or therapy if appropriate.
- Reinforce or teach about sexual functioning, alternative sexual practices, and necessary sexual precautions, and update teaching as client status changes; if the client or significant other has received information during an institutional stay, other stressors may have made the information a temporarily low priority or may have impaired learning. Depending on the

cause for dysfunction, the client may experience changing status or feelings about the problem.

Client/Family Teaching and Discharge Planning

• Refer to appropriate community agencies (e.g., certified sex counselor, Reach to Recovery, Ostomy Association, American Association of Sex Educators, Counselors, and Therapists).
• Provide information regarding self-care and sexuality for the woman who has cancer and her partner.
• Sexuality education is important to all populations, whether hearing or deaf, sighted or blind, disabled or not disabled. Discuss contraceptive choices as appropriate, and refer to a health professional (e.g., gynecologist, urologist, nurse practitioner).
• Teach safe sex to all clients including the elderly, including using latex condoms, washing with soap immediately after sexual contact, not ingesting semen, avoiding oral-genital contact, not exchanging saliva, avoiding multiple partners, abstaining from sexual activity when ill, and avoiding recreational drugs and alcohol when engaging in sexual activity.

S

Risk for Shock

NANDA-I Definition

At risk for an inadequate blood flow to the body's tissues which may lead to life-threatening cellular dysfunction

Risk Factors

Advanced age (greater than 65 years); comorbidities (e.g., angina, prior stroke, peripheral vascular disease, diabetes, cancer, renal insufficiency); emergency procedures related to traumatic events; hypotension; hypovolemia; hypoxemia; hypoxia; infection; sepsis; systemic inflammatory response syndrome (SIRS)

Client Outcomes

Client Will (Specify Time Frame):

• Discuss precautions to prevent complications of disease
• Maintain adherence to agreed upon medication regimens

● = Independent   ▲ = Collaborative

- Maintain adequate hydration
- Monitor for infection signs and symptoms
- Maintain a mean arterial pressure above 65 mm Hg
- Maintain a heart rate between 60 and 100 with a normal rhythm
- Maintain urine output greater than 0.5 mL/kg/hr
- Maintain warm, dry skin

Nursing Interventions

- Review data pertaining to client risk status including age, primary diseases, immunosuppression, antibiotic use, and presence of hemodynamic alterations.
- Review client's medical and surgical history, noting conditions that place the client at higher risk for shock, including trauma, myocardial infarction, pulmonary embolism, head injury, dehydration, and infection.
- Complete a full nursing physical examination.
- Monitor circulatory status (e.g., blood pressure [BP], mean arterial pressure [MAP], skin color, skin temperature, heart sounds, heart rate and rhythm, presence and quality of peripheral pulses, Doppler ultrasound, and pulse oximetry).
- Maintain IV access and provide isotonic IV fluids such as 0.9% normal saline or Ringer's lactate as ordered; these fluids are commonly used in the prevention and treatment of shock.
- Monitor for inadequate tissue oxygenation (e.g., apprehension, increased anxiety, changes in mental status, agitation, oliguria, cool/mottled periphery) and determinants of tissue oxygen delivery (e.g., PaO_2, SpO_2, $ScvO_2/SvO_2$, MAP, hemoglobin levels, lactate levels, cardiac output [CO]).
- ▲ Maintain vital signs (BP, pulse, respirations, and temperature), and pulse oximetry within normal parameters.
- ▲ Administer oxygen immediately to maintain SpO_2 greater than 90% and antibiotics and other medications as prescribed to any client presenting with symptoms of early shock.
- ▲ Monitor trends in noninvasive hemodynamic parameters (e.g., MAP) as appropriate.
- ▲ Monitor hydration status including skin turgor, daily weights, postural blood pressure changes, serum electrolytes (sodium, potassium, chloride, and blood urea nitrogen), and intake and output. Consider insertion of a Foley catheter as ordered to measure hourly output.

S

● = Independent   ▲ = Collaborative

▲ Monitor serum lactate levels, interpreting them within the context of each client.

▲ Monitor blood glucose levels frequently and administer insulin as prescribed to maintain normal blood sugar levels (blood glucose levels of 70 to 110 mg/dL [3.9 to 6.1 mmol/L]).

Critical Care

▲ Prepare the client for the placement of an additional IV line, central line, and/or a pulmonary artery catheter as prescribed.

▲ Monitor trends in hemodynamic parameters (e.g., CVP, CO, CI, SVR, PAOP, and MAP) as appropriate.

▲ Monitor electrocardiography.

▲ Monitor arterial blood gases, coagulation, chemistries, point-of-care blood glucose, cardiac enzymes, blood cultures, and hematology.

▲ Administer vasopressor agents as prescribed. If the client is in shock, refer to the care plan **Risk for ineffective Renal Perfusion** as needed. If the client is in shock, refer to the care plan **Risk for ineffective Gastrointestinal Perfusion** as needed. If the client is in shock, refer to the care plan **Impaired Gas Exchange** as needed. If the client is in shock and develops heart failure, refer to the care plan **Decreased Cardiac Output** as needed.

Client/Family Teaching and Discharge Planning

▲ Teach client and family or significant others about any medications prescribed. Instruct the client to report any adverse side effects to his/her health care provider.

• Instruct the client and family on disease process and rationale for care.

• Instruct clients and their family members on the signs and symptoms of low blood pressure to report to their health care provider (dizziness, lightheadedness, fainting, dehydration and unusual thirst, lack of concentration, blurred vision, nausea, cold, clammy, pale skin, rapid and shallow breathing, fatigue, depression).

• Implement educational initiatives to reduce health care–associated infections (HAIs).

• Promote a culture of client safety and individual accountability.

• = Independent   ▲ = Collaborative

Impaired Skin Integrity

NANDA-I Definition

Altered epidermis and/or dermis

Defining Characteristics

Destruction of skin layers; disruption of skin surface; invasion of body structures

Related Factors (r/t)

External

Chemical substance; extremes in age; humidity; hyperthermia; hypothermia; mechanical factors (e.g., friction, shearing forces, pressure, restraint); medications; moisture; physical immobilization; radiation

Internal

Changes in fluid status; changes in pigmentation; changes in turgor; developmental factors; imbalanced nutritional state (e.g., obesity, emaciation, chronic disease, vascular disease); immunological deficit; impaired circulation; impaired metabolic state; impaired sensation; skeletal prominence

Client Outcomes

Client Will (Specify Time Frame):

- Regain integrity of skin surface
- Report any altered sensation or pain at site of skin impairment
- Demonstrate understanding of plan to heal skin and prevent reinjury
- Describe measures to protect and heal the skin and to care for any skin lesion

Nursing Interventions

- Assess site of skin impairment and determine cause (e.g., acute or chronic wound, burn, dermatological lesion, pressure ulcer, skin tear).
- For clients with limited mobility, use a risk assessment tool to systematically assess immobility-related risk factors.
- Determine that skin impairment involves skin damage only (e.g., partial-thickness wound, stage I or stage II pressure

• = Independent   ▲ = Collaborative

ulcer). The following classification system is for pressure ulcers:

- **Category/Stage I:** Intact skin with nonblanchable erythema of a localized area, usually over a bony prominence. Darkly pigmented skin may not have visible blanching. The area may be painful, firm, soft, warmer, or cooler as compared to adjacent tissue.

- **Category/Stage II:** Partial-thickness skin loss of dermis presenting as a shallow open ulcer with a red-pink wound bed, without slough. May also present as an intact or open/ruptured serum-filled. Presents as a shiny or dry shallow ulcer without slough or bruising.[*]

- Inspect and monitor site of skin impairment at least once a day for color changes, redness, swelling, warmth, pain, or other signs of infection. Determine whether the client is experiencing changes in sensation or pain. Pay special attention to high-risk areas such as bony prominences, skin folds, the sacrum, and heels.

- Monitor the client's skin care practices, noting type of soap or other cleansing agents used, temperature of water, and frequency of skin cleansing.

- Consider using normal saline to clean the pressure ulcer or as ordered by physician.

- Individualize plan according to the client's skin condition, needs, and preferences.

- Monitor the client's continence status, and minimize exposure of skin impairment to other areas of moisture from perspiration or wound drainage.

▲ If the client is incontinent, implement an incontinence management plan to prevent exposure to chemicals in urine and stool that can strip or erode the skin. Utilize a skin protectant or cleanser protectant. Refer to a continence care specialist, urologist, or gastroenterologist for incontinence assessment.

- For clients with limited mobility, use a risk assessment tool to systematically assess immobility-related risk factors

---

[*]Bruising indicates suspected deep tissue injury. For wounds deeper into subcutaneous tissue; muscle, or bone (category/stage III or stage IV pressure ulcers), see the care plan for **Impaired Tissue Integrity.**

● = Independent   ▲ = Collaborative

- Do not position the client on site of skin impairment. If consistent with overall client management goals, reposition the client as determined by individualized tissue tolerance and overall condition. Reposition and transfer the client with care to protect against the adverse effects of external mechanical forces such as pressure, friction, and shear.
- Evaluate for use of support surfaces (specialty mattresses, beds), chair cushions, or devices as appropriate. Maintain the head of the bed at the lowest possible degree of elevation to reduce shear and friction, and use lift devices, pillows, foam wedges, and pressure-reducing devices in the bed.
- Implement a written treatment plan for topical treatment of the site of skin impairment.
- Select a topical treatment that will maintain a moist wound-healing environment (stage II) and that is balanced with the need to absorb exudate. Stage I pressure ulcers may be managed by keeping the client off of the area and using a protective dressing.
- Avoid massaging around the site of skin impairment and over bony prominences.
- ▲ Assess the client's nutritional status. Refer for a nutritional consult and/or institute dietary supplements as necessary.
- Identify the client's phase of wound healing (inflammation, proliferation, maturation) and stage of injury.

Home Care

- The interventions described previously may be adapted for home care use.
- Instruct and assist the client and caregivers in how to change dressings and maintain a clean environment. Provide written instructions and observe them completing the dressing change.
- Educate client and caregivers on proper nutrition, signs and symptoms of infection, and when to call the agency and/or physician with concerns.
- ▲ It may be beneficial to initiate a consultation in a case assignment with a wound, ostomy, continence (WOC) nurse (or wounds specialist) to establish a comprehensive plan for complex wounds.

S

• = Independent   ▲ = Collaborative

Client/Family Teaching and Discharge Planning

▲ Teach skin and wound assessment and ways to monitor for signs and symptoms of infection, complications, and healing.
▲ Teach the client why a topical treatment has been selected.
▲ If consistent with overall client management goals, teach how to reposition as client condition warrants.
▲ Teach the client to use pillows, foam wedges, chair cushions, and pressure-redistribution devices to prevent pressure injury.

Risk for impaired Skin Integrity

NANDA-I Definition

At risk for alteration in epidermis and/or dermis

Risk Factors

External

Chemical substance; excretions and/or secretions; extremes of age; humidity; hyperthermia; hypothermia; mechanical factors (e.g., friction, shearing forces, pressure, restraint); moisture; physical immobilization; radiation

Internal

Alterations in skin turgor (change in elasticity); altered circulation; altered metabolic state; altered nutritional state (e.g., obesity, emaciation); altered pigmentation; altered sensation; chronic disease, developmental factors; history of pressure ulcers, immunological deficit; medication; psychogenetic, immunological factors; skeletal prominence, vascular disease

NOTE: Risk should be determined by the use of a risk assessment tool (e.g., Norton scale, Braden scale).

Client Outcomes

Client Will (Specify Time Frame):

• Report altered sensation or pain at risk areas as soon as noted
• Demonstrate understanding of personal risk factors for impaired skin integrity
• Verbalize a personal plan for preventing impaired skin integrity

● = Independent   ▲ = Collaborative

Nursing Interventions

- Inspect and monitor skin condition at least once a day for color or texture changes, redness, localized heat, edema or induration, pressure damage, dermatological conditions, or lesions and any incontinence-associated dermatitis. Determine whether the client is experiencing loss of sensation or pain.
- Identify clients at risk for impaired skin integrity as a result of immobility, chronological age, malnutrition, incontinence, compromised perfusion, immunocompromised status, or chronic medical condition, such as diabetes mellitus, spinal cord injury, or renal failure.
- Monitor the client's skin care practices, noting type of soap or other cleansing agents used, temperature of water, and frequency of skin cleansing.
- Cleanse the skin gently with pH-balanced cleansers. Avoid harsh cleansing agents, hot water, extreme friction or force, or too-frequent cleansing.
- ▲ Monitor the client's continence status and minimize exposure of the site of skin impairment (incontinence-associated dermatitis) and other areas to moisture from incontinence, perspiration, or wound drainage. If the client is incontinent, implement an incontinence management plan to prevent exposure to chemicals in urine and stool that can strip or erode the skin. Use a barrier product to reduce risk of exposure; refer to a physician (e.g., continence care specialist, urologist, gastroenterologist) for an incontinence assessment.
- For clients with limited mobility, inspect and monitor condition of skin covering bony prominences.
- Use a risk assessment tool to systematically assess immobility-related risk factors.
- Implement a written prevention plan.
- The use of repositioning should be considered in all at-risk individuals. Frequency of repositioning will be influenced by variables concerning the individual and the support surface in use. Frequency of repositioning should be determined by the individual's tissue tolerance and medical condition. Reposition the client with care to protect against the adverse effects of external mechanical forces (e.g., pressure, friction, shear).

● = Independent   ▲ = Collaborative

- Evaluate for use of specialty mattresses, beds, or devices as appropriate.
- Avoid massaging over bony prominences.
- ▲ Assess the client's nutritional status; refer for a nutritional consult, and/or institute dietary supplements.

Geriatric

- Limit number of complete baths to two or three per week, and alternate them with partial baths. Use a tepid water temperature (between 90° and 105° F) for bathing.
- Use lotions and moisturizers to prevent skin from drying out, especially in the winter.
- Increase fluid intake within cardiac and renal limits to a minimum of 1500 mL per day.
- Increase humidity in the environment, especially during the winter, by using a humidifier or placing a container of water on a warm object.

Home Care

- Assess caregiver vigilance and ability
- ▲ Initiate a consultation in a case assignment with a wound care specialist or wound, ostomy, and continence (WOC) nurse to establish a comprehensive plan as soon as possible.
- See the care plan for **Impaired Skin Integrity.**

Client/Family Teaching and Discharge Planning

- Teach the client skin assessment and ways to monitor for impending skin breakdown.
- If consistent with overall client management goals, teach how to turn and reposition the client. Teach the client and or caregivers to use pillows, foam wedges, and pressure-reducing devices to prevent pressure injury.

Sleep deprivation

NANDA-I Definition

Prolonged periods of time without sleep (sustained natural, periodic suspension of relative consciousness)

• = Independent   ▲ = Collaborative

Defining Characteristics

Acute confusion, agitation, anxiety, apathy, combativeness, daytime drowsiness, decreased ability to function, fatigue, fleeting nystagmus, hallucinations, hand tremors, heightened sensitivity to pain, inability to concentrate, irritability, lethargy, listlessness, malaise, perceptual disorders (i.e., disturbed body sensation, delusions, feeling afloat), restlessness, slowed reaction, transient paranoia

Related Factors (r/t)

Aging-related sleep stage shifts, dementia, familial sleep paralysis, inadequate daytime activity, idiopathic central nervous system hypersomnolence, narcolepsy, nightmares, non–sleep-inducing parenting practices, periodic limb movement (e.g., restless leg syndrome, nocturnal myoclonus), prolonged discomfort (e.g., physical, psychological), sustained inadequate sleep hygiene, prolonged use of pharmacological or dietary antisoporifics, sleep apnea, sleep terror, sleep walking, sleep-related enuresis, sleep-related painful erections, sundowner's syndrome, sustained circadian asynchrony, sustained environmental stimulation, sustained uncomfortable sleep environment

Client Outcomes

Client Will (Specify Time Frame):

- Verbalize plan that provides adequate time for sleep
- Identify actions that can be taken to ensure adequate sleep time
- Awaken refreshed as soon as adequate time is spent sleeping
- Be less sleepy during the day as soon as adequate time is spent sleeping

Nursing Interventions

- Obtain a sleep history including amount of sleep obtained each night, use of medications and stimulants that may interfere with sleep amount, medical conditions and their treatment that limits sleep time, work and family responsibilities that limit sleep time, and daytime sequelae suggestive of sleep deprivation (e.g., drowsiness, inability to concentrate, slowed reactions).
  - From the history, assess degree of sleep deprivation.
  - From the history, identity factors leading to sleep deprivation.

● = Independent   ▲ = Collaborative

▲ Assess evening pain medication use and, when feasible, administer pain medications that promote rather than interfere with sleep. (See further Nursing Interventions for **Pain.**)

▲ Assess hypersensitivity to pain.

▲ Assess for underlying physiological illnesses causing sleep loss (e.g., cardiovascular, pulmonary, gastrointestinal, hyperthyroidism, nocturia occurring with benign hypertrophic prostatitis or pain).

▲ Assess for underlying psychiatric illnesses causing sleep loss (e.g., bipolar depression, anxiety disorders, schizophrenia).

▲ Monitor for nocturnal panic attacks. Refer for treatment as appropriate.

▲ Monitor for sleep disordered breathing (e.g., apneas and hypopneas) and accompanying daytime sleepiness. Refer for diagnosis by sleep specialists as appropriate.

▲ Monitor for presence of nocturnal symptoms of restless leg syndrome with uncomfortable restless sensations in legs that occur before sleep onset or during the night. Refer for treatment as appropriate.

▲ Monitor for symptoms of overactive bladder.

▲ Assess for chronic insomnia. See further Nursing Interventions for **Insomnia.**

• Monitor caffeine intake.

• Encourage napping as a way to compensate for sleep deprivation when severely restricted nighttime sleep cannot be avoided. Set a regular schedule for napping.

• Minimize factors that disturb the client's sleep by consolidating care. See Nursing Interventions for **Disturbed Sleep Pattern.**

• Keep the sleep environment quiet (e.g., avoid use of intercoms, lower the volume on radio and television, keep beepers on nonaudio mode, anticipate alarms on intravenous [IV] pumps, talk quietly on unit). See Nursing Interventions for **Disturbed Sleep Pattern.**

• Mask noise in sleep area if noise cannot be eliminated. See Nursing Interventions for **Readiness for enhanced Sleep.**

● = Independent   ▲ = Collaborative

Geriatric

- Interventions identified previously may be adapted for use with geriatric clients.
- In addition, see the Geriatric section of Nursing Interventions for **Disturbed Sleep Pattern.**

Home Care

- Interventions identified previously may be adapted for home care use. See the Home Care section of Nursing Interventions for **Disturbed Sleep Pattern.**
- Teach family about the short-term and long-term consequences of inadequate amounts of sleep.
- Teach client/family about the need for those with chronic conditions to avoid schedules and commitments that interfere with obtaining adequate amounts of sleep.
- Promote adoption of behaviors that ensure adequate amounts of sleep for all family members. See Nursing Interventions for **Readiness for enhanced Sleep.**
- Teach family about signs of sleep deprivation and how to avoid chronic sleep loss. See Nursing Interventions for **Disturbed Sleep Pattern.**
- Advise against the sleep deprived person's chronic use of stimulants (e.g., caffeine) to overcome daytime sequelae of sleep deprivation; focus on elimination of factors that lead to chronic sleep loss.

S

Readiness for enhanced Sleep

NANDA-I Definition

A pattern of natural, periodic suspension of consciousness that provides adequate rest, sustains a desired lifestyle, and can be strengthened

Defining Characteristics

Expresses willingness to enhance sleep; amount of sleep is congruent with developmental needs; reports being rested after sleep; follows sleep routines that promote sleep habits; occasional use of pharmaceutical agents to induce sleep

• = Independent   ▲ = Collaborative

Client Outcomes

Client Will (Specify Time Frame):

- Verbalize an interest in what constitutes normal sleep
- Verbalize an interest in nonpharmacological approaches to sleep promotion
- Establish an environment conducive to sleep initiation and maintenance throughout the night

Nursing Interventions

- Obtain a sleep history including bedtime routines, sleep patterns, use of medications and stimulants, and use of complementary/alternative medical practices for stress management and relaxation prior to bedtime.
  - From the history, assess the client's ability to initiate and maintain sleep, obtain adequate amounts of sleep, and manage daytime responsibilities free from fatigue and sleepiness.
- Based on assessment, teach one or more of the listed sleep promotion practices as appropriate.
  - Establish a regular schedule for sleep, exercise, napping, and mealtimes.
  - Avoid long periods of daytime sleep.
  - Arise at the same time each day even if sleep was poor during the previous night.
  - If not contraindicated have high-glycemic-index carbohydrate dinner and/or bedtime snack.
  - Limit caffeine.
  - Limit alcohol use.
  - Avoid long-term use of sleeping pills.
  - Engage in relaxing activities before bed.
  - Provide backrub or other forms of massage.
  - Teach relaxation techniques.
  - Teach complementary and alternative interventions as culturally congruent.
  - Lower lighting in sleep area.
  - Mask noise in sleep area when it cannot be eliminated.
  - For anxious clients consider use of a lavender oil preparation in the health care setting.

S

• = Independent   ▲ = Collaborative

Geriatric

- Interventions discussed previously may be adapted for use with geriatric clients.
- Counsel the older adult regarding normal age-related changes in sleep:
- Elicit the older adult's expectations for sleep and correct misconceptions.
- Assess and refer as appropriate if coexisting conditions may be disrupting sleep.
- Discuss appropriate and inappropriate self-help measures for improving sleep.
- Encourage walking and other exercise outdoors unless contraindicated.
- Help elderly clients engage with others who enjoy similar events.
- Combine strength training, walking, and social activities when feasible.

Home Care

- Interventions discussed previously may be adapted for home care use.
- Some complementary and alternative medicine interventions may be more easily tried at home than in health care facilities.
- Assess the conduciveness of the home environment for both caregivers and clients' sleep.

S

Disturbed Sleep Pattern

NANDA-I Definition

Time-limited interruptions of sleep amount and quality due to external factors

Defining Characteristics

Change in normal sleep pattern; reports not feeling well rested; dissatisfaction with sleep; decreased ability to function; reports being awakened; reports no difficulty falling asleep

• = Independent   ▲ = Collaborative

Related Factors

Ambient temperature; ambient humidity; caregiving responsibilities; change in daylight-darkness exposure; interruptions (e.g., for therapeutics, monitoring, lab tests), lack of sleep privacy/control; lighting; noise, noxious odors; physical restraint; sleep partner; unfamiliar sleep furnishings

Client Outcomes

Client Will (Specify Time Frame):

- Verbalize plan to implement sleep promotion routines
- Maintain a regular schedule of sleep and waking
- Fall asleep without difficulty
- Remain asleep throughout the night
- Awaken naturally, feeling refreshed and is not fatigued during day

Nursing Interventions

- Obtain a sleep history including bedtime routines, number of times awakened during the night, noise and light levels in the sleep environment, and activities occurring in the sleep environment during hours of sleep.
  - From the history, assess whether client has an opportunity for normal sleep.
  - From the history, assess environmental factors that interrupt sleep.
- Assess level of pain. (See further Nursing Interventions for **Pain.**)
- If client has recurring pain, provide pain relief shortly before bedtime and position client comfortably for sleep.
- Keep environment quiet, room lighting dim, and bedding supportive of comfortable body alignment. See Nursing Interventions for **Readiness for enhanced Sleep.**
- Offer earplugs and eye masks if feasible.
- Establish a sleeping and waking routine with regular times for sleeping and waking, including routines for preparing for sleep. See Nursing Interventions for **Readiness for enhanced Sleep.**
- For hospitalized stable clients, consider instituting the following sleep protocol to a regular sleep-wake routine:
  - Night shift: Give the client the opportunity for uninterrupted sleep the first 3 to 4 hours of the sleep period. Keep

environmental noise and light to a minimum. After major sleep period, allow 80 to 90 minutes between interruptions. (If client must be disturbed the first 3 to 4 hours, attempt to protect 90- to 110-minute blocks of time in between awakenings.)

■ Day shift: Encourage short morning and/or after-lunch naps as needed. Promote a physical activity regimen as appropriate. Schedule newly ordered medications to avoid the need to wake the client the first few hours of the night.

■ Evening shift: Limit napping. Encourage a suitable bedtime routine. At sleep time, lower intensity of room and unit lights and keep noise and conversation on the unit to a minimum.

Geriatric

• Most interventions identified previously are suitable for use with geriatric clients; however, be cautious about introducing earplugs and eye masks with ataxic clients and dementia clients, given that they may contribute to disorientation. Elderly clients should also be observed for nighttime safety risk due to increased incidence of sleep apnea with nocturia.

• Assessments for pain, anxiety, depression, sleep apnea, restless leg syndrome, and substance use/abuse are especially important in the elderly because sleep disruption is more common with the elderly and is made worse by these conditions.

• In addition see the Geriatric section of Nursing Interventions for **Readiness for enhanced Sleep.**

Home Care

• Interventions identified previously may be adapted for home care use.

• In addition, see the Home Care section of Nursing Interventions for **Readiness for enhanced Sleep.**

Client/Family Teaching and Discharge Planning

• Teach family about sleep and the importance of uninterrupted sleep during treatment and recovery.

• Teach family about signs of sleep deprivation, which may result from several environmental factors. See Nursing Interventions for **Sleep deprivation.**

• = Independent ▲ = Collaborative

Impaired Social Interaction

NANDA-I Definition

Insufficient or excessive quantity or ineffective quality of social exchange

Defining Characteristics

Discomfort in social situations; dysfunctional interaction with others; family report of changes in interaction (e.g., style, pattern); inability to communicate a satisfying sense of social engagement (e.g., belonging, caring, interest, or shared history); inability to receive a satisfying sense of social engagement (e.g., belonging, caring, interest, or shared history); use of unsuccessful social interaction behaviors

Related Factors (r/t)

Absence of significant others; communication barriers; deficit about ways to enhance mutuality (e.g., knowledge, skills); disturbed thought processes; environmental barriers; limited physical mobility; self-concept disturbance; sociocultural dissonance; therapeutic isolation

Client Outcomes

S

Client Will (Specify Time Frame):

* Identify barriers that cause impaired social interactions
* Discuss feelings that accompany impaired and successful social interactions
* Use available opportunities to practice interactions
* Use successful social interaction behaviors
* Report increased comfort in social situations
* Communicate, state feelings of belonging, demonstrate caring and interest in others
* Report effective interactions with others

Nursing Interventions

* Consider using a self-rating scale to assess social functioning.
* Monitor the client's use of defense mechanisms and support healthy defenses (e.g., the client focuses on present and avoids placing blame on others for personal behavior).
* Spend time with the client.

• = Independent ▲ = Collaborative

- Use active listening skills, including assessment and clarification of the client's verbal and nonverbal responses and interactions.
- Identify client strengths. Have the client make a list of strengths and refer to it when experiencing negative feelings. He or she may find it helpful to put the list on a note card to carry at all times.
- Have group members support each other in a group setting.
- Model appropriate social interactions. Give positive verbal and nonverbal feedback for appropriate behavior (e.g., make statements such as, "I'm proud that you made it to work on time and did all the tasks assigned to you without saying that your supervisor was picking on you"; make eye contact). If not contraindicated, touch the client's arm or hand when speaking.
- Use role playing to increase social skills.
- Use client-centered humor as appropriate.
- Consider use of animal therapy; arrange for visitation.
- Consider the use of the Internet and email to promote socialization.
- ▲ Refer client for behavioral interventions (life skills program) to increase social skills.
- Refer to care plans for **Risk for Loneliness** and **Social Isolation** for additional interventions.

Pediatric

- Encourage social support for clients with visual and hearing impairments.
- Provide computers and Internet access to children with chronic disabilities that limit socialization.
- Consider use of RAP therapy (therapy using rap music) in groups to advance social skills of urban adolescents.
- Consider residential wilderness treatment programs for adolescents with unsuccessfully treated mental health issues and antisocial behavior.

Geriatric

- Encourage socialization through education, support groups, and programs for the elderly in the community.

• = Independent   ▲ = Collaborative

▲ Assess the client's potential or actual sensory problems with hearing and vision and make appropriate referrals if a problem is identified.

• Monitor for depression, a particular risk in the elderly.

• Encourage group physical activity, such as aerobics or stretching and toning.

• Consider having clients participate in playing Wii.

• Have clients reminisce.

• Refer to care plans for **Adult Failure to Thrive, Risk for Loneliness,** and **Social Isolation** for additional interventions.

Multicultural

• Assess for the effect of racism on the client's perceptions of social interactions.

• Approach individuals of color with respect, warmth, and professional courtesy.

• Validate the client's feelings regarding social interaction.

• Use interpreters as needed.

• Refer to care plan **Social Isolation** for additional interventions.

Home Care

• Previously discussed interventions may be adapted for home care use.

▲ Refer to or support involvement with supportive groups and counseling.

Client/Family Teaching and Discharge Planning

▲ Refer to appropriate social agencies for assistance (e.g., family therapy, self-help groups, creative activities, crisis intervention), especially individuals who are seriously ill.

Social Isolation

NANDA-I Definition

Aloneness experienced by the individual and perceived as imposed by others and as a negative or threatening state

• = Independent   ▲ = Collaborative

Defining Characteristics

Objective

Absence of supportive significant other(s); developmentally inappropriate behaviors; dull affect; evidence of handicap (e.g., physical, mental); exists in a subculture; illness; meaningless actions; no eye contact; preoccupation with own thoughts; projects hostility; repetitive actions; sad affect; seeks to be alone; shows behavior unaccepted by dominant cultural group; uncommunicative; withdrawn

Subjective

Developmentally inappropriate interests; experiences feelings of differences from others; inability to meet expectations of others; insecurity in public; reports feelings of aloneness imposed by others; reports feelings of rejection; reports inadequate purpose in life; reports values unacceptable to the dominant cultural group

Related Factors (r/t)

Alterations in mental status; alterations in physical appearance; altered state of wellness; factors contributing to the absence of satisfying personal relationships (e.g., delay in accomplishing developmental tasks); immature interests; inability to engage in satisfying personal relationships; inadequate personal resources; unaccepted social behavior; unaccepted social values

Client Outcomes

Client Will (Specify Time Frame):

- Identify feelings of isolation
- Practice social and communication skills needed to interact with others
- Initiate interactions with others; set and meet goals
- Participate in activities and programs at level of ability and desire
- Describe feelings of self-worth

Nursing Interventions

- Establish a therapeutic relationship with the client.
- Observe for barriers to social interaction: physical, emotional, and environmental.
- Note risk factors.
- Discuss/assess causes of perceived or actual isolation

● = Independent   ▲ = Collaborative

- Allow the client opportunities to describe his or her daily life and to introduce any issues that may be of concern.
- Promote social interactions. Support the expression of feelings.
- Assist the client in identifying specific health and social problems and involve them in their resolution.
- Assist the client in identifying acceptable activities that encourage socialization.
- Identify available personal support systems and involve those individuals in the client's care.
▲ Refer clients to support groups as necessary.
- Encourage liberal visitation for a client who is hospitalized or in an extended care facility (ECF).
- Help the client identify role models and encourage interactions with others with similar interests. Technology may be helpful in finding others with similar interests.
- See the care plan for **Risk for Loneliness.**

Pediatric

▲ Refer obese adolescents for diet, exercise, and psychosocial support.
▲ Assess socially isolated adolescents for substance abuse. Refer to appropriate organizations for support and treatment.

Geriatric

- Assess physical and mental status to establish a firm basis for planning social activities.
- Assess for hearing deficit. Provide aids and use adaptive techniques.
- Encourage physical closeness if appropriate.
- Involve client in goal-setting and planning activities.
- Involve nonprofessionals in activities, projects, and goal setting with the client. Activities might include engaging in arts and crafts, reading, playing games, and music therapy.
- Suggest varied social activities that would decrease isolation and encourage participation.
- Position clients in group interventions according to abilities, age, life situations, preferences, and personal and cultural characteristics.

• = Independent   ▲ = Collaborative

- Consider the use of simulated presence therapy (see the care plan for **Hopelessness**) for clients with cognitive distress.
▲ Consider using computers and the Internet to alleviate or reduce loneliness and social isolation.

Multicultural

- Acknowledge racial/ethnic differences at the onset of care.
- Assess for the influence of cultural beliefs, norms, and values.
- Assess personal space needs, communication styles, acceptable body language, attitude toward eye contact, perception of touch, and paraverbal messages when communicating with the client.
- Use a culturally competent, professional approach when working with clients of various ethnic groups.
- Promote a sense of ethnic attachment.
- Assess the client's feelings regarding social isolation.
- Assist those ethnic minorities who are underserved to access essential health care.

Home Care

- The interventions described previously may be adapted for home care use.
- Confirm that the home setting has a health-safety communication system that is user friendly.
- Consider the use of the computer and Internet to decrease isolation.
- Assess options for living that allow the client privacy, but not isolation.
- Assist clients to interact with neighbors in the community when they move to supported housing.

Client/Family Teaching and Discharge Planning

- Assist the client in initiating contacts with self-help groups, counselors, and therapists.
- Provide information to the client about senior citizen services and community resources.
- Refer socially isolated caregivers to appropriate support groups as well.
- See the care plan for **Caregiver Role Strain.**

• = Independent   ▲ = Collaborative

Chronic Sorrow

NANDA-I Definition

Cyclical, recurring, and potentially progressive pattern of pervasive sadness experienced (by parent, caregiver, individual with chronic illness or disability) in response to continual loss throughout the trajectory of an illness or disability

Defining Characteristics

Reports feelings of sadness (e.g., periodic, recurrent); reports feelings that interfere with ability to reach highest level of personal well-being; reports feelings that interfere with ability to reach highest level of social well-being; reports negative feelings (e.g., anger, being misunderstood, confusion, depression, disappointment, emptiness, fear, frustration, guilt, helplessness, hopelessness, low self-esteem, being overwhelmed, recurring loss, self-blame)

Related Factors (r/t)

Crisis in management of the disability; crises in management of the illness; crises related to developmental stages; death of a loved one; experiences chronic disability (e.g., physical or mental); experiences chronic illness (e.g., physical or mental); missed opportunities; missed milestones; unending caregiving

Client Outcomes

Client Will (Specify Time Frame):
- Express appropriate feelings of guilt, fear, anger, or sadness
- Identify problems associated with sorrow (e.g., changes in appetite, insomnia, nightmares, loss of libido, decreased energy, alteration in activity levels)
- Seek help in dealing with grief-associated problems
- Plan for future one day at a time
- Function at normal developmental level

Nursing Interventions

- Determine the client's degree of sorrow. Use the Burke/NCRS Chronic Sorrow Questionnaire for the individual or caregiver as appropriate.

• = Independent   ▲ = Collaborative

- Identify problems of eating and sleeping; ensure that basic human needs are being met.
- Develop a trusting relationship with the client by using empathetic therapeutic communication techniques.
- Help the client to understand that sorrow may be ongoing. No timetable exists for grieving, despite popular thought. After loss, life is characterized by good times and bad times when sorrow is triggered by events.
- Help the client recognize that, although sadness will occur at intervals for the rest of his or her life, it will become bearable.
- Give anticipatory guidance about life events when the families might experience renewed feelings of loss.
- Encourage the use of positive coping techniques:
  - Taking action: Suggested strategies include keeping busy, keeping personal interests, going away, getting out of the house, doing something to gain a feeling of control over life.
  - Cognitive coping: Techniques include concentrating on the positive aspects of life, having a "can do" attitude, taking one day at a time, and taking responsibility for the quality of one's own life. Encourage the client to write about the experience.
  - Interpersonal coping: Techniques include talking to a close friend, a health care professional, or someone with the same condition or circumstance. Joining a support group can also help the sorrowful person to cope.
  - Emotional coping: Encourage the client to express feelings both to other people and to write out feelings, cry as desired, give thanks, and pray if desired.
- Expect the client to meet responsibilities; give positive reinforcement for planning how to meet responsibilities, and for accomplishing responsibilities.
- ▲ Encourage the client to make time to talk to family members about the loss with the help of professional support as needed and without criticizing or belittling each other's feelings about the loss.
- Help the client determine the best way and place to find social support.
- Monitor for symptoms of exhaustion, isolation, and, potentially, loss of hope and dreams as potential indicators of caregiving burden and burnout.

• = Independent   ▲ = Collaborative

▲ Identify available community resources, including grief coun-selors or support groups available for specific losses (e.g., Mul-tiple Sclerosis Society).

▲ Identify whether the client is experiencing depression, suicidal tendencies, or other emotional disorders. Refer for counseling as appropriate.

Pediatric

- Treat the child with respect, give him or her the opportunity to talk about concerns, and answer questions honestly.
- Listen to the child's expression of grief.
- Help parents recognize that the grieving child does not have to be "fixed"; instead, he needs support going through an experience of grieving just as adults do.
- Consider the use of art for children in hospice care who are dying or dealing with the death of a parent, sibling, or other family member.
- ▲ Refer grieving children and parents to a program to help facil-itate grieving if desired, especially if the death was traumatic.
- Help the adolescent determine sources of support and how to use them effectively.
- ▲ Encourage parents in chronic sorrow to seek mental health services as needed, learn stress reduction, and take good care of their health.
- Recognize that mothers who have a miscarriage grieve and experience sorrow because of loss of the child.

Geriatric

- Identify previous losses and assess the client for depression.
- Evaluate the social support system of the elderly client. If the support system is minimal, help the client determine how to increase available support.

Home Care

- The interventions described previously may be adapted for home care use.
- ▲ Assess the client for depression. Refer for mental health ser-vices as indicated.

● = Independent   ▲ = Collaborative

▲ When sorrow is focused around loss of a pregnancy, encourage the client to follow through on a counseling referral.

• Encourage the client to participate in activities that are diversionary and uplifting as tolerated (e.g., outdoor activities, hobby groups, church-related activities, pet care).

• Encourage the client to participate in support groups appropriate to the area of loss or illness (e.g., Crohn's disease support group or Widow to Widow).

• Provide psychological support for family/caregivers.

▲ In the presence of a psychiatric disorder, refer for psychiatric home health care services for client reassurance and implementation of a therapeutic regimen.

▲ See the care plans for **Chronic low Self-Esteem, Risk for Loneliness,** and **Hopelessness.**

Spiritual Distress

NANDA-I Definition

Impaired ability to experience and integrate meaning and purpose in life through connectedness with self, others, art, music, literature, nature, and/or a power greater than oneself

Defining Characteristics

Connections to Self

Anger; expresses lack of acceptance; expresses lack of courage; expresses lack of hope; expresses lack of love; expresses lack of meaning in life; expresses lack of purpose in life; expresses lack of self-forgiveness; expresses lack of serenity (e.g., peace); guilt; ineffective coping

Connections with Others

Expresses alienation; refuses interactions with significant others; refuses interactions with spiritual leaders; verbalizes being separated from support system

Connections with Art, Music, Literature, Nature

Disinterest in nature; disinterest in reading spiritual literature; inability to express previous state of creativity (e.g., singing/listening to music/writing)

• = Independent   ▲ = Collaborative

Connections with Power Greater Than Oneself

Expresses anger toward power greater than self; expresses being abandoned; expresses hopelessness; expresses suffering; inability for introspection; inability to experience the transcendent; inability to participate in religious activities; inability to pray; requests to see a spiritual leader; sudden changes in spiritual practices

Related Factors (r/t)

Active dying; anxiety; chronic illness; death; life change; loneliness; pain self-alienation; social alienation; sociocultural deprivation

Client Outcomes

Client Will (Specify Time Frame):

- Express meaning and purpose in life
- Express sense of hope in the future
- Express sense of connectedness with self
- Express sense of connectedness with family/friends
- Express ability to forgive
- Express acceptance of health status
- Find meaning in relationships with others
- Find meaning in relationship with Higher Power
- Find meaning in personal and health care treatment choices

Nursing Interventions

- Observe clients for cues indicating difficulties in finding meaning, purpose, or hope in life.
- Observe clients with chronic illness, poor prognosis, or life-changing conditions for loss of meaning, purpose, and hope in life.
- Offer spiritual care in disaster relief.
- Promote a sense of love, caring, and compassion in nursing encounters.
- Be physically present and actively listen to the client.
- Help the client find a reason for living, be available for support and promote hope.
- Listen to the client's feelings about suffering and/or death. Be nonjudgmental and allow time for grieving.
- Respect the client's beliefs; avoid imposing your own spiritual beliefs on the client. Be aware of your own belief systems and accept the client's spirituality.

• = Independent   ▲ = Collaborative

- Monitor and promote supportive social contacts.
- Integrate family into spiritual practices as appropriate.
- Assist family in searching for meaning in client's health care situation.
- Offer spiritual support to caregivers.
- ▲ Refer the client to a support group or counseling.
- Support meditation, guided imagery, journaling, relaxation, and involvement in art, music, or poetry. Support outdoor activities.
- Offer or suggest visits with spiritual and/or religious advisors.
- Provide privacy or a "sacred space."
- Allow time and a place for prayer.
- Coordinate or encourage attending spiritual retreats, courses, or programming.

Geriatric

- Identify the client's past spiritual practices that have been helpful. Help the client explore his or her life and identify those experiences that are noteworthy.
- Offer opportunities to practice one's religion.

Pediatric

- Offer adolescents opportunities for reflection and storytelling to express their spirituality.

Multicultural

- Recognize the importance of spirituality and provide culturally competent spiritual care to specific populations:
  - Arab Americans
  - Hawaiians
  - Latinos
  - African Americans
  - Domestic violence survivors
  - African women
  - Aborigine

Home Care

- All of the nursing interventions described previously apply in the home setting.

• = Independent   ▲ = Collaborative

Risk for Spiritual Distress

NANDA-I Definition

At risk for an impaired ability to experience and integrate meaning and purpose in life through connectedness with self, others, art, music, literature, nature, and/or a power greater than oneself

Risk Factors

Developmental
Life changes

Environmental
Environmental changes; natural disasters

Physical
Chronic illness; physical illness; substance abuse

Psychosocial
Anxiety; blocks to experiencing love; change in religious rituals; change in spiritual practices; cultural conflict; depression; inability to forgive; loss; low self-esteem; poor relationships; racial conflict; separated support systems; stress

Client Outcomes, Nursing Interventions, Client/Family Teaching and Discharge planning

Refer to care plan **Spiritual Distress.**

Readiness for enhanced Spiritual Well-Being

NANDA-I Definition

A pattern of experiencing and integrating meaning and purpose in life through connectedness with self, others, art, music, literature, nature, and/or a power greater than oneself that is sufficient for well-being and can be strengthened

Defining Characteristics

Connections to Self

Expresses desire for enhanced acceptance; expresses desire for enhanced coping; expresses desire for enhanced courage; expresses desire for

• = Independent   ▲ = Collaborative

enhanced hope; expresses desire for enhanced joy; expresses desire for enhanced love; expresses desire for enhanced meaning in life; expresses desire for enhanced purpose in life; expresses desire for enhanced satisfying philosophy of life; expresses desire for enhanced self-forgiveness; expresses desire for enhanced serenity (e.g., peace); expresses desire for enhanced surrender; meditation

Connections with Others

Provides service to others; requests forgiveness of others; requests interactions with significant others; requests interaction with spiritual leaders

Connections with Art, Music, Literature, Nature

Displays creative energy (e.g., writing, poetry, singing); listens to music; reads spiritual literature; spends time outdoors

Connection with Power Greater Than Self

Expresses awe; expresses reverence; participates in religious activities; prays; reports mystical experiences

Client Outcomes

Client Will (Specify Time Frame):

- Express hope
- Express sense of meaning and purpose in life
- Express peace and serenity
- Express love
- Express acceptance
- Express surrender
- Express forgiveness of self and others
- Express satisfaction with philosophy of life
- Express joy
- Express courage
- Describe being able to cope
- Describe use of spiritual practices
- Describe providing service to others
- Describe interaction with spiritual leaders, friends, and family
- Describe appreciation for art, music, literature, and nature

• – Independent ▲ = Collaborative

Nursing Interventions

- Perform a spiritual assessment that includes the client's relationship with God, meaning and purpose in life, religious affiliation, and any other significant beliefs.
- Be present and actively listen to the client.
- Encourage the client to pray or engage in other spiritual meditative practices.
- Coordinate or encourage attending spiritual retreats or courses.
- Promote hope.
- Encourage clients to reflect on what is meaningful to them in life.
- Encourage increased quality of life through social support and family relationships.
- Assist the client in identifying religious or spiritual beliefs that encourage integration of meaning and purpose in the client's life.
- Support meditation, guided imagery, journaling, relaxation, and involvement in art, music, or poetry. Support outdoor activities.
- Encourage outdoor activities.
- Encourage expressions of spirituality.
- Encourage integration of spirituality in healthy lifestyle choices.

Geriatric

- Identify the client's past spiritual practices that have been growth-filled. Help the client explore his or her life and identify those experiences that are noteworthy.
- Offer opportunities to practice one's religion.

Pediatric

- Offer adolescents opportunities for reflection and storytelling to express their spirituality.

Multicultural

- Recognize the importance of spirituality and provide culturally competent spiritual care to specific populations:
  - Arab Americans
  - Hawaiians
  - Latinos
  - African Americans
  - Integrate spiritual practices in health-promoting programs, particularly within the African American community

● = Independent   ▲ = Collaborative

- Domestic violence survivors
- African women
- Aborigine

Home Care

- All of the nursing interventions described previously apply in the home setting.

Stress overload

NANDA-I Definition

Excessive amounts and types of demands that require action

Defining Characteristics

Demonstrates increased feelings of anger; demonstrates increased feelings of impatience; reports a feeling of pressure; reports a feeling of tension; reports difficulty in functioning; reports excessive situational stress (e.g., rates stress level as 7 or above on a 10-point scale); reports increased feelings of anger; reports increased feelings of impatience; reports negative impact from stress (e.g., physical symptoms, psychological distress, feeling of being sick or of going to get sick); reports problems with decision-making

Related Factors (r/t)

Inadequate resources (e.g., financial, social, education/knowledge level); intense stressors (e.g., family violence, chronic illness, terminal illness); multiple coexisting stressors (e.g., environmental threats/demands, physical threats/demands, social threats/demands); repeated stressors (e.g., family violence, chronic illness, terminal Illness)

Client Outcomes

Client Will (Specify Time Frame):

- Review the amounts and types of stressors in daily living
- Identify stressors that can be modified or eliminated
- Mobilize social supports to facilitate lower stress levels
- Reduce stress levels through use of health promoting behaviors and other strategies

• = Independent   ▲ = Collaborative

Nursing Interventions

- Assist client in identification of stress overload during vulnerable life events.
- Listen actively to descriptions of stressors and the stress response.
- In younger adult women, assess interpersonal stressors.
- Categorize stressors as modifiable or nonmodifiable.
- Help clients distinguish among short-term, chronic, and secondary stressors.
- Provide information as needed to reduce stress responses to acute and chronic illnesses.
- Explore possible therapeutic approaches such as cognitive-behavioral therapy, biofeedback, neurofeedback, acupuncture, pharmacological agents, and complementary and alternative therapies.
- Help the client to reframe his or her perceptions of some of the stressors.
- Assist the client to mobilize social supports for dealing with recent stressors.

S Pediatric

- With children, nurses should work with parents to help them to reduce children's stressors.
- Help children to manage their feelings related to self-concept.
- Help children to deal with bullies and other sources of violence in schools and neighborhoods.
- Help young children to identify and mitigate the experience of "feeling sick."
- Help children to manage the complexities of chronic illnesses.

Geriatric

- Assess for chronic stress with older adults and provide a variety of stress relief techniques.
- ▲ Encourage older adults to seek appropriate counseling.

Multicultural

- Review cultural beliefs and acculturation level in relation to perceived stressors.

• = Independent   ▲ = Collaborative

Home Care

- The preceding interventions may be adapted for home care use.
- Develop community-based programs for stress management as needed for groups with increased risk of stress overload (e.g., firefighters, policemen, military personnel, and nurses).
- Support and encourage neighborhood stability.

Client/Family Teaching and Discharge Planning

- Diagnose the possibility of stress overload before teaching.
- Establish readiness for learning.
- Provide manageable amounts of information at the appropriate educational level.
- Evaluate the need for additional teaching and learning experiences.

Risk for Sudden Infant Death Syndrome

NANDA-I Definition

Presence of risk factors for sudden death of an infant under 1 year of age

Risk Factors

Modifiable

Delayed prenatal care; infant overheating; infant overwrapping; infants placed to sleep in the prone position; infants placed to sleep in the side-lying position; bed sharing; lack of prenatal care; postnatal infant smoke exposure; prenatal infant smoke exposure; soft underlayment (loose articles in the sleep environment)

Potentially Modifiable

Low birth weight, prematurity, young maternal age

Nonmodifiable

Ethnicity (e.g., African American or Native American), male gender, seasonality of SIDS deaths (e.g., winter and fall months), infant age of 2-4 months, possible gene mutation resulting in Brugada (QT) syndrome

• = Independent   ▲ = Collaborative

Client Outcomes

Client Will (Specify Time Frame):

- Explain appropriate measures to prevent SIDS
- Demonstrate correct techniques for positioning and blanketing the infant, protecting the infant from harm

Nursing Interventions

- Position the infant supine to sleep; do not position in the prone position or side-lying position.
- Lightly clothe the infant for sleep. Avoid overbundling and overheating the infant. The infant should not feel hot to touch.
- Provide the infant a certain amount of time in prone position while the infant is awake and observed. Change the direction that your baby lies in the crib from one week to the next; and avoid too much time in car seats, carriers, and bouncers.
- Consider offering the infant a pacifier during sleep times.
- ▲ Use electronic respiratory or cardiac monitors to detect cardiorespiratory arrest only if ordered.

S   Home Care

- Most of the interventions discussed previously are relevant to home care.
- Evaluate home for potential safety hazards, such as inappropriate cribs, cradles, or strollers.
- Determine where and how the child sleeps, and provide instructions on safe sleeping positions and environments as needed.

Multicultural

- Treat the parent with respect and caring.
- Encourage pregnant American Indian mothers to avoid drinking alcoholic beverages and to avoid wrapping infants in excessive blankets or clothing.
- Encourage African American mothers to find alternatives to bed sharing or placing infants for sleep on adult beds, sofas, or cots, and to avoid placing pillows, soft toys, and soft bedding in the sleep environment.

● = Independent   ▲ = Collaborative

Client/Family Teaching and Discharge Planning

- Teach families to position infants to sleep on their back rather than in the prone position or side position.
- Teach the parents the need for observed "tummy time."
- Recommend the following infant care practices to parents:
  - Infants should not be put to sleep on soft surfaces such as waterbeds, sofas, or soft mattresses.
  - Avoid placing soft materials in the infant's sleeping environment such as pillows, quilts, and comforters. Do not use sheepskins under a sleeping infant.
  - Avoid the use of loose bedding, such as blankets and sheets.
- Recommend breastfeeding.
- Teach parents the need to obtain a new crib that conforms to the safety standards of the Federal Safety Commission.
- Teach parents not to place the infant in an adult bed to sleep, or a sofa chair or other soft surface. Infants should sleep in a crib.
- Teach parents not to sleep with an infant, especially if alcohol or medications/illicit drugs are used by the parents.
- Recommend an alternative to sleeping with an infant; parents might consider placing the infant's crib near their bed to allow for more convenient breastfeeding and parent contact.
- Teach parents to avoid overbundling and overheating the infant.
- Teach the need to stop smoking during pregnancy and to not smoke around the infant. Smoking is a risk factor for SIDS.
- Recommend that parents with infants in child care make it very clear to the employees that the infant must always be placed in the supine position to sleep, not prone or in a side-lying position.
- ▲ Suggest speaking with a physician about genetic counseling if there is a family history of SIDS or if parents have lost an infant to SIDS.
- ▲ Involve family members in learning and practicing rescue techniques, including treatment of choking, breathing, and cardiopulmonary resuscitation (CPR). Initiate referral to formal training classes.

S

• = Independent   ▲ = Collaborative

Risk for Suffocation

NANDA-I Definition

Accentuated risk of accidental suffocation (inadequate air available for inhalation)

Risk Factors

External

Discarding refrigerators without removing doors; eating large mouthfuls of food; hanging a pacifier around infant's neck; household gas leaks; inserting small objects into airway; leaving children unattended in water; low-strung clothesline; pillow placed in infant's crib; playing with plastic bags; propped bottle placed in infant's crib; smoking in bed; use of fuel-burning heaters not vented to outside; vehicle warming in closed garage

Internal

Cognitive difficulties; disease process; emotional difficulties; injury process; lack of safety education; lack of safety precautions; reduced motor abilities; reduced olfactory sensation

Client Outcomes

Client Will (Specify Time Frame):

- Undertake appropriate measures to prevent suffocation
- Demonstrate correct techniques for emergency rescue maneuvers (e.g., Heimlich maneuver, rescue breathing, cardiopulmonary resuscitation [CPR]) and describe situations that require them

Nursing Interventions

- Identify hospitalized clients at particular risk for suffocation, including the following:
  - Clients with altered levels of consciousness
  - Infants or young children
  - Clients with developmental delays
  - Clients with mental illness, especially schizophrenia

Pediatric

- Counsel families on the following for care of an infant:
  - Position infants on their back to sleep; do not position them in the prone or side-lying position.

• = Independent   ▲ = Collaborative

- Obtain a new crib that conforms to the safety standards of the Federal Safety Commission.
- Place the infant in the crib only to sleep, not on an adult bed, sofa, chair, or playpen.
- Avoid use of loose bedding such as blankets and sheets for sleeping. If blankets are used, they should be tucked in around the crib mattress so the infant's face is less likely to become covered by bedding. The blanket should end at the level of the infant's chest.
- Assess for signs and symptoms of abuse such as Munchausen syndrome by proxy (MSBP).
- Conduct risk factor identification, noting special circumstances in which preventive or protective measures are indicated. Note the presence of environmental hazards, including the following: plastic bags/cribs with slats wider than 2 inches/ill-fitting crib mattresses that can allow the infant to become wedged between the mattress and crib/pillows in cribs/abandoned large appliances such as refrigerators, dishwashers, or freezers/clothing with cords or hoods that can become entangled/bibs, pacifiers on a string, drapery cords, pull-toy strings.
- Counsel families to evaluate household furniture for safety, including large dressers, televisions, and appliances that may need to be anchored to the wall, to prevent the child from climbing on the furniture, and it falling forward and suffocating the child.
- Counsel families to not serve these foods to the child younger than 4 years of age: nuts, hot dogs, popcorn, pretzels, chips, chunks of meat, hard pieces of fruit or vegetables, raisins, whole grapes, hard candies, and marshmallows.
- Counsel families to keep the following items away from infants and toddlers: balloons, coins, marbles, toys with small parts or toys that can be compressed to fit entirely into a child's mouth (small balls, pen or marker caps, small button-type batteries, medicine syringes).
- Stress water and pool safety precautions, including vigilant, uninterrupted parental supervision.
- Underscore the necessity of not allowing children to play with or near electric garage doors and of keeping garage door openers out of the reach of young children.
- For adolescents, watch for signs of depression that could result in suicide by suffocation.

● = Independent   ▲ = Collaborative

Geriatric

- Assess the status of the swallow reflex. Offer appropriate foods and beverages accordingly.
- Use care in pillow placement when positioning frail elderly clients who are on bed rest.
- Recognize that elderly clients in depression may use hanging, strangulation, and suffocation as a means of suicide.

Home Care

- Assess the home for potential safety hazards in systems that are not likely to be fixed (e.g., faulty pilot lights or gas leaks in gas stoves, carbon monoxide release from heating systems, kerosene fumes from portable heaters).
- Assist the family in having these areas assessed and making appropriate safety arrangements (e.g., installing detectors, making repairs).

Client/Family Teaching and Discharge Planning

- Recommend that families who are seeking day care or in-home care for children, geriatric family members, or at-risk family members with developmental or functional disabilities inspect the environment for hazards and examine the first aid preparation and vigilance of providers.
- Ensure family members learn and practice rescue techniques, including treatment of choking and lack of breathing, as well as CPR.

Risk for Suicide

NANDA-I Definition

At risk for self-inflicted, life-threatening injury

Related Factors (r/t)

Behavioral

Buying a gun; changing a will; giving away possessions; history of prior suicide attempt; impulsiveness; making a will; marked changes in attitude; marked changes in behavior; marked changes in school performance; stockpiling medicines; sudden euphoric recovery from major depression

Demographic
Age (e.g., elderly people, young adult males, adolescents); divorced; male gender; race (e.g., white, Native American); widowed

Physical
Chronic pain; physical illness; terminal illness

Psychological
Childhood abuse; family history of suicide; guilt; homosexual youth; psychiatric disorder; psychiatric illness; substance abuse

Situational
Adolescents living in nontraditional settings (e.g., juvenile detention center, prison, halfway house, group home); economic instability; institutionalization; living alone; loss of autonomy; loss of independence; presence of gun in home; relocation; retired

Social
Cluster suicides; disciplinary problems; disrupted family life; grieving; helplessness; hopelessness; legal problems; loneliness; loss of important relationship; poor support systems; social isolation

Verbal
States desire to die; threats of killing oneself

Client Outcomes

Client Will (Specify Time Frame):
* Not harm self
* Maintain connectedness in relationships
* Disclose and discuss suicidal ideas if present; seek help
* Express decreased anxiety and control of impulses
* Talk about feelings; express anger appropriately
* Refrain from using mood-altering substances
* Obtain no access to harmful objects
* Yield access to harmful objects
* Maintain self-control without supervision

• = Independent   ▲ = Collaborative

Nursing Interventions

NOTE: Before implementing interventions in the face of suicidal behavior, nurses should examine their own emotional responses to incidents of suicide to ensure that interventions will not be based on countertransference reactions.

- Assess for suicidal ideation when the history reveals the following: depression, substance abuse; bipolar disorder, schizophrenia, anxiety disorders, post-traumatic stress disorder, dissociative disorder, eating disorders, substance use disorders, antisocial or other personality disorders; attempted suicide, current or past; recent stressful life events (divorce and/or separation, relocation, problems with children); recent unemployment; recent bereavement; adult or childhood physical or sexual abuse; gay, lesbian, or bisexual gender orientation; family history of suicide, history of chronic trauma.
- Assess all medical clients and clients with chronic illnesses, traumatic injuries, or pain for their perception of health status and suicidal ideation.
- Assess the client's ability to enter into a no-suicide contract. Contract (verbally or in writing) with the client for no self-harm if the client is appropriate for a contract; recontract at appropriate intervals.
- Be alert for warning signs of suicide: making statements such as, "I can't go on," "Nothing matters anymore," "I wish I were dead"; becoming depressed or withdrawn; behaving recklessly; getting affairs in order and giving away valued possessions; showing a marked change in behavior, attitudes, or appearance; abusing drugs or alcohol; suffering a major loss or life change.
- Take suicide notes seriously and ask if a note was left in any previous suicide attempts. Consider themes of notes in determining appropriate interventions.
- Question family members regarding the preparatory actions mentioned.
- Determine the presence and degree of suicidal risk. A number of questions will elicit the necessary information: Have you been thinking about hurting or killing yourself? How often do you have these thoughts and how long do they last? Do you have a plan? What is it? Do you have access to the means to

carry out that plan? How likely is it that you could carry out the plan? Are there people or things that could prevent you from hurting yourself? What do you see in your future a year from now? Five years from now? What do you expect would happen if you died? What has kept you alive up to now?

- Observe, record, and report any changes in mood or behavior that may signify increasing suicide risk and document results of regular surveillance checks.
- Develop a positive therapeutic relationship with the clients; do not make promises that may not be kept.
▲ Refer for mental health counseling and possible hospitalization if evidence of suicidal intent exists, which may include evidence of preparatory actions (e.g., obtaining a weapon, making a plan, putting affairs in order, giving away prized possessions, preparing a suicide note).
- Assign a hospitalized client to a room located near the nursing station.
- Search the newly hospitalized client and the client's personal belongings for weapons or potential weapons and hoarded medications during the inpatient admission procedure, as appropriate. Remove dangerous items.
- Limit access to windows and exits unless locked and shatterproof, as appropriate.
- Monitor the client during the use of potential weapons (e.g., razor, scissors).
- Increase surveillance of a hospitalized client at times when staffing is predictably low (e.g., staff meetings, change of shift report, periods of unit disruption).
▲ If imminent suicide is suspected or an attempt has occurred, call for assistance and do not leave the client alone.
- Place the client in the least restrictive, safe, and monitored environment that allows for the necessary level of observation. Assess suicidal risk at least daily and more frequently as warranted.
- Consider strategies to decrease isolation and opportunity to act on harmful thoughts (e.g., use of a sitter).
- Explain suicide precautions and relevant safety issues to the client and family (e.g., purpose, duration, behavioral expectations, and behavioral consequences).

● = Independent   ▲ = Collaborative

▲ Refer for treatment and participate in the management of any psychiatric illness or symptoms that may be contributing to the client's suicidal ideation or behavior.

▲ Verify that the client has taken medications as ordered (e.g., conduct mouth checks after medication administration).

▲ Maintain increased surveillance of the client whenever use of an antidepressant has been initiated or the dose increased. Antidepressant medications take anywhere from 2 to 6 weeks to achieve full efficacy.

• Involve the client in treatment planning and self-care management of psychiatric disorders.

• Explore with the client all circumstances and motivations related to the suicidality. Listen to the client's own views on his or her problems.

• Explore with the client all perceived consequences that could act as a barrier to suicide (e.g., effect on family, religious beliefs).

• Keep discussion oriented to the present and future.

• Discuss plans for dealing with suicidal ideation in the future (e.g., how to identify precipitating factors, whom to contact, where to go for help, how to respond to desire for self-harm).

• Assist the client in identifying a network of supportive persons and resources (e.g., clergy, family, care providers).

▲ Refer family members and friends to local mental health agencies and crisis intervention centers if the client has suicidal ideation or a suspicion of suicidal thoughts exists.

▲ Document client behavior in detail to support outpatient commitment or an overnight psychiatric observation program for an actively suicidal client.

• Utilize cognitive-behavioral techniques that help the client to modify thinking styles that promote depression, hopelessness, and a belief that suicide is a valid means of escaping the current situation.

• Engage the client in group interventions that can be useful to address recurrent suicide attempts.

• With the client's consent, facilitate family-oriented crisis intervention. Family-oriented crisis intervention can clarify stresses and allow assessment of family dynamics.

• = Independent   ▲ = Collaborative

- Involve the family in discharge planning (e.g., illness/medication teaching, recognition of increasing suicidal risk, client's plan for dealing with recurring suicidal thoughts, community resources).
▲ Before discharge from the hospital, ensure that the client has a supply of ordered medications, has a plan for outpatient follow-up, understands the plan or has a caregiver able and willing to follow the plan, and has the ability to access outpatient treatment.
▲ In the event of successful suicide, refer the family to a therapy group for survivors of suicide.
- See the care plans for **Risk for self-directed Violence, Hopelessness,** and **Risk for Self-Mutilation.**

Pediatric

- The preceding interventions may be appropriate for pediatric clients.
- Use brief self-report measures to improve clinical management of at-risk cases.
- Recognize that the developmental issues of childhood and adolescence may heighten suicide risks and involve different issues from those with adults. Assess specific stressors for the adolescent client.
- Assess for exposure to suicide of a significant other.
- Be alert to the presence of school victimization around lesbian, gay, bisexual, and transgender issues and be prepared to advocate for the client.
- Evaluate for the presence of self-mutilation and related risk factors. Refer to care plan for **Risk for Self-Mutilation** for additional information.
- Be aware that complete overlap does not exist between suicidal behavior and self-mutilation. The motivation may be different (ending life rather than coping with difficult feelings), and the method is usually different.
- Involve the adolescent in multimodal treatment programs.
- Before discharge from the hospital, ensure that the client's parent has a supply of ordered medications, has a plan for outpatient follow-up, has a caregiver who understands the plan or is able and willing to follow the plan, and has the ability to access outpatient treatment.

● = Independent   ▲ = Collaborative

- Parental education groups can influence suicide risk factors.
- Support the implementation of school-based suicide prevention programs.

Geriatric

- Evaluate the older client's mental and physical health status and financial stressors.
- Explore with client any concerns or pressures (physical and financial) regarding ability to secure support of medical care, especially perceived pressures about being a burden on family.
- Conduct a thorough assessment of clients' medications.
- When assessing suicide risk factors, incorporate a higher degree of risk for older men and for some older adults who have lost a loved one in the previous year.
- Explore triggers of and barriers to suicidal behavior, with particular attention to real and perceived losses (e.g., professional role, health).
- An older adult who shows self-destructive behaviors should be evaluated for dementia.
- Anticipate overall responsiveness to treatment, but monitor for early relapse.
- ▲ Advocate for the older client with other professionals in securing treatment for suicidal states. Primary care physicians have been noted to underrecognize and undertreat older adult clients with depression.
- Encourage physical activity in older adults.
- ▲ Refer older adults in primary care settings for care management.
- Consider telephone contacts as an effective intervention for suicidal older adults.

Multicultural

- Assess for the influence of cultural beliefs, norms, and values on the individual's perceptions of suicide.
- Identify and acknowledge the stresses unique to culturally diverse individuals.
- Identify and acknowledge unique cultural responses to stressors in determining sensitive interventions to prevent suicide.

● = Independent   ▲ = Collaborative

- Encourage family members to demonstrate and offer caring and support to each other.
- Validate the individual's feelings regarding concerns about the current crisis and family functioning.

Home Care

- Communicate the degree of risk to family and caregivers; assess the family and caregiving situation for ability to protect the client and to understand the client's suicidal behavior. Provide the family and caregivers with guidelines on how to manage self-harm behaviors in the home environment.
- If the client's suicidal ideation intensifies, or if a suicide plan with access to means becomes evident, institute an emergency plan for mental health intervention
- Counsel parents and homeowners to restrict unauthorized access to potentially lethal prescription drugs and firearms within the home.
- Identify the client's concerns and implement interventions to address the consequences of disability in a client with medical illness. Refer to the care plans for **Hopelessness** and **Powerlessness.**
- ▲ Refer for homemaker or psychiatric home health care services for respite, client reassurance, and implementation of a therapeutic regimen.
- ▲ If the client is on psychotropic medications, assess the client's and family's knowledge of medication administration and side effects. Teach as necessary.
- ▲ Evaluate the effectiveness and side effects of medications and adherence to the medication regimen. Review with the client and family all medications kept in the home; encourage discarding of old prescriptions. Monitor the amount of medications ordered/provided by the physician; limiting the amount of medications to which the client has access may be necessary.

Client/Family Teaching and Discharge Planning

- Establish a supportive relationship with family members.

- Explain all relevant symptoms, procedures, treatments, and expected outcomes for suicidal ideation that is illness based (e.g., depression, bipolar disorder).
- Teach the family how to recognize that the client is at increased risk for suicide (changes in behavior and verbal and nonverbal communication, withdrawal, depression, or sudden lifting of depression).
- Provide written instructions for treatments and procedures for which the client will be responsible.
- Instruct the client in coping strategies (assertiveness training, impulse control training, deep breathing, progressive muscle relaxation).
- Role play (e.g., say, "Tell me how you will respond if a friend asks why you were in the hospital").
- Teach cognitive-behavioral activities, such as active problem solving, reframing (reappraising the situation from a different perspective), or thought stopping (in response to a negative thought, picturing a large stop sign and replacing the image with a prearranged positive alternative). Teach the client to confront his or her own negative thought patterns (or cognitive distortions), such as catastrophizing (expecting the very worst), dichotomous thinking (perceiving events in only one of two opposite categories), or magnification (placing distorted emphasis on a single event).
- Provide the client and family with phone numbers of appropriate community agencies for therapy and counseling. NAMI is an excellent resource for client and family support.

Delayed Surgical Recovery

NANDA-I Definition

Extension of the number of postoperative days required to initiate and perform activities that maintain life, health, and well-being

Defining Characteristics

Difficulty in moving about; evidence of interrupted healing of surgical area (e.g., red, indurated draining, immobilized); fatigue; loss of appetite with nausea; loss of appetite without nausea; perception that more time is needed to recover; postpones resumption of work/employment activities; requires help to complete self-care; report of discomfort; report of pain

Related Factors (r/t)

Extensive surgical procedure; obesity; pain; postoperative surgical site infection; preoperative expectations; prolonged surgical procedure

Client Outcomes

Client Will (Specify Time Frame):

- Have surgical area that shows evidence of healing: no redness, induration, draining, or immobility
- State that appetite is regained
- State that no nausea is present
- Demonstrate ability to move about
- Demonstrate ability to complete self-care activities
- State that no fatigue is present
- State that pain is controlled or relieved after nursing interventions
- Resume employment activities/activities of daily living (ADLs)

Nursing Interventions

- Perform a thorough assessment of the client, including risk factors. Allow time to be with the client.
- Assess for the presence of medical conditions and treat appropriately before surgery. If the client is diabetic, maintain normal blood glucose levels before surgery.
- Carefully assess client's use of dietary supplements such as feverfew, ginkgo biloba, garlic, ginseng, ginger, valerian, kava, St. John's wort, ephedra (Ma huang or metabolite), and echinacea. It is recommended that all clients be advised to stop all dietary supplements at least 1 week before major surgical or diagnostic procedures.
- Assess and treat for depression and anxiety in a client complaining of continuing fatigue after surgery.
- Play music of the client's choice preoperatively, intraoperatively, and postoperatively.
- Consider using healing touch and other mind-body-spirit interventions such as stress control and imagery in the perianesthesia setting.

S

• = Independent ▲ = Collaborative

- Use warmed cotton blankets to reduce heat loss during surgery.
- Use careful aseptic technique when caring for wounds.
- Suggest the use of a semipermeable dressing and suction drainage for selected orthopedic clients.
- Clients should be allowed to shower after surgery to maintain cleanliness if not contraindicated because of the presence of pacemaker wires.
- Promote early ambulation and deep breathing. Consider use of a transcutaneous electrical nerve stimulation (TENS) unit for pain relief.
- The client should be provided with a complete, balanced therapeutic diet after the immediately postoperative period (24 to 48 hours).
- Provide 20-minute foot and hand massage (5 minutes to each extremity), 1 to 4 hours after a dose of pain medication.
- ▲ Carefully consider the use of alternative therapy with a physician's order, such as application of aloe vera or aqueous cream to promote wound healing.
- Consider the use of noetic therapies: stress management, imagery, and touch therapy.
- Encourage the client to use prayer as a form of spiritual coping if this is comfortable for the client.
- See the care plans for **Anxiety, Acute Pain, Fatigue, Risk for deficient Fluid Volume, Risk for Perioperative Positioning Injury, Impaired physical Mobility,** and **Nausea.**

Pediatric

- Support information the parents have gotten from the Internet regarding their child's condition.
- Teach imagery and encourage distraction for children for postsurgical pain relief.
- Children who are at normal risk for aspiration/regurgitation should be allowed fluids prior to anesthesia.

Geriatric

- Perform a thorough preoperative assessment, including a cardiac and social support assessment.
- Assess for pain.

• = Independent   ▲ = Collaborative

- Carefully evaluate the client's temperature. Know what is normal and abnormal for each client. Check baseline temperature and monitor trends.
- Teach guided imagery for pain relief.
- Offer spiritual support.

Home Care

- The preceding interventions may be adapted for the home setting.
- Provide supportive telephone calls from nurse to client as a means of decreasing anxiety and providing the psychosocial support necessary for recovery from surgery.

Client/Family Teaching and Discharge Planning

- Provide preoperative teaching by a nurse to decrease postoperative problems of anxiety, pain, nausea, and lack of independence.
- Provide preoperative information in verbal and written form.
- Teach systematic muscle relaxation for pain relief.
- Provide individualized teaching plans for the client with an ostomy. Consider basic needs: (1) maintenance of a pouching seal for a consistent, predictable wear time; (2) maintenance of peristomal skin integrity; and (3) social and professional support of the client.

Impaired Swallowing

NANDA-I Definition

Abnormal functioning of the swallowing mechanism associated with deficits in oral, pharyngeal, or esophageal structure or function

Defining Characteristics

Esophageal Phase Impairment

Abnormality in esophageal phase by swallow study; acidic-smelling breath; bruxism; complaints of "something stuck"; epigastric pain; food refusal; heartburn or epigastric pain; hematemesis; hyperextension of head (e.g., arching during or after meals); nighttime awakening; nighttime coughing; observed evidence of difficulty in swallowing (e.g., stasis of food in oral cavity, coughing/choking); odynophagia; regurgitation of

• = Independent   ▲ = Collaborative

gastric contents (wet burps); repetitive swallowing; unexplained irritability surrounding mealtime; volume limiting; vomiting; vomitus on pillow

Oral Phase Impairment

Abnormality in oral phase of swallow study; choking, coughing, or gagging before a swallow; drooling; food falls from mouth; food pushed out of mouth; inability to clear oral cavity; incomplete lip closure; lack of chewing; lack of tongue action to form bolus; long meals with little consumption; nasal reflux; piecemeal deglutition; pooling in lateral sulci; premature entry of bolus; sialorrhea; slow bolus formation; weak suck resulting in inefficient nippling

Pharyngeal Phase Impairment

Abnormality in pharyngeal phase by swallowing study; altered head position; choking, coughing, or gagging; delayed swallow; food refusal; gurgly voice quality; inadequate laryngeal elevation; multiple swallows; nasal reflux; recurrent pulmonary infections; unexplained fevers

Related Factors (r/t)

Congenital Defects

Behavioral feeding problems; conditions with significant hypotonia; congenital heart disease; failure to thrive; history of tube feeding; mechanical obstruction (e.g., edema, tracheostomy tube, tumor); neuromuscular impairment (e.g., decreased or absent gag reflex, decreased strength or excursion of muscles involved in mastication, perceptual impairment, facial paralysis); protein energy malnutrition; respiratory disorders; self-injurious behavior; upper airway anomalies

Neurological Problems

Achalasia; acquired anatomic defects; cerebral palsy; cranial nerve involvement; developmental delay; esophageal defects; gastroesophageal reflux disease; laryngeal abnormalities; laryngeal defects; nasal defects; nasopharyngeal cavity defects; oropharynx abnormalities; prematurity; tracheal defects; traumas; traumatic head injury; upper airway anomalies

Client Outcomes

Client Will (Specify Time Frame):
- Demonstrate effective swallowing without signs of aspiration (see defining characteristics above)
- Remain free from aspiration (e.g., lungs clear, temperature within normal range)

● = Independent   ▲ = Collaborative

Nursing Interventions

▲ If the client has impaired swallowing, do not feed orally until an appropriate diagnostic workup is completed.

▲ Ensure proper nutrition by consulting with a physician regarding alternative nutrition and hydration when oral nutrition is not safe/adequate.

▲ Refer to a speech-language pathologist for bedside evaluation, and videofluoroscopy or fiberoptic endoscopic evaluation of swallowing (FEES) to determine swallowing problems and solutions as soon as oral and/or pharyngeal dysphagia is suspected.

▲ To manage impaired swallowing, use a dysphagia team composed of a rehabilitation nurse, speech pathologist, dietitian, physician, and radiologist.

▲ Observe the following feeding guidelines:

■ Prior to giving oral feedings, determine the client's readiness to eat (e.g., alert, able to hold head erect, follow instructions, move tongue in mouth, and manage oral secretions).

■ Monitor client during oral feedings and provide cueing as needed to ensure client follows swallowing guidelines/ aspiration precautions recommended by speech language pathologist or dysphagia specialist. NOTE: General aspiration precautions include: sit at 90 degrees for all oral feedings; take small bites/sips, slow rate, no straws. However, strategies for individual clients will be determined via bedside and/or instrumental swallowing evaluation performed by dysphagia specialist.

■ If older client or client with GERD, ensure client is kept in an upright posture for an hour after eating.

• During meals and all oral intake, observe for signs associated with swallowing problems such as coughing, choking, spitting of food, drooling, difficulty handling oral secretions, double swallowing or delay in swallowing, watering eyes, nasal discharge, wet or gurgly voice, decreased ability to move the tongue and lips, decreased mastication of food, decreased ability to move food to the back of the pharynx, slow or scanning speech.

S

• = Independent ▲ = Collaborative

▲ Watch for uncoordinated chewing or swallowing; coughing immediately after eating or delayed coughing; pocketing of food; wet-sounding voice; sneezing when eating; delay of more than 1 second in swallowing; or a change in respiratory patterns. If any of these signs is present, remove all food from the oral cavity, stop feedings, and consult with speech and language pathologist and dysphagia team.

▲ If signs of aspiration or pneumonia are present, auscultate lung sounds after feeding. Note new onset of crackles or wheezing, and note elevated temperature.

• Watch for signs of malnutrition and dehydration and keep a record of food intake.

▲ Evaluate nutritional status daily. Weigh the client weekly to help evaluate nutritional status. If the client is not adequately nourished, work with the dysphagia team to determine whether the client needs therapeutic feeding only or needs enteral feedings until the client can swallow adequately.

• If client is not eating a sufficient amount of food, recognize that the immune system may be impaired with resultant increased risk of infection.

▲ Document and notify the physician and dysphagia team of changes in medical, nutritional, or swallowing status.

▲ Work with the client on swallowing exercises prescribed by the dysphagia team.

• If needed, provide meals in a quiet environment away from excessive stimuli, such as a community dining room for some clients who are easily distracted.

▲ For many adult clients, if recommended by the speech therapist, avoid the use of straws if recommended by the speech pathologist.

• Recognize that the client can aspirate oral feedings, even if there are no symptoms of coughing or distress.

• Ensure that oral hygiene is maintained.

• Check the oral cavity for proper emptying after the client swallows and after the client finishes the meal. Provide oral care at the end of the meal. It may be necessary to manually remove food from the client's mouth. If this is the case, use gloves and keep the client's teeth apart with a padded tongue blade.

- Praise the client for successfully following directions and swallowing appropriately.
- Keep the client in an upright position for 45 minutes to an hour after a meal.
- Recognize that impaired swallowing may be caused by the medications the client is taking. Side effects of medications include xerostomia (antidepressants, anticholinergics, antihistamines, bronchodilators, antineoplastic, anti-parkinson), CNS depression (anticonvulsants, benzodiazepines, antispasmodics, antidepressants, antipsychotics), myopathy (corticosteroids, lipid-lowering agents, colchicines), and esophageal sphincter tone decrease (antihistamines, diuretics, opiates, antipsychotics, antihypertensives, anticholinergics).
▲ If client has a tracheostomy, ask for referral to speech pathologist for swallowing studies before attempting to feed. After evaluation, the decision should be made to have cuff either inflated or deflated when client eats.

Pediatric

▲ Refer to speech-language pathologist (or dysphagia specialist), and a dietitian for a child who has difficulty swallowing and symptoms such as difficulty manipulating food, delayed swallow response, and pocketing of a bolus of food.
▲ Consult with speech-language pathologist or dysphagia specialist regarding modifications to nipple; appropriate positioning and feeding strategies; and other therapeutic activities deemed most appropriate based on bedside and instrumental swallowing evaluation.
▲ The following are general feeding guidelines. Specific strategies to eliminate aspiration and maximize intake should be individualized and determined by swallowing specialist through bedside and instrumental swallowing assessment.
  ■ In preterm infant, provide opportunities for patterned nonnutritive sucking (NNS).
  ■ In preterm infant, alter nipple flow rate to one that is easily managed by infant to facilitate intake while achieving physiological stability.
  ■ Avoid feeding-induced apnea in preterm infant by pacing (offer respiratory break after 3 to 5 sucks).

- Watch for indicators of aspiration and physiological instability during feeding: coughing, a change in vocal quality or wet vocal quality, perspiration and color changes, sneezing, apnea, and/or increased heart rate and breathing.
- Watch for warning signs of reflux: sour-smelling breath after eating, sneezing, lack of interest in feeding, crying and fussing extraordinarily when feeding, pained expressions when feeding, and excessive chewing and swallowing after eating.
- Observe infant's behavior and cues and adjust feeding to promote a safe pleasurable feeding experience while eliminating aspiration and maximizing intake.

Geriatric

- Recognize that being elderly does not necessarily result in dysphagia, but having medical problems including such things as cerebrovascular and other neurological disease along with chronic medical problems can result in dysphagia.
- ▲ Evaluate medications the client is taking, especially if elderly. Consult with the pharmacist for assistance in monitoring for incorrect doses and drug interactions that could result in dysphagia.
- Recognize that the elderly client with dementia needs a longer time to eat.
- For the client with dementia, hydration and nutrition can be optimized using the following techniques:
  - Provide good oral hygiene.
  - Encourage six small meals and hydration breaks per day.
  - Offer foods that are sweet, spicy, or sour to increase sensory input.
  - Allow clients to touch food, and self-feed, with their hands if necessary.
  - Eliminate from the tray or table nonfoods such as salt and pepper, or anything that can be distracting.
  - Keep desserts out of sight until the end of the meal.
  - Offer finger foods to the client who has trouble holding still to eat.
  - Allow clients to eat immediately when they come for the meal.

• = Independent   ▲ = Collaborative

- Recognize that the client with advanced dementia, who is unable to swallow, may or may not benefit from enteral tube feedings.

Home Care

▲ Refer to speech therapy.

Client/Family Teaching and Discharge Planning

▲ Teach the client and family exercises prescribed by the dysphagia team.
▲ Teach the client a systematic method of swallowing effectively as prescribed by the dysphagia team.
- Educate the client, family, and all caregivers about rationales for food consistency and choices.
- Teach the family how to monitor the client to prevent and detect aspiration during eating.

Risk for imbalanced body Temperature

NANDA-I Definition

At risk for failure to maintain body temperature within a normal range

Risk Factors

Altered metabolic rate; dehydration; exposure to extremes of environmental temperature; extremes of age or weight; illness affecting temperature regulation; inactivity; inappropriate clothing for environmental temperature; medications causing vasoconstriction; medications causing vasodilation; sedation; trauma affecting temperature regulation; vigorous activity

Ineffective family Therapeutic Regimen Management

NANDA-I Definition

A pattern of regulating and integrating into family processes a program for the treatment of illness and its sequelae that is unsatisfactory for meeting specific health goals

• = Independent   ▲ = Collaborative

Defining Characteristics

Acceleration of illness symptoms of a family member; failure to take action to reduce risk factors; inappropriate family activities for meeting health goals; lack of attention to illness; reports desire to manage the illness; reports difficulty with prescribed regimen

Related Factors (r/t)

Complexity of health care system; complexity of therapeutic regimen; decisional conflicts; economic difficulties; excessive demands; family conflict

Family Outcomes

Family Will (Specify Time Frame):

- Make adjustments in usual activities (e.g., diet, activity, stress management) to incorporate therapeutic regimens of its members
- Reduce illness symptoms of family members
- Desire to manage therapeutic regimens of its members
- Describe a decrease in the difficulties of managing therapeutic regimens
- Describe actions to reduce risk factors

Nursing Interventions

- Base family interventions on knowledge of the family, family context, and family function.
- Use a family approach when helping an individual with a health problem that requires therapeutic management.
- Review with family members the congruence and incongruence of family behaviors and health-related goals.
- Acknowledge the challenge of integrating therapeutic regimens with family behaviors.
- Review the symptoms of specific illness(es) and work with the family toward development of greater self-efficacy in relation to these symptoms.
- Support family decisions to adjust therapeutic regimens as indicated.
- Advocate for the family in negotiating therapeutic regimens with health providers.
- Help the family mobilize social supports.
- Help family members modify perceptions as indicated.

• = Independent   ▲ = Collaborative

- Use one or more theories of family dynamics to describe, explain, or predict family behaviors (e.g., theories of Bowen, Satir, and Minuchin).
▲ Collaborate with expert nurses or other consultants regarding strategies for working with families.
- Coaching methods can be used to help families improve their health.

Pediatric

- Support kangaroo care for infants at risk at birth. Keep infants in an upright position in skin-to-skin contact until they no longer tolerate it.

Geriatric

- Recommend that clients use the "Ask Me 3" program when communicating with their pharmacist (What is my main problem? What do I need to do? Why is it important for me to do this?).

Multicultural

- Acknowledge racial and ethnic differences at the onset of care.
- Ensure that all strategies for working with the family are congruent with the culture of the family.
- Use a family-centered approach when working with Latino, Asian, African American, and Native American clients.
- Facilitate modeling and role playing for the family regarding healthy ways to communicate and interact.
- Use the nursing intervention of cultural brokerage to help families deal with the health care system.

Client/Family Teaching and Discharge Planning

- Teach about all aspects of therapeutic regimens. Provide as much knowledge as family members will accept, adjust instruction to account for what the family already knows, and provide information in a culturally congruent manner.
- Teach ways to adjust family behaviors to include therapeutic regimens, such as safety in taking medications and teaching family members to act as self-advocates with health providers who prescribe therapeutic regimens.

● = Independent   ▲ = Collaborative

Risk for Thermal Injury

NANDA-I Definition

At risk for damage to skin and mucous membranes due to extreme temperatures

Risk Factors

Cognitive impairment (e.g., dementia, psychoses); developmental level (infants, aged); exposure to extreme temperatures; fatigue; inadequate supervision; inattentiveness; intoxication (alcohol, drug); lack of knowledge (patient, caregiver); lack of protective clothing (e.g., flame-retardant sleepwear, gloves, ear covering); neuromuscular impairment (e.g., stroke, amyotrophic lateral sclerosis, multiple sclerosis); neuropathy; smoking; treatment-related side effects (e.g., pharmaceutical agents); unsafe environment

Client Outcomes

Client Will (Specify Time Frame)
- Be free of burned skin or tissue
- Explain actions can take to protect self, and family from burns
- Explain actions can take to protect self and others in the work environment

Nursing Interventions

- Teach the following interventions to prevent fires in the home, to handle any possible fire, and to have a readily available exit from the home:
  - Avoid plugging several appliance cords into the same electrical socket.
  - Do not use open candles or allow smoking in the home.
  - Keep a fire extinguisher within reach in case a fire should occur.
  - Install smoke alarms on every level of the home and in every sleeping area.
  - Keep furniture and other heavy objects out of the way of doors and windows.
  - Develop a fire escape plan that includes two ways out of every room and an outside meeting place. Practice the escape plan at least twice a year.

• = Independent ▲ = Collaborative

- Teach the following activities to homes with small children:
  - Lock up matches and lighters out of sight and reach.
  - Never leave a hot stove unattended.
  - Do not allow small children to use the microwave until they are at least 7 or 8 years of age.
  - Keep all portable heaters out of children's reach and at least 3 feet away from anything that can burn.
  - Install thermostatic mixer valves in hot water system to prevent extreme hot water causing scalding burns.
- Utilize sunscreen when out in the sun. Also use sun-blocking clothing, and stay in the shade if possible.
- Teach the following interventions to prevent fires in the home where medical oxygen is in use:
  - **Never smoke** in a home where medical oxygen is in use. "No smoking" signs should be posted inside and outside the home.
  - All ignition sources—matches, lighters, candles, gas stoves, appliances, electric razors and hair dryers—should be kept at least 10 feet away from the point where the oxygen comes out.
  - Do not wear oxygen while cooking. Oils, grease and petroleum products can spontaneously ignite when exposed to high levels of oxygen. Also, do not use oil-based lotions, lip balm, or aerosol sprays.
  - Homes with medical oxygen must have working smoke alarms that are tested monthly.
  - Keep a fire extinguisher within reach. If a fire occurs, turn off the oxygen and leave the home.
  - Develop a fire escape plan that includes two ways out of every room and an outside meeting place. Practice the escape plan at least twice a year.

Ineffective Thermoregulation

NANDA-I Definition

Temperature fluctuation between hypothermia and hyperthermia

• = Independent   ▲ = Collaborative

Defining Characteristics

Cool skin; cyanotic nail beds; fluctuations in body temperature above and below the normal range; flushed skin; hypertension; increased respiratory rate; shivering; moderate pallor; piloerection; seizures; slow capillary refill; tachycardia; warm to touch (adapted from the work of NANDA-I)

Related Factors (r/t)

Aging; fluctuating environmental temperature; illness; immaturity; infection; trauma; stress; medications

Client Outcomes

Client Will (Specify Time Frame):

* Maintain temperature within normal range
* Explain measures needed to maintain normal temperature
* Describe two to four symptoms of hypothermia or hyperthermia
* List two or three self-care measures to treat hypothermia or hyperthermia

Nursing Interventions

Temperature Measurement

* Measure and record the client's temperature using a consistent method of temperature measurement every 1 to 4 hours depending on severity of the situation or whenever a change in condition occurs (e.g., chills, change in mental status)
* Select core, near core, or peripheral temperature monitoring mode based on ability to obtain an accurate temperature from that site and clinical situation dictating the need for mode of temperature monitoring required for clinical treatment decisions.
* Caution should be taken in interpreting extreme values of temperature (less than 35° C or greater than 39° C) from a near core temperature site device.
* Evaluate the significance of a decreased or increased temperature.
▲ Notify the physician of temperature according to institutional standards or written orders, or when temperature reaches

---

• = Independent   ▲ = Collaborative

100.5° F (38.3° C) and above. Also notify the physician of the presence of a change in mental status and temperature greater than 38.3° C or less than 36° C.

Fever (Pyrexia)

- Recognize that fever is characterized as a temporary elevation in internal body temperature 1° to 2° C higher than the client's normal body temperature.
- Recognize that fever is a normal physiological response to a perceived threat by the body, frequently in response to an infection.
- ▲ Review client history to include current medical diagnosis, medications, recent procedures/interventions, and review of laboratory analysis for cause of ineffective thermoregulation.
- Recognize that fever may be low grade (36° C to 38° C) in response to an inflammatory process such as infection, allergy, trauma, illness, or surgery. Moderate to high-grade fever (38° C to 40° C) indicates a more concerted inflammatory response from a systemic infection. Hyperpyrexia (40° C and higher) occurs as a result of damage of the hypothalamus, bacteremia, or an extremely overheated room.
- Recognize that fever has a predictable physiological pattern.
- Monitor and intervene to provide comfort during a fever by:
  - Obtaining vital signs and accurate intake and output
  - Checking laboratory analysis trends of white blood cell counts and other infectious markers
  - Providing blankets when the client complains of being cold; but removing surplus of blankets when the client is too warm
  - Encouraging fluid and nutrition
  - Limiting activity to conserve energy
  - Providing frequent oral care

Hypothermia

- Take vital signs frequently, noting changes associated with hypothermia: increased blood pressure, pulse, and respirations which then advance to decreased values as hypothermia progresses.

• = Independent   ▲ = Collaborative

- Monitor the client for signs of hypothermia (e.g., shivering, cool skin, piloerection, pallor, slow capillary refill, cyanotic nailbeds, decreased mentation, dysrhythmias)
- See the care plan for **Hypothermia** as appropriate.

Hyperthermia

- Note changes in vital signs associated with hyperthermia: rapid, bounding pulse; increased respiratory rate; and decreased blood pressure, accompanied by orthostatic hypotension, and signs and symptoms of dehydration.
- Monitor the client for signs of hyperthermia (e.g., headache, nausea and vomiting, weakness, absence of sweating, delirium, and coma).
- Adjust clothing to facilitate passive warming or cooling as appropriate.
- See the care plan for **Hyperthermia** as appropriate.

Pediatric

- For routine measurement of temperature, use an electronic thermometer in the axilla in infants under the age of 4 weeks; for a child up to 5 years of age, use an electronic thermometer in the axilla, or an infrared tympanic thermometer.
- Recognize that pediatric clients have a decreased ability to adapt to temperature extremes. Take the following actions to maintain body temperature in the infant/child:
  - Keep the head covered.
  - Use blankets to keep the client warm.
  - Keep the client covered during procedures, transport, and diagnostic testing.
  - Keep the room temperature at 72° F (22.2° C).
- Recognize that the infant and small child are both vulnerable to develop heat stroke in hot weather; ensure that they receive sufficient fluids and are protected from hot environments.
- Antipyretic treatments typically are not indicated unless the child's temperature is higher than 38.3° C and may be given to provide comfort.

• = Independent ▲ = Collaborative

Geriatric

- Do not allow an elderly client to become chilled. Keep the client covered when giving a bath and offer socks to wear in bed. Be aware of factors such as room temperature (heating/air conditioning), clothing (layered/loose), and fluid intake.
- Recognize that the elderly client may have an infection without a significant rise in body temperature.
- Fever does not put the older adult at risk for long-term complications; thus, fever should not be treated with antipyretic agents or other external methods of cooling, unless there is serious heart disease present.
- Ensure that elderly clients receive sufficient fluids during hot days and stay out of the sun.
- Assess the medication profile for the potential risk of drug-related altered body temperature.

Home Care
Treating Fever

- Instruct client/parents on the physiological benefits of fever and provide interventions to treat fever symptoms, avoiding antipyretic agents and external cooling interventions.
- Ensure that client/parents know when to contact a health care provider for fever-related concerns.

Prevention of Hypothermia in Cold Weather

See the care plan **Hypothermia**.

Prevention of Hyperthermia in Hot Weather

See the care plan **Hyperthermia**.

Client/Family Teaching and Discharge Planning

- Teach the client and family the signs of fever, hypothermia, and hyperthermia and appropriate actions to take if either condition develops.
- Teach the client and family an age-appropriate method for taking the temperature.
- Teach the client to avoid alcohol and medications that depress cerebral function.

• = Independent   ▲ = Collaborative

Impaired Tissue Integrity

NANDA-I Definition

Damage to mucous membrane, corneal, integumentary, or subcutaneous tissues

Defining Characteristics

Damaged tissue (e.g., cornea, mucous membrane, integumentary or subcutaneous tissue); destroyed tissue

Related Factors (r/t)

Altered circulation; chemical irritants; fluid deficit; fluid excess; impaired physical mobility; knowledge deficit; mechanical factors (e.g., pressure, shear, friction); nutritional factors (e.g., deficit or excess); radiation; temperature extremes

Client Outcomes

Client Will (Specify Time Frame):

- Report any altered sensation or pain at site of tissue impairment
- Demonstrate understanding of plan to heal tissue and prevent reinjury
- Describe measures to protect and heal the tissue, including wound care
- Experience a wound that decreases in size and has increased granulation tissue

Nursing Interventions

- Assess the site of impaired tissue integrity and determine the cause (e.g., acute or chronic wound, burn, dermatological lesion, pressure ulcer, leg ulcer, skin failure).
- Determine the size (length, width) and depth of the wound (e.g., full-thickness wound, deep tissue injury, stage III or IV pressure ulcer).
- Classify pressure ulcers in the following manner:
  - **Category/Stage III:** Full-thickness tissue loss. Subcutaneous fat may be visible, but bone, tendon, or muscle is not exposed. Slough may be present but does not obscure the

• = Independent   ▲ = Collaborative

depth of tissue loss. May include undermining and tunneling. The depth of a Category/Stage III pressure ulcer varies by anatomic location. The bridge of the nose, ear, occiput, and malleolus do not have (adipose) subcutaneous tissue and can be shallow. In contrast, areas of significant adiposity can develop extremely deep Category/Stage III pressure ulcers. Bone/tendon is not visible or directly palpable.

- **Category/Stage IV:** Full-thickness tissue loss with exposed bone, tendon, or muscle. Slough or eschar may be present on some parts of the wound bed. Often include undermining and tunneling. The depth of a Category/Stage IV pressure ulcer varies by anatomic location. The bridge of the nose, ear, occiput, and malleolus do not have (adipose) subcutaneous tissue and can be shallow. Category IV ulcers can extend into muscle and/or supporting structures (e.g., fascia, tendon, or joint capsule) making osteomyelitis possible. Exposed bone/tendon is visible or directly palpable.

- **Suspected Deep Tissue Injury:** Purple or maroon localized area of discolored intact skin or blood-filled blister due to damage of underlying soft tissue from pressure and/or shear. The area may be preceded by tissue that is painful, firm, mushy, boggy, warmer, or cooler as compared to adjacent tissue. Deep tissue injury may be difficult to detect in individuals with dark skin tones. Evolution may include a thin blister over a dark wound bed. The wound may further evolve and become covered by thin eschar. Evolution may be rapid, exposing additional layers of tissue even with optimal treatment.

- **Unstageable (Depth Unknown):** Full-thickness tissue loss in which the base of the ulcer is covered by slough (yellow, tan, gray, green, or brown) and/or eschar (tan, brown, or black) in the wound bed. Until enough slough and/or eschar is removed to expose the base of the wound, the true depth and, therefore, category/stage cannot be determined. Stable (dry, adherent, intact without erythema or fluctuance) eschar on the heels serves as "the body's natural cover" and should not be removed.

- Inspect and monitor the site of impaired tissue integrity at least once daily for color changes, redness, swelling, warmth, pain, or other signs of infection or per facility/agency policy. Determine whether the client is experiencing changes in sensation or pain. Pay special attention to all high-risk areas such as bony prominences, skin folds, sacrum, and heels.

- Monitor the status of the skin around the wound. Monitor the client's skin care practices, noting type of soap or other cleansing agents used, temperature of water, and frequency of skin cleansing.

- Monitor the client's continence status and minimize exposure of the skin impairment site and other areas to moisture from urine or stool, perspiration, or wound drainage.

- Monitor for correct placement of tubes, catheters, and other devices. Assess the skin and tissue affected by the tape that secures these devices.

- In an orthopedic client, check every 2 hours for correct placement of foot boards, restraints, traction, casts, or other devices, and assess skin and tissue integrity. Be alert for symptoms of compartment syndrome (refer to the care plan for **Risk for Peripheral Neurovascular Dysfunction**).

- For a client with limited mobility, use a risk-assessment tool to assess immobility-related risk factors systematically.

- Implement a written treatment plan for the topical treatment of the skin impairment site.

▲ Identify a plan for debridement if necrotic tissue (eschar or slough) is present and if consistent with overall client management goals.

- Select a topical treatment that maintains a moist, wound-healing environment and also allows absorption of exudate and filling of dead space.

- Do not position the client on the site of impaired tissue integrity.

- Evaluate for the use of support surfaces (specialty mattresses, beds) chair cushion, or devices as appropriate.

- If the goal of care is to keep the client comfortable (e.g., for a terminally ill client), repositioning may not be appropriate.

- Avoid massaging around the site of impaired tissue integrity and over bony prominences.

▲ Assess the client's nutritional status. Refer for a nutritional consult and/or institute dietary supplements as necessary.

• = Independent   ▲ = Collaborative

▲ Develop a comprehensive plan of care that includes a thorough wound assessment, treatment interventions, support surfaces, nutritional products, adjunctive therapies, and evaluation of the outcome of care.

Home Care

- Some of the interventions previously described may be adapted for home care use.
- ▲ Assess the client's current phase of wound healing (inflammation, proliferation, maturation) and stage of injury; initiate appropriate wound management.
- Instruct and assist the client and caregivers in understanding how to change dressings and in the importance of maintaining a clean environment. Provide written instructions and observe them completing the dressing change.
- ▲ Initiate a consultation in a case assignment with a wound specialist or wound, ostomy, and continence nurse to establish a comprehensive plan as soon as possible. Plan case conferencing to promote optimal wound care.
- ▲ Consult with other health care disciplines to provide a thorough, comprehensive assessment.

Client/Family Teaching and Discharge Planning

- Teach skin and wound assessment and ways to monitor for signs and symptoms of infection, complications, and healing.
- Teach the client why a topical treatment has been selected. Explain wound bed changes that the caregiver can expect to see. Instruct on when the dressing needs to be changed.
- ▲ If it is consistent with overall client management goals, teach how to reposition the client, based on client's tissue tolerance and condition.
- Teach the use of pillows, foam wedges, and pressure-reducing devices to prevent pressure injury.

● = Independent ▲ = Collaborative

Ineffective peripheral Tissue Perfusion

NANDA-I Definition

Decrease in blood circulation to the periphery that may compromise health

Defining Characteristics

Absent pulses; altered motor function; altered skin characteristics (color, elasticity, hair, moisture, nails, sensation, temperature); blood pressure changes in extremities; claudication; color does not return to leg on lowering it; delayed peripheral wound healing; diminished pulses; edema; extremity pain; paresthesia; skin color pale on elevation

Related Factors (r/t)

Deficient knowledge of aggravating factors (e.g., smoking, sedentary lifestyle, trauma, obesity, salt intake, immobility); deficient knowledge of disease process (e.g., diabetes, hyperlipidemia); diabetes mellitus; hypertension; sedentary lifestyle; smoking

Client Outcomes

Client Will (Specify Time Frame):

- Demonstrate adequate tissue perfusion as evidenced by palpable peripheral pulses, warm and dry skin, adequate urine output, and absence of respiratory distress
- Verbalize knowledge of treatment regimen, including appropriate exercise and medications and their actions and possible side effects
- Identify changes in lifestyle needed to increase tissue perfusion

Nursing Interventions

- ▲ Check the brachial, radial, dorsalis pedis, posterior tibial, and popliteal pulses bilaterally. If unable to find them, use a Doppler stethoscope and notify the physician immediately if new onset of absence of pulses along with a cold extremity.
- Note skin color and feel the temperature of the skin. Assess for pain in the extremities, noting severity, quality, timing, and exacerbating and alleviating factors. Differentiate venous from arterial disease.

• = Independent   ▲ = Collaborative

- Check capillary refill.
- Note skin texture and the presence of hair, ulcers, or gangrenous areas on the legs or feet.
- Note the presence of edema in the extremities and rate severity on a four-point scale. Measure the circumference of the ankle and calf at the same time each day in the early morning.

Arterial Insufficiency

▲ Monitor peripheral pulses. If there is new onset of loss of pulses with bluish, purple, or black areas and extreme pain, notify the physician immediately.

▲ Measure ankle brachial index (ABI) via Doppler.

- Avoid elevating the legs above the level of the heart.

▲ For early arterial insufficiency, encourage exercise such as walking or riding an exercise bicycle from 30 to 60 minutes per day as ordered by the physician.

- Keep the client warm and have the client wear socks and shoes or sheepskin-lined slippers when mobile. Do not apply heat.
- Use a variety of leg positions after surgical intervention for PAD (either supine with legs extended, or sitting with legs extended) when getting this population out of bed.

▲ Pay meticulous attention to foot care.

- If the client has ischemic arterial ulcers, refer to the care plan for **Impaired Tissue Integrity.**

▲ If the client smokes, aggressively counsel the client to stop smoking and refer to the physician for medications to support nicotine withdrawal and a smoking withdrawal program.

Venous Insufficiency

▲ Elevate edematous legs as ordered and ensure no pressure under the knee and heels to prevent pressure ulcers.

▲ Apply graduated compression stockings as ordered. Ensure proper fit by measuring accurately. Remove the stockings at least twice a day, in the morning with the bath and in the evening, to assess the condition of the extremity, then reapply. Knee length is preferred rather than thigh length.

- Encourage the client to walk with compression stockings on and perform toe-up and point-flex exercises.

• = Independent   ▲ = Collaborative

- If the client is overweight, encourage weight loss to decrease venous disease.
- If the client has venous leg ulcers, encourage the client to avoid prolonged sitting, standing, and elevation of the involved leg. Encourage proper use of compression stockings.
- Discuss lifestyle with the client to determine if the client's occupation requires prolonged standing or sitting, which can result in chronic venous disease.
▲ If the client is mostly immobile, consult with the physician regarding use of a calf-high pneumatic compression device for prevention of deep vein thrombosis.
- Observe for signs of deep vein thrombosis, including pain, tenderness, swelling in the calf and thigh, and redness in the involved extremity. Take serial leg measurements of the thigh and calf circumferences. In some clients a tender venous cord can be felt in the popliteal fossa. Do not rely on Homans' sign.
▲ Note the results of a D-dimer test and ultrasounds.
- If deep vein thrombosis is present, observe for symptoms of a pulmonary embolism, including dyspnea, pleuritic chest pain, cough, and sometimes hemoptysis, especially with a history of trauma.
▲ If the client develops deep vein thrombosis, after treatment and hospital discharge recommend client wear below-the-knee elastic compression stockings during the day on the involved extremity.

Geriatric

- Change the client's position slowly when getting the client out of bed because of possible syncope.
- Recognize that the elderly have an increased risk of developing pulmonary embolism; if it is present, the symptoms are non-specific and often mimic those of heart failure or pneumonia.

Home Care

- The interventions previously described may be adapted for home care use.
- If arterial disease is present and the client smokes, aggressively encourage smoking cessation.
- Examine the feet carefully at frequent intervals for changes and new ulcerations.

• = Independent   ▲ = Collaborative

▲ Assess the client's nutritional status, paying special attention to obesity, hyperlipidemia, and malnutrition. Refer to a dietitian if appropriate.

• Monitor for development of gangrene, venous ulceration, and symptoms of cellulitis (redness, pain, and increased swelling in an extremity).

• Assess pain management strategies and their effectiveness.

• Assess support systems available at home and in the community.

Client/Family Teaching and Discharge Planning

• Explain the importance of good foot care. Teach the client and family to wash and inspect the feet daily. Recommend that the diabetic client wear comfortable shoes and break them in slowly, watching for blisters.

▲ Teach the diabetic client that he or she should have a comprehensive foot examination at least annually (which includes an analysis for predicting foot ulceration risk), also including assessment of sensation using the Semmes-Weinstein monofilaments. If good sensation is not present, refer to a footwear professional for fitting of therapeutic shoes and inserts, the cost of which is covered by Medicare.

• For arterial disease, stress the importance of not smoking, following a weight loss program (if the client is obese), carefully controlling a diabetic condition, controlling hyperlipidemia and hypertension, maintaining intake of antiplatelet therapy, and reducing stress.

• Teach the client to avoid exposure to cold; limit exposure to brief periods if going out in cold weather and wear warm clothing.

• For venous disease, teach the importance of wearing compression stockings as ordered, elevating the legs at intervals, and watching for skin breakdown on the legs.

• Teach the client to recognize the signs and symptoms that should be reported to a physician (e.g., change in skin temperature, color, or sensation or the presence of a new lesion on the foot).

• Provide clear, simple instructions about plan of care.

NOTE: If the client is receiving anticoagulant therapy, see the care plan for **Risk for Bleeding.**

• = Independent   ▲ = Collaborative

Risk for ineffective peripheral Tissue Perfusion

NANDA-I Definition

At risk for a decrease in blood circulation to the periphery that may compromise health

Risk Factors

Age greater than 60 years; deficient knowledge of aggravating factors (e.g., smoking, sedentary lifestyle, trauma, obesity, salt intake, immobility); deficient knowledge of disease process (e.g., diabetes, hyperlipidemia); diabetes mellitus; endovascular procedures; hypertension; sedentary lifestyle; smoking

Impaired Transfer Ability

NANDA-I Definition

Limitation of independent movement between two nearby surfaces

Defining Characteristics

Inability to transfer: between uneven levels; from bed to chair; from chair to bed; on or off a toilet; on or off a commode; in or out of tub; in or out of shower; from chair to car; from car to chair; from chair to floor; from floor to chair; from standing to floor; from floor to standing; from bed to standing; from standing to bed; from chair to standing; from standing to chair

Related Factors (r/t)

Cognitive impairment; insufficient muscle strength; musculoskeletal impairment (e.g., contractures); neuromuscular impairment; obesity; pain

NOTE: Specify level of independence using a standardized functional scale

Client Outcomes

Client Will (Specify Time Frame):
• Transfer from bed to chair and back successfully
• Transfer from chair to chair successfully
• Transfer from wheelchair to toilet and back successfully
• Transfer from wheelchair to car and back successfully

• = Independent ▲ = Collaborative

Nursing Interventions

- ▲ Request consult for a physical and/or occupational therapist (PT and OT) to develop exercise and strengthening program early in the client's recovery.
- ▲ Obtain a consult for a PT, OT, or orthotist to evaluate and fit clients with proper orthoses, braces, collars, and walking aids before helping them stand.
- • Help client put on/take off collars, braces, prostheses in bed, as well as antiembolism stockings and abdominal binders. Apply antiembolism stockings and abdominal binders while the client is in bed, as these appliances may help prevent or reduce hypotension.
- • Assess clients' dependence, weight, strength, balance, tolerance to position change, cooperation, fatigue level, and cognition plus available equipment and staff ratio/experience to decide whether to do a manual or device-assisted transfer.
- ▲ Collaborate with PT and use algorithms to identify technological aids to handle and transfer dependent and obese clients; do not use under-axilla method.
- • Implement and document type of transfer (such as slide board, pivot), weight-bearing status (non-weight-bearing, partial), equipment (walker, sling lift), and level of assistance (standby, moderate) on care plan and white board in room.
- • Apply a gait belt with handles before transferring clients with partial weight-bearing abilities; keep the belt and client close to provider during the transfer.
- • Help clients don shoes with nonskid soles and socks/hose.
- • Nursing staff should wear positive-grip shoe covers or nonslip shoes when transferring clients off shower chairs on tile floors.
- • Remove or swivel wheelchair armrests, leg rests, and footplates to the side, especially with squat or slide board transfers.
- • Adjust transfer surfaces so they are similar in height. For example, lower a hospital bed to about an inch higher than commode height.
- • Place wheelchair and commode at a slight angle toward the surface onto which client will transfer.
- • Teach client to consistently lock brakes on wheelchair/commode/shower chair before transferring.

T

• = Independent   ▲ = Collaborative

- Give clear, simple instructions, allow client time to process information, and let him or her do as much of the transfer as possible.
▲ Remind clients to comply with weight-bearing restrictions ordered by their physician.
- Place client in set position before standing him or her—for example, sitting on edge of surface with bilateral weight bearing on buttocks and hips, with knees flexed, balls of feet aligned under knees, and head in midline.
- Support and stabilize client's weak knee(s) by placing one or both of your knees next to or encircling client's knee(s), rather than blocking them.
  - Squat transfer: client leans well forward, slightly raises flexed hips off the surface, pivots, and sits down on new surface.
  - Standing pivot transfer: client leans forward with hips flexed and pushes up with hands from seat surface (or arms of chair), then stands erect, pivots, and sits down on new surface.
  - Slide board transfer: client should have on pants or have a pillowcase over the board. Remove arm and leg rest from wheelchair on one side, then slightly angle chair toward new surface. Help client lean sideways, thus shifting his or her weight so transfer board can be placed well under the upper thigh of the leg next to new surface. Make sure board is safely angled across both surfaces. Help client to sit upright and place one hand on board and the other hand on surface. Remind and help client perform a series of pushups with arms while leaning slightly forward and lifting (not sliding) hips in small increments across board with each pushup.
- Position walking aids appropriately so a standing client can grasp and use them once he or she is upright.
- Reinforce to clients who use walkers, to place one hand on walker and push with opposite hand against chair arm or surface from which they are arising to stand up.
- Use ceiling-mounted or bedside mechanical bariatric lifts to transfer dependent bariatric (extremely obese) clients.

● = Independent   ▲ = Collaborative

▲ Assist therapists to transfer bariatric clients who can support their own weight with minimal assistance. Position locked beds against a corner wall. Before sitting client, inflate air mattress overlay if applicable and place a friction-reducing sheet underneath client, then "flat spin" client with the transfer sheet so he/she is lying supine perpendicular to the bed. Deflate all air devices and pad bed edge where posterior thighs will dig in if skin is fragile. Place both knees level with thighs (put feet on a footstool if needed) while client is still supine and assist client to arise to sitting. If client starts sliding, lay client back supine.

• Use bariatric devices and utilize available safe patient handling equipment for lifting, transferring, positioning, and sliding client.

• Place a mechanical lift sling in the wheelchair preventatively. Place two transfer sheets or a slide board under bariatric client. Reinforce that head should be leaning forward and that knees should be level with hips; help hold wheelchair in place as therapist directs/helps client with a scoot transfer.

• Perform initial and subsequent fall risk assessment.

▲ Collaborate with PT, OT, and pharmacy for individualized preventative/postfall plans, for example, scheduled toileting, balance and strength training, removal of hazards, chair alarms, call system/phone in reach, and review of medications.

• Encourage an exercise component such as tai chi, physical therapy, or other exercise for balance, gait, and strength training in group programs or at home.

• Modify environment for safety; recommend vision assessment and consideration for cataract removal.

• Recommend polypharmacy assessment with special consideration to sedatives, antidepressants, and drugs affecting the CNS; recommend evaluation for orthostatic hypotension and irregular heartbeats; and recommend vitamin D supplementation 800 IU per day.

Home Care

▲ Obtain referral for OT and PT to teach home exercises and balance as well as fall prevention and recovery. They also evaluate for potential modifications such as an entry ramp,

• = Independent ▲ = Collaborative

elevated toilet seat/toilevator (raised base under toilet), tub seat or shower chair, need for shower stall with built-in seat or wheel-in shower stall without a curb/threshold, handheld flexible shower head, lever-type facets, pull-out drawers with loop handles versus cupboards, standing lift, and so on.

- Assess for adequate lighting and hazards such as throw/area rugs, clutter, cords, and unfitted bedspreads. Suggest safe floor surfaces, such as use of adhesive nonslip strips in tubs/thresholds/areas where floor height changes; removal of wax from slippery floors; and installing low-pile carpet/nonglazed or nonglossy tiles/wood/linoleum coverings. Stress relocating commonly used items to shelves/drawers in reach, applying remote controls to appliances, and optimizing furniture placement for function, maneuverability, and stability.

- Nurses can provide further safety assessments by suggesting installing hand rails in bathrooms and by stairs, ensuring client's slippers and clothes fit properly, and recommending repairing or discarding broken equipment in the home.

▲ Involve social worker or case manager to educate clients about potential assistive technology, financial cost and benefits, regulations of payers, and local resources.

▲ Implement approaches for home care staff and family to safely handle and transfer clients.

- For further information, refer to care plans for **Impaired physical Mobility** and **Impaired Walking.**

Client/Family Teaching and Discharge Planning

- Assess for readiness to learn and use teaching modalities conducive to personal learning styles, including written instructions for home use.

- Supervise practice sessions in which client and family apply items such as gait belts, braces, and orthoses. Check skin once aids are removed.

- Teach and monitor client/family for consistent use of safety precautions for transfers (e.g., nonskid shoes, correctly placed equipment/chairs, locked brakes, leg rests swiveled away, and so forth) and for correct performance of transfer or use of lifts/slings.

- Teach client/family how to check brakes on chairs to ensure they engage and how to check tires for adequate air pressure; advise routine inspection and annual tune-up of devices.
- Offer information on safe use of shower and commode chairs to prevent discomfort, pressure, and falls during transfer, transport, care, and hygiene.
- For further information, refer to the care plans for **Impaired physical Mobility, Impaired Walking, and Impaired wheelchair Mobility.**

Risk for Trauma

NANDA-I Definition

At risk of accidental tissue injury (e.g., wound, burn, fracture)

Risk Factors

External

Accessibility of guns; bathing in very hot water (e.g., unsupervised bathing of young children); children playing with dangerous objects; children riding in the front seat in car; contact with corrosives; contact with intense cold; contact with rapidly moving machinery; defective appliances; delayed lighting of gas appliances; driving a mechanically unsafe vehicle; driving at excessive speeds; driving while intoxicated; driving without necessary visual aids; entering unlighted rooms; experimenting with chemicals; exposure to dangerous machinery; faulty electrical plugs; flammable children's toys; frayed wires; grease waste collected on stoves; high beds; high-crime neighborhood; inadequate stair rails; inadequately stored combustibles (e.g., matches, oily rags); inadequately stored corrosives (e.g., lye); inappropriate call-for-aid mechanisms for bed-bound client; knives stored uncovered; lack of gate at top of stairs; lack of protection from heat source; lacks antislip material in bath; lacks antislip material in shower; large icicles hanging from roof; misuse of necessary headgear; misuse of seat restraints; nonuse of seat restraints; obstructed passageways; overexposure to radiation; overloaded electrical outlets; overloaded fuse boxes; physical proximity to vehicle pathways (e.g., driveways, lanes, railroad track); playing with explosives; pot

● = Independent   ▲ = Collaborative

handles facing toward the stove; potential igniting of gas leaks; slippery floor (e.g., wet or highly waxed); smoking in bed; smoking near oxygen; struggling with restraints; throw rugs; unanchored electric wires; unsafe road; unsafe walkways; unsafe window protection in homes with young children; use of cracked dishware; use of unsteady chairs; use of unsteady ladders; wearing flowing clothes around open flame

Internal
Balancing difficulties; cognitive difficulties; deficient knowledge regarding safe procedures; deficient knowledge regarding safety precautions; economically disadvantaged; emotional difficulties; history of previous trauma; poor vision; reduced hand-eye coordination; reduced muscle coordination; reduced sensation; weakness

Related Factors (r/t)
See Risk Factors.

Client Outcomes

Client Will (Specify Time Frame):
- Remain free from trauma
- Explain actions that can be taken to prevent trauma

Nursing Interventions

- Screen clients with a fall risk factor assessment tool to identify those at risk for falls.
- Provide vision aids for visually impaired clients.
- Assist the client with ambulation. Encourage the client to use assistive devices in ADLs as needed.
- Educate and provide clients and family with hip protector devices.
- Have a family member evaluate water temperature for the client.
- Assess the client for causes of impaired cognition.
- Provide assistive devices in the home, especially in bathrooms (e.g., hand rails, nonslip decals on the floor of the shower and bathtub).
- Ensure that call light systems are functioning and that the client is able to use them in conjunction with the nurse making hourly rounds.

• = Independent   ▲ = Collaborative

- Use a nightlight after dark to assist in orientation and improve visual acuity.
- Teach the client to observe safety precautions, especially in high-crime area neighborhoods (e.g., lock doors, do not leave home at night without a companion; keep entryways well lighted).
▲ Instruct the client not to drive under the influence of alcohol or drugs. Assess for a substance abuse problem and refer to appropriate resources for drug and alcohol education.
▲ Review drug profile for potential side effects that may inhibit performance of ADLs.
- See care plans for **Risk for Aspiration, Impaired Home Maintenance, Risk for Injury, Risk for Poisoning,** and **Risk for Suffocation.**

Pediatric

- Assess the client's socioeconomic status.
- Assess family interests in safety topics to identify priority areas for counseling.
- Never leave young children unsupervised around water or cooking areas.
- Keep flammable and potentially flammable articles out of the reach of young children.
- Lock up harmful objects such as guns.

Geriatric

- Assess the geriatric client's cognitive level of functioning both at admission and periodically.
- Assess for routine eye examinations and use of appropriate prescription glasses.
- Perform a home safety assessment and recommend the following preventive measures: keep electrical cords out of the flow of traffic; remove small rugs or make sure they are slip resistant; increase lighting in hallways and other dark areas; place a light in the bathroom; keep towels, curtains, and other items that might catch fire away from the stove; store harmful products away from food products; provide at least one grab bar in tubs and showers; check prescribed medications for

● = Independent   ▲ = Collaborative

appropriate labels; and store medications in original containers or in a dispenser of some type (e.g., egg carton, 7-day plastic dispenser). If the client cannot administer medications according to directions, secure someone to administer medications.
- Mark stove knobs with bright colors (yellow or red) and outline the borders of steps.
- Discourage driving at night.
- Encourage the client to participate in resistance and impact exercise programs as tolerated.
- Implement fall and injury prevention strategies in residential care facilities.
- Attend a fall prevention screening clinic.

Client/Family Teaching and Discharge Planning

- Educate the family regarding age-appropriate child safety precautions, environmental safety precautions, and intervention in an emergency
- Teach the family to assess the child care provider's knowledge regarding child safety, environmental safety precautions, and assistance of a child in an emergency.
- Educate the client and family regarding helmet use during recreation and sports activities.
- Encourage the proper use of car seats and safety belts.
- Teach parents to restrict nighttime driving after 10 PM for young drivers.
- Teach how to plan safe prom and graduation parties.
- Teach parents the importance of monitoring youths after school.
- Teach firearm safety. Encourage the family to keep firearms and ammunition in locked storage.
▲ Educate that the use of psychotropic medications may increase the risk of falls and that withdrawal of psychotropic medications should be considered.
- For further information, refer to care plans for **Risk for Aspiration, Impaired Home Maintenance, Risk for Injury, Risk for Poisoning,** and **Risk for Suffocation.**

• = Independent   ▲ = Collaborative

Unilateral Neglect

NANDA-I Definition

Impairment in sensory and motor response, mental representation, and spatial attention of the body and the corresponding environment characterized by inattention to one side and overattention to the opposite side; left-side neglect is more severe and persistent than right-side neglect

Defining Characteristics

Appears unaware of positioning of neglected limb; difficulty remembering details of internally represented familiar scenes that are on the neglected side; displacement of sounds to the nonneglected side; distortion of drawing on the half of the page on the neglected side; failure to cancel lines on the half of the page on the neglected side; failure to eat food from portion of the plate on the neglected side; failure to dress neglected side; failure to groom neglected side; failure to move eyes, head, limbs, trunk in the neglected hemispace, despite being aware of a stimulus in that space; failure to notice people approaching from the neglected side; lack of safety precautions with regard to the neglected side; marked deviation of the eyes to the nonneglected side to stimuli and activities on that side; marked deviation of the head to the nonneglected side to stimuli and activities on that side; marked deviation of the trunk to the nonneglected side to stimuli and activities on that side; omission of drawing on the half of the page on the neglected side; perseveration of visual motor tasks on nonneglected side; substitution of letters to form alternative words that are similar to the original in length when reading; transfer of pain sensation to the nonneglected side; use of only vertical half of page when writing

Related Factors (r/t)

Brain injury from cerebrovascular problems; brain injury from neurological illness; brain injury from trauma; brain injury from tumor, hemianopsia

NOTE: Because the right hemisphere plays a role in focusing attention while the left hemisphere specializes in global attention, unilateral neglect is more common if neurological pathology occurs in the right hemisphere of the brain, which results in left-sided neglect.

• = Independent   ▲ = Collaborative

Client Outcomes

Client Will (Specify Time Frame)

- Use techniques that can be used to minimize unilateral neglect
- Care for both sides of the body appropriately and keep affected side free from harm
- Return to the highest functioning level possible based on personal goals and abilities
- Remain free from injury

Nursing Interventions

- Assess the client for signs of unilateral neglect (UN; e.g., not washing, shaving, or dressing one side of the body; sitting or lying inappropriately on affected arm or leg; failing to respond to environmental stimuli contralateral to the side of lesion; eating food on only one side of plate; or failing to look to one side of the body).
- ▲ Collaborate with physician for referral to a rehabilitation team (including, but not limited to, rehabilitation clinical nurse specialist, physical medicine and rehabilitation physician, neuropsychologist, occupational therapist, physical therapist, and speech and language pathologist) for continued help in dealing with UN.
- Use the principles of rehabilitation to progressively increase the client's ability to compensate for UN by using assistive devices, feedback, and support.
- Set up the environment so that essential activity is on the unaffected side:
  - Place the client's personal items within view and on the unaffected side.
  - Position the bed so that client is approached from the unaffected side.
  - Monitor and assist the client to achieve adequate food and fluid intake.
- Implement fall prevention interventions.
- Position affected extremity in a safe and functional manner.
- Teach the client to be aware of the problem and modify behavior and environment.

● = Independent   ▲ = Collaborative

Home Care

- Many of the previously listed interventions may be adapted for use in the home care setting.
- Position bed at home so that client gets out of bed on unaffected side.

Client/Family Teaching and Discharge Planning

- Engage discharge planning specialists for comprehensive assessment and planning early in the client's stay.
- Encourage family participation in care and exercise.
- Explain pathology and symptoms of unilateral neglect to both the client and family.
- Teach the client how to scan regularly to check the position of body parts and to regularly turn head from side to side for safety when ambulating, using a wheelchair, or doing self-care tasks.
- Reinforce the client's use of adaptive devices such as prisms prescribed by rehabilitation professionals.
- Teach caregivers to cue the client to the environment

Impaired Urinary Elimination

NANDA-I Definition

U

Dysfunction in urine elimination

Defining Characteristics

Dysuria; frequency; hesitancy; incontinence; nocturia; retention; urgency

Related Factors

Anatomic obstruction; multiple causality; sensory motor impairment; urinary tract infection

Client Outcomes

Client Will (Specify Time Frame):

- State absence of pain or excessive urgency during urination
- Demonstrate voiding frequency no more than every 2 hours

● = Independent   ▲ = Collaborative

Nursing Interventions

- Question the client regarding the following:
  - Presence of bothersome symptoms such as incontinence, dribbling, frequency, urgency, dysuria, and nocturia
  - Presence of pain in the area of the bladder
  - The pattern of urination, and approximate amount
  - Possible aggravating and alleviating factors for urinary problems
- Ask the client to keep a bladder diary/bladder log.
- For interventions on urinary incontinence, refer to the following nursing diagnosis care plans as appropriate: **Stress Incontinence, Urge urinary Incontinence, Reflex Incontinence, Overflow Incontinence,** or **Functional Incontinence.**
- ▲ Perform a focused physical assessment including inspecting the perineal skin integrity, percussion, and palpation of the lower abdomen looking for obvious bladder distention or an enlarged kidney.
- ▲ Check for costovertebral tenderness.
- ▲ Review results of urinalysis for the presence of urinary infection: WBCs, RBCs, bacteria, positive nitrites. If urinalysis results are not available, request a midstream specimen of urine (urine obtained during voiding, discarding the first and last portions) for a urinalysis.
- ▲ If blood or protein is present in the urine, recognize that both hematuria and proteinuria are serious symptoms, and the client should be referred to a urologist to receive a workup to rule out pathology.

Urinary Tract Infection

- ▲ Consult the physician for a culture and sensitivity testing and antibiotic treatment in the individual with evidence of a symptomatic urinary tract infection.
- ▲ Teach the client to recognize symptoms of UTI: dysuria that crescendos as the bladder nears complete evacuation; urgency to urinate followed by micturition of only a few drops; suprapubic aching discomfort; malaise; voiding frequency; sudden exacerbation of urinary incontinence with or without fever, chills, and flank pain.

● = Independent   ▲ = Collaborative

▲ Recognize that a cloudy or malodorous urine, in the absence of other lower urinary tract symptoms, may not indicate the presence of a urinary tract infection and that asymptomatic bacteriuria, in the elderly, does not justify a course of antibiotics.

▲ Refer the individual with chronic lower urinary tract pain to a urologist or specialist in the management of pelvic pain.

Geriatric

▲ Perform urinalysis in all elderly persons who experience a sudden change in urine elimination patterns such as new-onset incontinence, lower abdominal discomfort, acute confusion, or a fever of unclear origin.

• Encourage elderly women to drink at least 10 oz of cranberry juice daily, regularly consume one to two servings of fresh blueberries, or supplement the diet with cranberry concentrate capsules as ordered.

▲ Refer the elderly woman with recurrent urinary tract infections to her physician for possible use of topical estrogen creams for treatment of atrophic vaginal mucosa from decreased hormonal stimulation, which can predispose to UTIs.

▲ Recognize that UTIs in elderly men are typically associated with prostatic hyperplasia, or strictures of the urethra. Refer to a urologist.

Client/Family Teaching and Discharge Planning

• Teach the client/family methods to keep the urinary tract healthy. Refer to Client/Family Teaching in the care plan **Readiness for enhanced Urinary Elimination.**

• Teach the following measures to women to decrease the incidence of urinary tract infections:
  ■ Urinate at appropriate intervals. Do not ignore need to void, which can result in stasis of urine.
  ■ Drink plenty of liquids, especially water.
  ■ Wipe from front to back.
  ■ Wear panties with a cotton crotch.
  ■ Avoid potentially irritating feminine products.

U

• = Independent   ▲ = Collaborative

- Recommend that cranberry juice, cranberry tablets, or blue-berries be used to prevent recurrent UTIs (see the geriatric interventions discussed previously).
- Teach the sexually active woman with recurrent urinary tract infections prevention measures including:
  - Void after intercourse to flush bacteria out of the urethra and bladder.
  - Use a lubricating agent as needed during intercourse to protect the vagina from trauma and decrease the incidence of vaginitis.
  - Watch for signs of vaginitis and seek treatment as needed.
  - Avoid use of diaphragms with spermicide.
- Teach clients with spinal cord injury and neurogenic bladder dysfunction to consume cranberry extract tablets or cranberry juice on a daily basis.
- Teach all persons to recognize hematuria and to promptly seek care if this symptom occurs.

Readiness for enhanced Urinary Elimination

NANDA-I Definition

A pattern of urinary functions that is sufficient for meeting eliminatory needs and can be strengthened

Defining Characteristics

Amount of output is within normal limits; expresses willingness to enhance urinary elimination; fluid intake is adequate for daily needs; positions self for emptying of bladder; specific gravity is within normal limits; urine is odorless; urine is straw colored

Client Outcomes

Client Will (Specify Time Frame):

- Urinate every 3 to 4 hours while awake
- Remain free of undetected symptoms of a urinary tract infection or cancer of the kidney or bladder
- Drink fluids at a sufficient level to have straw-colored urine

• = Independent   ▲ = Collaborative

Nursing Interventions

- Question the client regarding any bothersome urinary symptoms such as frequency, nocturia, urgency, dysuria, or retention of urine.
- Question the client regarding presence of incontinence. If incontinence is present, refer to the appropriate care plan: **Stress urinary Incontinence, Urge urinary Incontinence, Functional urinary Incontinence,** or **Reflex urinary Incontinence.**
- Question the client regarding history of UTIs. If she has had UTIs in the past, provide teaching for prevention as outlined in the care plan **Impaired Urinary Elimination.**
- Ask the client to complete a bladder diary of diurnal and nocturnal urine elimination patterns and patterns of urinary leakage.

Pediatric

- Encourage children and adolescents to maintain normal weight because obesity has been related to cancers of the urinary tract.

Geriatric

- Encourage elderly women to drink at least 10 oz of cranberry juice daily, regularly consume one to two servings of fresh blueberries, or supplement the diet with cranberry concentrate capsules (usually taken in 500-mg doses with each meal).

Client/Family Teaching and Discharge Planning

- Teach the client general guidelines for health of the urinary system:
  - Ensure good hydration. Total daily fluid intake should be approximately 2.7 L per day for women, and 3.7 L per day for men
  - Recommend the client have a physical exam, a metabolic panel of laboratory tests, and a urinalysis done yearly.
  - Recommend the client not hold urine for long periods of time before emptying the bladder. It is normal to urinate every 3 to 4 hours.

U

- Recommend that the client with frequency, urgency in the morning, or possible incontinence consider reducing or eliminating caffeine intake.
- If the client has constipation at intervals, share measures to alleviate or prevent constipation, including adequate consumption of dietary fluids, dietary fiber, exercise, and regular bowel elimination patterns. See care plan for **Constipation.**
- Advise to stop smoking because of the association with damage to the kidney and bladder, including chronic kidney disease, bladder cancer, urinary incontinence, and bothersome lower urinary tract symptoms in men.
- Encourage the client to eat a healthy diet, avoiding processed meats, with sodium nitrate as a preservative, to decrease incidence of cancer of the bladder.

Urinary Retention

NANDA-I Definition

Incomplete emptying of the bladder

Defining Characteristics

Absence of urine output; bladder distention; dribbling; dysuria; frequent voiding; overflow incontinence; residual urine; sensation of bladder fullness; small voiding

Related Factors (r/t)

Blockage; high urethral pressure; inhibition of reflex arc; strong sphincter

Client Outcomes

Client Will (Specify Time Frame):

- Demonstrate consistent ability to urinate when desire to void is perceived
- Measured urinary residual volume of <200 to 250 mL
- Experience correction or relief from dysuria, nocturia, postvoid dribbling, and voiding frequently
- Be free of a urinary tract infection

● = Independent   ▲ = Collaborative

Nursing Interventions

- Obtain a focused urinary history including questioning the client about episodes of acute urinary retention (complete inability to void) or chronic retention (documented elevated postvoid residual volumes), also symptoms such as dysuria, nocturia, postvoid dribbling, and voiding frequently.
- Question the client concerning specific risk factors for urinary retention including:
  - Spinal cord injuries
  - Ischemic stroke
  - Metabolic disorders such as diabetes mellitus, chronic alcoholism, and related conditions associated with polyuria and peripheral polyneuropathies
  - Herpetic infection
  - Heavy-metal poisoning (lead, mercury) causing peripheral polyneuropathies
  - Advanced-stage human immunodeficiency virus (HIV)
  - Medications including antispasmodics/parasympatholytics, alpha-adrenergic agonists, antidepressants, sedatives, narcotics, psychotropic medications, illicit drugs
  - Recent surgery requiring general or spinal anesthesia
  - Vaginal delivery within the past 48 hours
  - Bowel elimination patterns, history of fecal impaction, encopresis
  - Recent surgical procedures
  - Recent prostatic biopsy
- Complete a pain assessment including pain intensity using a self-report pain tool, such as the 0-10 numerical pain rating scale. Also determine location, quality, onset/duration, intensity, aggravating and alleviating factors, and effects of pain on function and quality of life.
- ▲ Perform a focused physical assessment including perineal skin integrity and inspection, percussion, and palpation of the lower abdomen looking for obvious bladder distention or an enlarged kidney.
- ▲ Recognize that unrelieved obstruction of urine can result in renal damage and, if severe, renal failure. Urinary retention can be a medical emergency and should be reported to the primary provider as soon as possible.

• = Independent   ▲ = Collaborative

▲ Note results of laboratory tests including serum electrolytes, and BUN/creatinine, along with calcium, phosphate, magnesium, uric acid, and albumin.

▲ Monitor for signs of dehydration, peripheral edema, elevating blood pressure, and heart failure.

• Ask the client to complete a bladder diary including patterns of urine elimination, urine loss (if present), nocturia, and volume and type of fluids consumed for a period of 3 to 7 days.

▲ Consult with the physician concerning eliminating or altering medications suspected of producing or exacerbating urinary retention.

• Advise the male client with urinary retention related to BPH to avoid risk factors associated with acute urinary retention as follows:

  ■ Avoid over-the-counter cold remedies containing a decongestant (alpha-adrenergic agonist) or antihistamine such as diphenhydramine that has anticholinergic effects.

  ■ Avoid taking over-the-counter dietary medications (frequently contain alpha-adrenergic agonists).

  ■ Discuss voiding problems with a health care provider before beginning new prescription medications.

  ■ After prolonged exposure to cool weather, warm the body before attempting to urinate.

  ■ Avoid overfilling the bladder by regular urination patterns and refrain from excessive intake of alcohol.

• Advise the client who is unable to void specific strategies to manage this potential medical emergency as follows:

  ■ Attempt urination in complete privacy.

  ■ Place the feet solidly on the floor.

  ■ If unable to void using these strategies, take a warm sitz bath or shower and void (if possible) while still in the tub or shower.

  ■ Drink a warm cup of caffeinated coffee or tea to stimulate the bladder, which may promote voiding.

  ■ If unable to void within 6 hours or if bladder distention is producing significant pain, seek urgent or emergency care.

• = Independent   ▲ = Collaborative

- ■ Perform sterile (in acute care) or clean intermittent catheterization at home as ordered for clients with urinary retention.
- • For more information about intermittent catheterization, see care plan **Reflex urinary Incontinence.**
- • Insert an indwelling catheter only as ordered for the individual with urinary retention who is not a suitable candidate for intermittent catheterization, recognizing that the catheter can be a significant cause of harm to the client through development of a catheter-associated urinary tract infection (CAUTI), or through genitourinary trauma when the catheter is pulled on.
- ▲ Utilize a silver alloy-coated urinary catheter if possible.
- • Advise clients with indwelling catheters that bacteria in the urine is an almost universal finding after the catheter has remained in place for more than 1 week and that only symptomatic infections warrant treatment.
- • Use the following strategies to reduce the risk for CAUTI whenever feasible:
  - ■ Insert the indwelling catheter with sterile technique, only when insertion is indicated.
  - ■ Remove the indwelling catheter as soon as possible; acute care facilities should institute a policy for regular review of the necessity of an indwelling catheter.
  - ■ Insert a silver alloy catheter for short-term indwelling catheterization (<14 days).
  - ■ Maintain a closed drainage system whenever feasible.
  - ■ Maintain unobstructed urine flow, avoiding kinks in the tubing, and keeping the collecting bag below the level of the bladder at all times.
  - ■ Regularly cleanse the urethral meatus with a gentle cleanser to remove apparent soiling.
  - ■ Change the long-term catheter every 4 weeks; more frequent catheter changes should be reserved for clients who experience catheter encrustation and blockage.
  - ■ Place clients managed in an acute or long-term care facility with a CAUTI in a separate room from others managed by an indwelling catheter to reduce the risk of spreading the offending pathogen.

U

● = Independent   ▲ = Collaborative

▲ Educate staff about the risks of CAUTI and specific strategies to reduce this risk.

Postoperative Urinary Retention

- Recognize that urinary retention can follow many kinds of surgery and is commonly associated with use of anesthesia and opioid pain medications.
- ▲ Remove the indwelling urethral catheter at midnight in the hospitalized postoperative client to reduce the risk of acute urinary retention.
- ▲ Perform a bladder scan of the bladder before considering inserting a catheter to determine postvoid residual volume following surgery.

Geriatric

- Aggressively assess elderly clients, particularly those with dribbling urinary incontinence, UTI, and related conditions for urinary retention.
- Assess elderly clients for impaction when urinary retention is documented or suspected.
- Monitor elderly male clients for retention related to prostatic enlargement (BPH or prostate cancer).

Home Care

- Encourage the client to report any inability to void.
- ▲ Maintain an up-to-date medication list; evaluate side effect profiles for risk of urinary retention.
- ▲ Refer the client for physician evaluation if urinary retention occurs.

Client/Family Teaching and Discharge Planning

- Teach the client with mild to moderate obstructive symptoms to double void by urinating, resting in the bathroom for 3 to 5 minutes, and then trying again to urinate.
- Teach the client with urinary retention and infrequent voiding to urinate by the clock.
- Teach the client with an indwelling catheter to assess the tube for patency, maintain the drainage system below the level of

• = Independent   ▲ = Collaborative

the symphysis pubis, and routinely cleanse the bedside bag as directed.
- Teach the client with an indwelling catheter or undergoing intermittent catheterization the symptoms of a significant urinary infection, including hematuria, acute-onset incontinence, dysuria, flank pain, or fever.

Risk for Vascular Trauma

NANDA-I Definition

At risk for damage to a vein and its surrounding tissues related to the presence of a catheter and/or infused solutions

Risk Factors

Catheter type; catheter width; impaired ability to visualize the insertion site; inadequate catheter fixation; infusion rate; insertion site; length of insertion time; nature of solution (e.g., concentration, chemical irritant, temperature, pH)

Client Outcomes

Client Will (Specify Time Frame):
- Remain free from vascular trauma
- Remain free from signs and symptoms that indicate vascular trauma
- Remain free from impaired tissue and/or skin
- Maintain skin integrity, tissue perfusion, usual tissue temperature, color and pigment
- Report any altered sensation or pain
- State site is comfortable

Nursing Interventions

Client Preparation
- ▲ Verify objective and estimate duration of treatment. Check physician's order.
- Assess client's clinical situation when venous infusion is indicated.

• = Independent   ▲ = Collaborative

- Assess if client is prepared for an IV procedure. Explain the procedure if necessary to decrease stress.
- Provide privacy and make the client comfortable during the intravenous insertion.
- Teach the client what symptoms of possible vascular trauma he should be alert to and to immediately inform staff if they notice any of these symptoms.

Insertion

- Wash hands before and after touching the client, as well as when inserting, replacing, accessing, repairing, or dressing an intravascular catheter.
- Maintain aseptic technique for the insertion and care of intravascular catheters. Use gloves and always reduce the number of staff present in the environment during the procedure if possible.
- Assess the condition of the client's veins, possible age-related influence, and previous intravenous site use.
- In cases of hard-to-access veins, consider strategies such as the use of ultrasound (US) to assist in vein localization and safe venipuncture.
- Avoid areas of joint flexion or bony prominences.
- Choose an appropriate vascular access device (VAD) based on the types and characteristics of the devices and insertion site. Consider the following:
  - **Peripheral cannulae:** short devices that are placed into a peripheral vein; can be straight, winged, or ported and winged
  - **Midline catheters or peripherally inserted catheters (PICs)** with ranges from 7.5 to 20 cm
  - **Central venous access devices (CVADs):** terminated in the central venous circulation; are available in a range of gauge sizes; they can be nontunneled catheters, skin-tunneled catheters, implantable injection ports, or peripherally inserted central catheters/PICCs.
  - **Polyurethane venous devices and silicone rubber** may cause less friction and consequently less risk of mechanical phlebitis compared to the polytetrafluoroethylene devices.

V

▲ Choose a device with consideration of the nature, volume, and flow of prescribed solution.

- If possible, choose the venous access site considering the client's preference.
- Select the gauge of the venous device according to the duration of treatment, purpose of the procedure, and size of the vein.
- Verify if client is allergic to fixation or device material.
- Disinfect the venipuncture site.
- Provide a comfortable, safe, hypoallergenic, easily removable stabilization dressing, allowing for visualization of the access site.
- Use either sterile gauze or sterile, transparent, semipermeable dressing to cover catheter site. Replace dressing used on short-term CVC sites every 2 days for gauze dressings and replace it at least every 7 days for transparent dressings.
- Document insertion date, site, type of VAD, number of punctures performed, other occurrences, and measures/arrangements taken.
- Always decontaminate the device before infusing medication or manipulating IV equipment.

▲ Verify the sequence of drugs to be administrated

Monitoring Infusion

- Monitor permeability and flow rate at regular intervals.
- Monitor catheter-skin junction and surrounding tissues at regular intervals, observing possible appearance of burning, pain, erythema, altered local temperature, infiltration, extravasation, edema, secretion, tenderness, or induration. Remove promptly.

▲ Replace device according to institution protocol.

▲ Flush vascular access according to organizational policies and procedures, and as recommended by the manufacturer.

- Remove catheter on suspected contamination, if the client develops signs of phlebitis, infection, or a malfunctioning catheter, or when no longer required.
- Clients need to be encouraged to report any discomfort such as pain, burning, swelling, or bleeding.

Pediatric

- The preceding interventions may be adapted for the pediatric client.
- Inform the client and family about the IV procedure, obtain permissions, maintain client's comfort, and perform appropriate assessment prior to venipuncture. Assess the client for any allergies or sensitivities to tape, antiseptics, or latex. Choose a healthy vein and appropriate site for insertion of selected device.
- The use of an appropriate device to obtain blood samples reduces discomfort in the pediatric client. However, this procedure needs to be effective and safe.
- Avoid areas of joint flexion or bony prominences.
- ▲ Consider if sedation or the use of local anesthetic is suitable for insertion of a catheter, taking into consideration the age of the pediatric client.
- Use diversion while carrying out the procedure

Geriatric

- The preceding interventions may be adapted for the geriatric client.
- Consider the physical, emotional, and cognitive changes related to older adults.
- Use strict aseptic technique for venipuncture of older clients.

Home Care

- Some devices can be kept after discharge. Inform client and family members about care of the selected device.
- Help in the choice of actions that support self-care.
- Select, with the client, the insertion site most compatible with the development of activities of daily living.
- Avoid the use of the dominant hands as an IV placement site.
- Minimize the use of continuous IV therapy whenever possible.

Impaired spontaneous Ventilation

NANDA-I Definition

Decreased energy reserves result in an individual's inability to maintain breathing adequate to support life

Defining Characteristics

Apprehension; decreased cooperation; decreased PO_2; decreased SaO_2; decreased tidal volume; dyspnea; increased heart rate; increased metabolic rate; increased PCO_2; increased restlessness; increased use of accessory muscles

Related Factors (r/t)

Metabolic factors; respiratory muscle fatigue

Client Outcomes

Client Will (Specify Time Frame):

- Maintain arterial blood gases within safe parameters
- Remain free of dyspnea or restlessness
- Effectively maintain airway
- Effectively mobilize secretions

Nursing Interventions

- ▲ Collaborate with the client, family, and physician regarding possible intubation and ventilation. Ask whether the client has advance directives and, if so, integrate them into the plan of care with clinical data regarding overall health and reversibility of the medical condition.
- • Assess and respond to changes in the client's respiratory status. Monitor the client for dyspnea, increase in respiratory rate, use of accessory muscles, retraction of intercostal muscles, flaring of nostrils, decrease in O_2 saturation, and subjective complaints.
- • Have the client use a numerical scale (0-10) to self-report his rating of dyspnea before and after interventions.
- • Assess for history of chronic respiratory disorders when administering oxygen. With chronic obstructive pulmonary

disease (COPD), the respiratory drive is primarily in response to hypoxia, not hypercarbia; oxygenating too aggressively can result in respiratory depression. When managing acute respiratory failure in clients with COPD, use caution in administering oxygen because hyperoxygenation can lead to respiratory depression.

▲ Collaborate with the physician and respiratory therapists in determining the appropriateness of noninvasive positive pressure ventilation (NPPV/NIV) for the decompensated client with COPD.

▲ Assist with implementation, client support, and monitoring if NPPV is used.

• If the client has apnea, pH less than 7.25, $PaCO_2$ greater than 50 mm Hg, PaO_2 less than 50 mm Hg, respiratory muscle fatigue, or somnolence, prepare the client for possible intubation and mechanical ventilation.

Ventilator Support

▲ Explain the intubation and mechanical ventilation process to the client and family as appropriate, and during intubation administer sedation for client comfort according to the physician's orders.

• Secure the endotracheal tube in place using either tape or a commercially available device, auscultate bilateral breath sounds, use a CO_2 detector, and obtain a chest radiograph to confirm endotracheal tube placement.

• Ensure that ventilator settings are appropriate to meet the client's minute ventilation requirements.

▲ Suction as needed and hyperoxygenate according to unit policy. Refer to the care plan **Ineffective Airway Clearance** for further information on suctioning.

• Check that monitor alarms are set appropriately at the start of each shift.

• Respond to ventilator alarms promptly. If unable to immediately locate the source/cause of an alarm, use a manual self-inflating resuscitation bag to ventilate the client while waiting for assistance.

• Prevent unplanned extubation by maintaining stability of endotracheal tube with careful taping or use of a device for

V

stabilization of the tube, also use of restraints if needed with physician's order.
- Drain collected fluid from condensation out of ventilator tubing as needed.
- Note ventilator settings of flow of inspired oxygen, peak inspiratory pressure, tidal volume, and alarm activation at intervals and when removing the client from the ventilator for any reason.
▲ Administer analgesics and sedatives as needed to facilitate client comfort and rest. Pain and sedation scales provide a consistent way of monitoring sedation levels and ensuring that therapeutic outcomes are being met.
▲ Initiate a "sedation vacation" daily, with lightening of analgesics and sedatives until the client becomes awake. During this time carefully monitor the client to protect from inadvertent self-extubation, pain and anxiety, and periods of desaturation from asynchrony of breathing with the ventilator.
- Utilize tools such as the Riker Sedation-Agitation Scale, the Motor Activity Assessment Scale, the Ramsey Scale, or the Richmond Agitation-Sedation Scale because they can be useful in monitoring levels of sedation.
- Alternatives to medications for decreasing anxiety should be attempted, such as music therapy with selections of the client's choice played on headphones at intervals.
- Analyze and respond to arterial blood gas results, end-tidal CO_2 levels, and pulse oximetry values.
- Use an effective means of verbal and nonverbal communication with the client such as an alphabet board, picture board, electronic voice output communication aids, computers, and writing slates. Ask the client for input into his or her care as appropriate. Barriers to communication include endotracheal tubes, sedation, and general weakness associated with a critical illness.
- Move the endotracheal tube from side to side every 24 hours, and tape it or secure it with a commercially available device. Assess and document client's skin condition, and ensure correct tube placement at lip line.

V

- Implement steps to prevent ventilator-associated pneumonia (VAP), including continuous removal of subglottic secretions, elevation of the head of bed to 30 to 45 degrees unless medically contraindicated, change of the ventilator circuit no more than every 48 hours, and handwashing before and after contact with each client. See details in the sections that follow.
▲ Use endotracheal tubes that allow for the continuous aspiration of subglottic secretions.
- Position the client in a semirecumbent position with the head of the bed at a 30- to 45-degree angle to decrease the aspiration of gastric, oral, and nasal secretions.
- Consider use of kinetic therapy, using a kinetic bed that slowly moves the client with 40-degree turns.
- Perform handwashing using both soap and water and alcohol-based solution before and after all mechanically ventilated client contact to prevent VAP.
- Provide routine oral care using toothbrushing and oral rinsing with an antimicrobial agent if needed.
- Maintain proper cuff inflation for both endotracheal tubes and cuffed tracheostomy tubes with minimal leak volume or minimal occlusion volume to decrease risk of aspiration and reduce incidence of ventilator-associated pneumonia.
- Reposition the client as needed. Use rotational bed or kinetic bed therapy in clients for whom side-to-side turning is contraindicated or difficult.
▲ If the client is intubated and is stable, consider getting the client up to sit at the edge of the bed, transfer to a chair, or walk as appropriate, if an effective interdisciplinary team is developed to keep the client safe.
- Assess bilateral anterior and posterior breath sounds every 2 to 4 hours and PRN; respond to any relevant changes.
- Assess responsiveness to ventilator support; monitor for subjective complaints and sensation of dyspnea.
▲ Collaborate with the interdisciplinary team in treating clients with acute respiratory failure. Collaborate with the health care team to meet ventilator care needs and avoid complications.

V

• = Independent   ▲ = Collaborative

Geriatric

- Recognize that critically ill older adults have a high rate of morbidity when mechanically ventilated.

Home Care

▲ Some of the interventions listed previously may be adapted for home care use. Begin discharge planning as soon as possible with the case manager or social worker to assess the need for home support systems, assistive devices, and community or home health services.

▲ With help from a medical social worker, assist the client and family to determine the fiscal effect of care in the home versus an extended care facility.

- Assess the home setting during the discharge process to ensure the home can safely accommodate ventilator support (e.g., adequate space and electricity).

- Have the family contact the electric company and place the client's residence on a high-risk list in case of a power outage.

- Assess the caregivers for commitment to supporting a ventilator-dependent client in the home.

- Be sure that the client and family or caregivers are familiar with operation of all ventilation devices, know how to suction secretions if needed, are competent in doing tracheostomy care, and know schedules for cleaning equipment. Have the designated caregiver or caregivers demonstrate care before discharge.

- Assess client and caregiver knowledge of the disease, client needs, and medications to be administered via ventilation-assistive devices. Avoid analgesics. Assess knowledge of how to use equipment. Teach as necessary.

- Establish an emergency plan and criteria for use. Identify emergency procedures to be used until medical assistance arrives. Teach and role play emergency care.

Client/Family Teaching and Discharge Planning

- Explain to the client the potential sensations that will be experienced, including relief of dyspnea, the feeling of lung inflations, the noise of the ventilator, and the reality of alarms.

V

- Explain to the client and family about being unable to speak, and work out an alternative system of communication. See previously mentioned interventions.
- Demonstrate to the family how to perform simple procedures, such as suctioning secretions in the mouth with a tonsil-tip catheter, providing range-of-motion exercises, and reconnecting the ventilator immediately if it becomes disconnected.
- Offer both the client and family explanations of how the ventilator works and answer any questions.

Dysfunctional Ventilatory Weaning Response

NANDA-I Definition

Inability to adjust to lowered levels of mechanical ventilator support that interrupts and prolongs the weaning process

Defining Characteristics

Mild

Breathing discomfort; expressed feelings of increased need for oxygen; fatigue; increased concentration on breathing; queries about possible machine malfunction; restlessness; slight increase of respiratory rate from baseline; warmth

Moderate

Apprehension; baseline increase in respiratory rate (<5 breaths/min); color changes; decreased air entry on auscultation; diaphoresis; hypervigilance to activities; inability to cooperate; inability to respond to coaching; pale; slight cyanosis; slight increase from baseline blood pressure (<20 mm Hg); slight increase from baseline heart rate (<20 beats/min); light respiratory accessory muscle use; wide-eyed look

Severe

Adventitious breath sounds; agitation; asynchronized breathing with the ventilator; audible airway secretions; cyanosis; decreased level of consciousness; deterioration in arterial blood gases from current baseline; full respiratory accessory muscle use; gasping breaths; increase from baseline blood pressure (≥20 mm Hg); increase from baseline heart rate (≥20 breaths/min); paradoxical abdominal breathing; profuse diaphoresis; respiratory rate increases significantly from baseline; shallow breaths

Related Factors (r/t)

Physiological
Inadequate nutrition; ineffective airway clearance; sleep pattern disturbance; uncontrolled pain

Psychological
Anxiety; decreased motivation; decreased self-esteem; fear; hopelessness; insufficient trust in the nurse; knowledge deficit of the weaning process; client-perceived inefficacy about ability to wean; powerlessness

Situational
Adverse environment (e.g., noisy, active environment; negative events in the room; low nurse:client ratio, unfamiliar nursing staff; history of ventilator dependence longer than 4 days; inadequate social support; inappropriate pacing of diminished ventilator support; uncontrolled episodic energy demands)

Client Outcomes

Client Will (Specify Time Frame):
- Wean from ventilator with adequate arterial blood gases
- Remain free of unresolved dyspnea or restlessness
- Effectively clear secretions

Nursing Interventions

- Assess client's readiness for weaning as evidenced by the following:
  - Physiological readiness
  - Resolution of initial medical problem that led to ventilator dependence
  - Hemodynamic stability
  - Normal hemoglobin levels
  - Absence of fever
  - Normal state of consciousness
  - Metabolic, fluid, and electrolyte balance

• = Independent   ▲ = Collaborative

- Adequate nutritional status with serum albumin levels >2.5 g/dL
- Adequate sleep
- Adequate pain management and sedation

• For best results ensure that the client is in an optimal physiological and psychological state before introducing the stress of weaning.

• Involve family as appropriate to help the client provide a maximal effort during weaning readiness measurements.

• Provide adequate nutrition to ventilated clients, using enteral feeding when possible.

• Use evidence-based weaning and extubation protocols as appropriate.

• Identify reasons for previous unsuccessful weaning attempts and include that information in development of the weaning plan.

▲ Collaborate with an interdisciplinary team (physician, nurse, respiratory therapist, physical therapist, and dietitian) to develop a weaning plan with a time line and goals; revise this plan throughout the weaning period. Use a communication device, such as a weaning board or flow sheet.

• Assist client to identify personal strategies that result in relaxation and comfort (e.g., music, visualization, relaxation techniques, reading, television, family visits). Support implementation of these strategies. Music intervention can be used to allay anxiety and can be a powerful distractor from distressful sounds and thoughts in the ICU.

• Provide a safe and comfortable environment. Stay with the client during weaning if possible. If unable to stay, make the call light button readily available and assure the client that needs will be met responsively. Presence entails a focus by the nurse to engage attentively with the client.

▲ Coordinate pain and sedation medications to minimize sedative effects.

• Schedule weaning periods for the time of day when the client is most rested. Cluster care activities to promote successful weaning. Avoid other procedures during weaning: keep the

V

• = Independent   ▲ = Collaborative

environment quiet and promote restful activities between weaning periods.

- Promote a normal sleep-wake cycle, allowing uninterrupted periods of nighttime sleep.
- During weaning, monitor the client's physiological and psychological responses; acknowledge and respond to fears and subjective complaints. Validate the client's efforts during the weaning process.
- Monitor subjective and objective data (breath sounds, respiratory pattern, respiratory effort, heart rate, blood pressure, oxygen saturation per oximetry, amount and type of secretions, anxiety, and energy level) throughout weaning to determine client tolerance and responses.
- Involve the client and family in the weaning plan. Inform them of the weaning plan and possible client responses to the weaning process (e.g., potential feelings of dyspnea). Foster a partnership between clients and nurses in care planning for weaning.
- Coach the client through episodes of increased anxiety. Remain with the client or place a supportive and calm significant other in this role. Give positive reinforcement, and with permission, use touch to communicate support and concern.
- Terminate weaning when the client demonstrates predetermined criteria or when the following signs of weaning intolerance occur:
  - Tachypnea, dyspnea, or chest and abdominal asynchrony
  - Agitation or mental status changes
  - Decreased oxygen saturation: SaO_2 less than 90%
  - Increased $PaCO_2$ or $ETCO_2$
  - Change in pulse rate or blood pressure or onset of new dysrhythmias
- ▲ If the dysfunctional weaning response is severe, consider slowing weaning to brief periods (e.g., 5 minutes). Continue to collaborate with the team to determine whether an untreated physiological cause for the dysfunctional weaning pattern remains. Consult with physician regarding use of noninvasive ventilation immediately after discontinuing ventilation.

V

Consider an alternative care setting (subacute, rehabilitation facility, home) for clients with prolonged ventilator dependence as a strategy that can positively affect outcomes.

Geriatric

- Recognize that older clients may require longer periods to wean.

Home Care

- Weaning from a ventilator at home should be based on client stability and comfort of the client and caregivers under an intermittent care plan.

Risk for other-directed Violence

NANDA-I Definition

At risk for behaviors in which an individual demonstrates that he or she can be physically, emotionally, and/or sexually harmful to others

Risk Factors

Availability of weapon(s); body language (e.g., rigid posture, clenching of fists and jaw, hyperactivity, pacing, breathlessness, threatening stances); cognitive impairment (e.g., learning disabilities, attention deficit disorder, decreased intellectual functioning); cruelty to animals; fire setting; history of childhood abuse; history of indirect violence (e.g., tearing off clothes, ripping objects off walls, writing on walls, urinating on floor, defecating on floor, stamping feet, temper tantrum, running in corridors, yelling, throwing objects, breaking a window, slamming doors, making sexual advances); history of other-directed violence (e.g., hitting someone, kicking someone, spitting at someone, scratching someone, throwing objects at someone, biting someone, attempted rape, rape/sexual molestation, urinating/defecating on a person); history of substance abuse; history of threats of violence (e.g., verbal threats against property, verbal threats against person, social threats, cursing, threatening notes/letters, threatening gestures, sexual threats); history of

• = Independent   ▲ = Collaborative

violent antisocial behavior (e.g., stealing, insistent borrowing, insistent demands for privileges, insistent interruption of meetings, refusal to eat, refusal to take medication, ignoring instructions); history of witnessing family violence; impulsivity; motor vehicle offense (e.g., frequent traffic violations, use of a motor vehicle to release anger); neurological impairment (e.g., positive EEG, computed tomography, or magnetic resonance imaging scan, neurological findings, head trauma, seizure disorders); pathological intoxication; perinatal complications; psychotic symptomatology (e.g., auditory, visual, command hallucinations; paranoid delusions; loose, rambling, or illogical thought processes; suicidal behavior)

Client Outcomes

Client Will (Specify Time Frame):

- Stop all forms of abuse (physical, emotional, sexual; neglect; financial exploitation)
- Have cessation of abuse reported by victim
- Display no aggressive activity
- Refrain from verbal outbursts
- Refrain from violating others' personal space
- Refrain from antisocial behaviors
- Maintain relaxed body language and decreased motor activity
- Identify factors contributing to abusive/aggressive behavior
- Demonstrate impulse control or state feelings of control
- Identify impulsive behaviors
- Identify feelings/behaviors that lead to impulsive actions
- Identify consequences of impulsive actions to self or others
- Avoid high-risk environments and situations
- Identify and talk about feelings; express anger appropriately
- Express decreased anxiety and control of hallucinations as applicable
- Displace anger to meaningful activities
- Communicate needs appropriately
- Identify responsibility to maintain control
- Express empathy for victim
- Obtain no access or yield access to harmful objects
- Use alternative coping mechanisms for stress
- Obtain and follow through with counseling
- Demonstrate knowledge of correct role behaviors

V

• = Independent   ▲ = Collaborative

Victim (and Children if Applicable) Will (Specify Time Frame):
* Have safe plan for leaving situation or avoiding abuse
* Resolve depression or traumatic response

Parent Will (Specify Time Frame):
* Monitor social/play contacts
* Provide supervision and nurturing environment
* Intervene to prevent high-risk social behaviors

Nursing Interventions

Client Violence

▲ Monitor the environment, evaluate situations that could become violent, and intervene early to deescalate the situation. Know and follow institution's policies and procedures concerning violence. Consider that family members or other staff may initiate violence in all settings. Enlist support from other staff rather than attempting to handle the situation alone.

* Assess causes of aggression: social versus biological.

* Assess the client for risk factors of violence, including those in the following categories: personal history (e.g., past violent behavior); psychiatric disorders (particularly psychoses, paranoid or bipolar disorders, substance abuse, PTSD, antisocial personality or borderline personality disorder); neurological disorders (e.g., head injury, temporal lobe epilepsy, CVA, dementia or senility), medical disorders (e.g., hypoxia, hypo- or hyperglycemia), psychological precursors (e.g., low tolerance for stress, impulsivity), coping difficulties (e.g., inability to plan solutions or see long-term consequences of behavior), and childhood or adolescent disorders (e.g., conduct disorders, hyperactivity, autism, learning disability).

* Measures of violence may be useful in predicting or tracking behavior, and serving as outcome measures.

* Assess the client with a history of previous assaults. Listen to and acknowledge feelings of anger, observe for increased motor activity, and prepare to intervene if the client becomes aggressive.

V

• = Independent   ▲ = Collaborative

- Assess the client for physiological signs and external signs of anger.
- Assess for the presence of hallucinations.
- Apply STAMPEDAR as an acronym for assessing the immediate potential for violence.
- Determine the presence and degree of homicidal or suicidal risk. A number of questions will elicit the necessary information. "Have you been thinking about harming someone? If yes, who? How often do you have these thoughts, and how long do they last? Do you have a plan? What is it? Do you have access to the means to carry out that plan? What has kept you from hurting the person until now?" Refer to the care plan for **Risk for Suicide.**
- Take action to minimize personal risk: Use nonthreatening body language. Respect personal space and boundaries. Maintain at least an arm's length distance from the client; do not touch the client without permission (unless physical restraint is the goal). Do not allow the client to block access to an exit. If speaking with the client alone, keep the door to the room open. Be aware of where other staff is at all times. Notify other staff of where you are at all times. Take verbal threats seriously and notify other staff. Wear clothing and accessories that are not restricting and that will not be dangerous (e.g., sandals or shoes with heels can lead to twisted ankles; necklaces or dangling earrings could be grabbed).
- Remove potential weapons from the environment. Be prepared to remove obstructions to staff response from the environment. Search the client and his or her belongings for weapons or potential weapons on admission to the hospital as appropriate.
- Inform the client of unit expectations for appropriate behavior and the consequences of not meeting these expectations. Emphasize that the client must comply with the rules of the unit. Give positive reinforcement for compliance. Increase surveillance of the hospitalized client at smoking, meal, and medication times.
- Assign a single room to the client with a potential for violence toward others.

● = Independent   ▲ = Collaborative

- Maintain a calm attitude in response to the client. Provide a low level of stimulation in the client's environment; place the client in a safe, quiet place, and speak slowly and quietly.
- Redirect possible violent behaviors into physical activities (e.g., walking, jogging) if the client is physically able.
- Provide sufficient staff if a show of force is necessary to demonstrate control to the client.
- Protect other clients in the environment from harm. Remove other individuals from the vicinity of a violent or potentially violent client. Follow safety protocols of the department.
- Maintain a secluded area for the client to be placed when violent. Ensure that staff are continuously present and available to client during seclusion.
- ▲ Recognize legal requirements that the least restrictive alternative of treatment should be used with aggressive clients. The hierarchy of intervention is: promote a milieu that provides structure and calmness, with negotiation and collaboration taking precedence over control; maintain vigilance of the unit and respond to behavioral changes early; talk with client to calm and promote understanding of emotional state; use chemical restraints as ordered; increase to manual restraint if needed; increase to mechanical restraint and seclusion as a last resort.
- ▲ Use mechanical restraints if ordered and as necessary. Physical restraint can be therapeutic to keep the client and others safe.
- ▲ Follow the institution's protocol for releasing restraints. Observe the client closely, remain calm, and provide positive feedback as the client's behavior becomes controlled.
- ▲ After a violent event on a unit, debriefing and support of both staff and clients should be made available.
- Form a therapeutic alliance with the client, remaining calm, identifying the source of anger as external to both nurse and client, and using the therapeutic relationship to prevent the need for seclusion or restraint.
- Allow, encourage, and assist the client to verbalize feelings appropriately either one-on-one or in a group setting. Actively listen to the client; explore the source of the client's anger, and negotiate resolution when possible. Teach healthy ways to

V

• = Independent   ▲ = Collaborative

express feelings/anger, appropriate gender roles, and how to communicate needs appropriately.
- Identify with client the stimuli that initiate violence and the means of dealing with the stimuli. Have the client keep an anger diary and discuss alternative responses together. Teach cognitive-behavioral techniques.
▲ Initiate and promote staff attendance at aggression management training programs.

Intimate Partner Violence (IPV)/Domestic Violence

NOTE: Before implementation of interventions in the face of domestic violence, nurses should examine their own emotional responses to abuse, their knowledge base about abuse, and systemic elements within the emergency department (ED) to ensure that interventions will be compassionate and appropriate.
- Screen for possible abuse in women or children with a pattern of multiple injuries, particularly if any suspicion exists that the physical findings are inconsistent with the explanation of how the injuries were incurred.
▲ Report suspected child abuse to Child Protective Services.
▲ Refer women suspected of being in a spousal abuse situation to an area crisis center and provide phone number of area crisis hotline.
- Assess for physical and mental concerns of women, including risk of HIV.
- Assist the client in negotiating the health care system and overcoming barriers.
- With women who repeatedly experience injuries from domestic violence, maintain a nonjudgmental approach and continue to offer resources/referrals. If the woman voices a willingness to leave her situation, assist with developing an emergency plan that will consider all contingencies possible (e.g., safe location, financial resources, care of children, when to leave safely).
- Maintain a nonjudgmental response when clients return to husbands or refuse to leave them.
- Focus on providing support, ensuring safety, and promoting self-efficacy while encouraging disclosure about IPV events.

- Screen pregnant women for the potential for domestic violence during pregnancy, especially with teenage pregnancies.
- Screen women and children for effects of domestic violence during the postpartum period.
- Women with physical or mental disabilities require extended assessment, including a comprehensive functional assessment, with attention to cultural issues, the nature of the disability, and needed resources. Women with disabilities may experience abuse from multiple sources, and particular attention should be paid to the additional emotional stressors present.
- ▲ Referral for spiritual counseling may be considered, but be aware that clergy vary in their helpfulness.
- Identify risk factors such as ongoing mental illness of a parent, and monitor family closely.
- ▲ In cases where spouse or child abuse accompanies substance abuse, refer the abusive client to a substance abuse treatment program. Refer the spouse receiving abuse to Al-Anon and the children to Alateen.
- ▲ In cases where an adult reveals a history of unresolved/untreated sexual abuse as a child, referral to a local Adults Molested as Children (AMAC) group may be helpful.
- ▲ Referral of women for psychiatric/psychological treatment or parenting classes should be considered as an appropriate intervention.
- ▲ Referral of children for psychiatric/psychological treatment should be considered as an appropriate intervention.
- ▲ Batterer intervention programs are often available and may be court mandated.

Social Violence

- Assess for acute stress disorder (ASD) and post-traumatic stress disorder (PTSD) among victims of violence.
- ▲ Assess the support network of women who become victims of violent crime and refer for appropriate levels of assistance.
- Be aware that hate crime is increasing, particularly toward gay and transgendered individuals, and it requires support and advocacy for victims.

• = Independent ▲ = Collaborative

▲ Victims of violence seen in the ED should receive an assessment for needed services and assignment to case management.

Rape-Trauma Syndrome

- Assist client to cope with potential stalking activity.
- Approach client with sensitivity.
- ▲ Monitor for paradoxical drug reactions, and report any to the physician.
- Assess for brain insults, such as recent falls or injuries, strokes, or transient ischemic attacks.
- Decrease environmental stimuli if violence is directed at others.
- Assess holistic needs of the client.
- Discuss with client her wishes regarding use of an emergency contraceptive.
- ▲ If abuse or neglect of an elderly client is suspected, report the suspicion to an adult protective services agency with jurisdiction over the geographical area where the client lives.

Pediatric

- Assess for predictors of anger that can lead to violent behavior.
- Be alert for both shaken baby syndrome and exposure of children to violence.
- Pregnant teens should be assessed for abuse, particularly if they are with an older partner.
- ▲ In the case of child abuse or neglect, refer for early childhood home visitation.

Geriatric

- Be alert to the potential for elder abuse in clients, including the possibility of psychological abuse.
- Assess for changes in physiological functions (e.g., constipation, dehydration) or impairment of the ability to meet basic needs (e.g., inadequate toileting, decreased mobility). Observe for signs of fear, anxiety, anger, and agitation, and intervene immediately.
- Observe for dementia and delirium.

V

- Be aware that IPV may arise or continue under circumstances of medical illness.
- Be alert for the potential of sexual abuse of elders.

Multicultural

- Exercise cultural competence when dealing with domestic violence.
- Identify and respond to unique needs of immigrant women who experience IPV.
- Assist with acculturation and activating social support.

Home Care

- Be alert to the potential for violent behavior in the home setting. Respond to verbal aggression with interventions to deescalate negative emotional states.
- Assess family members or caregivers for their ability to protect the client and themselves.
- Include an initial and ongoing assessment and evaluation of potential abuse and neglect. Photograph evidence of abuse or neglect when possible.
▲ If neglect or abuse is suspected, identify an emergency plan that addresses the problem immediately, ensures client safety, and includes a report to the appropriate authorities. Discuss when to use hotlines and 911. Role-play access to emergency resources with the client and caregivers.
- Encourage appropriate safety behaviors in abused women; call the client at intervals during a 6-month period to determine whether safety behaviors are being carried out.
- Assess the home environment for harmful objects. Have the family remove or lock objects as able.
▲ Refer for homemaker or psychiatric home health care services for respite, client reassurance, and implementation of a therapeutic regimen.
▲ If the client is taking psychotropic medications, assess client and family knowledge of medication and its administration and side effects. Teach as necessary.
▲ Evaluate effectiveness and side effects of medications.

- If client displays mildly intensifying aggressive behavior, attempt to diffuse anger or violence (e.g., ask for a glass of water to distract client). Later in the visit, explain that aggressive behavior is not acceptable and present consequences of continued aggressive behavior (i.e., right of agency to discontinue services).
- Document all acts or verbalizations of aggression.
▲ If client verbalizes or displays threatening behavior, notify your supervisor and plan to make joint visits with another staff person or a security escort.
- If the client's behavior is not overtly threatening but makes the nurse uncomfortable, a meeting may be held outside the home in sight of others (e.g., front porch).
- Never enter a home or remain in a home if aggression threatens your well-being.
▲ Never challenge a show of force, such as a gun threat. Leave and notify your supervisor and the appropriate authorities. Document the incident.
▲ If client behaviors intensify, refer for immediate mental health intervention.

Client/Family Teaching and Discharge Planning

- Instruct victims of IPV in the dynamics and prognosis of domestic violence behavior.
- Instruct victims of IPV in the outcomes for children who witness or are victims of domestic violence.
- Teach relaxation and exercise as ways to release anger and deal with stress.
- Teach cognitive-behavioral activities, such as active problem solving, reframing (reappraising the situation from a different perspective), or thought stopping (in response to a negative thought, picture a large stop sign and replace the image with a prearranged positive alternative). Teach the client to confront his or her own negative thought patterns (or cognitive distortions), such as catastrophizing (expecting the very worst), dichotomous thinking (perceiving events in only one of two opposite categories), magnification (placing distorted

V

emphasis on a single event), or unrealistic expectations (e.g., "I should get what I want when I want it").

▲ Refer to individual or group therapy.

• Teach the adolescent client violence prevention, and encourage him or her to become involved in community service activities.

• Teach the use of appropriate community resources in emergency situations (e.g., hotline, community mental health agency, ED, 911 in most places in the United States, the toll-free National Domestic Violence Hotline [1-800-799-SAFE]).

• Encourage the use of self-help groups in nonemergency situations.

• Inform the client and family about medication actions, side effects, target symptoms, and toxic reactions.

Risk for self-directed Violence

NANDA-I Definition

At risk for behaviors in which an individual demonstrates that he or she can be physically, emotionally and/or sexually harmful to self

Risk Factors

Ages 15 to 19; age 45 or older; behavioral cues (e.g., writing forlorn love notes, directing angry messages at a significant other who has rejected the person, giving away personal items, taking out a large life insurance policy); conflictual interpersonal relationships; emotional problems (e.g., hopelessness, despair, increased anxiety, panic, anger, hostility); employment problems (e.g., unemployed, recent job loss/failure); engagement in autoerotic sexual acts; family background (e.g., chaotic or conflictual, history of suicide); history of multiple suicide attempts; lack of personal resources (e.g., poor achievement, poor insight, affect unavailable and poorly controlled); lack of social resources (e.g., poor rapport, socially isolated, unresponsive family); marital status (single, widowed, divorced); mental health problems (e.g., severe depression, psychosis, severe personality disorder, alcoholism or drug abuse); occupation (executive, administrator/owner of business, professional, semiskilled worker); physical health problems (e.g., hypochondriasis, chronic or terminal illness); sexual orientation (bisexual [active], homosexual [inactive]); suicidal ideation; suicidal plan; verbal cues (e.g., talking about death, "better off without me," asking questions about lethal dosages of drugs)

Impaired Walking

NANDA-I Definition

Limitation of independent movement within the environment on foot (or artificial limb)

Defining Characteristics

Impaired ability to: climb stairs, walk on uneven surface, walk required distances, walk on even surfaces, walk on an incline or decline, navigate curbs

Related Factors (r/t)

Cognitive impairment; deconditioning; depressed mood; environmental constraints (e.g., stairs, inclines, uneven surfaces, unsafe obstacles, distances, lack of assistive devices or person, restraints); fear of falling; impaired balance; impaired vision; insufficient muscle strength; lack of knowledge; limited endurance; musculoskeletal impairment (e.g., contractures); neuromuscular impairment; obesity; pain

Client Outcomes/Goals

Client Will (Specify Time Frame):

* Demonstrate optimal independence and safety in walking
* Demonstrate the ability to direct others on how to assist with walking
* Demonstrate the ability to properly and safely use and care for assistive walking devices

W

Nursing Interventions

* Progressively mobilize clients (gradual elevation of head of bed [HOB], sitting in reclined chair, standing, etc.).
* Assist clients to apply orthosis, immobilizers, splints, and braces before walking.

● = Independent   ▲ = Collaborative

- Eat frequent small, low-carbohydrate meals.
- Maintain partial head elevation when resting in bed for orthostatic hypotension.
▲ Compare morning lying/sitting/standing blood pressures. If systolic pressure falls 20 mm Hg or diastolic pressure falls 10 mm Hg from lying to standing within 3 minutes, and/or if lightheadedness, dizziness, syncope, or unexplained falls occur, consult a physician.
- Apply thromboembolic deterrent (TED) stockings and/or elastic leg wraps and abdominal binders; raise HOB slowly in small increments to sitting, have client move feet/legs up and down, then stand slowly; avoid prolonged standing.
▲ Give prescribed hydration and medications to treat orthostatic hypotension; also consider leg wraps and abdominal binders; client should perform warm-up bed exercises as well as a medication review for possible contributing factors such as blood pressure medicine.
- Screen for deep vein thrombosis (DVT), vigilantly apply compression stockings (TEDs), and give medications as prescribed to persons at risk for/with DVT. Refer to care plan for **Ineffective peripheral Tissue Perfusion.**
▲ Apply compression stockings and assist persons with DVT to walk as ordered.
▲ Recognize that ambulating as ordered after diagnosis of DVT as opposed to initial bed rest is recommended when feasible and helps prevent further thromboses.
- Reinforce correct use of prescribed mobility devices and remind clients of weight-bearing restrictions.
- Teach clients with leg amputations to correctly don stump socks, liner, immediate postoperative prostheses (IPOP), or traditional prosthesis before standing/walking.
- Teach client with an amputation the importance of avoiding prolonged hip and knee flexion. If contractures occur, the client may experience difficulty with fit of prosthesis and have difficulty using a prosthesis.
- Emphasize the importance of wearing properly fitting, low-heeled shoes with nonskid soles, and socks/hose, and of

W

● = Independent   ▲ = Collaborative

seeking medical care for foot pain or problems with abnormal toenails, corns, calluses, or diabetes.

▲ Use a snug gait belt with handles and assistive devices while walking clients, as recommended by the physical therapist (PT).

• Walk clients frequently with an appropriate number of people; have one team member state short, simple motor instructions.

• Cue and manually guide clients with neglect as they walk.

• Document the number of helpers, level of assistance (maximum, standby, etc.), type of assistance, and devices needed on the care plan and room white board.

▲ Take pulse rate/rhythm, respiratory rate, and pulse oximetry before walking clients, and reassess within 5 minutes of walking, then ongoing as needed. If abnormal, have the client sit 5 minutes, then remeasure. If still abnormal, walk clients more slowly and with more help or for a shorter time, or notify physician. If uncontrolled diabetes/angina/arrhythmias/tachycardia (100 bpm or more) or resting SBP at or above 200 mm Hg or DBP at or above 110 mm Hg occur, do not initiate walking exercise. Refer to the care plan **Activity Intolerance.**

▲ Perform initial/ongoing screening for risk of falling and perform postfall assessments including meds and lab results to prevent further falls.

• Individualize interventions to prevent falls such as scheduled toileting, monitored rooms, bed alarms, wheelchair alarms, balance/strength training, sleep hygiene, education on risk of medication/alcohol use, removal of hazards, and attention to safe handling during any transfers, toileting, showering/bathing.

Geriatric

▲ Assess for swaying, poor balance, weakness, and fear of falling while elders stand/walk. If present, implement fall protection precautions and refer to physical therapy (PT).

▲ Review medications for polypharmacy (more than five drugs) and medications that increase the risk of falls, including sedatives, antidepressants, and drugs affecting the CNS.

• = Independent   ▲ = Collaborative

- Encourage tai chi, physical therapy, or other exercise for balance, gait, and strength training in group programs or at home.
- Recommend vision assessment and consideration for cataract removal if needed.

Home Care

- Establish a support system for emergency and contingency care (e.g., Lifeline)
- Assess for and modify any barriers to walking in the home environment.
- ▲ Obtain orders for PT home visits for individualized strength, balance retraining, and an exercise plan.
- ▲ Make referrals for home health services for support and assistance with activities of daily living (ADLs).

Client/Family Teaching and Discharge Planning

- Teach clients to check ambulation devices weekly for cracks, loose nuts, or worn tips and to clean dust and dirt on tips.
- Teach diabetics that they are at risk for foot ulcers and teach them preventive interventions. See care plan **Ineffective peripheral Tissue Perfusion.**
- ▲ Instruct men/women at risk for osteoporosis or hip fractures to bear weight, walk, engage in resistance exercise (with appropriate adjustments for conditions), ensure good nutrition (especially adequate intake of calcium and vitamin D), drink milk, stop smoking, monitor alcohol intake, and consult a physician for appropriate medications.

W

Wandering

NANDA-I Definition

Meandering; aimless or repetitive locomotion that exposes the individual to harm; frequently incongruent with boundaries, limits, or obstacles

● = Independent   ▲ = Collaborative

Defining Characteristics

Frequent or continuous movement from place to place, often revisiting the same destinations; persistent locomotion in search of "missing" or unattainable people or places; haphazard locomotion; locomotion in unauthorized or private spaces; locomotion resulting in unintended leaving of a premise; long periods of locomotion without an apparent destination; fretful locomotion or pacing; inability to locate significant landmarks in a familiar setting; locomotion that cannot be easily dissuaded or redirected; following behind or shadowing a caregiver's locomotion; trespassing; hyperactivity; scanning, seeking, or searching behaviors; periods of locomotion interspersed with periods of nonlocomotion (e.g., sitting, standing, sleeping); getting lost

Related Factors (r/t)

Cognitive impairment, specifically memory and recall deficits, disorientation, poor visuoconstructive (or visuospatial) ability, and language (primarily expressive) defects; cortical atrophy; premorbid behavior (e.g., outgoing, sociable personality); separation from familiar people and places; sedation; emotional state, especially fear, anxiety, boredom, or depression (agitation); overstimulating/understimulating social or physical environment; physiological state or need (e.g., hunger/thirst, pain, urination, constipation); time of day

Client Outcomes

Client Will (Specify Time Frame):
- Maintain psychological well-being
- Decrease the amount of time getting lost
- Engage in meaningful activities daily
- Remain safe and free from falls and clopement
- Maintain physical activity and remain comfortable and free of pain
- Maintain appropriate body weight and be well nourished and well hydrated

Caregiver Will (Specify Time Frame):
- Be able to explain interventions he or she can use to provide a safe environment for a care receiver who displays wandering behavior
- Develop strategies to reduce caregiver stress levels

• = Independent ▲ = Collaborative

W

Nursing Interventions

Nursing Care Facilities: Wandering

- Assess and document the amount (frequency and duration), percentage of hours with wandering, and 24-hour distribution of wandering behavior over 3 days.
- Assess and document the quantity and qualities of wandering behaviors (e.g., persistent walking, repetitive walking, eloping behaviors, spatial disorientation, goal directed, negative outcomes).
- Obtain a history of personality characteristics and behavioral responses to stress.
- Evaluate for neurocognitive strengths and limitations, particularly language, attention, and visuospatial skills.
- Assess for changes in cognition and signs and symptoms of medical illness such as pneumonia or cardiovascular disease.
- Assess and monitor for drug-induced akathisia (motor restlessness).
- Discontinue use of medications and physical restraints that are used for the sole purpose of controlling wandering behavior.
- Assess for emotional or psychological distress, such as anxiety, fear, or feeling lost.
- Assess for physical distress or unmet needs (e.g., hunger, thirst, pain discomfort, elimination) with the Need-Driven Dementia-Compromised Behaviors model.
- Observe wandering episodes for antecedents and consequences.
- Observe the location where and environmental conditions in which wandering is occurring and modify those that appear to induce wandering.
- Assess regularly for the presence of or potential for negative outcomes of wandering (e.g., elopement, declining social skills, onset of falls, becoming lost, and injuries).
- For the client who displays wandering behavior during mealtimes, use behavioral interventions to shape behavior, including verbal statements, nonverbal social behavior, and systematic extinguishing of undesirable client behavior.
- Provide for safe ambulation with comfortable and well-fitting clothes, shoes with nonskid soles and foot support, and any necessary walking aids (e.g., a cane or walker).

W

• = Independent ▲ = Collaborative

- Refer to physical therapy for core therapeutic exercise, balance, gait, and assistive device training.
- Provide safe and secure surroundings that deter accidental elopements, using perimeter control devices or electronic tracking systems.
- During periods of inactivity, position the wanderer so that desirable destinations (e.g., bathroom) are within the client's line of vision and undesirable destinations (e.g., exits or stair-wells) are out of sight.
- Facilitate way-finding through therapeutic environmental design.
- Enhance the physical environment by increasing visual appeal and provide interesting views and opportunities to sit.
- Engage wanderers in social interaction and structured activity such as painting or coloring, especially when wanderers appear distressed or otherwise uncomfortable, or their wandering presents a challenge to others in the setting.
- Provide headphones and iPod with individualized preferred music while the person with dementia is wandering, or encourage the person to participate in a music group.
- If wandering has a pacing quality, attempt to identify and address any underlying problems or concerns. Offer stress-reducing approaches, such as music, massage, or rocking. Attempts to distract or redirect the pacing wanderer may worsen wandering.
- Provide a regularly scheduled and supervised exercise or walking program, particularly if wandering occurs excessively during the night or at times that are inconvenient in the setting.
- Use soft tactile hand massage before the times of day or events that induce wandering.

Multicultural

- Recognize that wandering occurs with little variation in expression among individuals with dementia regardless of culture or ethnicity.
- Assess for the influence of cultural beliefs, norms, and values on the family's understanding of wandering behavior.

• = Independent   ▲ = Collaborative

▲ Refer the family to social services or other supportive services to assist with the impact of caregiving for the wandering client.
• Encourage the family to use support groups or other service programs.

Home Care

• Help the caregiver set up a plan to deal with wandering behavior using the interventions mentioned earlier.
• Assess the home environment for modifications that will protect the client and prevent elopement.
• Assist the family to set up a plan of exercise for the client, including safe walking.
• Enroll wanderers in the Safe Return Program of the Alzheimer's Association, and help the caregiver develop a plan of action to use if the client elopes.
• Help the caregiver develop a plan of action to use if the client elopes.
▲ Refer for homemaker or psychiatric home health care services for respite, client reassurance, and implementation of a therapeutic regimen. Refer to the care plan for **Caregiver Role Strain.**

Client/Family Teaching and Discharge Planning

• Inform the client and family of the meaning of and reasons for wandering behavior.
• Teach the caregiver/family methods to deal with wandering behavior using the interventions mentioned in Nursing Interventions.

W

Bibliography

Abrams P, et al: The standardization of terminology of lower urinary tract function: report from the Standardization Sub-committee of the International Continence Society, *Am J Obstet Gynecol* 187(1):116–126, 2002.

Abrams P, et al: Fourth International Consultation on Incontinence Recommendations of the International Scientific Committee: evaluation and treatment of urinary incontinence, pelvic organ prolapse, and fecal incontinence, *Neurourol Urodynam* 29(1):213–240, 2010.

American College of Sports Medicine (ACSM): *American College of Sports Medicine's guidelines for exercise testing and prescription*, ed 8, Philadelphia, 2010, Lippincott Williams & Wilkins.

Akers AL, et al: InReach: connecting NICU infants and their parents with community early intervention services, *Zero Three* 27(3), 2007.

Altena T: *DIY: How a smartphone can benefit your health*, 2012. Retrieved from http://www.acsm.org/docs/other-documents/2012winterfspn_diyexercise.pdf.

American Academy of Nursing's Expert Panel on Acute and Critical Care: *Reducing functional decline in older adults during hospitalization: A best practice approach,* 2012. Retrieved from http://www.hartfordign.org.

American Academy of Pediatrics (AAP): *Reduce the risk of SIDS*, 2010. Retrieved July 22, 2011, from http://www.healthychildren.org/English/ages-stages/baby/sleep/pages/Preventing-SIDS.aspx.

American College of Sports Medicine (ACSM): *American College of Sports Medicine's guidelines for exercise testing and prescription*, ed 8, Philadelphia, 2010, Wolters Kluwer/Lippincott Williams & Wilkins.

American College of Sports Medicine (ACSM): *Selecting and effectively using a walking program,* 2011a. Retrieved from http://www.acsm.org/docs/brochures/.

American College of Sports Medicine (ACSM): Quantity and quality of exercise for developing and maintaining cardiorespiratory, musculoskeletal, and neuromotor fitness in apparently healthy adults: guidance for prescribing exercise, *Med Sci Sports Exerc* 43(7):1334–1359, 2011b.

American Dental Association (ADA): *Oral health topics A-Z*. Retrieved July 3, 2009, from http://www.ada.org/public/index.asp.

American Pain Society (APS): *Principles of analgesic use in acute and chronic pain*, ed 6, Glenview, IL, 2008, American Pain Society.

Anderson JL, et al: ACC/AHA 2007 guidelines for the management of patients with unstable angina/non-ST elevation myocardial infarction, *J Am Coll Cardiol* 50(7):e1–e157.

Antman EM, et al: 2007 Focused update of the ACC/AHA 2004 guidelines for the management of patients with ST-elevation myocardial infarction, *J Am Coll Cardiol* 51(2):210–247, 2008.

AORN: Recommended practices for positioning the patient in the perioperative practice setting, *AORN Standards and Recommended Practices for
Perioperative Nursing*, 2012.

Auger L: *Vivre avec sa tête ou avec son cœur (Live with your head or with your
heart)*, Quebec, 2006, Centre la Pensée Réaliste, republication par Pierre
Bovo.

Bankhead R, Boullata J, Brantley S, et al: Aspen enteral nutrition practice
recommendations, *J Parenteral Enteral Nutr* 33(2):122–167, 2009.

Baranoski S, Ayello EA, editors: *Wound care essentials: practice principles*, ed 3,
Ambler, PA, 2012, Lippincott Williams & Wilkins.

Barclay L: *Updated guidelines to prevent falls in elderly*, 2011, . Medscape Education
Clinical Briefs. Retrieved December 7, 2011, from http://www.medscape.org/
viewarticle/735899.

Beaumont T, Leadbeater M: Treatment and care of patients with metastatic
breast cancer, *Nurs Stand* 25(40):49–56, 2011.

Becker JH, Wu SC: Fever: an update, *J Am Podiatr Med Assoc* 100(4):281–290,
2010.

Bhowmik A, Chahal K, Austin G, et al: Improving mucociliary clearance in
chronic obstructive pulmonary disease, *Respir Med* 103(4):496–502, 2009.

Bickley LS, Szilagyi P: *Guide to physical examination*, ed 10, Philadelphia, 2009,
Lippincott.

Bliss DZ, Norton C: Conservative management of fecal incontinence, *Am J
Nurs* 110(9):30–40, 2010.

Borchert K, et al: The incontinence-associated dermatitis and its severity instrument, *J Wound Ostomy Continence Nurs* 37(5):527–535, 2010.

Brennan C, Mazanec P: Dyspnea management across the palliative care continuum, *J Hosp Palliat Nurs* 13(3):130–139, 2011.

Breitbart W, Alici Y: Agitation and delirium at the end of life: "We couldn't
manage him," *JAMA* 300(24):2898–2910, 2008.

Boudrias J, Gaudreau P, Laschinger HKS: Testing the structure of psychological empowerment: does gender make a difference? *Educ Psychol Meas*
64:861, 2004.

Bourne RS: Delirium and use of sedation agents in intensive care, *Crit Care
Nurs* 13(4):195–202, 2008.

Brienza DM, et al: Pressure redistribution: seating, positioning, and support
surfaces. In Baranoski S, Ayello EA, editors: *Wound care essentials: practice
principles*, ed 3, Ambler, PA, 2012, Lippincott Williams & Wilkins.

Bruckenthal P: Integrating nonpharmacologic and alternative strategies into
a comprehensive management approach for older adults with pain, *Pain
Manag Nurs* 11(2):S23–S31, 2010.

Buck HG, Zambroski CH: Upstreaming palliative care for patients with heart
failure, *J Cardiovasc Nurs* 27(2):147–153, 2012.

Buhr GT, Genao L, White HI: Urinary tract infections in long-term care
residents, *Clin Geriatr Med* 27(2):229–239, 2011.

Burns SM: Invasive mechanical ventilation (through an artificial airway): volume and pressure modes. In Lynn-McHale DJ, editor: *AACN procedure manual for critical care*, ed 6, Philadelphia, 2011, Saunders Elsevier.

Burns SM: Weaning from mechanical ventilation. In Burns SM, editor: *AACN protocols for practice: care of mechanically ventilated patients*, ed 2, Sudbury, MA, 2007, Jones & Bartlett.

Camden S: Obesity: an emerging concern for patients and nurses, *Online J Issues Nurs* 14(1):5–17, 2009.

Cameron ID, et al: Interventions for preventing falls in older people in nursing care facilities and hospitals, *Cochrane Database Syst Rev*(1):CD005465, 2010.

Campbell-Taylor I: Oropharyngeal dysphagia in long-term care: misperceptions of treatment efficacy, *J Am Med Dir Assoc* 9(7):523–531, 2008.

Castelhano N, Roque L: The integration of the computer-mediated ludic experience in multisensory environments. In *Breaking new ground: innovation in games, play, practice and theory, Proceedings of DiGRA 2009*.

Centers for Disease Control and Prevention (CDC): Childhood lead poisoning associated with lead dust contamination of family vehicles and child safety seats—Maine, 2008, *MMWR Morb Mortal Wkly Rep* 58(32):890–893, 2009.

Centers for Disease Control and Prevention: Prevention and control of influenza: recommendations of the Advisory Committee on Immunization Practices (ACIP), 2011, *MMWR Recomm Rep* 60(33):1128–1132, 2011b.

Centers for Disease Control and Prevention (CDC): Healthy weight, it is not a diet, it is a lifestyle, *BMI calculator*, 2011. Retrieved June 10, 2012, from http://www.cdc.gov/healthyweight/assessing/bmi/index.html.

Chang CC, Roberts B: Strategies for feeding patients with dementia, *Am J Nurs* 11(4):36–44, 2011.

Chulay M, Seckel M: Suctioning: Endotracheal tube or tracheostomy tube. In Lynn-McHale DJ, editor: *AACN procedure manual for critical care*, ed 6, Philadelphia, 2011, Saunders Elsevier.

Cohen MH, et al: *Patient handling and movement assessments: a white paper*, April 2010, The Facility Guideline Institute.

Coss E, Geske JB, Mueller PS: 57-year old woman with acute lower extremity pain and swelling, *Mayo Clin Proc* 84(10):e1–e4, 2009.

De Almeida LM, Braga CG: Construction and validation of an instrument to assess powerlessness, *Int J Nurs Terminol Classif* 17:67, 2006.

Deeken J, et al: Care for the caregivers: a review of self-report instruments developed to measure the burden, needs, and quality of life of informal caregivers, *J Pain Symptom Manage* 26(4):922–953, 2003.

Devroey D, Van Casteren V: Signs for early diagnosis of heart failure in primary health care, *Vasc Health Risk Manag* 7:591–596, 2011.

Dienstag J: Toxic and drug-induced hepatitis. In Longo DL, et al, editor: *Harrison's principles of internal medicine*, ed 18, New York, 2011, McGraw-Hill.

Dwyer T, Ponsonby AL: Sudden infant death syndrome and prone sleeping position, *Ann Epidemiol* 19(4):245–249, 2009.

Easterling CS, Robbins E: Dementia and dysphagia, *Geriatr Nurs* 29(4): 275–285, 2008.

Eisenstadt ES: Dysphagia and aspiration pneumonia in older adults, *J Am Acad Nurse Pract* 22(1):17–22, 2010.

European Pressure Ulcer Advisory Panel and National Pressure Ulcer Advisory Panel (EPUAP/NPUAP): *Prevention and treatment of pressure ulcers*, Washington, DC, 2009, National Pressure Ulcer Advisory Panel.

Fletcher SG, et al: Sexual dysfunction in patients with multiple sclerosis: a multidisciplinary approach to evaluation and management, *Nat Clin Pract Urol* 6(2):96–107, 2009.

Flinn DR, et al: Prevention, diagnosis, and management of postoperative delirium in older adults, *J Am Coll Surg* 209(2):261–268, 2009.

Gabriel J: Infusion therapy part one: minimising the risks, *Nurs Stand* 22(31):51–56, 2008.

Gallagher PF, O'Mahony D, Quigley MM: Management of chronic constipation in the elderly, *Drugs Aging* 25(10):807–821, 2008.

Geerts WH, et al: Prevention of venous thromboembolism: American College of Chest Physicians evidence-based clinical practice guidelines, ed 8, *Chest* 133(suppl 6):381S–453S, 2008.

Gershon R, et al: *Home health care patients and safety hazards in the home: preliminary findings*, Rockville, MD, 2008, Agency for Healthcare Research and Quality (AHRQ).

Gibbons S, Lauder W, Ludwick R: Self-neglect: a proposed new NANDA diagnosis, *I nt J Nurs Terminol Classif* 17(1):10–18, 2006.

Girard TD, et al: Efficacy and safety of a paired sedation and ventilator weaning protocol for mechanically ventilated patients in intensive care (Awakening and Breathing Controlled Trial): a randomized controlled trial, *Lancet* 371(9607):126–134, 2008.

Grap M: Not-so-trivial pursuit: mechanical ventilation risk reduction, *Am J Crit Care* 18(4):299–309, 2009.

GOLD: *Global strategy for the diagnosis, management, and prevention of COPD (revised 2011)*, Global Initiative for Chronic Obstructive Lung Disease, 2011.

Gorski LA: Total parenteral nutrition administration. In Ackley B, et al, editor: *Evidence-based nursing care guidelines: medical-surgical interventions*, Philadelphia, 2008, Mosby.

Grossbach I, Stanberg S, Chlan L: Promoting effective communication for patients receiving mechanical ventilation, *Crit Care Nurse* 31(3):46–61, 2011.

Gosselink R, Bott J, Johnson M, et al: J: Physiotherapy for adult patients with critical illness: recommendations of the European respiratory society and European society of critical care medicine task force on physiotherapy for critically ill patients, *Intensive Care Med* 34:1188–1199, 2008.

Guenter P: Safe practices for enteral nutrition in critically ill patients, *Crit Care Nurs Clin North Am* 22(2):197–208, 2010.

Hansson L, Bjorkman T: Empowerment in people with a mental illness: reliability and validity of the Swedish version of an empowerment scale, *Scand J Caring Sci* 19:32, 2005.

Harris DJ, et al: Putting evidence into practice: evidence-based interventions for the management of oral mucositis, *Clin J Oncol Nurs* 12(1):141–152, 2008.

Harvard Health Letter: Keep a lookout for sodium, 37(4):1, 2012.

Hauck FR, et al: Breastfeeding and reduced risk of sudden infant death syndrome: a meta-analysis, *Pediatrics* 128(1):103–110, 2011.

Healing Touch International, Inc. Retrieved November 2, 2009, from http://www.healingtouchinternational.org.

Hipp B, Letizia MJ: Understanding and responding to the death rattle in dying patients, *Medsurg Nurs* 18(1):17–21, 2009.

Hooper VD, et al: ASPAN's evidence-based clinical practice guideline for the promotion of perioperative normothermia, *J PeriAnesth Nurs* 24(5): 217–287, 2009.

Hurnauth C: Management of faecal incontinence in acutely ill patients, *Nurs Stand* 25(2):48–56, 2011.

Ignoffo RJ: Current research on PONV/PDNV: practical implications for today's pharmacist, *Am J Health Syst Pharmacist* 66(1, suppl 1):S19–S24, 2009.

Ickenstein GW, et al: Prediction of outcome in neurogenic oropharyngeal dysphagia within 72 hours of acute stroke, *J Stroke Cerebrovasc Dis* 21(7):569–576, 2012.

Infusion Nurses Society (INS): Infusion nursing standards of practice, *J Infus Nurs* 34(1S):S1–S110, 2011.

Institute of Medicine: *Dietary reference intakes for calcium and vitamin D,* 2010. http://www.iom.edu/Reports/2010/Dietary-Reference-Intakes-for-Calcium-and-Vitamin-D/~/media/Files/Report%20Files/2010/Dietary-Reference-Intakes-for-Calcium-and-Vitamin-D/calciumvitdlg.jpg, Sept 19, 2012.

International Critical Incident Stress Foundation: *Critical incident stress information, signs and symptoms,* 2011. Retrieved September 26, 2011, from http://www.icisf.or/articles/CISInfoSheet.pdf.

Jarvis C: *Physical examination and health,* ed 6, St. Louis, 2012, Saunders.

Jarzyna D, et al: American Society for Pain Management Nursing evidence-based consensus guideline on monitoring of opioid-induced sedation and respiratory depression, *Pain Manag Nurs* 12(3):118–145, 2011.

Jakobsen JN, Herrstedt J: Prevention of chemotherapy-induced nausea and vomiting in elderly cancer patients, *Crit Rev Oncol Hematol* 71(3): 214–221, 2009.

Jepson R, Despain K, Keller DC: Unilateral neglect: assessment in nursing practice, *J Neurosci Nurs* 40(3):142–149, 2008.

Joanna Briggs Institute: Management of peripheral intravascular devices, *Aust Nurs J* 16(3):25–28, 2008.

Johnson DM, Worell J, Chandler RK: Assessing psychological health and empowerment in women: The Personal Progress Scale Revised, *Women Health* 41(1):109, 2005.

Joyner D: *Home oxygen can raise burn risk. HealthDay News*, 2012. Retrieved May 30, 2012, from http://consumer.healthday.com/Article.asp? AID=661193.

Kahn S, et al: *Antithrombotic therapy and prevention of thrombosis*, ed 9, American College of Chest Physician Evidence-Based Clinical Practice Guidelines Online Only Articles, *Chest* 141 (suppl 2):e195S-e226S, 2012:doi.10.1378.

Keefe DM, et al: Updated clinical practice guidelines for the prevention and treatment of mucositis, *Am Cancer Soc* 109(5):820–831, 2007.

Kellicker PG, Schub T: *Renal failure, acute: an overview*, 2010. Nursing reference center. Retrieved April 9, 2011, from http://0-search.ebscohost.com. topcat.switchinc.org/login.aspx?direct=true&db=nrc&AN=5000004704& site=nrc-live.

Kemmer H, et al: Obstructive sleep apnea syndrome is associated with overactive bladder and urgency incontinence in men, *Sleep* 32(2):271–275, 2009.

Keske L, Letizia MJ: *Clostridium difficile* infection: essential information for nurses, *Med Surg Nurs* 19(6):329–332, 2010.

Klein S: Protein-energy malnutrition. In Goldman L, Schafer A, editors: *Goldman's Cecil medicine*, ed 24, St Louis, 2011, Saunders.

Koenig S, Teixeira J, Yetzer E: Promoting mobility and function. In Mauk KL, editor: *Rehabilitation nursing, a contemporary approach to practice*, Sudbury, MA, 2012, Jones & Bartlett Learning.

Kolcaba K: *Comfort theory and practice: a holistic vision for health care*, New York, 2003, Springer.

Kolcaba K, et al: Efficacy of hand massage for enhancing comfort of hospice patients, *J Hospice Palliat Care* 6(2):91–101, 2004.

Krieger D: *Therapeutic touch inner workbook*, Santa Fe, NM, 1997, Bear and Company.

Kuntz D, Krieger D: *The spiritual dimension of therapeutic work*, 2004, Inner Traditions International, Limited.

Kranke P, Eberhart L: Possibilities and limitations in the pharmacological management of postoperative nausea and vomiting, *Eur J Anaesthesiol* 28(11):758–765, 2011.

Lacherade JC, et al: Intermittent subglottic secretion drainage and ventilator-associated pneumonia: a multicenter trial, *Am J Respir Crit Care Med* 182:910–917, 2010.

Lamm J, et al: Obtaining a thorough sleep history and routinely screening for obstructive sleep apnea, *J Am Acad Nurs Pract* 20:225, 2008.

Langemo D, et al: Incontinence and incontinence-associated dermatitis, *Adv Skin Wound Care* 24(3):126–140, 2011.

Larson J, et al: Spouse's life situation after partner's stroke: psychometric testing of a questionnaire, *J Adv Nurs* 52:300, 2005.

Lavery I, Smith E: Peripheral vascular access devices: risk prevention and management, *Br J Nurs* 16(22):1378–1383, 2007.

Leininger MM, McFarland MR: *Transcultural nursing: concepts, theories, research and practices*, ed 3, New York, 2002, McGraw-Hill.

Lerret SM, Skelton JA: Pediatric nonalcoholic fatty liver disease, *Gastroenterol Nurs* 31(2):115–119, 2008.

Lindenfeld J, et al: Executive summary: HFSA comprehensive heart failure practice guidelines, *J Card Fail* 16(6):475–539, 2010.

Logan C: Substantial solutions: creating safe and sensitive care pathways for bariatric patients, *Rehabil Manag* 21(5):23–25, 2008.

Long F: Safe lift strategy, *Rehabil Manag* 21(6):28–30, 2008.

Longo D, Fauci A, Kasper D, et al: *Harrison's principles of internal medicine*, ed 18, New York, 2011, McGraw-Hill.

Lowenstein L, et al: The relationship between obstructive sleep apnea, nocturia, and daytime overactive bladder syndrome in women, *Am J Obstet Gynecol* 198(5):598, e1-e5, 2008.

Lutz C, Przytulski K: *Nutrition and diet therapy*, ed 5, Philadelphia, 2011, FA Davis.

Madden M: Responding to pediatric poisoning, *Nursing* 38(8):52–55, 2008.

Makic MBF, et al: Evidence-based practice habits: putting more sacred cows out to pasture, *Crit Care Nurse* 31:38–62, 2011.

Makic MB: Management of nausea, vomiting and diarrhea during critical illness, *Adv Crit Care Nurs* 22(3):265–274, 2011.

Marshall SJ, et al: Translating physical activity recommendations into a pedometer-based step goal: 3000 steps in 30 minutes, *Am J Prev Med* 36(5):410–415, 2009.

Masterson M: *Chronic sorrow in mothers of adult children with cerebral palsy: an exploratory study*, 2010. Unpublished dissertation.

Matteucci R, Schub T, Pravikoff D: Shock, hypovolemic. *CINAHL nursing guide*, 2011, Nursing Reference Center.

Matthews EE: Sleep disturbances and fatigue in critically ill patients, *AACN Adv Crit Care* 22(3):204, 2011.

Mayo Clinic Health Letter: Risks of vitamin supplements, March, 2012.

McCaffery M, Herr K, Pasero C: Assessment. In Pasero C, McCaffery M, editors: *Pain assessment and pharmacologic management*, St Louis, 2011, Mosby Elsevier.

Mickler PA: Neonatal and pediatric perspectives in PICC placement, *J Infus Nurs* 31(5):282–285, 2008.

Mitchell A, Skraida TJ, Kim Y, et al: Depression, anxiety and quality of life in suicide survivors, *Arch Psychiatr Nurs* 23(1):2–10, 2009.

Mishra GD, et al: Body weight through adult life and risk of urinary incontinence in middle-aged women: results from a British prospective cohort, *Int J Obesity* 32(9):1415–1422, 2008.

Moody L: E-health web portals: delivering holistic healthcare and making home the point of care, *Holist Nurs Pract* 19(4):156–160, 2005.

National Cancer Institute: *Posttraumatic stress disorder*, 2011. Retrieved September 26, 2011, from http://www.cancer.gov/cancer topics/pdq/supportivecare/post-traumatic-stress/HealthProfessional.

National Diabetes Information Clearing House, U.S. Department of Health and Human Services: *How can I take care of my feet? 2011*. Retrieved December 13, 2011, from http://diabetes.niddk.nih.gov/dm/pubs/complications_feet/#feet.

National Stroke Association: *Warning signs of a stroke*, 2012. http://www.stroke.org/site/PageServer?pagename=symp. Accessed August 27, 2012.

NICE: *CG 116, Food allergy in children and young people: diagnosis and assessment of food allergy in children and young people in primary care and community settings*, 2011. Retrieved May 2, 2012, from http://publications.nice.org.uk/food-allergy-in-children-and-young-people-cg116/guidance.

Nelson A, et al: Myths and facts about safe patient handling in rehabilitation, *Rehabil Nurs* 33(1):10–17, 2008b.

Newman AM: Arthritis and sexuality, *Nurs Clin North Am* 42(4):605–619, 2007.

Newman D, Willson M: Review of intermittent catheterization and current best practices, *Urol Nurs* 31(1):12–48, 2011.

Norrby SR: Approach to the patient with urinary tract infection. In Goldman L, Schafer A, editors: *Goldman's Cecil medicine*, ed 24, St Louis, 2011, Saunders/Elsevier.

Nurko S, Scott SM: Coexistence of constipation and incontinence in children and adults, *Best Pract Res Clin Gastroenterol* 25:29–41, 2011.

Nutrition Action Health Letter: *Eat smart: which foods are good for what*, December, 2011.

Oerther SE: Plant poisonings: common plants that contain cardiac glycosides, *J Emerg Nurs* 37(1):102–103, 2011.

O'Grady NP, et al: Guidelines for evaluation of new fever in critically ill adult patients: 2008 update from the American College of Critical Care Medicine and the Infectious Diseases Society of America, *Crit Care Med* 36(4):1330–1349, 2008.

O'Grady NP, et al: *Guidelines for the prevention of intravascular catheter-related infections*, 2011. Retrieved from http://www.cdc.gov/hicpac/pdf/guidelines/bsi-guidelines-2011.pdf.

Ostaszkiewicz J, et al: The effects of conservative treatment for constipation on symptom severity and quality of life in community-dwelling adults, *J Wound Ostomy Continence Nurs* 37(2):193–198, 2010.

Paquette A, Gou P, Tannenbaum C: Systematic review and meta-analysis: do clinical trials testing antimuscarinic agents for overactive bladder adequately measure central nervous system adverse events? *J Am Geriatr Soc* 59(7):1332–1339, 2011.

Pasero C, McCaffrey M: Comfort-function goals, *Am J Nurs* 104(9):77–81, 2004.

Pasero C: Challenges in pain assessment, *J Perianesth Nurs* 24(1):50–54, 2009a.

Pasero C: Assessment of sedation during opioid administration for pain management, *J Perianesth Nurs* 24(3):186–190, 2009b.

Pasero C: Safe IV opioid titration for severe acute pain, *J PeriAnesth Nurs* 25(5):314–318, 2010c.

Pasero C: Persistent post-surgical and post-trauma pain, *J PeriAnesth Nurs* 26(1):38–41, 2011.

Pasero C, Portenoy RK, McCaffery M: Nonopioid analgesics. In Pasero C, McCaffery M, editors: *Pain assessment and pharmacologic management*, St Louis, 2011, Mosby Elsevier.

Pasero C, et al: Opioid analgesics. In Pasero C, McCaffery M, editors: *Pain assessment and pharmacologic management*, St. Louis, 2011b, Mosby Elsevier, pp 277–622.

Pattison N, Watson J: Ventilatory weaning: a case study of protracted weaning, *Nurs Crit Care* 14(2):75–85, 2009.

Paulus RA, Davis K, Steele GD: Continuous innovation in health care: implication of the Geisinger experience, *Health Aff* 27(5):1235–1245, 2008.

Peavy GM, et al: Effects of chronic stress on memory decline in cognitively normal and mildly impaired older adults, *Am J Psychiatry* 166(12):1384–1391, 2009.

Pender NJ, Murdaugh CL, Parsons MA: *Health promotion in nursing practice*, ed 6, Upper Saddle River, NJ, 2010, Prentice Hall.

Phillips BA: Obstructive sleep apnea in the elderly. In Kryger MH, Roth T, Dement WC, editors: *Principles and practice of sleep medicine*, ed 5, St Louis, 2011, Saunders.

Pierson FM, Fairchild SL: Features and activities of wheeled mobility aids. In Pierson FM, Fairchild SL, editors: *Principles & techniques of patient care*, ed 4, St Louis, 2008, Saunders.

Pierson FM, Fairchild SL: Ambulation aids, patterns, and activities. In Pierson FM, Fairchild SL, editors: *Principles & techniques of patient care*, ed 4, St Louis, 2008, Saunders.

Pitoni S, Sinclair HL, Andrews PJD: Aspects of thermoregulation physiology, *Curr Opin Crit Care* 17:115–121, 2011.

Policastro M, et al: *Urinary obstruction*, 2011 Medscape Reference. Retrieved April 18, 2012, from http://emedicine.medscape.com/article/778456-overview.

Prigerson HG, et al: Prolonged grief disorder: psychometric validation of criteria proposed for DSM-V and ICD-11, *PLoS Med* 6(8):e1000121, 2009.

Pye J: Travel-related health and safety considerations for children, *Nurs Stand* 25(39):50–56, 2011.

Resnick B, et al: Nursing home resident outcomes from the Res-Care Intervention, *J Am Geriatr Soc* 57(7):1156–1165, 2009.

Resnick B, D'Adamo C: Factors associated with exercise among older adults in a continuing care retirement community, *Rehabil Nurs* 36(2):47–53, 82, 2011.

Resnick B, Jenkins LS: Testing the reliability and validity of the self-efficacy for exercise scale, *Nurs Res* 49(3):154–159, 2000.

Resnick B, Zimmerman S, Orwig D: Model testing for reliability and validity of the outcome expectations for exercise scale, *Nurs Res* 50:5, 2001.

Roach M, Christie JA: Fecal incontinence in the elderly, *Geriatrics* 63(2):13–21, 2008.

Rodgers C, et al: Nausea and vomiting perspectives among children receiving moderate to highly emetogenic chemotherapy treatment, *Cancer Nurs* 35(3):203–210, 2012.

Rodgers GB, Franklin RL, Midgett JD: Unintentional paediatric ingestion poisonings and the role of imitative behavior, *Inj Prev* 18(2):103–108, 2012.

Safe Kids: *USA: Toy safety*, 2007. Retrieved from http://sk.convio.net/site/Page Navigator/-Campaigns/ToySafety/campaignToySafetyGuide.

Sargent S: Hepatic nursing: pathophysiology and management of hepatic encephalopathy, *Br J Nurs* 16(6):335–339, 2007.

Sateia MJ: Update on sleep and psychiatric disorders, *Chest* 135(5):1370, 2009.

Scales K: Intravenous therapy: a guide to good practice, *Br J Nurs IV Suppl* 17(19):S4–S10, 2008.

Schub T, Grose S, Pravikoff D: Xerostomia. *Nursing Reference Center: CINAHL Nursing Guide*, Sept 3, 2010.

Scott-Williams S: Materials that help reduce pressure injuries, *Outpatient Surg Mag*, November, 2009.

Scrase W, Tranter S: Improving evidence-based care for patients with pyrexia, *Nurs Stand* 25(29):37–41, 2011.

Sedlak CA, et al: Development of the National Association of Orthopaedic Nurses guidance statement on safe patient handling and movement in the orthopaedic setting, *Orthop Nurs* 28(Suppl 2):S2–S8, 2009.

Sendelbach S, Guthrie PF: *Acute confusion/delirium evidence-based guideline*, Ames, IA, 2009, John A. Hartford Foundation Center of Geriatric Nursing Excellence, University of Iowa.

Shah A, Buckley L: The current status of methods used by the elderly for suicides in England and Wales, *J Inj Violence Res* 3(2):68–73, 2011.

Shiraishi H, et al: Long-term effects of prism adaptation on chronic neglect after stroke, *Neuro Rehabilitation* 23(2):137–151, 200.

Siela D: Evaluation standards for management of artificial airways, *Crit Care Nurse* 30(4):76–78, 2010.

Skillings K, Curtis B: Tracheal tube cuff care. In Lynn-McHale DJ, editor: *AACN procedure manual for critical care*, ed 6, Philadelphia, 2011, Saunders Elsevier.

Smith R: Devising a system: new tools help therapists find seating solutions, *Rehabil Manag* 21(3):10, 12–15, 2008.

Smith N, Grose S: *Accidental, accidental: response, Nursing Reference Center*. CINAHL Nursing Guide, October 29, 2010.

Sole M, et al: Assessment of endotracheal cuff pressure by continuous monitoring: a pilot study, *Am J Crit Care* 18(2):133–143, 2009.

Steinke EE, et al: Sexual concerns and educational needs after an implantable cardioverter defibrillator, *Heart Lung* 34(5):299–308, 2005.

Steinke EE, Jaarsma T: Impact of cardiovascular disease on sexuality. In Moser D, Riegel B, editors: *Cardiac nursing: a companion to Braunwald's heart disease*, St Louis, 2008, Saunders.

Stevens RD, et al: A framework for diagnosing and classifying intensive care unit–acquired weakness, *Crit Care Med* 37(10):S299–S308, 2009.

Stewart WF, et al: Prevalence and burden of overactive bladder in the United States, *World J Urol* 20(6):327–336, 2003.

Stiles AS: A pilot study to test the feasibility and effectiveness of an intervention to help teen mothers and their mothers clarify relational boundaries, *J Pediatr Nurs* 23(6):415–428, 2008.

Taylor CR, et al: Safety, security and emergency preparedness. In Taylor CR, et al, editor: *Fundamentals of nursing, the art and science of nursing care*, ed 7, Philadelphia, 2011, Lippincott Williams &Wilkins.

Tizzard S, Yiannouzis K: Yellow alert! How to identify neonatal liver disease, *J Fam Health Care* 18(3):98–100, 2008.

Tracy MF, Chlan L: Nonpharmacological interventions to manage common symptoms in patients receiving mechanical ventilation, *Crit Care Nurse* 31(3):19–29, 2011.

United States Department of Agriculture (USDA): *USDA U.S. dietary guidelines: executive summary*, 2010, Retrieved June 10, 2012, from http://www.cnpp. usda.gov/Publications/DietaryGuidelines/2010/PolicyDoc/ExecSumm. pdf.

United States Department of Agriculture: *Supertracker, my food, my fitness, my health*, 2010. Accessed May 25, 2012, from https://www.choosemyplate. gov/SuperTracker/default.aspx.

U.S. Department of Health and Human Services: *Physical activity guidelines for Americans, 2008*, Washington, DC, 2008, Author.

U.S. Department of Health and Human Services: *Guidelines for the use of anti-retroviral agents in HIV-1-infected adults and adolescents, 1–166*. Retrieved January 10, 2011, from http://www.aidsinfo.nih.gov/ContentFiles/ AdultandAdolescentGL.pdf.

U.S. Food and Drug Administration: *Public health advisory: FDA recommends that over-the-counter (OTC) cough and cold products not be used for infants and children under 2 years of age*, 2010. Retrieved January 18, 2011, from http:// www.fda.gov/drugs/drugsafety/publichealthadvisories/ucm051137.html.

Vitaliano P, et al: The screen for caregiver burden, *Gerontologist* 31(1):76–83, 1991.

Vollman K, Sole M: Endotracheal tube and oral care. In Lynn-McHale DJ, editor: *AACN procedure manual for critical care*, ed 6, Philadelphia, 2011, Saunders Elsevier.

Walton-Geer PS: Prevention of pressure ulcers in the surgical patient, *AORN J* 89(3), 2009.

Wardell D, et al: Pilot study of healing touch and progressive relaxation for chronic neuropathic pain in persons with spinal cord injury, *J Holist Nurs* 24(4):231–240, 2006.

Weimer LH, Zadeh P: Neurological aspects of syncope and orthostatic intolerance, *Med Clin North Am* 93(2):427–449, 2009.

Weitz J: Pulmonary embolism. In Goldman L, Schafer A, editors: *Goldman's Cecil medicine*, ed 24, St Louis, 2011, Saunders/Elsevier.

Weikel DS, et al: Oral health maintenance guideline. In Ackley B, editor: *Evidence-based nursing care guidelines: medical-surgical interventions*, Philadelphia, 2008, Mosby.

White C: Atherosclerotic peripheral arterial disease. In Goldman L, Schafer A, editors: *Goldman's Cecil medicine*, ed 24, St Louis, 2011, Saunders/Elsevier.

White J, Guenter P, Gordon J: Consensus statement of the Academy of Nutrition and Dietetics/American Society for Parenteral and Enteral Nutrition: characteristics recommended for the identification and documentation of adult malnutrition, *J Acad Nutr Dietetics* 112:730–738, 2012.

Wieseke A, Bantz D, Siktberg L: Assessment and early diagnosis of dysphagia, *Geriatr Nurs* 29(6):376–383, 2008.

Wilson B: Contrast media-induced compartment syndrome, *Radiol Technol* 83(1):63–77, 2011.

Workeneh BT, et al: *Acute renal failure*, 2012. Medscape Reference. Retrieved February 11, 2012, from http://emedicine.medscape.com/article/243492-overview.

Wound, Ostomy, and Continence Nurses Society (WOCN): *Pressure ulcer assessment: best practice for clinicians*, Mt Laurel, NJ, 2009, Author.

Wound, Ostomy, and Continence Nurses Society (WOCN): *Guideline for prevention and management of pressure ulcers, WOCN clinical practice guideline series no 2*, Mount Laurel, NJ, 2010, Author.

Wyngarden K, DeWys M, Padnos P: Learnings from the field: the impact of using two new nursing diagnoses, organized infant behavior and disorganized infant behavior [abstract]. *Classification of Nursing Diagnoses: Proceedings of the Thirteenth Conference*, 1999, NANDA.

Yeom HA, Keller C, Fleury J: Interventions for promoting mobility in community-dwelling older adults, *J Am Acad Nurse Pract* 21(2):95–100, 2009.

Index